250
CASES IN
CLINICAL
MEDICINE

Commissioning Editor: Laurence Hunter
Project Manager: Ruth Swan
Production Manager: Nancy Arnott
Designer: Erik Bigland

250
CASES IN CLINICAL MEDICINE

Ragavendra R. Baliga MBBS MD DNB MRCP(UK)

Assistant Professor of Medicine
Division of Cardiology
University of Michigan
Ann Arbor
Michigan
USA

(Formerly, Harvard Medical School, Boston,
and Hammersmith Hospital, Royal Postgraduate
Medical School and Imperial College of Medicine, London)

THIRD EDITION

W. B. SAUNDERS COMPANY LTD

Edinburgh • London • New York • Oxford • Philadelphia • St Louis • Sydney • Toronto

W.B. SAUNDERS
An imprint of Elsevier Limited

Third Edition
(Second Edition published under the title '250 Short Cases in Clinical Medicine')

ISBN 0-7020-2624-7
Reprinted 2002, 2003, 2004

International Student Edition ISBN 0-7020-2625-5
Reprinted 2002, 2003, 2004

British Library Cataloguing in Publication Data
A catalogue record for this book is available from the British Library

Library of Congress Cataloging in Publication Data
A catalog record for this book is available from the Library of Congress

Note
Medical knowledge is constantly changing. As new information becomes available, changes in treatment, procedures, equipment and the use of drugs become necessary. The authors and the publishers have taken care to ensure that the information given in this text is accurate and up to date. However, readers are strongly advised to confirm that the information, especially with regard to drug usage, complies with the latest legislation and standards of practice.

ELSEVIER SCIENCE
your source for books, journals and multimedia in the health sciences
www.elsevierhealth.com

The publisher's policy is to use paper manufactured from sustainable forests

Printed in China
N/04

PREFACE

The new MRCP Part 2 clinical examination, Practical Assessment of Clinical Examination Skills (PACES), aims to test several aspects of clinical care including clinical skills of history taking, immediate and long-term management plans and communication of clinical information to colleagues, patients or their relatives, and ethical issues. In addition, it covers aspects tested in the old examination which include examination of the patient to detect the absence or presence of physical signs, interpretation of physical signs, and making appropriate diagnoses. These changes in the structure of the MRCP Clinical Examination mean that the candidate will be expected to know aspects of the history and management in greater detail. Keeping this in mind, the book has been reorganized. The goals of this book, however, remain the same: to provide strategies to satisfy the requirements of a clinical examination in general internal medicine. Each candidate will have to mix and match these strategies depending on a given examination situation.

This book should be useful for MBBS, PLAB, LRCP, MRCP (UK), MRCPI, postgraduate clinical examinations in the US, Australia (FRACP) and Canada (FCCP), and MD (New Zealand, Malaysia, Singapore, India, Pakistan, Sri Lanka and Bangladesh). The current organization of this book should also be appropriate for medical students in the US taking the USMLE and is best used as a guide by the patient's bedside. Cases for examinations are drawn from the same pool for both undergraduate and postgraduate examinations, although in the latter the candidate's performance has to be faultless and he or she will be expected to know certain aspects in greater detail.

Each case is discussed under the following headings:

Instruction: This allows the candidate to know what sort of instruction or command may be expected from an examiner.

Salient Features: This section includes important features in each case including aspects in history, physical signs, guidelines on how to proceed when faced with these signs and what to tell the examiner, in order to satisfy the examiner that the candidate is 'safe and sound' to be a junior doctor.

Diagnosis: Most candidates are unable to present their diagnosis in a succinct manner, although they are able to elicit the clinical signs. This heading has been included to help candidates present their diagnosis in a crisp and confident fashion.

Questions: This section supplies the questions (with answers) that a candidate can expect in a given case. These are also useful for the viva component of the examination.

Footnotes: Many of the cases have footnotes giving historical aspects relevant to that particular case. Although examiners will not deduct marks for ignorance of things that have little relevance to patient welfare, candidates who know the facts can expect a congratulatory glow to pervade the examiner, so that the rest of the questions may be softened accordingly.

R.R.B.

Ann Arbor
2002

ACKNOWLEDGEMENTS

I would like to thank Dr James Rasmussen, Professor of Dermatology, and Dr Csaba Martonyi, Associate Professor of Opthalmic Photography, for providing illustrations for this edition; Laurence Hunter, Commissioning Editor, W.B. Saunders UK for inviting me to write this Third Edition and Ruth Swan for copy editing this book. I thank Shari Voisard for her secretarial assistance.

Finally I thank my wife Jayashree for doing my share of the domestic chores while I worked on this book and my children Anoop and Neena for their patience.

CONTENTS

FUNDUS   517

MISCELLANEOUS   553

HISTORY AND EXAMINATION OF THE CARDIOVASCULAR SYSTEM

HISTORY

1. Chest pain: exertional, at rest (when angina is present, comment on the Canadian Cardiovascular Angina class, p. 42).
2. Shortness of breath: exertional, at rest (when dyspnoea is present, comment on the New York Heart Association class, p. 2), paroxysmal nocturnal dyspnoea.
3. Palpitations (see pp 35–6)
4. Dizziness, pre-syncope, syncope.
5. Swelling of feet.

EXAMINATION OF THE CARDIOVASCULAR SYSTEM

1. Introduce yourself: 'I am Dr/Mr/Ms............ May I examine your heart?'.
2. Ensure adequate exposure of the precordium: 'Would you take your top off, please?'. However, be sensitive of the feelings of female patients.
3. Get the patient to sit at 45 degrees – use pillows to support the neck.
4. Inspection: comment on the patient's decubitus (whether he or she is comfortable at rest or obviously short of breath); comment on malar flush (seen in mitral stenosis).
5. Examine the pulse: rate (count for 15 s), rhythm, character, volume; lift the arm to feel for the collapsing pulse. Feel the other radial pulse simultaneously.
6. Comment on the scar at antecubital fossa (cardiac catheterization scars).
7. Look at the tongue for pallor, central cyanosis.
8. Look at the eye for pallor, Argyll Robertson pupil.
9. Examine the jugular venous pulse: comment on the wave form and height from the sternal angle. Check the abdominojugular reflux.
10. Comment on any carotid pulsations (Corrigan's sign of aortic regurgitation).
11. Examine the precordium: comment on surgical scars (midline sternotomy scars, thoracotomy scars for mitral valvotomy may be missed under the female breast).
12. Feel the apex beat – position and character.
13. Feel for left parasternal heave and thrills at the apex and on either side of the sternum.
14. Listen to the heart, beginning from the apex: take care to palpate the right carotid pulse simultaneously so that the examiner notices that you are timing the various cardiac events.
    - Always comment on the first and second heart sounds. Mention any additional heart sounds (*Am J Med* 1959; **27**: 360).
    - If you do not hear the mid-diastolic murmur of mitral stenosis, make sure you listen to the apex in the left lateral position with the bell of the stethoscope.
    - If you hear a murmur at the apex, ensure that you get the patient to breathe in and out – the examiner will be observing whether or not you are listening for the variation in intensity with respiration.
    - If you hear a pansystolic murmur, listen at the axilla (mitral regurgitant murmurs are conducted to the axilla).

15. Using the diaphragm of your stethoscope, listen at the apex, below the sternum, along the left sternal edge, the second right intercostal space and the neck (for ejection systolic murmur of aortic stenosis, aortic sclerosis).
16. Request the patient to sit forward and listen with the diaphragm along the left sternal edge in the 3rd intercostal area with the patient's breath held in expiration for early diastolic murmur of aortic regurgitation.
17. Tell the examiner that you would like to do the following:
    • Listen to lung bases for signs of cardiac failure.
    • Check for sacral and leg oedema.
    • Examine the liver (tender liver of cardiac failure), splenomegaly (endocarditis).
    • Check the blood pressure.
    • Check the peripheral pulses and also check for radiofemoral delay.

The New York Heart Association classification of dyspnoea:
• Class I: Asymptomatic (shortness of breath on unaccustomed exertion).
• Class II: There is slight limitation of physical activity and patients develop shortness of breath on accustomed exertion.
• Class III: Marked limitation of physical activity; patients develop shortness of breath on activities of daily living such as having a shower, etc.
• Class IV: Inability to carry out physical activity; shortness of breath at rest.

René Theophile Hyacinthe Laennec invented the stethoscope in 1816 and reported his early experience with auscultation in a two-volume book published 3 years later (Laennec RTH 1821 *A Treatise on the Diseases of the Chest*. London: T and G Underwood. Translated by and with a preface and notes by John Forbes).

British physician Sir John Forbes (1787–1861) is best remembered for popularizing the stethoscope among English-speaking doctors. Forbes was born in Banff in the north east of Scotland. He studied at Marischal College, Aberdeen, before he went to Edinburgh where he received his medical education. Forbes translated Laennec's monograph in English in 1821 and published his own book on the subject in 1824 (Forbes J 1824 *Original Cases with Dissections and Observations Illustrating the Use of the Stethoscope and Percussion in the Diagnosis of the Diseases of the Chest*. London: T and G Underwood). The latter included a brief biographical sketch of the Austrian physician Leopald Auenbrugger and the first English translation of his essay (which was in Latin) on percussion. It also contained a summary of Parisian physician Victor Collin's recent manual on cardiac physical diagnosis.

Case 1

MITRAL STENOSIS

INSTRUCTION

This patient developed dyspnoea and orthopnoea during pregnancy, please examine her.
This 55-year old patient has atrial fibrillation, please perform the relevant clinical examination.

SALIENT FEATURES

History

- Symptoms of left-sided heart failure: exertional dyspnoea, orthopnoea, paroxysmal dyspnoea.
- Less frequent symptoms: haemoptysis, hoarseness of voice, symptoms of right-sided failure (these symptoms are somewhat more specific for mitral stenosis).
- Obtain a history of rheumatic fever in childhood.

Examination

- Pulse regular or irregularly irregular (due to atrial fibrillation).
- Jugular venous pressure (JVP) may be raised.
- Malar flush.
- Tapping apex beat in the 5th intercostal space just medial to midclavicular line.
- Left parasternal heave (indicating right ventricular enlargement).
- Loud first heart sound.
- Opening snap (often difficult to hear; a high-pitched sound that can vary from 0.04 to 0.10 s after the second sound, and is best heard at the apex with the patient in the lateral decubitus position).
- Rumbling, low-pitched, mid-diastolic murmur – best heard in the left lateral position on expiration. In sinus rhythm there may be presystolic accentuation of the murmur. If you are not sure about the murmur, tell the examiner that you want the patient to perform sit-ups or hop on one foot to increase the heart rate. This will increase the flow across the mitral valve and the murmur is better heard.
- Pulmonary component of second sound (P2) is loud.

Remember. The signs of pulmonary hypertension include loud P2, right ventricular lift, elevated neck veins, ascites and oedema. This is an ominous sign of the disease progression because pulmonary hypertension increases the risk associated with surgery (*Br Heart J* 1975; **37:** 74–8).

Note

- In patients with valvular lesions the candidate would be expected to comment on rhythm, the presence of heart failure and signs of pulmonary hypertension.
- In atrial septal defect, large flow murmurs across the tricuspid valve can cause mid-diastolic murmurs. The presence of wide, fixed splitting of second sound,

absence of loud first heart sound, and an opening snap and incomplete right bundle branch block should indicate the correct diagnosis. However, about 4% of patients with atrial septal defect have mitral stenosis, a combination called Lutembacher's syndrome.

DIAGNOSIS

This patient has mitral stenosis (lesion) which is almost always due to rheumatic heart disease (aetiology), and has atrial fibrillation, pulmonary hypertension and congestive cardiac failure (functional status).

QUESTIONS

What is the commonest cause of mitral stenosis?
Rheumatic heart disease.

What is the mechanism of tapping apex beat?
It is due to an accentuated first heart sound.

What does the opening snap indicate?
The opening snap is caused by the opening of the stenosed mitral valve and indicates that the leaflets are pliable. The opening snap is usually accompanied by a loud first heart sound. It is absent when the valve is diffusely calcified. When only the tips of the leaflets are calcified, the opening snap persists.

What is the mechanism of a loud first heart sound?
The loud first heart sound occurs when the valve leaflets are mobile. The valve is open during diastole and is suddenly slammed shut by ventricular contraction in systole.

What is the mechanism of presystolic accentuation of the murmur?
In sinus rhythm it is due to the atrial systole which increases flow across the stenotic valve from the left atrium to the left ventricle; this causes accentuation of the loudness of the murmur. This may also be seen in atrial fibrillation and is explained by the turbulent flow caused by the mitral valve starting to close with the onset of ventricular systole. This occurs before the first heart sound and gives the impression of falling in late diastole; it is, however, due to the start of ventricular systole.

What are the complications?
- Left atrial enlargement and atrial fibrillation.
- Systemic embolization, usually of the cerebral hemispheres.
- Pulmonary hypertension.
- Tricuspid regurgitation.
- Right heart failure.

How does one determine clinically the severity of the stenosis?
- The narrower the distance between the second sound and the opening snap, the greater the severity. The converse is not true. (**Note.** This time interval between the second sound and opening snap is said to be inversely related to the left atrial pressure.)
- The longer the duration of the diastolic murmur, the greater the severity. Note that in tight mitral stenosis the murmur may be less prominent or inaudible and the findings may be primarily those of pulmonary hypertension.

ADVANCED-LEVEL QUESTIONS

What are the investigations you would perform?

ECG
Broad bifid P wave (P mitrale); atrial fibrillation in advanced disease.

Chest radiography
- Congested upper lobe veins.
- Double silhouette due to enlarged left atrium.
- Straightening of the left border of the heart due to prominent pulmonary conus and filling of the pulmonary bay by the enlarged left atrium.
- Kerley B lines (horizontal lines in the regions of the costophrenic angles).
- Uncommonly the left bronchus may be horizontal due to an enlarged left atrium.
- Mottling due to secondary pulmonary haemosiderosis.

Echocardiography
2D and Doppler echocardiography is the diagnostic tool of choice for assessing the severity of mitral stenosis and for judging the applicability of balloon mitral valvotomy (*N Engl J Med* 1997; **337**: 32–41).

- It is able to identify restricted diastolic opening of the mitral valve leaflets due to 'doming' of the anterior leaflet and immobility of the posterior leaflet.
- It also allows assessment of the mitral valve apparatus and left atrial enlargement.
- Echocardiography usually permits an accurate planimetric calculation of the valve area (*Am J Cardiol* 1979; **43**: 560–8).
- It can also be used to assess the severity of stenosis by measuring the decay of the transvalvular gradient or the 'pressure half-time', an empirical measurement (*Br Heart J* 1978; **40**: 131–40).
- The mean transmitral gradient can be accurately and reproducibly measured from continuous wave Doppler signal across the mitral valve with the modified Bernoulli equation.
- The mitral valve area can be non-invasively derived from Doppler echocardiography with either the diastolic half-time method or the continuity equation. The continuity equation should be used when the area derived from the half-time does not correlate with the mean transmitral gradient.
- Doppler also allows estimation of pulmonary artery systolic pressure from the TR velocity signal and assessment of the severity of concomitant MR or AR.
- Trans-oesophageal echocardiography is not required unless a question about diagnosis remains after transthoracic echocardiography.

Cardiac catheterization
- Shows raised right heart pressures and an end-diastolic gradient from pulmonary artery wedge pressure (or left atrium if trans-septal puncture has been done) to the left ventricle.
- Left and right heart cardiac catheterization is indicated when percutaneous mitral balloon valvotomy is being considered.
- Cardiac catheterization is also indicated when there is a discrepancy between Doppler-derived haemodynamics and the clinical status of a symptomatic patient.
- Coronary angiography may be required in selected patients who need intervention.

- Exercise haemodynamics should be performed when the symptoms are out of proportion to the calculated mitral valve gradient area.

What is the normal cross-sectional area of the mitral valve?

It ranges from 4 to 6 cm^2; turbulent flow occurs when this area is less than 2 cm^2.

What is the area in 'tight' mitral stenosis?

It is usually less than 1 cm^2 and consequently the gradient across the valve is >10 mmHg.

How would you manage the patient?

- Asymptomatic patient in sinus rhythm: prophylaxis against infective endocarditis only.
- Mild symptoms: diuretics to reduce left atrial pressure and therefore symptoms.
- Atrial fibrillation: (1) rate control (digitalis, beta-blocker or calcium channel blocker); (2) anticoagulants (*Eur Heart J* 1988; **9:** 291–4).
- Moderate to severe symptoms or pulmonary hypertension is beginning to develop: mechanical relief of valve stenosis including (1) balloon valvotomy (*N Engl J Med* 1994; **331:** 961–7; *Br Heart J* 1988; **60:** 299–308) – percutaneous mitral balloon valvuloplasty is usually the procedure of choice when there is a non-calcified pliable valve; (2) surgery.

What are the indications for surgery?

- Patients with severe symptoms of pulmonary congestion and significant mitral stenosis.
- Patients with pulmonary hypertension or haemoptysis, even if minimally symptomatic.
- Recurrent thromboembolic events despite therapeutic anticoagulation.

Which surgical procedures are used to treat mitral stenosis?

Closed commissurotomy

- Closed mitral valvotomy – involves the use of mechanical dilators, inserted through the apex of the left ventricle. It is complicated by mitral regurgitation, systemic embolization and restenosis.
- Balloon valvuloplasty (a form of closed commissurotomy) – percutaneous trans-septal balloon mitral valvotomy (or valvuloplasty). Remember, percutaneous balloon dilatation of the mitral valve is a useful option in patients who are unable to undergo cardiac surgery, as in late pregnancy or when too ill (severe respiratory disease, non-mitral cardiac disease, multiorgan failure).

Open commissurotomy

Requires cardiopulmonary bypass and allows surgical repair of the valve under direct vision, resulting in more effective and safer valvotomy than the closed procedure.

Valve replacement

Entails risks including thromboembolism, endocarditis and primary valve failure.

What factors determine the success of balloon valvuloplasty?

- Good mobility of the valves.
- Little calcification.

- Minimal subvalvular disease.
- Mild mitral regurgitation.

In which trimester do patients with mitral stenosis usually become symptomatic?

Patients usually become symptomatic in the second trimester of pregnancy, when blood volume increases significantly and increases pulmonary pressures. As the blood volume diminishes late in the third trimester, the symptoms might slightly improve.

Mention some rarer causes of mitral stenosis.

- Calcification of mitral annulus and leaflets.
- Rheumatoid arthritis.
- Systemic lupus erythematosus.
- Malignant carcinoid.
- Congenital stenosis.

Which conditions simulate mitral stenosis?

- Left atrial myxoma.
- Ball valve thrombus in the left atrium.
- Cor triatriatum (a rare congenital heart condition where a thin membrane across the left atrium obstructs pulmonary venous flow).

Have you heard of Ortner's syndrome?

It refers to the hoarseness of voice caused by left vocal cord paralysis associated with enlarged left atrium in mitral stenosis.

> N. Ortner (1865–1935), Professor of Medicine, Vienna, described the syndrome in 1897. He believed in laboratory research and its application to bedside clinical work and said that the clinician's motto ought to be 'übers laboratorium dauernd zur Klinik' (translated: 'always via the laboratory to the clinic').
>
> P.J. Kerley (1900–1978), British radiologist.
>
> Paul Wood was a cardiologist at the Hammersmith and National Heart Hospitals. His clinical skills are legendary and he had a profound influence on British cardiology.
>
> Elliott Cutler, in 1923 in Boston, was the first to attempt surgical treatment of mitral stenosis by inserting a knife through the apex of the left ventricle and blindly cutting the valve at right angles to its natural orifice.
>
> Henry Souttar, in 1925, relieved mitral stenosis with a finger inserted through the atrial appendage.
>
> In 1948, four surgeons working independently performed successful valvotomies: Horace Smithy, Charles Bailey, Dwight Harken and Russell Brock.
>
> In 1984, Kanji Inoue from Japan and in 1985, James E Lock, contemporary Professor of Pediatric Cardiology, Harvard Medical School, and colleagues introduced balloon valvuloplasty for mitral stenosis.

Case 2

MITRAL REGURGITATION

INSTRUCTION

Examine this patient's heart.

SALIENT FEATURES

History

- Asymptomatic or mild symptoms: often.
- Dyspnoea (due to pulmonary congestion).
- Fatigue (due to low cardiac output).
- Palpitation (due to atrial fibrillation or LV dysfunction).
- Fluid retention (in late-stage disease).
- Obtain a history of myocardial infarction, rheumatic fever, connective tissue disorder, infective endocarditis.

Examination

- Peripheral pulse may be normal or jerky (i.e. rapid upstroke with a short duration).
- Apex beat will be displaced downwards and outwards and will be forceful in character.
- First heart sound will be soft.
- Third heart sound is common (left ventricular gallop sound).
- Pansystolic murmur (Hope murmur) conducted to the axilla, best detected with the diaphragm and on expiration. (**Note.** It is important to be sure that there is no associated tricuspid regurgitation.)
- Loud pulmonary second sound and left parasternal heave when there is associated pulmonary hypertension.

Note. When mitral regurgitation is caused by left ventricular dilatation and diminished cardiac contractility, the systolic murmur may be mid, late or pansystolic. Other causes of short systolic murmurs at the apex include mitral valve prolapse, papillary muscle dysfunction and aortic stenosis. In calcific aortic stenosis of the elderly, the murmur may be more prominent in the apex and may be confused with mitral regurgitation. In such instances try to listen to the murmur after a pause with premature beat or listen to the beat after a pause with atrial fibrillation. The murmur of aortic stenosis becomes louder, whereas that of mitral regurgitation shows little change.

DIAGNOSIS

This patient has mitral regurgitation (lesion) as evidenced by grade III/VI pansystolic murmur, which is probably due to ischaemic or rheumatic heart disease (aetiology), and is in cardiac failure as evidenced by bibasal crackles (functional status). The patient is in NYHA class III heart failure.

QUESTIONS

Mention some causes of chronic mitral regurgitation.

- Mitral valve prolapse.
- Rheumatic heart disease.
- Left ventricular dilatation.
- Coronary artery disease.
- Annular calcification.
- Infective endocarditis.
- Papillary muscle dysfunction.
- Cardiomyopathy.
- Connective tissue disorders.

Mention a few causes of acute mitral regurgitation.

- Acute myocardial infarction (rupture of the papillary muscle).
- Endocarditis (due to perforation of the mitral valve leaflet or the chordae).
- Trauma.
- Myxomatous degeneration of the valve.

How would you investigate this patient?

- Electrocardiography (ECG), looking for broad bifid P waves (P mitrale), left ventricular hypertrophy, atrial fibrillation. When coronary artery disease is the cause, there is often evidence of inferior or posterior wall myocardial infarction.
- Chest radiograph, looking for pulmonary congestion, large heart, left atrial enlargement and pulmonary artery enlargement (if severe and longstanding).
- Echocardiogram to determine the anatomy of the mitral valve apparatus, left atrial and left ventricular size and function (typical features include large left atrium, large left ventricle, increased fractional shortening, regurgitant jet on colour Doppler, leaflet prolapse, floppy valve or flail leaflet). The echocardiogram provides baseline estimation of left ventricle and left atrial volume, an estimation of left ventricular ejection fraction, and an approximation of the severity of regurgitation. It can be helpful to determine the anatomic cause of MR. In the presence of even mild TR, an estimate of pulmonary artery pressure can be obtained.
- Trans-oesophageal echocardiography is useful in those in whom transthoracic echocardiography provides non-diagnostic images. It may give better visualization of mitral valve prolapse. It is useful intraoperatively to establish the anatomic basis for MR and to guide repair.
- Cardiac catheterization is useful to determine coexistent coronary artery or aortic valve disease. Large 'v' waves are seen in the wedge tracing. Left ventriculogram and haemodynamic measurements are indicated when non-invasive tests are inconclusive regarding the severity of MR, LV function, or the need for surgery.

How would you differentiate between mitral regurgitation and tricuspid regurgitation?

	Mitral regurgitation	Tricuspid regurgitation
Pulse	Jerky or normal pulse	Normal pulse
JVP		Prominent 'v' wave
Palpation	Left ventricular heave	Left parasternal heave
Auscultation	Pansystolic murmur	Pansystolic murmur
	Intensity increases with expiration	Intensity increases with inspiration
	Radiates to the axilla	
Other signs		Hepatic pulsations

Why may these patients have a jerky pulse?
Because of reduced systolic ejection time, secondary to a large volume of blood regurgitating into the left atrium.

When does the murmur of mitral regurgitation radiate to the neck (i.e. base of the heart)?
Rarely, due to involvement of the posterior mitral leaflet or to ruptured chordae tendineae, the regurgitant jet strikes the left atrial wall adjacent to the aortic root and the murmur radiates to the base of the heart, and therefore may be confused with the murmur of aortic stenosis.

How do you grade systolic murmurs?
Levine's grading of systolic murmurs (*Ann Intern Med* 1933; **6**: 1371):

- Grade 1: Murmur is so faint that it is heard only with special effort.
- Grade 2: Murmur is faint but readily detected.
- Grade 3: Murmur is prominent but not loud.
- Grade 4: Murmur is loud.
- Grade 5: Murmur is very loud.
- Grade 6: Murmur is loud enough to be heard with the stethoscope just removed from contact with the chest wall.

What are the causes of pansystolic murmur over the precordium?
- Mitral regurgitation.
- Tricuspid regurgitation.
- Ventricular septal defect (this generally radiates to the right of the sternum).

ADVANCED-LEVEL QUESTIONS

Which congenital cardiac conditions can be associated with mitral valve regurgitation?
- Ostium primum atrial septal defect (due to cleft mitral valve).
- Partial atrioventricular canal.
- Corrected transposition of the great arteries.

How would you determine the severity of the lesion?
- The larger the left ventricle on clinical examination, the greater the severity.
- An S3 suggests that the disease is severe.
- Colour Doppler ultrasonography quantifies the severity of the regurgitant jet, usually into three grades. However, echocardiography provides only a semi-quantitative estimate of the severity of regurgitation. Left ventriculography performed during cardiac catheterization provides an additional but also imperfect estimate of the severity of mitral regurgitation.
- Prognosis is worsened if right ventricular function is reduced, and patients with a right ventricular ejection fraction of <30% are particularly at high risk (*Circulation* 1986; **73**: 900–12).

What is the significance of third heart sounds in mitral regurgitation?
The prevalence of third heart sounds increases with the severity of mitral regurgitation. However, in patients with mitral regurgitation, the third heart sound is due to rapid ventricular filling and does not necessarily reflect left ventricular systolic

dysfunction or increased filling pressure. In this situation S3 is caused by rapid filling of the left ventricle by the large volume of blood stored in the left atrium in diastole.

What is the medical management of such patients?
- Asymptomatic patients: antibiotic prophylaxis for endocarditis.
- When atrial fibrillation develops: digitalis to slow ventricular response.
- Heart failure: diuretics and inotropes, but major consideration should be given to surgery.

What are the indications for surgery in this patient?
- Moderate to severe symptoms despite medical therapy (NYHA functional class III or IV), provided that left ventricular function is adequate.
- Patients with minimal or no symptoms should be followed up every 6 months by echocardiographic or radionuclide assessment of left ventricular size and systolic function. When the ejection fraction falls to 60% (*Circulation* 1994; **90:** 830–7), or when left ventricular end-systolic dimension is greater than 45 mm (*J Am Coll Cardiol* 1984; **3:** 235–42), mitral valve repair or replacement should be considered even in the absence of symptoms.

Remember that ischaemic mitral regurgitation carries the worse prognosis: operative mortality is 10–20% and long-term survival is substantially lower than with non-ischaemic mitral regurgitation (*J Thorac Cardiovasc Surg* 1986; **91:** 379–88; *Ann Thorac Surg* 1994; **58:** 668–75).

When is successful valve repair less likely?
It is less likely when the aetiology is ischaemic, infectious or rheumatic, when there is significant calcification, when the prolapse is bileaflet or anterior.

What do you know about mitral regurgitation due to flail leaflet?
In patients with mitral regurgitation due to flail leaflet, the lesion usually results in high degrees of regurgitation (*J Am Coll Cardiol* 1990; **16:** 232–9). In Western countries flail leaflet is the most frequent cause of mitral regurgitation requiring surgical correction (*Mayo Clinic Proc* 1987; **62:** 22–34; *Eur Heart J* 1991; **12** suppl B: 2–4). When treated medically, mitral regurgitation due to flail leaflet is associated with excess mortality and high morbidity. Surgery is almost unavoidable within 10 years after the diagnosis and appears to be associated with an improved prognosis, suggesting that surgery should be considered early in the course of the disease (*N Engl J Med* 1996; **335:** 1417–23).

Samuel A. Levine was Professor of Cardiology at Harvard Medical School and Peter Bent Brigham Hospital in Boston.

James Hope (1801–1841) was an English physician who worked at St George's Hospital, London, and wrote a book in 1831 entitled *Diseases of the Heart and Great Vessels.*

Case 3

MIXED MITRAL VALVE DISEASE

INSTRUCTION

Listen to this patient's heart.

SALIENT FEATURES

- The patient will have signs of both mitral stenosis and regurgitation.
- The candidate will be expected to indicate the dominant lesion (see below).

Proceed as follows:
Look carefully for surgical scars of mitral valvotomy in all patients (scars under the left breast in female patients are often missed). Patients with previous valvotomy may have regurgitation and restenosis.

	Dominant mitral stenosis	Dominant mitral regurgitation
Apex beat	Tapping, not displaced	Heaving and displaced
First heart sound	Loud	Soft
Third heart sound	Absent	Present

A third heart sound in mitral regurgitation indicates that any associated mitral stenosis is insignificant.

Note. There may be patients who do not have clear-cut signs such as a loud first heart sound with a displaced apex; in such cases you must say that it is difficult to ascertain clinically the dominant lesion and that cardiac catheterization should resolve the issue.

DIAGNOSIS

This patient has mitral stenosis with mitral regurgitation (lesion), with the dominant lesion being stenosis due to rheumatic heart disease (aetiology), and is in cardiac failure (functional status).

Read these papers for further information: *Circulation* 1973; **48**: 357; *Ann Intern Med* 1972; **77**: 939.

QUESTIONS

What is the cause of mitral stenosis with regurgitation?
Mixed mitral valve disease is usually caused by chronic rheumatic heart disease.

What are the approximate frequencies with which various valves are affected by rheumatic heart disease?
- Mitral valve disease, 80%.
- Aortic valve, 50%.

- Combined mitral and aortic valve lesion, 20%.
- Tricuspid valve, 10%.
- Pulmonary valve, <1%.

What is the significance of a diastolic rumble in mitral regurgitation?

It signifies the presence of coexistent mitral stenosis. In the absence of mitral stenosis it suggests that there is high diastolic transmitral flow and severe mitral regurgitation. Inhalation of amyl nitrate increases both the duration and intensity of the diastolic murmur due to mitral stenosis whereas it decreases them if the diastolic rumble is caused solely by mitral regurgitation. Also the presence of an opening snap suggests mitral stenosis as the cause of the diastolic rumble.

In patients with mitral regurgitation and a diastolic rumble, what does the presence of a giant left atrium indicate?

It indicates that there is no significant mitral stenosis.

> Joseph K. Perloff is contemporary Professor of Cardiology, Los Angeles; his chief interest is congenital heart disease.
>
> William C. Roberts is a contemporary US cardiac pathologist and Editor of the *American Journal of Cardiology*.

Case 4

AORTIC REGURGITATION

INSTRUCTION

Examine this patient's cardiovascular system.
Examine this patient's heart.

SALIENT FEATURES

History

- Asymptomatic (but may have normal or depressed left ventricular function).
- Dyspnoea and fatigue (due to left ventricular impairment and low cardiac output initially on exertion).
- Symptoms of left ventricular failure in later stages.
- Angina pectoris is less common than in aortic stenosis; it usually indicates coronary artery disease.

Examination

Pulse
- Collapsing pulse (large volume, rapid fall with low diastolic pressure).
- Visible carotid pulsation in neck (dancing carotids or Corrigan's sign).
- Capillary pulsation in fingernails (Quincke's sign).

- A booming sound heard over femorals ('pistol-shot' femorals or Traube's sign).
- To and fro systolic and diastolic murmur produced by compression of femorals by stethoscope (Duroziez's sign or murmur).

Heart

- Heart sounds are usually normal.
- Apex beat is displaced outwards and is forceful.
- Third heart sound (in early systole with bicuspid aortic valve).
- Early diastolic, high-pitched murmur is heard at the left sternal edge with the diaphragm – if not readily apparent, it is important to sit the patient forward and auscultate with the patient's breath held at the end of expiration. When the ascending aorta is dilated and displaced to the right, the murmur may be heard along the right sternal border as well.
- An ejection systolic murmur may be heard at the base of the heart in severe aortic regurgitation (without aortic stenosis). This murmur may be as loud as grade 5 or 6, and underlying organic stenosis can be ruled out only by investigations.
- Ejection click suggests underlying bicuspid aortic valve.
- Mid-diastolic murmur of Austin Flint may be heard at the apex. It is typically low-pitched, similar to the murmur of mitral stenosis but without a preceding opening snap.
- Loud pulmonary component of second sound (suggests pulmonary hypertension).

General examination

- Head nodding in time with the heart beat (de Musset's sign) may be present.
- Visible carotid pulsation may be obvious in the neck – dancing carotids or Corrigan's sign.
- Check the blood pressure (wide pulse pressure).
- Look for systolic pulsations of the uvula (Muller's sign).
- Check pupils for Argyll Robertson pupil of syphilis.
- Look for stigmata of Marfan's syndrome – high arched palate, arm span greater than height.
- Check joints for ankylosing spondylitis and rheumatoid arthritis.

DIAGNOSIS

This patient has pure aortic regurgitation (lesion), which is due to associated ankylosing spondylitis (aetiology), and is in cardiac failure (functional status).

QUESTIONS

Mention a few causes of chronic aortic regurgitation.

- Rheumatic fever.
- Hypertension (accentuated tambour quality of second sound).
- Atherosclerosis.
- Bacterial endocarditis.
- Idiopathic dilatation of the aortic root and annulus.
- Syphilis.

- Marfan's syndrome.
- Rheumatoid arthritis.
- Cystic medial necrosis.
- Seronegative arthritis (ankylosing spondylitis, Reiter's syndrome).
- Bicuspid aortic valve.

How would you investigate a patient with aortic regurgitation?

- Chest radiograph is usually normal in mild aortic regurgitation; there may be valvular calcification or cardiomegaly.
- ECG typically shows features of left ventricular hypertrophy and strain (increased QRS amplitude and ST/T wave changes in precordial leads) and left atrial hypertrophy (wide P wave in lead II and biphasic P in lead V1).
- Echocardiography is indicated to: confirm the diagnosis of AR; determine aetiology; assess valve morphology; determine a semiquantitative estimate of severity of regurgitation; assess LV dimension, mass and systolic function; assess aortic size; estimate the degree of pulmonary hypertension (when TR is present); determine whether there is rapid equilibration of aortic and LV diastolic pressure. Doppler is the best method for detecting aortic regurgitation
- Exercise testing: is useful to assess functional capacity, symptomatic responses and haemodynamic effects of exercise in patients with severe AR with equivocal symptoms.
- Radionuclide angiography is useful in asymptomatic patients with poor quality echocardiographic images.
- Cardiac catheterization is necessary when coronary artery disease is suspected (e.g. in patients >40 years) and when the severity of aortic regurgitation is doubted; injection of contrast into aortic root gives information on degree of regurgitation and state of aortic root (presence of dilatation, dissection, root abscesses).
- MRI or spiral CT scan for assessment of aortic root size.

ADVANCED-LEVEL QUESTIONS

What is the prevalence of aortic regurgitation in the elderly?

According to the Helsinki Ageing Study, 13% of persons aged 75–86 years have moderate to severe aortic regurgitation (*J Am Coll Cardiol* 1993; **21**: 1220–5).

What are the clinical signs of severity?

- Wide pulse pressure.
- Soft second heart sound.
- Duration of the decrescendo diastolic murmur.
- Presence of the left ventricular third heart sound.
- Austin Flint murmur.
- Signs of left ventricular failure.

What do you know of Hill's sign?

Hill's sign is the presence of higher systolic pressure in the leg than in the arm, and is said to be an indicator of the severity of aortic regurgitation.

In mild aortic regurgitation the difference is less than 20 mmHg, in moderate regurgitation it is between 20 and 40 mmHg and in severe regurgitation it is over 60 mmHg.

Do characteristics of the early diastolic murmur correlate with severity?

Yes. In mild aortic regurgitation the murmur is short but, as the severity of the regurgitation increases, the murmur becomes longer and louder. In very severe regurgitation the murmur may extend throughout diastole.

What is an Austin Flint murmur?

It is an apical, low-pitched, diastolic murmur caused by vibration of the anterior mitral cusp in the regurgitant jet, and is heard at the apex.

Mention a few causes of acute aortic regurgitation.

- Infective endocarditis.
- Aortic dissection.
- Trauma.
- Failure of prosthetic valve.
- Rupture of sinus of Valsalva.

What do you know about the natural history of asymptomatic aortic regurgitation?

About 4% of patients develop symptoms, left ventricular dysfunction, or both, every year.

What do you understand by the term cor bovinum?

In chronic aortic regurgitation there is slow and progressive left ventricular dilatation and hypertrophy in an attempt to normalize wall stress. The heart may thus become larger and heavier than in any other form of chronic heart disease – cor bovinum (bovine or ox heart).

What is the role of vasodilators in aortic regurgitation?

- Long-term vasodilator therapy with nifedipine reduces or delays the need for aortic valve replacement in asymptomatic patients with severe aortic regurgitation (*N Engl J Med* 1994; **331**: 689). Patients in whom left ventricular dysfunction developed when treated with nifedipine respond favourably to valve replacement in terms of both survival and normalization of ejection fraction.
- Long-term treatment of patients with severe AR who have symptoms and/or LV dysfunction who are considered poor candidates for surgery due to other factors.
- Long-term vasodilator therapy should not be recommended for patients with left ventricular dysfunction.
- Patients with subnormal left ventricular ejection fractions should be considered candidates for aortic valve replacement rather than vasodilator therapy, since valve replacement remains the more definitive therapy to reduce volume overload.
- Vasodilator therapy is not recommended for asymptomatic patients with mild AR and normal LV function in the absence of systemic hypertension, as these patients have an excellent outcome with no therapy.
- The goal of vasodilator therapy is to reduce systolic blood pressure. However, it is rarely possible to reduce systolic blood pressure to normal because of increased LV stroke volume, and hence drug dosage should not be increased excessively in an attempt to achieve this goal. The benefit of vasodilator therapy in patients with normal blood pressure and/or normal LV cavity size is not known and hence is not recommended in these patients (*Circulation* 1998; **98**: 1949–84).

How is aortic regurgitation treated?

Aortic regurgitation is usually treated surgically. The timing of surgery is important and depends on severity of symptoms and extent of left ventricular dysfunction (*Circulation* 1998; **98:** 1949–84). Valve replacement should be performed as soon as possible after the onset of ventricular dysfunction. Indications for surgery include:

- Symptoms of heart failure and diminished left ventricular function (an ejection fraction of less than 50% but more than 20–30%).
- Concomitant angina and severe AR.
- A reduction in exercise ejection fraction (as estimated with radionuclide ventriculography and exercise testing) of 5% or more is considered by some to be an indication for surgery, even in the absence of symptoms.
- Several investigators have suggested an end-systolic dimension of 55 mm to represent the limit of surgically reversible dilatation of the left ventricle, so that aortic valve replacement is performed before this chamber size is exceeded. Others have challenged the validity of the 55 mm systolic limit, as postoperative reduction in chamber size remains variable.
- When aortic root dilatation reaches or exceeds 50 mm by echocardiography, AVR and aortic root reconstruction are indicated in patients with disease of the proximal aorta and AR of any severity (*Circulation* 1998; **98:** 1949–84).

Note

1. In the young, mechanical prostheses are used as the valves are more durable.
2. Tissue valves are prone to calcification and degeneration. In the elderly and in those for whom anticoagulants are contraindicated, tissue valves are preferred.

How would you follow up a patient with AR?

- Asymptomatic patients with mild AR, little or no LV dilatation, and normal systolic LV function may be followed on an annual basis with the advice to alert the physician if symptoms develop between appointments (*Circulation* 1998; **98:** 1949–84).
- Asymptomatic patients with normal systolic function but severe AR and significant LV dilatation should be followed up at least every 6 months, preferably with an echocardiogram (*Circulation* 1998; **98:** 1949–84).
- Asymptomatic patients with normal systolic function but severe AR and with more severe LV dilatation (end-diastolic dimension >70 mm or end-systolic dimension >50 mm) have a 10–20% risk of developing symptoms and hence should have serial echocardiograms every 4 months (*Circulation* 1998; **98:** 1949–84).
- Patients who have had valve replacement should also be seen regularly and monitored for signs of failure of the aortic valve prosthesis (particularly in patients with biological valves) and endocarditis (*Circulation* 1998; **98:** 1949–84).

Alfred de Musset was a French poet whose nodding movements were described by his brother in a biography. When told of this, Alfred put his thumb and forefinger on his neck and his head stopped bobbing.

Austin Flint (1812–1886) was one of the founders of Buffalo Medical College, New York, and reported the murmur in two patients with aortic regurgitation, confirmed by autopsy. He also held chairs at New Orleans, Chicago, Louisville and New York.

H.I. Quincke (1842–1922) was a German physician who described angioneurotic oedema and benign intracranial hypertension.

P.I. Duroziez (1826–1897), a French physician, was widely acclaimed for his articles on mitral stenosis.

L. Traube (1818–1876), a German physician, was the first to describe pulsus bigeminus.

Antonio Maria Valsalva (1666–1723) was an Italian anatomist and surgeon who discovered the labyrinth and developed the Valsalva manoeuvre to remove foreign bodies from the ear.

Case 5

AORTIC STENOSIS

INSTRUCTION

Examine this patient's heart.

SALIENT FEATURES

History

- Asymptomatic (many patients do not have symptoms).
- Fatigue.
- Angina (in ~70% of adults average survival after onset of angina is 5 years).
- Syncope (in 25% of patients, during or immediately after exercise; average survival after onset of syncope is 3 years).
- Dyspnoea is a common presenting symptom (suggests left ventricular dysfunction; heart failure reduces life expectancy to less than 2 years).

Examination

Pulse

- Low volume pulse. It is reduced in volume with a delayed upstroke (pulsus parvus et tardus). This is due to a reduction in systolic pressure and a gradual decline in diastolic pressure.
- Normal pulse in mild aortic stenosis when the gradient is <50 mmHg.
- Slow rise with diminished volume, sometimes with a notch on the upstroke, is an 'anacrotic pulse', suggesting severe aortic stenosis. When aortic stenosis is associated with aortic regurgitation, a double or 'bisferious' pulse may be felt.

Heart

- Apex beat is heaving in nature but is not displaced. (A displaced apex beat indicates left ventricular dilatation and severe disease.)
- Palpable systolic vibrations over the primary aortic area, with the patient in the sitting position during full expiration (often correlates with a gradient of more than 40 mmHg).
- Systolic thrill over the aortic area and the carotids.

- Soft second heart sound.
- Ejection click heard 0.1 s after first heart sound, along the left sternal border (indicates valvular stenosis). An ejection sound that moves with respiration is not aortic in origin.
- An atrial (S4) sound may be heard.
- Ejection systolic murmur at the base of the heart conducted to the carotids and the right clavicle. (Listen carefully for an early diastolic murmur as mild aortic regurgitation often accompanies aortic stenosis.)
- Third heart sound: in patients with aortic stenosis, third heart sounds are uncommon but usually indicate the presence of systolic dysfunction and raised filling pressures.

General examination
- Check the blood pressure, keeping in mind that the pulse pressure is low in moderate to severe stenosis.

DIAGNOSIS

This patient has pure aortic stenosis (lesion) which may be due to rheumatic aetiology or a bicuspid aortic valve (aetiology); he has severe aortic stenosis as he gives a history of recurrent syncope (functional status).

QUESTIONS

How would you differentiate aortic stenosis from aortic sclerosis?
Aortic sclerosis is seen in the elderly; the pulse is normal volume, the apex beat is not shifted and the murmur is localized.

Mention some causes of aortic stenosis.
- Under the age of 60 years: rheumatic, congenital.
- Between 60 and 75 years: calcified bicuspid aortic valve, especially in men.
- Over the age of 75 years: degenerative calcification.

What does the second heart sound tell us in this condition?
- A soft second heart sound indicates valvular stenosis (except in calcific stenosis of the elderly, where the margins of the leaflets usually maintain their mobility).
- A single second heart sound may be heard when there is fibrosis and fusion of the valve leaflets.
- Reversed splitting of the second sound indicates mechanical or electrical prolongation of ventricular systole.
- A perfectly normal second heart sound (i.e. normal splitting with A2 of normal intensity) is strong evidence against the presence of critical aortic stenosis.

What do you understand by the term ejection systolic murmur?
It is a crescendo–decrescendo murmur which begins after the first heart sound (or after the ejection click when present), peaks in mid or late systole and ends before the second heart sound. This peak is delayed with increasing severity of aortic stenosis.

ADVANCED-LEVEL QUESTIONS

Does the loudness of the murmur reflect the severity of the aortic stenosis?

No, the loudness of the murmur is related more to the cardiac output and the systolic turbulence surrounding the valve than to the severity of the stenosis. Thus, a loud murmur may be associated with trivial stenosis and, in severe heart failure, the murmur may be soft because of decreased flow across the valve from the diminished cardiac output.

Mention other causes of ejection systolic murmur at the base of the heart.

* Pulmonary stenosis.
* Hypertrophic obstructive cardiomyopathy.
* Supravalvular aortic stenosis.

What is the prevalence of aortic stenosis in the elderly?

According to the Helsinki Ageing Study, almost 3% of individuals aged between 75 and 86 years have critical aortic stenosis (*J Am Coll Cardiol* 1993; **21**: 1220–5).

What is the mechanism of syncope in aortic stenosis?

* The left ventricle is suddenly unable to contract (transient electro-mechanical dissociation) against the stenosed valve.
* Cardiac arrhythmias (bradycardia, ventricular tachycardia or fibrillation).
* Marked peripheral vasodilatation without a concomitant increase in cardiac output, particularly after exercise.

What investigations would you perform?

ECG

ECG usually shows left ventricular hypertrophy, ST–T changes, possibly left axis deviation, later left atrial hypertrophy (negative P waves in V1), conduction abnormalities due to calcification of conducting tissues (first-degree heart block, left bundle branch block).

Chest radiograph

May show cardiac enlargement, post-stenotic dilatation of aorta (a bicuspid valve should be suspected if the proximal aorta is greatly enlarged), calcification of aortic valve (particularly in older patients).

Echocardiography is useful in:

* The diagnosis and assessment of severity of aortic stenosis: estimates valve gradient, normal valve appearance excludes significant aortic stenosis in adults; also helps to define the level of obstruction (i.e. valvar, supravalvar, subvalvar); calcified valves can be identified.
* The assessment of left ventricular size, function and/or haemodynamics.
* The re-evaluation of patients with known AS with changing symptoms and signs.
* The re-evaluation of asymptomatic patients with severe AS and the assessment of patients with known AS during pregnancy.

Note. The degree of aortic stenosis is graded as: mild (valve area >1.5 cm^2), moderate (area >1.0 to 1.5 cm^2) or severe (area ≤ 1.0 cm^2).

Exercise testing

Exercise testing in adults with AS has been discouraged largely because of safety; it should not be performed in symptomatic patients as it may be fatal; in asymptomatic patients an abnormal haemodynamic response (e.g. hypotension) is sufficient to consider AVR. In selected patients it may be useful to provide a basis for advice about physical activity.

Cardiac catheterization

This is done to assess the coronary circulation and to confirm or clarify the diagnosis. When the echocardiogram is inadequate, cardiac haemodynamics using both left and right heart catheterization is indicated and requires: (1) measurement of transvalvular flow, (2) determination of transvalvular pressure gradient and (3) calculation of the effective valve area.

What are the complications of aortic stenosis?

- Left ventricular failure indicates poor prognosis unless the valve is replaced.
- Sudden death occurs in 10–20% of adults and 1% of children. It has been rarely documented to occur without prior symptoms. It is an uncommon event – probably <1% per year.
- Arrhythmias and conduction abnormalities include ventricular arrhythmias (more common than supraventricular arrhythmias) and heart block (may occur because of calcification of conducting tissues).
- Systemic embolization is caused by disintegration of the aortic valve apparatus or by concomitant aortic atheroma.
- Infective endocarditis (in 10% of cases) should be considered when these patients present with unexplained illness.
- Haemolytic anaemia.

What are the clinical signs of severity of aortic stenosis?

- Narrow pulse pressure.
- Soft second sound.
- Narrow or reverse split second sound.
- Systolic thrill and heaving apex beat.
- Fourth heart sound.
- Cardiac failure.

How would you manage this patient?

If the patient is *asymptomatic* and the valvular gradient is less than 50 mmHg, then observe the patient. Surgery is not recommended in asymptomatic patients.

Valve replacement in the following circumstances:

- The patient is *symptomatic* or the valvular gradient is more than 50 mmHg. Surgery is mandatory in symptomatic patients.
- Valve replacement should be considered in asymptomatic patients with severe aortic stenosis (peak-to-peak gradient >50 mmHg) particularly when any one or more of the following features is present: left ventricular systolic dysfunction; abnormal response to exercise (e.g. hypotension), ventricular tachycardia; marked excessive left ventricular hypertrophy (≥ 15 mm); valve area <0.6 cm^2.
- In asymptomatic patients with moderate AS it is generally acceptable to perform aortic valve replacement in those who are undergoing mitral valve or aortic root surgery or coronary artery bypass surgery.

- Severe aortic stenosis with low mean systolic aortic valve gradient (≤ 30 mmHg) and severe LV dysfunction (*Circulation* 2000; **101:** 1940–6).
- Valve area less than 0.8 cm^2 (normal area 2.5–3.0 cm^2). Patients with severe aortic stenosis should have valve replacement early to avoid deterioration.
- Patients with severe AS, with or without symptoms, who are undergoing coronary artery bypass surgery, surgery on the aorta or other heart valves should undergo AVR at the time of their surgery.
- Patients often require **coronary artery bypass grafts** during aortic valve replacement.

Balloon valvuloplasty should be limited to moribund patients requiring emergency intervention or those with a very poor life expectancy due to other pathology. In one study, although in-hospital mortality rates were similar to those following conventional surgical replacement, there were more deaths in the valvuloplasty group in the subsequent follow-up period (*J Am Coll Cardiol* 1992; **20:** 796–801).

If a young person presents with signs and symptoms of aortic stenosis but the aortic valve is normal on echocardiography which condition would you suspect?

Supravalvular or subvalvular aortic stenosis.

What are the genetics of supravalvular stenosis?

Studies suggest that mutation in the elastin gene causes supravalvular stenosis (*Cell* 1993; **73:** 159).

If this patient had bleeding per rectum what unusual cause would come to mind?

Angiodysplasia of the colon (*Radiology* 1974; **113:** 11).

If the patient was icteric and had haemolytic anaemia, what would the mechanism be?

Microangiopathic haemolysis has been described in severe calcified aortic stenosis manifesting with anaemia and icterus (*Semin Hematol* 1969; **6:** 133).

What do you understand by the term 'Gallavardin phenomenon'?

The high-frequency components of the ejection systolic murmur may radiate to the apex, falsely suggesting mitral regurgitation. This is known as the Gallavardin phenomenon (*Lyons Med* 1925; **135:** 523).

Williams' syndrome is characterized by elfin facies, supravalvular aortic stenosis and hypercalcaemia (J.C.P. Williams, New Zealand physician).

Case 6

MIXED AORTIC VALVE LESION

INSTRUCTION

Examine this patient's heart.
Examine this patient's cardiovascular system.
Examine this patient's pulse.

SALIENT FEATURES

- Pulse may be bisferious, small volume or large volume, depending on the dominant lesion.
- Displaced apex beat (remember, a small left ventricle is inconsistent with chronic severe AR).
- Early diastolic murmur of aortic regurgitation.
- Ejection systolic murmur of aortic stenosis.

Proceed as follows:

Tell the examiner that you would like to check the blood pressure, in particular to determine the pulse pressure (systolic minus diastolic pressure).

DIAGNOSIS

This patient has mixed aortic stenosis with aortic regurgitation (lesion) due to rheumatic heart disease (aetiology). He has a dominant stenosis and is in cardiac failure (functional status).

Note
In *dominant aortic stenosis*:

- Pulse volume is small.
- Blood pressure is normal and pulse pressure is narrow.

In *dominant aortic regurgitation*:

- Pulse is collapsing.
- Pulse pressure is wide.

QUESTIONS

What are common causes of mixed aortic lesions?
- Rheumatic heart disease.
- Bicuspid aortic valve.

What is the pathophysiology of mixed aortic valve disease?
- In mixed aortic valve disease, one lesion usually predominates over the other and the pathophysiology resembles that of the pure dominant lesion. When aortic

stenosis predominates, the pathophysiology and, therefore, the management resembles that of pure aortic stenosis (*J Am Coll Cardiol* 1998; **32:** 1486–588). The LV in these patients develops concentric hypertrophy rather than dilatation. The timing of aortic valve replacement (as in pure aortic stenosis) depends on symptoms (*Circulation* 1998; **98:** 1949–84).

- When AR is more than mild and the AS is predominant, the concentrically hypertrophied and non-compliant left ventricle is on the steeper portion of the diastolic pressure–volume curve, resulting in pulmonary congestion. Therefore, although neither lesion by itself is sufficiently severe to merit surgery, both together produce substantial haemodynamic compromise and require surgery (*Circulation* 1998; **98:** 1949–84).

- When the AR is severe and the AS is mild, the high total stroke volume from extensive regurgitation may produce a substantial transvalvular gradient. Because the transvalvular gradient varies with the square of the transvalvular flow (*Am Heart J* 1951; **41:** 1–29), a high gradient in predominant regurgitation may be predicted primarily on excess transvalvular flow rather than on a severely compromised orifice area (*Circulation* 1998; **98:** 1949–84).

In mixed aortic valve disease is cardiac catheterization more accurate than Doppler echocardiography to measure valve area?

Aortic valve area will be measured inaccurately at the time of cardiac catheterization in mixed aortic valve lesions if the cardiac output is measured either by the Fick or the thermodilution method as both these methods usually underestimate total valve flow. The valve area can be measured more accurately using Doppler echocardiography (by continuity equation) in mixed aortic stenosis and aortic regurgitation. However, the confusing nature of mixed valve disease makes cardiac catheterization necessary to obtain additional haemodynamic information in most patients (including coronary anatomy) (*Circulation* 1998; **98:** 1949–84).

How would you manage such a patient?

- Surgical correction of disease that produces more than mild symptoms.
- When the AS is dominant: operate in the presence of even mild symptoms.
- When the AR is dominant: surgery can be delayed until symptoms develop or asymptomatic LV dysfunction becomes apparent on echocardiography.

Case 7

MIXED MITRAL AND AORTIC VALVE DISEASE

INSTRUCTION

Examine this patient's precordium.
Examine this patient's cardiovascular system.
Examine this patient's heart.

SALIENT FEATURES

- Pulse may be small volume (due to either dominant aortic stenosis or mitral stenosis), regular or irregularly irregular.
- Apex beat may be displaced.
- Left parasternal heave.
- Mid-diastolic murmur of mitral stenosis.
- Pansystolic murmur of mitral regurgitation.
- Ejection systolic murmur of aortic stenosis at the base of the heart.
- Early diastolic murmur of aortic regurgitation heard on end expiration with the patient sitting forward.

Note

If the apex beat is not displaced in such mixed lesions then mitral stenosis is the dominant lesion. (However, if the mitral stenosis developed earlier it can mask the signs of a significant stenosis.)

In aortic stenosis, the murmur of mitral stenosis may be diminished or absent. The presence of the following features should alert the clinician to a coexisting mitral stenosis because they are not commonly associated with isolated aortic stenosis:

- Atrial fibrillation.
- Absence of left ventricular hypertrophy in patients with left heart failure.
- Female sex.
- Giant-sized left atrium.
- Calcification of the mitral valve.
- Absence of aortic valve calcification in the symptomatic patient.

Combined mitral stenosis and aortic stenosis

- Severe mitral stenosis and low cardiac output may mask moderate to severe aortic stenosis. A history of angina, syncope or ECG evidence of left ventricular hypertrophy or calcification of the aortic valve on the chest radiograph suggests the presence of aortic stenosis (*Circulation* 1998; **98:** 1949–84).
- The murmur of aortic stenosis is occasionally better heard at the apex than at the base, particularly in the elderly (Gallavardin phenomenon). When this occurs in younger individuals with a coexisting mitral stenosis, the murmur of aortic stenosis may be mistaken for mitral regurgitation (*Circulation* 1998; **98:** 1949–84).
- In patients with significant aortic stenosis and mitral stenosis, the physical findings of aortic stenosis generally dominate and those of mitral stenosis may be missed, whereas the symptoms are usually those of mitral stenosis. 'Combination stenosis' is almost always the result of rheumatic heart disease (*Circulation* 1998; **98:** 1949–84).

Combined mitral stenosis and aortic regurgitation

The combination of severe mitral stenosis and severe aortic regurgitation may present with confusing pathophysiology and often leads to misdiagnosis. Mitral stenosis restricts left ventricular filling and so diminishes the impact of the aortic regurgitation on left ventricular volume (*J Am Coll Cardiol* 1984; **3:** 703–11). Thus, even severe aortic regurgitation may fail to cause a hyperdynamic circulation, causing typical signs of aortic regurgitation to be absent during physical examination (*Circulation* 1998; **98:** 1949–84).

Combined mitral and aortic regurgitation

Both lesions cause left ventricular dilatation, but aortic regurgitation causes systolic hypertension and mild left ventricular thickness. Treatment depends on the dominant lesion and consists of treating primarily that lesion.

Combined aortic stenosis and mitral regurgitation

The aetiology includes rheumatic heart disease, congenital AS with mitral valve prolapse in young patients and degenerative AS and MR in the elderly, when severe AS will worsen the degree of MR. MR may also cause difficulty in assessing the severity of AS because of reduced forward flow. MR will also enhance LV ejection performance, thereby masking the early development of LV systolic dysfunction caused by AS (*J Am Coll Cardiol* 1998; **32:** 1486–588).

Treatment:

- In patients with severe AS and severe MR with symptoms, LV dysfunction or pulmonary hypertension: combined AVR and MVR or mitral valve repair.
- In patients with severe AS and milder degrees of MR, the severity of mitral regurgitation may improve with isolated AVR, particularly when there is normal mitral valve morphology.
- In patients with mild to moderate aortic stenosis and severe mitral regurgitation in whom surgery on mitral valve is indicated because of symptoms of LV dysfunction, or pulmonary hypertension, preoperative assessment of the severity of aortic stenosis may be difficult because of reduced forward stroke volume. If the mean aortic valve gradient is ≥ 30 mmHg, AVR should be performed. In patients with less severe gradients, intraoperative TEE and visual assessment by the surgeon may be necessary to determine the need for AVR (*Circulation* 1998; **98:** 1949–84).

DIAGNOSIS

This patient has mixed mitral valve and aortic valve disease (lesion) of rheumatic aetiology with a dominant mitral regurgitation as evidenced by the hyperdynamic circulation. The patient is in cardiac failure (functional status).

QUESTIONS

Mention a few causes of combined aortic and mitral valve disease.

- Rheumatic valvular disease.
- Infective endocarditis.
- Collagen degenerative disorder, e.g. Marfan's syndrome.
- Calcific changes in the aortic and mitral valve apparatus.

What are the indications for surgery?

- New York Heart Association (NYHA) class III status.
- Class II status where there is volume overload of the left ventricle, e.g. in severe aortic regurgitation with moderate mitral valve disease or severe mitral regurgitation with moderate aortic stenosis and regurgitation.

Case 8

HYPERTENSION

INSTRUCTION

This patient has hypertension; would you like to examine her?

SALIENT FEATURES

History

- Chest pain or shortness of breath.
- Intermittent claudication.
- Headaches or visual disturbances (in accelerated or severe hypertension).
- Family history of hypertension.
- Ask about hypertension during pregnancy.
- Medications.

Examination

Look for aetiology:
- Comment on Cushingoid facies if present.
- Look for radiofemoral delay of coarctation of aorta.
- Examine blood pressure in both upper arms.
- Listen for renal artery bruit of renal artery stenosis and feel for polycystic kidneys.

Look for target organ damage:
- Palpate the apex for left ventricular hypertrophy.
- Look for signs of cardiac failure.
- Examine the fundus for changes of hypertensive retinopathy.
- Tell the examiner that you would like to check urine for protein (renal failure) and sugar (associated diabetes).

DIAGNOSIS

This patient has retinopathy (lesion) caused by hypertension, which is probably renovascular (aetiology) as evidenced by the renal artery bruit. She probably has damage to other target organs (functional status).

QUESTIONS

How would you record the blood pressure?

- Using a device whose accuracy has been validated and one that has been recently calibrated.
- The patient should be seated with the arm at the level of the heart. The blood pressure cuff should be appropriate for the size of the arm and the cuff should be deflated at 2 mm/s and the diastolic blood pressure is measured to the nearest

2 mmHg. Diastolic blood pressure is recorded as disappearance of the sounds (phase V).

- At least two recordings of blood pressure should be made at each of the several visits to determine blood pressure thresholds (*BMJ* 1999; **319**: 630–5).

What are the causes of blood pressure discrepancy between the arms or between the arms and legs?
- Coarctation of aorta (see pp 84–7).
- Patent ductus arteriosus (see pp 78–80).
- Dissecting aortic aneurysm.
- Arterial occlusion or stenosis of any cause.
- Supravalvular aortic stenosis (see pp 18–22).
- Thoracic outlet syndrome.

How would you investigate a patient with hypertension in outpatients?
- Full blood count (FBC).
- Urine for sugar, albumin and specific gravity.
- Urea, electrolytes and serum creatinine.
- Fasting lipids, fasting blood sugar, serum uric acid.
- Serum total:HDL cholesterol ratio.
- ECG.
- Chest radiograph.
- 24-hour urine collection to measure vanillylmandelic acid.

What are the indications for ambulatory blood pressure recording?
- When clinic blood pressure shows unusual variability.
- When hypertension is resistant to drug treatment with three or more agents.
- When symptoms suggest that the patient may have hypotension.
- To exclude 'white-coat hypertension'.

What are causes of hypertension?
- Unknown or idiopathic (in 90% of cases).
- Renal: glomerulonephritis, diabetic nephropathy, renal artery stenosis, pyelonephritis.
- Endocrine: Cushing's syndrome, steroid therapy, phaeochromocytoma.
- Others: coarctation of aorta, contraceptives, toxaemia of pregnancy.

What special investigations would you perform to screen for an underlying cause?
- Renal digital subtraction angiography.
- 24-hour urinary catecholamines – at least three samples (phaeochromocytoma).
- Overnight dexamethasone suppression test.

What are the British Hypertension Society Guidelines for initiating hypertensive agents?
- Sustained systolic blood pressure ≥ 160 mmHg or sustained diastolic blood pressure ≥ 100 mmHg.
- To determine the need for treatment in those with mild hypertension (systolic blood pressure between 140 and 159 mmHg or sustained diastolic blood pressure between 90 and 99 mmHg) according to the presence of target organ damage, cardiovascular disease, diabetes or a 10-year coronary heart disease risk of

$\geq 15\%$, according to the Joint British Societies Coronary Heart Disease Risk Assessment Program (*BMJ* 1999; **319**: 630–5).

What are the optimal treatment targets?

The optimal treatment targets are systolic blood pressure ≤ 140 mmHg and diastolic blood pressure ≤ 85 mmHg. The minimum acceptable level of control is 150/90 mmHg (*BMJ* 1999; **319**: 630–5).

What is the purpose of treatment in hypertension?

The purpose is to reduce the risk of devastating hypertensive complications such as myocardial infarction, stroke and heart failure.

How would you manage a patient with mild hypertension?

General measures
- Diet: weight reduction in obese patients, low-cholesterol diets for associated hyperlipidaemia, salt restriction. Increased consumption of fruit and vegetables.
- Regular physical exercise that should be predominantly dynamic (for example brisk walking) rather than isometric (weight lifting).
- Limit alcohol consumption (<14 units per week for women and <21 units/week for men).
- Stop smoking.

Antihypertensives
Beta-blockers or low-dose thiazides.

Other drugs
Aspirin, statins.

Why are diuretics and beta-blockers recommended as first-line agents in the management of hypertension?

Until recently, evidence about the effects of blood pressure lowering agents on the risks of cardiovascular complications came exclusively from trials of diuretic-based or beta-blocker based regimens in the hypertensive population. Those trials collectively showed reductions in risk of stroke and coronary heart disease of about 38% and 16% respectively (*Br Med Bull* 1994; **50**: 272–98) and reductions in the risk of heart failure of about 40% (*Hypertension* 1989; **13** (5 suppl): 174–9; *JAMA* 1997; **278**: 212–16).

What is the role of alpha-blocker based regimens in the control of blood pressure?

The Antihypertensive and Lipid Lowering Treatment to Prevent Heart Attack (ALLHAT) trial showed that an alpha-blocker based regimen is less effective than a diuretic-based regimen in preventing heart failure (*JAMA* 2000; **283**: 1967–75). Additionally, there was a marginally significant excess of stroke in the alpha-blocker group. Although poorer blood pressure control might account for the higher risk of stroke, it does not entirely explain the two-fold greater risk of heart failure.

What is the role of calcium channel blockers in the treatment of hypertension?

- In the SYST-EUR study nitrendipine showed a reduction in the risk of stroke in isolated systolic hypertension when compared to diuretics (*Lancet* 1997; **350:** 757–64).

- In the Swedish Trial in Old Patients with Hypertension-2 (STOP-2) study, there was some evidence that the risks of myocardial infarction and of heart failure were greater with calcium antagonist based therapy than with ACE-inhibitor based therapy, but there were no clear differences between either of these regimens and a third based on diuretics and beta-blockers (*Lancet* 1999; **354:** 1751–6). In this study 34–39% of patients withdrew from the three treatment regimens.
- The International Nifedipine GITS Study: Intervention as a Goal in Hypertension Treatment (INSIGHT) trial compared long-acting nifedipine with a diuretic (hydrochlorothiazide and amiloride combination) and found that the calcium channel antagonist was as effective as diuretics in preventing overall cardiovascular or cerebrovascular complications (*Lancet* 2000; **356:** 366–72). There was a marginally significant excess of heart failure with nifedipine-based treatment. Fatal myocardial infarctions were more common in the nifedipine group. There was an 8% excess withdrawal of drug in the nifedipine group because of peripheral oedema whereas serious adverse events were more frequent in the diuretic group.
- In the Nordic Diltiazem Study (NORDIL) from Sweden diltiazem was compared with diuretics, beta-blockers or both (*Lancet* 2000; **356:** 359–65). This study found that diltiazem was as effective as treatment based on diuretics, beta-blockers or both in preventing the primary end point of all stroke, myocardial infarction and other cardiovascular deaths. There was a marginally significant lower risk of stroke in the diltiazem group despite a lesser reduction in blood pressure. In this study, 23% of the patients withdrew from the diltiazem-based group and 7% withdrew from diuretic-based and beta-blocker based therapy.

What is the role of ACE inhibitors in hypertension?

- In the HOPE (Heart Outcomes Prevention Evaluation) study the use of ramipril was associated with reductions of stroke, coronary artery disease and heart failure in both hypertensive and non-hypertensive groups as compared to placebo (*N Engl J Med* 2000; **342:** 145–53).
- In the Captopril Prevention Project (CAPPP) the risk of stroke was slightly greater with ACE inhibitor based therapy than with diuretic-based or beta-blocker based therapy but the higher baseline and follow-up blood pressure among patients assigned the ACE inhibitor regimen may largely or entirely account for the excess risk of stroke (*Lancet* 1998; **353:** 611–16).

What are the indications for specialist referral?

- Hypertensive emergency: malignant hypertension, impending complications.
- To investigate possible aetiology when evaluation suggests this possibility.
- To evaluate therapeutic problems or failures.
- Special circumstances: unusually variable blood pressure, possible white-coat hypertension, pregnancy (*BMJ* 1999; **319:** 630–5).

Case 9

ATRIAL FIBRILLATION

INSTRUCTION

Examine this patient's pulse.

SALIENT FEATURES

History

- Palpitations.
- Pre-syncope, dizziness.
- Fatigue.
- Dyspnoea.
- Asymptomatic and atrial fibrillation is discovered incidentally.
- History of ischaemic heart disease, hypertension, valvular heart disease, rheumatic heart disease, COPD, congenital heart disease (atrial septal defect, ventricular septal defect), thyrotoxicosis (pp 355–9).
- History of consumption of caffeine, digitalis, theophylline.

Examination

- Irregularly irregular pulse (patients are often digitalized and in slow atrial fibrillation).
- Look for:
  - malar flush (mitral stenosis)
  - mitral valvotomy scar
  - warm hands, goitre, pretibial myxoedema (thyrotoxicosis).
- Elevated JVP without 'a' waves.
- Varying intensity of first heart sound (the intensity is inversely related to the previous RR cycle length; a longer cycle length produces a softer S1).
- Pulse deficit, which is the difference between the rate of the apex and the pulse rate (because varying stroke volumes result from varying periods of diastolic filling, not all ventricular beats produce a palpable peripheral pulse). The pulse deficit is greater when the ventricular rate is high.
- If you are not sure, tell the examiner that you would like to differentiate from ventricular ectopics by exercising the patient; after exercise, ventricular ectopics diminish in frequency whereas there is no change in the rhythm of atrial fibrillation.
- Look for the underlying cause:
  - Examine the heart for mitral valvular lesion.
  - Check the blood pressure for hypertension.
  - Ask the patient for history of ischaemic heart disease.
  - Check the patient's thyroid status for thyrotoxicosis.

DIAGNOSIS

This patient has fast atrial fibrillation (lesion) which is commonly caused by ischaemic heart disease (aetiology). The patient is short of breath, indicating that he may be in cardiac failure (functional status).

Read this recent review: *N Engl J Med* 2001; **344:** 1067.

QUESTIONS

What are the common causes of atrial fibrillation?

- Mitral valvular disease in the young and middle-aged.
- Ischaemic heart disease or hypertension in the elderly.
- Thyrotoxicosis (atrial fibrillation may be the only clinical feature in the elderly).
- Constrictive pericarditis.
- Chronic pulmonary disease.

Mention common sites of systemic embolization.

Brain, leg, kidney, superior mesenteric artery, coronary artery and spleen.

At the bedside, how would you differentiate atrial fibrillation from multiple ventricular ectopics?

If the patient is not in heart failure, exercise the patient; after exercise, ventricular ectopics tend to diminish in frequency whereas there is no change in the rhythm of atrial fibrillation.

How would you investigate this patient?

Electrocardiogram

P waves are absent. Fibrillatory or 'f' waves are present at a rate that may vary between 350 and 600 beats/minute and the 'f' waves vary in shape, amplitude and intervals. The RR interval is irregularly irregular. Narrow QRS complex with varying RR interval (regular unless there is an underlying ventricular conduction defect).

Echocardiogram

Useful to determine left atrial size and left ventricular systolic function, and to exclude underlying valvular heart disease and intracardiac thromboemboli.

Test of thyroid function

To exclude thyrotoxicosis.

Exercise treadmill

When atrial fibrillation is precipitated by exercise.

Holter monitor

Useful in paroxysmal atrial fibrillation to determine whether it was triggered by another arrhythmia such as when a premature atrial complex during a rapid paroxysmal atrial tachycardia may cause the immediate onset of atrial fibrillation.

ADVANCED-LEVEL QUESTIONS

Mention a few causes of irregularly irregular pulse.

- Atrial fibrillation.

- Multiple ventricular ectopics.
- Atrial flutter with varying block.
- Complete heart block (there is associated bradycardia).

In which congenital disorders is atrial fibrillation common?
Atrial septal defect, Ebstein's anomaly.

What do you understand by the term 'atrial fibrillation'?
Lone atrial fibrillation occurs in the absence of cardiopulmonary disease or a history of hypertension and before the age of 60 years. Such patients have a low risk of stroke (0.5% per year).

How would you treat a patient with atrial fibrillation?

Attempt to restore slow ventricular rate:
- In the hypertensive patient use calcium antagonists (verapamil, diltiazem).
- In thyroid disease use a beta-blocker (e.g. propranolol).
- In ischaemic heart disease use a beta-blocker or diltiazem, verapamil.
- In heart failure use digoxin or verapamil.
- In hypertrophic cardiomyopathy use a beta-blocker or calcium antagonists.
- In those who are intolerant of or do not respond to drugs, radiofrequency catheter ablation of the atrioventricular node (with a cardiac pacemaker) may provide symptomatic relief; however, it does not change the risk of systemic emboli or the need for anticoagulation (*N Engl J Med* 1999; **340:** 534).
- More recently, radiofrequency ablation of the pulmonary veins has been shown to be effective in paroxysmal atrial fibrillation when the ectopic focus is in the pulmonary veins.

Attempt to restore sinus rhythm by cardioversion if the following conditions apply:
- Left atrial size by echocardiogram is less than 4.5 cm (left atrial size >4.5 cm is not associated with long-term maintenance of sinus rhythm).
- Short duration of the arrhythmia (acute atrial fibrillation is likely to remain in sinus rhythm).
- Drugs used to restore sinus rhythm or prevent recurrence include quinidine, procainamide, disopyramide, propafenone, sotalol, flecainide, amiodarone and ibutilide (*N Engl J Med* 2000; **342:** 913–20; *Circulation* 1996; **94:** 1613).

Anticoagulation with warfarin is advised for certain patients:
- Undergoing cardioversion (electrical or drug).
- With underlying mitral valve disease.
- In left ventricular failure.
- With cardiomyopathy.
- Above the age of 60 years.

Mention a few drugs used to restore sinus rhythm.
Procainamide, disopyramide or quinidine for 2–3 days restores sinus rhythm in up to 30% of patients.

What is the role of oral anticoagulants in chronic atrial fibrillation?
Non-rheumatic atrial fibrillation is an important risk factor for stroke, even though it is recognized that only 80% of strokes in such patients result from embolism from

the heart. All patients with non-rheumatic atrial fibrillation should be anticoagulated with warfarin unless there are contraindications (*Br J Hosp Med* 1993; **50**: 452–7).

What is the role of surgery in the treatment of atrial fibrillation?

- A novel surgical technique, the Maze procedure, has recently been described in which multiple incisions are made in the atria to prevent re-entrant loops (*Clin Cardiol* 1991; **14**: 827–34). This procedure is highly effective in preventing atrial fibrillation: only one patient out of 65 suffered a clinical recurrence of the arrhythmia three or more months after the procedure. Although the long-term outcome is not known, it remains a promising procedure when atrial fibrillation is not controlled by medical therapy or in those cases complicated by recurrent thromboembolism.

- The 'corridor' procedure effectively isolates both the left and right atrium, leaving a strip of myocardium connecting the sinus node to the atrioventricular node. This procedure does not prevent atrial fibrillation but isolates the fibrillating atria. Although a 70% 'cure' rate is reported, sequential atrioventricular contraction is not restored (with the consequent haemodynamic effects and the risk of thromboembolism).

What do you know about holiday heart syndrome?

It is the occurrence of supraventricular arrhythmias, usually atrial fibrillation and atrial flutter, following an acute alcoholic binge in chronic alcoholics. These are usually transient.

It was James Mackenzie, a Scottish general practitioner working in Burnley, England, utilizing an ink-polygraph to record and label jugular venous pulses, who pioneered the deciphering of normal and abnormal cardiac rhythms. His key observation that the jugular 'a' wave disappeared in a patient who went from a normal to an irregular rhythm provided the first insight into the mechanism of atrial fibrillation.

In 1924, Willem Einthoven (1860–1927) of Leyden University, The Netherlands, was awarded the Nobel Prize for his discovery of the mechanism of electrocardiography (*Am J Cardiol* 1994; **73**: 384–9).

In 1909, Lewis in England and Rothberger and Winterberg in Vienna, taking advantage of Einthoven's newly developed string galvanometer, were the first to establish electrocardiographically that auricular fibrillation was the cause of pulsus irregularis perpetuus.

Rodney Falk is Professor of Cardiology at Boston University. He trained in England and his main interests are amyloidosis and atrial fibrillation.

Case 10

PALPITATIONS

INSTRUCTION

This patient has palpitations: would you like to ask her a few questions?

SALIENT FEATURES

History

- Are the palpitations regular or irregular? (Rapid regular rhythms suggest SVT or VT whereas rapid, irregular rhythms suggest atrial fibrillation, atrial flutter or tachycardia with varying block.)
- Is the onset abrupt (paroxysmal tachyarrhythmias)?
- How frequent are the palpitations?
- What is the duration of each episode?
- Is each episode followed by polyuria (seen in supraventricular tachycardia)?
- Is there any relation to exercise (e.g. polymorphic VT in long QT syndrome)?
- What happens on standing (postural hypotension, atrioventricular nodal tachycardia)?
- Are there any precipitating factors such as coffee, tea, alcohol or medications such as thyroid extract, ephedrine, aminophylline, monoamine oxidase inhibitors?
- Are there any associated symptoms such as chest pain or shortness of breath?
- Is there associated syncope? (Dizziness or syncope accompanying palpitations should prompt a search for ventricular tachycardia.)
- Are the palpitations associated with anxiety or panic attacks? (Anxiety or panic can result in palpitations.)

Note. Palpitations are a common complaint in up to 16% of outpatients. They are non-specific and in only 15% of patients do they correlate with cardiac arrhythmia.

Examination

- Pulse for arrhythmia.
- JVP is distended in heart failure and 'frog' sign (where prominent jugular venous pulsations match the rate of tachycardia) in atrioventricular nodal re-entrant tachycardia (*Lancet* 1993; **341**: 1254–8).
- Auscultate the heart for murmurs (mitral valve prolapse, valvular heart disease, harsh systolic murmur of hypertrophic cardiomyopathy), split second heart sound (atrial fibrillation).
- Look for signs of atrial fibrillation.
- Although palpitations may not be present at rest, when the ventricular response is slow, a brisk walk down the corridor may result in palpitations.

Tell the examiner that you would like to examine the ECG for:

- Presence of Q waves typical of old myocardial infarction, prompting a search for non-sustained ventricular tachycardia.
- LVH with left atrial enlargement (as suggested by notched P wave in lead II or terminal P wave force in lead V1 more negative than 0.04 s) as this is a likely substrate for atrial fibrillation.

- Short PR interval and delta waves, which suggests ventricular pre-excitation and substrate for SVT (Wolff–Parkinson–White syndrome).
- Marked left ventricular hypertrophy with deep septal Q waves in I, L and V4 through V6, which suggests hypertrophic cardiomyopathy.
- Prolonged QT interval and abnormal T wave morphology, suggesting the presence of long QT syndrome.
- Bradycardias and complete heart block since they may be associated with ventricular premature depolarizations, long QT syndrome and torsade de pointes.
- Abnormal morphology of a ventricular ectopic, suggesting that one of the two types of idiopathic ventricular tachycardia is present.

DIAGNOSIS

This patient has palpitations (lesion) accompanied by polyuria, indicating a supraventricular tachycardia (aetiology).

QUESTIONS

What are the causes?
- Extrasystole.
- Tachycardia or bradycardia.
- Drugs (see above).
- Other: thyrotoxicosis, hypoglycaemia, unaccustomed exertion, phaeochromocytoma, fever.
- Anxiety state (also known as da Costa's syndrome or cardiac neurosis).

How would you investigate a patient suspected of having a disorder of cardiac rhythm?
- 12-lead ECG (look for evidence of a rhythm disturbance and pre-excitation syndrome).
- Continuous ambulatory (Holter) echocardiography (many patients with palpitations may have stable sinus rhythm).
- Exercise ECG.

J.M. da Costa (1833–1900) was Professor of Medicine at Jefferson Medical College, Philadelphia.

Case 11

SLOW PULSE RATE

INSTRUCTION

Examine this patient's pulse.

SALIENT FEATURES

History

- Drug history: beta-blockers, digoxin, verapamil.
- Is the patient an athlete?
- Symptoms which are usually non-specific (e.g. dizziness, fatigue, weakness, heart failure).
- History of recent myocardial infarction.
- Ask if the bradycardia is episodic. If so, enquire about precipitating factors and associated symptoms or signs.
- Ask about nocturnal bradycardia (a feature of obstructive sleep apnoea).

Examination

- Pulse rate of less than 60 beats per minute (*N Engl J Med* 2000; **342:** 703–9).
- Pulse rate may be either regular or irregular.
- If the pulse is irregular, get the patient to stand and then count his pulse rate (in complete heart block there is no increase in rate).
- Look at the JVP for cannon 'a' waves.
- Auscultate the heart for cannon first heart sound.
- Look for signs of hypothyroidism, particularly in the elderly.

DIAGNOSIS

This patient has a complete heart block (lesion) probably due to ischaemic heart disease (aetiology) and is disabled by syncopal attacks (functional status).

QUESTIONS

What are the causes of bradycardia?

- Physical fitness in athletes.
- Idiopathic degeneration (ageing).
- Acute myocardial infarction.
- Drugs (beta-blockers, digitalis, calcium channel blockers).
- Hypothyroidism.
- Obstructive jaundice.
- Increased intracranial pressure.
- Hypothermia.
- Hyperkalaemia.

ADVANCED-LEVEL QUESTIONS

How would you investigate this patient?
- 12-lead ECG to confirm bradycardia.
- 24–48-hour ambulatory ECG recording is useful in patients with frequent or continuous symptoms.
- Exercise ECG or ambulatory monitoring for chronotropic incompetence.
- Tilt-table testing when neurocardiogenic syncope is suspected.

What are the indications for temporary cardiac pacing in bradyarrhythmias?
- Symptomatic second- or third-degree heart block due to transient drug intoxication or electrolyte disturbance.
- Complete heart block, Mobitz II or bifascicular block in the setting of an acute myocardial infarct.
- Symptomatic sinus bradycardia, atrial fibrillation with slow ventricular response.

What are the indications for permanent pacing in bradyarrhythmias?
- Symptomatic congenital heart block.
- Symptomatic sinus bradycardia.
- Symptomatic second- or third-degree heart block.

Which drug would you use to treat sinus bradycardia seen in the setting of an acute myocardial infarction?
Intravenous atropine.

What do you understand by the term chronotropic incompetence?
Failure to reach a heart rate that is 85% of the age-predicted maximum (220 − age in years) at peak exercise, the failure to achieve a heart rate of 100 beats per minute, or a maximal heart rate more than 2 SD below that in a control population (*N Engl J Med* 2000; **342:** 703–9).

What do you know about Stokes–Adams syndrome?
It refers to syncope or fits occurring during complete heart block.

W. Stokes (1804–1878), Regius Professor of Medicine in Dublin, graduated from Edinburgh.

R. Adams (1791–1875), Professor of Surgery in Dublin, was an authority on gout and arthritis.

Case 12

GALLOP RHYTHM

INSTRUCTION

Listen to the precordium.
Examine this patient's heart.

SALIENT FEATURES

History

- Dyspnoea and determine NYHA class.
- Paroxysmal nocturnal dysnoea.
- Swelling of the feet.

Examination

- Presence of an abnormal third or fourth heart sound with tachycardia (the presence of a normal third or fourth heart sound does not connote a gallop rhythm unless there is associated tachycardia).
- Auscultate with the bell as third and fourth heart sounds are low pitched.
- Gallop rhythm due to third heart sound seems to sound like 'Kentucky', whereas that due to the fourth heart sound sounds like 'Tennessee'.

Note
- A left ventricular third heart sound is best heard at the apex, whereas the right ventricular third heart sound is best heard along the left sternal border.
- In emphysematous patients the gallop is better heard when listening over the xiphoid or epigastric area.

DIAGNOSIS

This patient has gallop rhythm (lesion) which indicates that he is in cardiac failure (functional status).

QUESTIONS

What is the expression used when both the third and fourth heart sounds are heard with tachycardia?
This is known as the summation gallop. It can sometimes be mistaken for a diastolic rumbling murmur.

ADVANCED-LEVEL QUESTIONS

What is the mechanism of production of the third heart sound?
It is caused by rapid ventricular filling in early diastole.

What is the mechanism of production of the fourth heart sound?

It is caused by vigorous contraction of the atria (atrial systole) and hence is heard towards the end of diastole.

How do you differentiate between the fourth heart sound, a split first heart sound and an ejection click?

The fourth heart sound is not heard when pressure is applied on the chest piece of the stethoscope, but pressure does not eliminate the ejection sound or the splitting of the first heart sound.

What are the causes of a third heart sound?

Physiological: in normal children and young adults.

Pathological:

- Heart failure.
- Left ventricular dilatation without failure: mitral regurgitation, ventricular septal defect, patent ductus arteriosus.
- Right ventricular S3 in right ventricular failure, tricuspid regurgitation.

What are the implications of a third heart sound in patients with valvular heart disease?

- In patients with mitral regurgitation, they are common but do not necessarily reflect ventricular systolic dysfunction or increased filling pressure (*N Engl J Med* 1992; **327**: 458–62).
- In patients with aortic stenosis, third heart sounds are uncommon but usually indicate the presence of systolic dysfunction and raised filling pressure.

What are the causes of a fourth heart sound?

Normal: in the elderly.

Pathological:

- Acute myocardial infarction.
- Aortic stenosis (the presence of S4 in individuals below the age of 40 indicates significant obstruction).
- Hypertension. (It is a constant finding in hypertension.)
- Hypertrophic cardiomyopathy.
- Pulmonary stenosis.

Note. The fourth heart sound does not denote heart failure, unlike the S3 gallop.

Potain credited Jean Baptiste Bouillaud (1786–1881), Professor of Medicine in Paris, as being the first person to describe gallop rhythm (Jean Baptiste Bouillaud. *Proc R Soc Med* 1931; **24**: 1253–1931).

Pierre Carl Edouard Potain (1825–1901), Parisian physician, was the first to distinguish between various types of gallop in a short account titled *Théorie du Bruit de Gallop* in 1885.

Case 13

ANGINA PECTORIS

INSTRUCTION

This patient is suspected to have angina pectoris. Would you like to ask her a few questions and perform a relevant examination, to confirm these suspicions?

SALIENT FEATURES

History

- Have you ever had any pain or discomfort in the chest?
- How would you describe the chest discomfort (heavy, burning, tightness, stabbing, pressure)?
- Do you get this on walking at ordinary pace on the level or does it come on when you walk uphill or hurry?
- When you get the pain/discomfort, do you stop, slow down or continue at the same pace?
- Does the pain/discomfort go away when you stand still? (It is typically relieved by rest or nitroglycerine within 10 minutes.)
- Where do you get this pain? (Angina is a visceral sensation and is poorly localized, therefore patients rarely point to the location of their discomfort with one finger.)
- Does it radiate elsewhere (e.g. arms, jaw, epigastrium)?
- Does food or cold weather bring on the pain?
- Ask about risk factors such as smoking, diabetes, hypertension, family history of ischaemic heart disease.

Examination

Typically no signs are manifest, but patients should be examined for evidence of the following:

- Hypertension (see pp 27–30).
- Hyperlipidaemia (see pp 440–1).
- Diabetes (see pp 518–23).
- Left ventricular outflow obstruction (aortic stenosis, hypertrophic cardiomyopathy).
- Previous myocardial infarction (see pp 45–52).

DIAGNOSIS

This patient has angina pectoris (lesion) which is due to atherosclerotic coronary artery disease (aetiology). She is in Canadian Cardiovascular Society functional class II (functional status).

QUESTIONS

How is angina graded by the Canadian Cardiovascular Society?
There are four functional classes:

- Class I: Angina occurs only with strenuous or rapid or prolonged exertion.
- Class II: There is slight limitation of ordinary activity (e.g. climbing more than one flight of ordinary stairs at a normal pace and in normal conditions).
- Class III: There is marked limitation of ordinary activity (e.g. climbing more than one flight in normal conditions).
- Class IV: Inability to carry out any physical activity without discomfort – anginal syndrome may be present at rest.

What is the mechanism of angina pectoris?
It commonly results from increased myocardial oxygen demand triggered by physical activity, but it can also be caused by transient decreases in oxygen delivery due to coronary vasospasm. Unstable angina is caused by non-occlusive intra-coronary thrombi.

How would you investigate a patient with angina pectoris?
- Haemoglobin: anaemia aggravates angina.
- Rest ECG: to detect left ventricular hypertrophy, prior Q-wave MI or ST–T changes.
- Rest echocardiogram: done only when there is clinical suspicion of aortic stenosis or hypertrophic cardiomyopathy.
- Exercise ECG: to precipitate symptoms, to document workload at onset and to record any associated ECG abnormality (≥ 1 mm of horizontal or downsloping ST-segment depression or elevation for ≥ 60 to 80 ms after the end of the QRS complex) or arrhythmia.
- Exercise myocardial perfusion imaging or exercise echocardiography in patients who have one of the following baseline ECG abnormalities: (a) LBBB, (b) more than 1 mm of rest ST depression, (c) electronically paced ventricular rhythm, and in patients with prior revascularization (PTCA or CABG) or in whom considerations of functional significance of lesions or myocardial viability are important.
- Coronary angiography: provides detailed anatomical information about site and severity of luminal narrowing due to coronary atherosclerosis and less common non-atherosclerotic causes such as coronary artery spasm, coronary anomaly, primary coronary artery dissection and radiation-induced coronary vasculopathy.

How would you treat a patient with chronic stable angina pectoris?

Mnemonic ABCDE (Circulation 1999; 99: 2829–48):

- **A**spirin, **A**nti-anginal therapy and **A**CE-inhibitor therapy. Aspirin has been shown to reduce the incidence of non-fatal myocardial infarction and the overall incidence of cardiac events, although overall death rate and the incidence of fatal myocardial infarction were similar to those obtained with placebo in the Swedish Angina Pectoris Aspirin Trial (SAPAT) study. Ramipril up to 10 mg once a day should be offered to all patients in view of the new HOPE trial.
- **B**eta-blocker and **B**lood pressure.
- **C**igarette smoking and **C**holesterol.
- **D**iet and **D**iabetes.
- **E**ducation and **E**xercise.

Percutaneous transluminal coronary angioplasty (with or without coronary stent)

- Complementary to drug treatment and surgery; no improvement in survival.
- Best results are achieved in discrete single-vessel coronary artery disease.
- The restenosis rate is ~30% at 6 months; for balloon angioplasty with stenting, restenosis is lower, ~20%.
- The ACME (Angioplasty Compared to Medicine) study showed that PTCA can offer better symptomatic relief than medical therapy in patients with single-vessel coronary artery disease, but is a much more expensive procedure and is associated with complications (including emergency and elective coronary by-pass and second PTCA).
- The RITA (Randomized Intervention Treatment of Angina) study compared PTCA with coronary artery bypass graft (CABG) and found that both procedures have similar prognostic implications with risk of death or myocardial infarction similar in the two groups, but more patients in the PTCA group required a second revascularization procedure and more antianginal therapy.

Coronary artery bypass grafting

- This has prognostic value in patients with left main-stem coronary stenosis or three-vessel coronary artery disease and impaired left ventricular function.
- The risk of surgery is related to the degree of impairment of left ventricular function.

Neurostimulation

This is useful in refractory cases and involves the use of percutaneous electric nerve stimulation (TENS) or spinal cord stimulation (SCS).

Transmyocardial revascularization

A laser is used to drill tiny holes into the heart, providing symptomatic relief from refractory angina, but does not improve cardiovascular function or reduce adverse ischaemic events.

ADVANCED-LEVEL QUESTIONS

What is the prognosis of patients with angina?

- Fourteen per cent of patients with newly diagnosed angina pectoris progress to unstable angina, myocardial infarction, or death within 1 year.
- Mortality at coronary artery bypass grafting with normal ventricular function is 1%.

What is the significance and the mechanism of postprandial angina?

The presence of postprandial angina indicates severe coronary artery disease; one mechanism is 'intramyocardial steal' with blood being distributed from the stenotic territories to the normal territories (*Circulation* 1998; **97:** 1144–9). It results from the carbohydrate content of the meal (*Am J Cardiol* 1997; **79:** 1397–1400) and can be ameliorated by prior treatment with octreotide (*Circulation* 1996; **94:** 1–730), which prevents postprandial vasodilatation of the superior mesenteric artery.

How would you follow a patient with stable angina in your clinic?

- Patients with successfully treated chronic stable angina pectoris should have a follow-up evaluation every 4–12 months. During the first year of therapy evaluations every 4–6 months are recommended. After the first year of therapy, annual evaluations are recommended provided the patient is stable and reliable enough to call or make an appointment when anginal symptoms become worse or other symptoms occur. Patients who are co-managed by their general practitioner and cardiologist may alternate these visits (*Circulation* 1999; **99**: 2829–48).

- The ACC/AHA 'five questions' that must be answered regularly during the follow-up of the patient who is receiving treatment for chronic stable angina (*Circulation* 1999; **99**: 2829–48):
  1. Has the patient decreased the level of physical activity since the last visit?
  2. Have the patient's anginal symptoms increased in frequency and become more severe since the last visit? If the symptoms have worsened or the patient has decreased physical activity to avoid precipitating angina, then he or she should be evaluated and treated according to either the unstable angina or chronic stable angina guidelines, as appropriate.
  3. How well is the patient tolerating therapy?
  4. How successful has the patient been in reducing modifiable risk factors and improving knowledge about ischaemic heart disease?
  5. Has the patient developed any new comorbid illnesses or has the severity or treatment of known comorbid illnesses worsened the patient's angina?

What do you understand by the term unstable angina?

This includes patients with more severe or frequent angina superimposed on chronic stable angina, angina at rest or minimal exertion, or angina of new onset (within 1 month) which is brought about by minimal exertion.

It is a potentially dangerous condition and patients should be admitted to a coronary care unit and begun on antianginal therapy including beta-blockers, aspirin and intravenous nitrates. Intravenous heparin should be started in patients with rest angina of 48 hours duration and in those with chest pain and ischaemic ECG changes on admission. Most patients stabilize with this treatment, although some may require intra-aortic balloon counterpulsation before cardiac catheterization. A monoclonal antibody $7E_3$ against platelet glycoprotein IIb/IIIa, which prevents platelet adhesion and degranulation, is undergoing evaluation in the treatment of unstable angina.

What is Prinzmetal's angina?

It is angina occurring at rest, unpredictably, and associated with transient ST segment elevation on the ECG. Coronary vasospasm is the cause, often in the presence of atherosclerosis.

How is exercise testing useful in determining the prognosis of chest pain?

A study at Duke University used exercise testing to determine high- and low-risk subsets in patients with chest pain suggestive of ischaemic heart disease:

- Low-risk subset: subjects who could complete 9 minutes of exercise using the Bruce protocol without evidence of ischaemic ST segment changes and achieve a maximal sinus heart rate in excess of 160 beats per minute. These were found to have a 1-year survival rate of 99% and a 4-year survival rate of 93%. This means that cardiac catheterization and CABG can be deferred.
- High-risk subset: those who were forced to stop exercising in stages I or II (under 6 minutes); survival rate was 85% at 1 year and 63% at 4 years.

What do you understand by the term 'syndrome X'?

- Syndrome X, or microvascular angina, is the presence of classic angina and ST depression on exercise stress testing and a normal coronary angiogram in the absence of any other demonstrable cardiac abnormalities.
- Reaven's syndrome or 'endocrine' syndrome X is the association of insulin resistance, hypertension, and increased very low density lipoprotein (VLDL) and decreased high density lipoprotein (HDL) cholesterol concentrations in the plasma.

Coronary artery bypass grafting was introduced by R.G. Favalaro in 1969 while he was at the Cleveland Clinic, USA (*J Thorac Cardiovasc Surg* 1969; **58**: 178–85).

Balloon angioplasty was introduced by Arthur Gruntzig, a Swiss cardiologist, in 1977 (*Lancet* 1978; **i**: 263).

Case 14

ACUTE MYOCARDIAL INFARCTION

INSTRUCTION

This patient had a myocardial infarction 2 days ago; would you like to take a short history and examine him?

SALIENT FEATURES

History

- Post-infarct angina.
- Shortness of breath.
- Palpitations.
- Dizziness or syncope.
- Family history of cardiovascular disease, hyperlipidaemia, gout.
- Smoking.
- Past history of diabetes mellitus, hypertension, stroke, myocardial infarction, intermittent claudication and hyperlipidaemia.
- History of oral contraceptives in young women.

Examination

- Hands: nicotine staining of fingers.
- Pulse: check pulse rate (keeping in mind heart block and tachycardia), rhythm (keeping in mind atrial fibrillation, ventricular arrhythmias).
- Check blood pressure.
- JVP may be raised in cardiac failure or right ventricular infarction.
- Eyes: look for arcus senilis, xanthelasma.
- Cardiac apex: look for double apical impulse (ventricular aneurysm).
- Auscultate for fourth heart sound, pericardial rub, pansystolic murmur of papillary muscle dysfunction (or ventricular septal defect).

Examine:
- The chest for crackles and pleural effusion
- The abdomen for tender liver of cardiac failure
- The legs for deep venous thrombosis and peripheral pulses.

DIAGNOSIS

This patient with myocardial infarction (aetiology) has papillary muscle dysfunction (lesion) and is in NYHA class II cardiac failure (functional status).

QUESTIONS

What is Levine's sign?

In acute myocardial infarction the patient often describes the pain by illustrating a clenched fist.

What are the major risk factors for an acute MI?
- Smoking.
- Hypercholesterolaemia.
- Diabetes.
- Hypertension.

How would you manage a patient with acute MI?

Treatment of MI includes (*BMJ* 1998; **316:** 280–4):

- In the A&E department, a patient with chest pain should have a quick clinical examination and an ECG performed within 10 minutes of arrival in hospital.
- Aspirin: chewable non-coated 160–325 mg should be administered immediately and then 160–325 mg daily. In the ISIS-2 and ISIS-3 trials 160 mg dosage was effective whereas a 325 mg dose was used successfully in GISSI-2. An initial large dose of aspirin of 325 mg orally or 160 mg chewable aspirin is preferred because lower doses may still allow significant thromboxane activity and may take a few days to become effective.
- Pain relief: immediate relief of pain should be a top priority because severe pain can cause autonomic disturbances that can result in sudden death.
- Reperfusion strategies: either thrombolysis or primary PTCA should be performed within 30 minutes of the patient's arrival in hospital.
- Beta-blockers: the patient should receive beta-blockers when there are no contraindications within 12 hours of onset of infarction, irrespective of administration of concomitant thrombolytic therapy or performance of primary angioplasty.
- ACE inhibitors: should be administered within the first 24 hours of a suspected acute myocardial infarction with ST segment elevation in ≥ 2 anterior precordial leads or with clinical heart failure in the absence of hypotension (systolic blood pressure <100 mmHg) or known contraindications to use of ACE inhibitors.

What are the complications of myocardial infarction?
- Extension of infarct and post-infarct ischaemia.
- Rhythm disorders: tachycardia, bradycardia, ventricular ectopics, ventricular fibrillation, atrial fibrillation and tachycardia.
- Heart failure: acute pulmonary oedema.

- Circulatory failure: cardiogenic shock.
- Infarction of papillary muscle: mitral regurgitation and acute pulmonary oedema.
- Rupture of interventricular septum.
- Left ventricular aneurysm.
- Mural thrombus.
- Thromboembolism: cerebral or peripheral.
- Venous thrombosis.
- Pericarditis.
- Dressler's syndrome, characterized by persistent pyrexia, pericarditis, pleurisy. It was first described in 1956 when Dressler recognized that chest pain following myocardial infarction is not caused by coronary artery insufficiency.

What is a silent myocardial infarct?

A painless infarct, common in diabetics and the elderly; it may present with complications of myocardial infarction.

What are TIMI grades?

Grades determined in the Thrombolysis in Myocardial Infarction trial (TIMI) that measure coronary blood flow and luminal narrowing:

- Grade 0: no flow of contrast beyond the point of occlusion.
- Grade 1: penetration with minimal perfusion (contrast fails to opacify the entire coronary bed distal to the stenosis for the duration of investigation).
- Grade 2: partial perfusion (contrast opacifies the entire distal coronary artery, but the rate of entry or clearance or both is slower in the previously blocked artery than in nearby normally perfused vessels).
- Grade 3: Complete perfusion (contrast filling and clearance are as rapid in the previously blocked vessel as in normally perfused vessels).

Which thrombolytic agent is preferred?

Three thrombolytic agents (which reduce mortality) are commonly available in the UK: streptokinase, anistreplase and tissue plasminogen activator (tPA), of which streptokinase is the cheapest and tPA the most expensive. In ISIS-3 (Third International Study of Infarct Survival) all three agents were found to be equally effective and in the GISSI-2 (Gruppo Italiano per lo Studio della Sopraviviena nell Infarcto Micocardioco) study both tPA and streptokinase were equally effective. However, in both these studies there was increased risk of haemorrhage with tPA. In the GUSTO (Global Utilization of Streptokinase and Tissue Plasminogen Activator) trial, tPA given in an accelerated manner was particularly useful in young men with anterior wall myocardial infarction. tPA is now given to patients previously treated with streptokinase because the development of anti-streptokinase antibodies puts them at risk of allergic reactions and reduces the effectiveness of thrombolysis.

The best thrombolytic treatment currently available – accelerated tPA – achieves grade 3 patency in only 54% of patients, which is better than streptokinase (30% of patients had TIMI grade 3). The difference in vessel patency achieved by tissue plasminogen activator and streptokinase treatment has not resulted in a significant difference in mortality in most trials. Although the GUSTO-1 trial showed reduced mortality with tissue plasminogen activator treatment, this benefit was partly offset by an excess of strokes in this treatment group. The current contender for the primary position held by accelerated tPA seems to be reteplase. Reteplase differs from tissue plasminogen activator at two molecular points, and deletion of these molecular domains contributes to its longer half-life. Reteplase is conveniently administered: two 10 unit boluses are given 30 minutes apart. It has been shown to be comparable with tPA. In the INJECT (International Joint Efficacy Comparison of Thrombolytics) trial patients in the reteplase group had significantly fewer side-effects such as atrial fibrillation and cardiogenic shock when compared to the streptokinase group.

What is the relation between thrombolysis and onset of symptoms?

Thrombolytic therapy reduces mortality and limits infarct size. The shorter the interval between the onset of symptoms and the initiation of thrombolysis, the greater is the survival. The greatest benefit occurs if the treatment is initiated within the first three hours, when a 50% or greater reduction in mortality rate can be achieved. The magnitude of benefit declines rapidly thereafter, but a 10% mortality reduction can be achieved up to 12 hours after the onset of pain.

Duration (hours) from onset of symptoms to initiation of thrombolysis	No of lives saved per 1000 treated
Within 60 minutes	65
2–3 hours	27
4–6 hours	25
7–12 hours	8

What is the benefit of late administration of thrombolytic therapy?

ISIS-2 (*Lancet* 1988; **ii:** 349–60) showed benefit for up to 24 hours (after onset of symptoms) with thrombolysis, but more recent studies – LATE (Late Assessment of Thrombolytic Therapy) and EMRAS (Estudio Multicentrico Esteptoquinasa Republicas de America del Sur) – have shown no benefit for treatment given beyond 12 hours.

What is the role of heparin with thrombolysis?

In the ISIS-3 (*Lancet* 1992; **339:** 753–70) and GISSI-2 (*Lancet* 1990; **336:** 65–75) studies heparin therapy with streptokinase or anistreplase was not beneficial, and it is believed that it may even be harmful. The GUSTO trial showed that, with tPA, early intravenous heparin results in a further reduction in the mortality rate compared with that found with a combination of heparin and streptokinase.

What is the role of pre-hospital thrombolysis?

Two studies – GREAT (Grampian Region Early Administration of Thrombolysis) and EMIP (European Myocardial Infarction Project) – showed that a single bolus dose of anistreplase reduced the total mortality rate. These results suggest that early thrombolysis has greater benefit, hence the importance in many hospitals of 'door to needle time'.

What is the role of angiotensin converting enzyme inhibitors (ACE) inhibitors following myocardial infarction?

Several large trials (SAVE, AIRE, SMILE, TRACE, GISSI-III and ISIS-IV) have shown both short- and long-term improvement in survival with ACE inhibitor therapy. The benefits are greatest in patients with low ejection fractions, large infarctions or clinical evidence of heart failure.

- The AIRE (Acute Infarction Ramipril Efficacy) and the AIREX (AIRE Extension) trials assessed the long-term (mean follow-up 59 months) efficacy of ramipril compared with placebo in 603 patients with heart failure after myocardial infarction. Treatment with ramipril resulted in a large and sustained reduction in mortality (relative risk reduction 36%).
- The SAVE (Survival and Ventricular Enlargement) Trial compared the effect of captopril or placebo in 2231 patients up to 16 days post myocardial infarction with an asymptomatic ejection fraction ≤40%. Captopril reduced overall and cardiovascular mortality, and also reduced the risk of requiring hospitalization or treatment for heart failure (*N Engl J Med* 1992; **327:** 685–91). At 5-year follow-up a substantial reduction in the risk of stroke was observed. Decreased ejection fraction and older age were independent risk factors (*N Engl J Med* 1997; **336:** 251–7).
- In the recent HOPE trial, ramipril has been shown to reduce significantly the rates of death, myocardial infarction and stroke in a broad range of high-risk patients who are not known to have a low ejection fraction or heart failure (*N Engl J Med* 2000; **342:** 145–53).

What is the role of primary angioplasty in acute infarction?

Angioplasty results in both lower mortality rates and a reduction in the incidence of recurrent ischaemic events. Also, angioplasty is associated with lower enzyme rise, better left ventricular function, and less reinfarction. Angioplasty led to shorter hospital stay, fewer re-admissions and lower follow-up costs. However, the major limitation of this approach is the access to both facilities and personnel to carry out the procedure.

Angioplasty should be considered in patients who have recognized contra-indications to thrombolysis (even if this means transferring the patient) or who are considered high risk and present with their infarction to a hospital where angioplasty can be performed. Patients who have received thrombolysis and who seem on clinical grounds (reduction in maximal ST segment elevation by 50% and resolution of chest pain) not to have reperfused at 90-minute review should be seriously considered for rescue angioplasty, again even if this means transferring the patient.

Is intravenous nitrate therapy routinely administered in acute myocardial infarction?

Routine administration of nitrates is not recommended since the ISIS-4 and GISSI-3 trials (in which >70 000 patients were randomized to nitrates or placebo) showed no improvement in outcome. However, nitroglycerine is the agent of choice for recurrent ischaemic pain and is useful in lowering blood pressure or relieving pulmonary congestion.

Why is the Asian population in Britain susceptible to premature myocardial infarction?

Premature ischaemic heart disease in migrants from the Indian subcontinent is associated with insulin resistance. The site of this defective insulin action has been localized to the skeletal muscle by means of positron emission tomography (Baliga RR et al. Positron emission tomography localizes insulin resistance to skeletal muscle in premature coronary heart disease. *Circulation* 1995; **92:** 1–16).

What is the role of troponins in the diagnosis of myocardial infarction?

Raised concentrations of the myocardial regulatory protein troponin I are highly specific for myocardial injury. Estimation of troponin I concentration may be particularly useful in patients with acute or chronic skeletal muscle disease or those with renal failure in whom the CK-MB (MB isoenzyme of creatine kinase) level may be raised in the absence of myocardial infarction. The measurement of troponin I is a sensitive and specific method (more specific than CK-MB) in the setting of perioperative myocardial infarction. Troponin T is also useful because it has a large diagnostic window, as it is increased from 12 hours to 10 days after myocardial infarction.

What do you know about right ventricular infarction?

Right ventricular infarction presents with retrosternal chest discomfort, nausea, vomiting and diaphoresis, unlike left ventricular infarction which presents with dyspnoea. On examination in right ventricular infarction, there is a raised jugular venous pressure with no evidence of pulmonary congestion; the patient often has a low cardiac output with hypotension. The patient typically presents with ST elevation in the inferior leads (II, III and aVF) and in one or more right-sided leads, particularly V_{4R}. The cornerstones of therapy include restoration of infarct artery patency, intravascular volume expansion and inotropic support.

What do you know about the open infarct-related coronary artery hypothesis?

This hypothesis holds that early reperfusion of the infarct-related coronary artery results in myocardial salvage, which preserves left ventricular function and is responsible for improved survival. Patients with complete occlusion of the coronary artery (TIMI grade 0) 90 minutes following thrombolysis had a 30-day mortality of 8.4%, whereas mortality was 4% in patients with TIMI grade 3 flow (complete perfusion).

What is the role of glycoprotein IIb/IIIa antagonists as adjuncts to thrombolytic therapy in acute MI?

After thrombolytic therapy for acute MI, full anterograde perfusion (TIMI grade 3 flow) occurs in only 29–54% of patients at 90 minutes while reocclusion occurs in at least 12%, with increased morbidity and mortality. Thrombolytic therapy may itself be prothrombotic by releasing clot-bound thrombin, which in turn stimulates platelet activation. Preclinical and early clinical trials have suggested that glycoprotein IIb/IIIa receptor blockers (which prevent fibrinogen binding to platelets) used as adjuncts to thrombolytic therapy may improve early patency and reduce the incidence of reocclusion. A large randomized trial has recently confirmed the early findings on patency and suggests that adjunctive treatment with glycoprotein IIb/IIIa receptor blockers may hold promise for better management of acute MI. The results from the GUSTO-AMI phase III trial using abciximab with reduced dose reteplase are awaited.

What do you know about post-MI risk stratification?

- Risk stratification before hospital discharge is an important aspect of management and determines whether coronary angiography is indicated.

- The first step is to determine whether the clinical variables indicating a relatively high risk for future cardiac events are present:
  1. Patients who have recurrent ischaemia at rest or with mild activity, who have had evidence of congestive heart failure or who are known to have an ejection fraction below 40% and in whom there are no contraindications for revascularization should undergo cardiac catheterization and coronary angiography. Revascularization should then be carried out if the coronary anatomy is suitable and there are no contraindications.
  2. Patients who have had an episode of ventricular fibrillation or sustained ventricular tachycardia more than 48 hours after acute MI should be considered for electrophysiological study or amiodarone therapy, or both.
  3. In patients with non-ST segment elevation MI or unstable angina who appear on clinical grounds to be candidates for coronary revascularization, coronary vascularization should be performed. Revascularization may then be carried out if the coronary anatomy is appropriate.
- Patients without these clinical indicators of high risk should undergo an assessment of left ventricular function (echocardiogram or radionuclide angiogram and submaximal stress) before hospital discharge. If the test is negative the patient may return for a symptom-limited exercise test at 3–6 weeks. If that too is negative he or she can remain on medical therapy and risk factor reduction. If the resting ejection fraction is <40% or if the stress is markedly abnormal (>2 mm ST segment depression, hypotension at peak exercise or low working capacity) then coronary angiography should be carried out if there are no contraindications to revascularization.
- In patients in whom the ECG is not intepretable because of resting ST–T wave abnormalities, digitalis therapy or left bundle branch block, rest and exercise radionuclide myocardial perfusion scintigraphy (with thallium or sestamibi) or rest and exercise echocardiography should be performed. Patients who cannot exercise should undergo a pharmacologic stress imaging study such as adenosine or dipyridamole myocardial perfusion scintigraphy or echocardiography with dobutamine or dipyridamole stress. A marked abnormality in any of these tests or a resting ejection fraction below 40%, measured by echocardiography or a radionuclide technique, should be followed by coronary angiography.

What advice would you give this patient on discharge?

Secondary prevention of myocardial infarction includes (*BMJ* 1998; **316:** 838–42):

- **Smoking cessation.** It should be emphasized to the patient that within 2 years of discontinuing smoking the risk of a non-fatal recurrent MI falls to the level observed in a patient who has never smoked.
- **Lipid profile.** A lipid profile should be obtained in all patients with acute MI. Since cholesterol may fall after 24–48 hours, it is important that these measurements be obtained on admission, otherwise a 6-week wait is necessary for cholesterol to reach pre-MI levels. It is desirable to fractionate the cholesterol, and patients with LDL cholesterol >3.37 mmol/l should be treated with lipid lowering agents (see pp 440–1).
- **Cardiac rehabilitation.** All discharged patients should be referred for outpatient cardiac rehabilitation. Patients should be encouraged to increase activity gradually over 1–2 months.

- **Risk factors.** Diabetes and hypertension should be aggressively controlled. Oestrogen replacement should be considered in postmenopausal women after MI without greater than usual risks of breast cancer (a family history of breast cancer).

- **Aspirin.** Aspirin led to a 12% reduction in death, a 31% reduction in reinfarction and a 42% reduction in non-fatal stroke in a study of 19 791 patients who had myocardial infarctions reviewed by the Antiplatelet Therapy Trialists. Low to medium doses (75–325 mg/day) seem to be as effective as high doses (1200 mg/day).

- **Beta-blockers.** Several controlled trials in more than 35 000 survivors of myocardial infarction have shown the benefit of long-term treatment with beta-blockers in reducing the incidence of recurrent myocardial infarction, sudden death and all-cause mortality. Beta-blockers reduce myocardial workload and oxygen consumption by reducing the heart rate, blood pressure and contractility, and they increase the threshold for ventricular fibrillation. The beneficial effect of beta-blockers seems to be a class effect, but those with agonist activity do not show a beneficial effect on mortality, and their use cannot be recommended at present.

- **ACE inhibitors.** Low-dose ramipril should be considered in all patients with uncomplicated myocardial infarction (*N Engl J Med* 2000; **342:** 145–53). Treatment with full-dose ACE inhibitors is recommended for an indefinite period in all patients with congestive heart failure, an ejection fraction <40% or a large regional wall motion abnormality.

- Avoid calcium channel blockers or prophylactic use of anti-arrhythmic drugs to suppress ventricular ectopy.

- The patient should not drive for at least one month after the event.

Eugene Braunwald (b. 1929) was consecutively Chair and Professor of Medicine in San Diego and Harvard Medical School, Boston. His research interests included heart failure, factors influencing cardiac contraction and hypertrophic cardiomyopathy. He was responsible for the idea that late patency of an occluded artery can lead to clinical benefit. His wife, Nina H. Starr Braunwald, was a cardiothoracic surgeon who made important contributions to heart valve replacement.

Case 15

JUGULAR VENOUS PULSE

INSTRUCTION

Examine this patient's neck.
Examine this patient's cardiovascular system.

SALIENT FEATURES

History
- Dyspnoea.
- Symptoms of right heart failure (leg oedema, ascites).

Examination
- The JVP is raised … cm above the angle of Louis (manubriosternal angle). Remember that the JVP may be raised to the level of the ear lobes.
- Comment on the waveform (timing it with the carotid pulse):
  - 'v' Waves of tricuspid regurgitation.
  - Cannon waves of heart block.
  - Absent 'a' waves in atrial fibrillation (irregular carotid pulse).
  - Large 'a' waves of pulmonary hypertension, pulmonary stenosis, tricuspid stenosis.
- Check the hepatojugular reflex.
- Tell the examiner that you would like to look for other signs of heart failure:
  - Basal crackles and pleural effusion.
  - Dependent oedema (ankle and sacral oedema).
  - Tender hepatomegaly.

DIAGNOSIS

This patient has raised jugular venous pulse with 'v' waves (lesion) due to tricuspid regurgitation and is in heart failure (functional status).

QUESTIONS

What are the causes of a raised JVP?
- Congestive cardiac failure.
- Cor pulmonale.
- Tricuspid regurgitation (prominent 'v' waves).
- Tricuspid stenosis (prominent 'a' waves).
- Complete heart block (cannon waves).
- Non-pulsatile neck veins seen in superior venal caval obstruction (see pp 593–4).

How do you differentiate jugular venous pulsations from carotid artery pulsations?
Unlike the arterial pulse, the venous pulse has a definite upper level which falls during inspiration and changes with posture. The venous pulse is seen to have a dominant inward motion, towards the midline (the 'y' descent), whereas the arterial pulse exhibits a dominant outward wave. The venous pulse is better seen than felt, whereas the arterial pulse is readily felt by very slight pressure of the clinician's finger.

What do you know about the hepatojugular reflux?
A positive hepatojugular (abdominojugular) reflux is a feature of left ventricular systolic failure with secondary pulmonary hypertension. It is elicited by upper abdominal compression for ~10 seconds. An abnormal response is one where there

is an increase followed by an abrupt fall. The hepatojugular manoeuvre is often useful in eliciting venous pulsations when they are not readily visible.

ADVANCED-LEVEL QUESTIONS

What do you know about the waveforms in the jugular pulse?

There are two outward-moving waves (the a and v wave) and two inward-moving waves (the x and y descent).

- The 'a' wave is caused by atrial contraction and is presystolic. It can be identified by simultaneous auscultation of the heart and the examination of the jugular venous pulse. The 'a' wave occurs at about the first heart sound.
- The 'c' wave is due to closure of the tricuspid valve and is not readily visible.
- The 'v' wave results from venous return to the right heart (*not* due to ventricular contraction) and occurs nearer to the second heart sound.
- The 'x' descent is due to atrial relaxation (sometimes referred to as systolic collapse).
- The 'y' descent is produced by opening of the tricuspid valve and rapid inflow of blood into the right ventricle.

What is Kussmaul's sign?

Normally there is an inspiratory decrease in JVP. In constrictive pericarditis there is an inspiratory increase in JVP. Kussmaul's sign is also seen in severe right heart failure regardless of aetiology. It is caused by the inability of the heart to accept the increase in right ventricular volume without a marked increase in the filling pressure.

Adolf Kussmaul (1822–1902) was Professor of Medicine successively at Heidelberg, Enlargen, Freiburg and Strasbourg, and coined the term 'polyarteritis nodosa' (*Berl Klin Wochnschr* 1873; **10**: 433). Kussmaul breathing is deep sighing respiration seen when the arterial pH is low.

Case 16

CONGESTIVE CARDIAC FAILURE

INSTRUCTION

Examine this patient's cardiovascular system.

SALIENT FEATURES

History

- Dyspnoea on exertion.
- Past history of hypertension, ischaemic heart disease or cardiomyopathy.

Examination

- Signs of fluid retention: raised jugular venous pressure, lung crepitations, pitting leg oedema, tender hepatomegaly.
- Signs of impaired perfusion: cold clammy skin, low blood pressure.
- Signs of ventricular dysfunction: displaced left ventricular apex, right ventricular heave, third or fourth heart sound, functional mitral or tricuspid regurgitation, tachycardia.

Look for the aetiology:

- Valvular disease.
- Atherosclerotic vascular disease.
- Severe hypertension.
- Severe anaemia or volume overload, e.g. arteriovenous shunt.
- Pathological arrhythmia.
- Evidence of generalized myopathy or poisoning.

DIAGNOSIS

This patient has congestive cardiac failure due to hypertension and is severely limited with NYHA class IV dyspnoea.

QUESTIONS

How would you investigate this patient?

- Chest radiography, echocardiogram, cardiopulmonary exercise testing to confirm diagnosis.
- Exercise testing is useful to identify ischaemic heart disease.
- Cardiopulmonary exercise testing is useful to determine functional capacity before cardiac rehabilitation and to determine eligibility for cardiac transplantation.
- ECG to look for underlying cause, e.g. ischaemia or infarction, left ventricular hypertrophy, arrhythmia, other causes of pathological Q waves.
- Echocardiogram to detect valvular disease; determines whether left ventricle function is globally impaired (e.g. idiopathic dilated cardiomyopathy) or whether there are segmental wall motion abnormalities (e.g. in ischaemic heart disease). Ejection fraction can be estimated and usually treatment is initiated when ejection fraction is ≤40. Doppler echocardiography allows determination of diastolic dysfunction.
- Blood tests for associated disease: renal, liver and electrolyte disturbances common; for metabolic causes, e.g. haemochromatosis, hypocalcaemic cardiomyopathy, thyroid heart disease, anaemia, heavy metal poisons, amyloid (serum electrophoresis, rectal biopsy), sarcoid (serum angiotensin converting enzyme).
- Coronary angiography to identify ischaemic heart disease.
- Ventricular biopsy for specific myocarditis, especially viral, and to exclude infiltrative diseases such as cardiac sarcoidosis and amyloidosis.
- Radionuclide ventriculography or echocardiography: to quantitate severity of systolic dysfunction (ejection fraction).
- 24-Holter ECG monitoring: for ventricular arrhythmias.

What is the pharmacological treatment of left ventricular systolic dysfunction?

- Diuretics for symptomatic patients to maintain appropriate fluid balance.
- For patients with systolic dysfunction (EF <40%) who have no contraindications:
  - ACE inhibitors for all patients.
  - Beta-blockers for all patients except those who are haemodynamically unstable or who are intolerant.
  - Spironolactone for patients with rest dyspnoea or with a history of rest dypnoea.
  - Digoxin both for patients who remain symptomatic despite diuretics, ACE inhibitors and beta-blockers and patients with rest dyspnoea or who have a history of rest dyspnoea.

Trial	Conclusions
Ve-HFT (N Engl J Med 1986; **314**: 1547–52)	
Ve-HFT-II (N Engl J Med 1991; **325**: 303–10)	Enalapril is superior to hydralazine–isosorbide nitrate combination
CONSENSUS (N Engl J Med 1987; **316**: 1429–35)	Enalapril resulted in a 27% reduction in all-cause mortality
SOLVD (Treatment arm; N Engl J Med 1991; **325**: 293–302)	Enalapril caused a 16% reduction in all-cause mortality in class II–III CHF
SOLVD (Prevention arm; N Engl J Med 1992; **327**: 685–91)	Enalapril reduced hospitalizations due to CHF and although it caused a 8% reduction in mortality it did not reduce statistical significance
ELITE-II (Lancet 2000; **355**: 1582–7)	No difference in all-cause mortality between captopril and losartan (angiotensin receptor blocker) in class II–IV CHF
DIG (N Engl J Med 1997; **336**: 525–33)	Digoxin does not reduce overall mortality in patients with chronic heart failure and normal sinus rhythm but it reduces the rate of hospitalization
RALES (N Engl J Med 1999; **341**: 709–717)	Blockade of aldosterone receptors by spironolactone in severe heart failure reduces the risk of death by 30% and reduces the risk of hospitalization for heart failure by 35%
US Carvedilol Trials (N Engl J Med 1996; **94**: 2793)	65% reduction in all-cause mortality by carvedilol in class II–III CHF; hence was prematurely terminated
COPERNICUS	35% reduction in all-cause mortality in class IV CHF; hence prematurely terminated
MERIT-CHF (Lancet 1999; **353**: 2001–7)	34% reduction in all-cause mortality with metoprolol; hence prematurely terminated
CIBIS-II (Lancet 1999; **353**: 9–13)	34% reduction in all-cause mortality with bisoprolol in class III–IV CHF
BEST (N Engl J Med 2001; **334**: 1659–67)	Bucindolol resulted in no survival benefit in patients with class III–IV CHF

ADVANCED-LEVEL QUESTIONS

What is diastolic dysfunction?

It is excessive stiffness of the heart resulting in an inability of the heart to fill properly (*Eur Heart J* 1998; **19:** 990–1003). This is in contrast to systolic dysfunction, where contractility is impaired. Patients have clinical features of left heart failure but normal systolic function by echocardiography or radionuclide ventriculography. It is a feature of hypertrophic cardiomyopathy, severe left ventricular hypertrophy (e.g. aortic stenosis or hypertension) and restrictive cardiomyopathy (e.g. amyloidosis). Treatment is directed towards the underlying cause.

What are the indications for heart transplantation?

When patients are refractory to treatment, both medical and surgical (such as valve replacement), and are in New York Heart Association class IV, then they are unlikely to survive for 1 year and should be considered for heart transplantation. The survival rate is about 69% at 5 years, although most patients have one episode of rejection and 25% have multiple episodes. They are also prone to accelerated coronary atherosclerosis.

In 1967, Christiaan Barnard, a South African surgeon, was the first to perform cardiac transplantation in humans.

Sir Magdi Yacoub, contemporary Professor of Cardiology at University of London and Royal Brompton Hospital and Harefield Hospital is an Egyptian-born surgeon who performed several pioneering cardiac operations.

R. Sanders Williams, MD, Professor of Medicine and contemporary Dean, Duke University Medical School and Vice Chancellor, Duke University, has worked successively at Duke, Harvard, Oxford, and UT Southwestern in Dallas. He has made major contributions to the understanding of molecular mechanisms of cardiac function.

Case 17

INFECTIVE ENDOCARDITIS

INSTRUCTION

This patient is suspected to have endocarditis; would you like to examine him?

SALIENT FEATURES

History

- Fever, malaise, anorexia, weight loss, rigors: non-specific symptoms of inflammation.
- Progressive heart failure: due to valve destruction (can be dramatic).
- Stroke, pulseless limb, renal infarct, pulmonary infarct: caused by embolization of vegetations.
- Arthralgia, loin pain: due to immune-complex deposition.
- Obtain a history of recent dental procedures.
- History of valvular heart disease, history of intravenous drug abuse.

Examination

- Look for the following signs:
  - Anaemia.
  - Clubbing (seen in one fifth of the cases).
  - Splinter haemorrhages in the nails (vasculitic phenomenon; probably due to embolic phenomena in the nail bed).
  - Osler's nodes (vasculitic phenomenon; tender, erythematous, pea-sized nodules seen in the pulp of the fingers; caused by inflammation around the site of the infected emboli lodged in distal arterioles).
  - Janeway lesions (vasculitic phenomenon; flat, non-tender red spots found on the palms and soles; they blanch on pressure).
  - Petechiae – conjunctiva, palate and skin.
- Record the temperature.
- Listen to the heart for murmurs and look for signs of cardiac failure.
- Examine the fundus for Roth's spots (vasculitic phenomena).
- Examine the abdomen for splenomegaly.
- Look for embolic phenomena: stroke, viscera or occlusion of peripheral arteries
- Test urine for microscopic haematuria (vasculitic phenomena).

Remember that ostium secundum atrial septal defects almost never have infective endocarditis.

DIAGNOSIS

This patient has Janeway lesions and Roth's spots (lesions) confirming infective endocarditis and is in severe heart failure (functional status).

QUESTIONS

How would you investigate such a patient?

- Test the urine for microscopic haematuria.
- Take a full blood count (FBC) to show normocytic, normochromic anaemia and raised white cell count.
- Test for raised erythrocyte sedimentation rate (ESR).
- Blood culture: take three samples from different sites in 24 hours. It is the most important test for diagnosing endocarditis and cultures are negative in more than 50% of cases of fungal aetiology.
- Echocardiography may show vegetations. A negative study does not rule out endocarditis as vegetations less than 3–4 mm in size cannot be detected. Furthermore, all the leaflets of the aortic, tricuspid and pulmonary valves may not be visualized in every patient.

What are the major manifestations of bacterial endocarditis?

- Manifestations of a systemic infection: fever, weight loss, pallor, splenomegaly.
- Manifestations of a vasculitic phenomenon: cardiac failure, changing murmurs, petechiae, Roth's spots, Osler's nodes, Janeway lesions, splinter haemorrhages, stroke, infarction of viscera, mycotic aneurysm.
- Manifestations of immunological reactions: arthralgia, finger clubbing, uraemia.

Name the common organisms found in infective endocarditis.
Streptococcus viridans, Staphylococcus aureus, Strep. faecalis, fungi.

What precautions would you take to prevent bacterial endocarditis?
Antibiotic prophylaxis before any dental, gastrointestinal, urological or gynaeco-
logical procedure is recommended in rheumatic valvular disease, most congenital
heart lesions (except uncomplicated atrial septal defect of secundum type), valvular
aortic stenosis, prosthetic heart valve, previously documented infective endocarditis
and calcified mitral valve annulus (*Circulation* 1997; **96:** 358–66).

How would you treat a patient suspected to have endocarditis?
Until the bacteriology results are available, with intravenous benzylpenicillin and
gentamicin. In severely ill patients intravenous cloxacillin would be added to this
regimen (*Circulation* 1998; **98:** 2936–48).

ADVANCED-LEVEL QUESTIONS

Mention a few prognostic factors.
- Heart failure.
- Non-streptococcal endocarditis, especially *Staph. aureus,* fungal endocarditis.
- Infection of a prosthetic valve.
- Elderly patients.
- Valve ring or myocardial abscess.

Mention a few conditions that can simulate clinical manifestations of
infective endocarditis.
- Atrial myxoma.
- Non-bacterial endocarditis.
- Systemic lupus erythematosus (SLE).
- Sickle cell disease.

What do you know of prosthetic valve endocarditis (PVE)?
About 3% of patients will develop PVE by the end of the first year after valve
replacement; thereafter, the incidence is lower. PVE is classified into two groups:

- Early: occurring within 2 months of surgery. It develops as a result of intraoperative contamination of the prosthetic valve or as a consequence of a postoperative nosocomial infection, such as sternotomy infection, postoperative
pneumonia, urinary tract infection or intravenous cathether-related insertion. The
clinical features may be masked by the ordinary events in the postoperative
course or by another infection. Cutaneous signs are not common.
- Late PVE: develops more than 2 months after valve surgery. It can occur after
transient bacteraemia as in minor skin or upper respiratory tract infections or
following dental or urinary manipulations. The non-cardiac manifestations
resemble those of native valve infective endocarditis.

Although this classification is convenient, the high prevalence of *Staph. epidermidis*
and diphtheroids among patients suggests that this division is not absolute.

What are the complications of infective endocarditis?
- Congestive heart failure: may develop acutely or insidiously; it portends a grave
prognosis.

- Conduction disturbances caused by abscesses in ventricular septum.
- Valve destruction: acute regurgitation, pulmonary oedema, heart failure.
- Embolism: occurs in 22–50% of cases, leading to infarction in any vascular bed including lungs, coronary arteries, spleen, bowel, and extremities; renal: flank pain and haematuria.
- Local extension of infection: purulent pericarditis, aortic root abscess (may cause sinus Valsalva fistula), myocardial abscess (conduction disturbance).
- Septic emboli to vasa vasorum: may lead to mycotic aneurysms anywhere in vascular tree; most worrying in cerebral vessels, resulting in cerebral haemorrhage.
- Distal infection (metastatic): due to septic emboli, e.g. brain abscess, cerebritis.
- Candidal endocarditis: may be manifest by fungal endophthalmitis.
- Glomerulonephritis: the renal lesions of SBE are of two kinds, (a) a diffuse proliferative glomerulonephritis and (b) focal embolic glomerulonephritis. This is associated with low complement levels and immune complexes.

What are the indications for surgery?
- Positive blood cultures or relapse after several days of the best available antibiotic therapy indicate the need for valve replacement.
- Drainage of myocardial or valve ring abscesses.
- Patients with aortic valve endocarditis who develop second- or third-degree heart block.
- Prosthetic valve replacement for non-streptococcal endocarditis, valve dysfunction, valve dehiscence or myocardial invasion.
- Development of a new aneurysm of the sinus of Valsalva.
- Fungal endocarditis.

What do you understand by the term 'marantic endocarditis'?
Marantic or Libman–Sacks endocarditis is seen in SLE and is a post-mortem diagnosis. It is rarely clinically significant.

Sir William Osler (1849–1919) was successively Professor of Medicine in Montreal, Pennsylvania, Baltimore and Oxford. He was reputed to be a brilliant clinician and educationalist.

M. Roth (1839–1914), Professor of Pathology in Basel, Switzerland.

E.G. Janeway (1841–1911) followed Austin Flint as Professor of Medicine at Bellevue Hospital, New York.

E. Libman (1872–1946), US physician.

B. Sacks (1873–1939), US physician who wrote on Hindu medicine.

Case 18

PROSTHETIC HEART VALVES

INSTRUCTION

Listen to this patient's heart.

SALIENT FEATURES

- *Mitral* valve prostheses can be recognized by their site, metallic first heart sound, normal second heart sound and metallic opening snap. Systolic murmurs are often also present and it is important to note that this does not indicate valve malfunction. Diastolic flow murmurs may be heard normally over the disc valves.
- *Aortic* valve prostheses may be recognized by their site, normal first heart sound and metallic second heart sound.
- Both *mitral and aortic* valves may be replaced and both the first and second heart sounds will be metallic. The presence of a systolic murmur does not indicate valve dysfunction. However, the presence of an early diastolic murmur indicates a malfunctioning aortic valve.

Note. Comment on the mid-sternal, vertical thoracotomy scar, and state whether or not the metallic valve sounds are audible to the unaided ear (they are most often audible). Some mechanical valves cause so many clicks that it may not be possible to determine which valve has been replaced solely by auscultation. Porcine and cadaveric heterografts do not cause metallic clicking or plopping sounds.

DIAGNOSIS

This patient has both first and second heart sounds with a metallic quality, indicating that both mitral and aortic valves are artificial valves (lesion) and the patient is not in heart failure (functional status).

QUESTIONS

What are the complications of prosthetic valves?

- Thromboembolism.
- Valve dysfunction, including valve leakage, valve dehiscence and valve obstruction due to thrombosis and clogging. Perivalvular leak is always abnormal. 'Built-in' transvalvular leakage should be less than 10 ml per beat. The loss of expected valve sounds is an important sign of mechanical valve thrombosis.
- Bleeding (such as upper gastrointestinal haemorrhage) due to anticoagulants.
- Haemolysis at the valve, causing anaemia.
- Endocarditis, which carries a mortality rate of up to 60%; patients should be urgently referred to a tertiary cardiothoracic centre (see pp 57–60).
- Structural dysfunction: fracture, poppet escape, cuspal tear, calcification.
- Non-structural dysfunction: paravalvular leak, suture/tissue entrapment, noise.

What are the causes of anaemia in such a patient?
- Bleeding due to anticoagulants.
- Haemolytic anaemia.
- Secondary to bacterial endocarditis.

What are the advantages of a porcine heart valve?
There is no need for chronic anticoagulation; hence it is safe in women of child-bearing age and in the elderly.

What are the complications of a porcine heart valve?
- Degeneration with time.
- Calcification.

ADVANCED-LEVEL QUESTIONS

What are the indications for valve replacement?
- Mitral stenosis (see pp 3–7).
- Mitral regurgitation (see pp 8–11).
- Aortic regurgitation (see pp 13–18).
- Aortic stenosis (see pp 18–22).

What are the different kinds of mechanical valves?

Mechanical valves
- The Starr–Edwards valve is a caged ball device and, because blood flows around the ball, there is a high incidence of haemolysis. This valve was introduced in 1960. The Silastic ball is specially cured to prevent lipid accumulation (which can result in ball variance). The struts of the modern Starr–Edwards prosthesis are not covered with cloth.
- The Medtronic–Hall valve is a tilting disc valve made of pyrolytic carbon. The disc tilts to an opening of 75° for aortic prostheses and 70° for mitral prostheses.
- The Bjork–Shiley pivoted single-tilting disc valve has laminar flow and hence a lower incidence of haemolysis. It was introduced in 1969. In the current model the entire ring and struts are machined from one piece (i.e. there are no welds). This is referred to as the 'monostrut valve'.
- The St Jude valve is a double-tilting disc valve (bileaflet valve). Other examples of bileaflet prostheses include the Carbomedics and Duromedics valves.

Xenografts
- Porcine valves (Carpentier–Edwards, Hancock Modified Orifice, C/E Duraflex, Medtronic Intact).
- Pericardial valves mounted on a frame (Mitroflow, Carpentier–Edwards pericardial, Ionescu–Shiley, Hancock). A design flaw predisposed the Ionescu–Shiley valve to sudden rupture of the cusps. Currently, the Baxter pericardial valve is being used but its long-term durability remains to be ascertained.

Homografts
These are cadaveric aortic or pulmonary valves. Homografts are considered the valve of first choice in a young patient requiring aortic valve replacement. They are useful in replacing infected aortic valves as they are more resistant to reinfection than other prosthetic valves.

What kind of valve would you use to replace the mitral valve?

A mechanical prosthesis. Patients in whom the risk posed by anticoagulants is unacceptably high may receive a bioprosthesis, but at the increased risk of further operation at a later date.

What kind of valve would you use to replace the aortic valve?

Mechanical valves are used in younger patients in whom the risk of porcine valve failure is higher and for whom durability of the valve is of paramount importance. Porcine valves may be considered for elderly patients whose life expectancy may not exceed that of the prosthesis.

Why are mechanical valves increasingly preferred over bioprosthetic valves?

Two randomized controlled trials have shown a lower rate of reoperation with mechanical prostheses than with porcine prostheses, and a smaller increased risk of anticoagulant-related bleeding.

What do you know about the convexo-concave model for the Bjork–Shiley prosthesis?

This was a modification of the previously reliable design which resulted in the strut retaining the tilting disc becoming liable to fracture several years after implantation, causing fatality. All Bjork–Shiley valves manufactured after 1975 have a radio-opaque ring marker in the edge of a tilting disc. This ring marker is missing if the strut is fractured. The disc may be spotted in the peripheral circulation. About two thirds of the patients with strut fracture die acutely. The risk of strut fracture is 7 per 10 000 per year, but the risk of another mitral valve replacement exceeds this. This risk is greatest in patients with a large-size mitral prosthesis (31 and 33 mm) and a weld date between 1 January 1981 and 30 July 1982.

Is there any difference between the lifespan of a porcine mitral prosthesis and that of a porcine aortic prosthesis?

Porcine mitral bioprostheses usually fail after about 7 years whereas those in the aortic position fail in about 10 years owing to degeneration of the valve leaflets. In younger patients, these prostheses tend to degenerate more rapidly.

Which patients should receive a bioprosthetic valve?

- Those unable to take anticoagulants and those not expected to live longer than the predicted lifespan of the prosthesis.
- Patients over the age of 70 years who require an aortic valve replacement as the rate of degeneration is relatively slow in these patients.

In a woman of childbearing age, which kind of valve – bioprosthetic or mechanical – do you prefer?

Until recently, bioprosthetic valves were advocated in women of childbearing age to avoid the adverse effects of warfarin on the fetus. More recently, it has been found that the risk of fetal abnormalities is very low in pregnant women receiving warfarin, although there is an increased risk of spontaneous abortion. There also appears to be an accelerated risk of bioprosthetic valve degeneration during pregnancy. Thus the risks of spontaneous abortion have to be weighed against the operative mortality rate of 10% during reoperation following valve failure. It is increasingly believed that, if valve replacement is needed, a mechanical prosthesis should be used (*Br Heart J* 1994; **71**: 196–201).

If a patient with atrial fibrillation requires a prosthetic mitral valve, which kind of valve would you prefer?

A mechanical valve, as these patients need warfarin treatment for atrial fibrillation.

The first aortic valve replacement (caged ball device) was performed by Dr Dwight Harken in March 1960 at Peter Bent Brigham Hospital in Boston. Shortly thereafter, Dr Nina Braunwald, at the National Institutes for Health, USA, performed a total mitral valve replacement with an artificial flexible leaflet valve.

A. Starr and M.L. Edwards, both US physicians.

Case 19

TRICUSPID REGURGITATION

INSTRUCTION

Examine this patient's heart.
Examine this patient's cardiovascular system.

SALIENT FEATURES

History

- Intravenous drug abuse.
- Trauma to the chest.
- Rheumatic fever.
- Chronic obstructive pulmonary disease.

Examination

- Peripheral cyanosis.
- Large 'v' waves in the jugular venous pulse.
- Left parasternal heave.
- Palpable or loud P2.
- Pansystolic murmur at the left lower sternal border which increases in inspiration – Carvallo's sign.
- Right ventricular third heart sound may be present.
- Atrial fibrillation may be present.

Look for:

- Mid-diastolic murmur of mitral stenosis.
- Systolic pulsations of an enlarged liver.
- Ascites and ankle oedema.

DIAGNOSIS

This patient has tricuspid regurgitation (lesion) secondary to chronic lung disease and cor pulmonale (aetiology of the lesion) and is in cardiac failure (functional status).

QUESTIONS

What are the causes of tricuspid regurgitation?

- Functional: pulmonary hypertension, congestive cardiac failure.
- Rheumatic (associated with mitral and/or aortic valve disease).
- Right heart endocarditis as in drug addicts.
- Uncommon causes: carcinoid syndrome, Ebstein's anomaly, endomyocardial fibrosis, infarction of right ventricular papillary muscles, tricuspid valve prolapse, blunt trauma to the heart.

How would you treat organic tricuspid regurgitation?

Surgically, by valve plication or annuloplasty, or valve replacement.

> J.M.R. Carvallo, Mexican cardiologist who worked in Mexico City (Rivero-Carvallo JM 1946 Signo para el diagnostico de las insuficiencias tricuspideas. *Arch Inst Cardiol Mex* **16**: 531).

Case 20

MITRAL VALVE PROLAPSE

INSTRUCTION

Examine this patient's heart.

SALIENT FEATURES

History

- Palpitations associated with mild tachyarrhythmias.
- Increased adrenergic symptoms.
- Chest pain.
- Anxiety or fatigue.

Examination

- Mid-systolic click followed by late or mid-systolic murmur. **Note.** Squatting will bring the click closer to the second heart sound and decrease the duration of the murmur. A Valsalva manoeuvre and standing have the opposite effect.
- Look for features of Marfan's syndrome (high-arched palate, arm span greater than height).

DIAGNOSIS

This patient has mitral valve prolapse (lesion) and a long pansystolic murmur, indicating significant mitral regurgitation which will require prophylaxis for infective endocarditis (functional status).

QUESTIONS

What are eponyms for mitral valve prolapse (MVP)?

Barlow's syndrome (*Br Heart J* 1968; **30:** 203), click–murmur syndrome, floppy mitral valve.

What is the prevalence in the normal population?

The exact prevalence is not known but is between 2 and 10% of the population. It is present in about 7% of females aged between 14 and 30 years (*N Engl J Med* 1976; **294:** 1986).

What are the complications of MVP?

- Severe mitral regurgitation.
- Arrhythmias: ventricular premature contractions, ventricular tachycardia, paroxysmal supraventricular tachycardia.
- Atypical chest pain.
- Transient ischaemic attacks (TIAs), embolism.
- Infective endocarditis in those with mitral regurgitation.
- Sudden death.

Mention a few associated conditions.

- Marfan's syndrome.
- Chronic rheumatic heart disease.
- Ischaemic heart disease.
- Cardiomyopathies.
- 20% of patients with atrial septal defects – secundum type.
- Ehlers–Danlos syndrome.
- Psoriatic arthritis.
- Ebstein's anomaly.
- SLE.

How would you manage such patients?

- Reassure the asymptomatic patient.
- Advise prophylaxis for infective endocarditis in those with the murmur.
- Relief of atypical chest pain with analgesics or beta-blockers (empirical treatment).
- Aspirin or anticoagulants in those with TIAs.
- Antiarrhythmics in those with frequent tachyarrhythmias or ventricular premature contractions.

ADVANCED-LEVEL QUESTIONS

What is the mechanism of the click in MVP?

Clicks result from sudden tensing of the mitral valve apparatus as the leaflets prolapse into the left atrium during systole.

What are the echocardiographic features of MVP?

- M-mode: abrupt posterior displacement of the posterior or sometimes both valve leaflets in mid or late systole.
- 2D: systolic displacement of one or both mitral valve leaflets into the left atrium.

John Barlow, South African Professor of Cardiology.

Celia Oakley, Professor of Cardiology, Hammersmith Hospital, London (*Q J Med* 1985; **219**: 317).

Case 21

VENTRICULAR SEPTAL DEFECT

INSTRUCTION

Listen to this patient's heart.

SALIENT FEATURES

History

- Small defects are usually asymptomatic.
- Large defects with shunts: repeated respiratory tract infections, debilitating dyspnoea and exercise intolerance.
- Symptoms of infective endocarditis or past history of endocarditis.
- Symptoms of Eisenmenger syndrome (see pp 88–90).

Examination

- Normal pulse.
- Normal findings on palpation (there may be either left or right ventricular enlargement).
- With substantial left-to-right shunting and little or no pulmonary hypertension, the left ventricular impulse is dynamic and laterally displaced, and the right ventricular impulse may not be felt. The murmur of a moderate or large defect is pansystolic, loudest at the lower left sternal border, and usually accompanied by a palpable thrill.
- A short mid-diastolic apical rumble (caused by increased flow through the mitral valve) may be heard.
- A decrescendo diastolic murmur of aortic regurgitation may be present if the ventricular septal defect undermines the aortic valve annulus.
- Small, muscular ventricular septal defects may produce high-frequency systolic ejection murmurs that terminate before the end of systole (when the defect is occluded by contracting heart muscle).
- If pulmonary hypertension develops, a right ventricular heave and a pulsation over the pulmonary trunk may be palpated. The pansystolic murmur and thrill

diminish and eventually disappear as flow through the defect decreases, and a murmur of pulmonary regurgitation (Graham Steell's murmur) may appear. Finally, cyanosis and clubbing are present.
- The second sound may be normal when the defect is small. A2 is obscured by the pansystolic murmur of large defects. A single second sound indicates that the ventricular pressures are equal and a loud P2 indicates pulmonary hypertension.
- Look for signs of cardiac failure.

Note. VSD is the most common congenital cardiac anomaly, occurring in 2 per 1000 births. VSD is a feature of Down's syndrome (see pp 600–2).

DIAGNOSIS

This patient has a ventricular septal defect (lesion) of congenital origin (aetiology) and has pulmonary hypertension (functional status).

QUESTIONS

Is the loudness of the murmur related to the size of the VSD?
No; in fact, very small defects (maladie de Roger) cause loud murmurs (*Bulletin de l'Académie de Médicine* 1879; **2 (VIII)**: 1074–94).

What are the causes of a VSD?
- Congenital.
- Rupture of the interventricular septum as a complication of myocardial infarction.

Where is the defect usually situated?
In the membranous portion of the interventricular septum.

Can such defects close spontaneously?
Spontaneous closure usually occurs in a small defect, in early childhood in about 50% of the patients.

What are the complications of a VSD?
- Congestive cardiac failure.
- Right ventricular outflow tract obstruction (muscular infundibular obstruction develops in about 5% of VSDs).
- Aortic regurgitation.
- Infective endocarditis.
- Pulmonary hypertension and reversal of shunt (Eisenmenger complex).

How would you investigate this patient?
- Electrocardiography and chest radiography provide insight into the magnitude of the haemodynamic impairment:
  - With a small ventricular septal defect, both ECG and chest radiograph are normal.
  - With a large defect, there is ECG evidence of left atrial and ventricular enlargement, and left ventricular enlargement and 'shunt vascularity' are evident on the chest radiograph.
  - If pulmonary hypertension occurs, the QRS axis shifts to the right, and right

atrial and ventricular enlargement are noted on the ECG. The chest radiograph of a patient with pulmonary hypertension shows marked enlargement of the proximal pulmonary arteries, rapid tapering of the peripheral pulmonary arteries, and oligaemic lung fields.

- Doppler echocardiography can identify the presence and location of the ventricular septal defect, and Doppler colour-flow mapping can identify the magnitude and direction of shunting.
- Cardiac catheterization and angiography can confirm the presence and location of the ventricular septal defect, as well as determine the magnitude of shunting and the pulmonary vascular resistance.

ADVANCED-LEVEL QUESTIONS

What types of VSD do you know of?

The *supracristal type* (above the crista supraventricularis) is a high defect just below the pulmonary valve and the right coronary cusp of the aortic valve. The latter may not be adequately supported, resulting in aortic regurgitation. In Fallot's tetralogy this defect is associated with a rightward shift of the interventricular septum, and in double-outlet left ventricle with subaortic stenosis the supracristal defect is associated with a leftward shift of the septum.

The *infracristal defect*, which may be in either the upper membranous portion of the interventricular septum, or the lower muscular part (less than 5% of the defects):

- Small defects (maladie de Roger).
- Swiss cheese appearance (multiple small defects).
- Large defects.
- Gerbode defect (defect opening into the right atrium; *Ann Surg* 1958; **148**: 433).

Note. The crista supraventricularis is a muscular ridge that separates the main portion of the right ventricular cavity from the infundibular or outflow portion.

Mention other cardiac lesions that may be associated with a VSD.

Conditions in which VSD is an essential part of the syndrome:
- Fallot's tetralogy.
- Truncus arteriosus.
- Double-outlet right ventricle.
- AV canal defects.

Conditions frequently associated with a VSD but not an essential part of the syndrome:
- Patent ductus arteriosus.
- Pulmonary stenosis.
- Secundum atrial septal defects.
- Coarctation of aorta.
- Tricuspid atresia.
- Transposition of the great arteries.
- Pulmonary atresia.

What is the effect of pregnancy in women with VSD?
- Small defects should present no problems.

- Patients with moderate sized defects and moderate pulmonary hypertension are at risk of developing acute right ventricular failure and rapidly worsening pulmonary hypertension in pregnancy.
- Pregnancy should be avoided in patients with pulmonary hypertension.

What is the management of patients with VSD?

The natural history of ventricular septal defect depends on: (a) the size of the defect and (b) the pulmonary vascular resistance:

- Adults with small defects and normal pulmonary arterial pressure are usually asymptomatic, and pulmonary vascular disease is unlikely to develop. Such patients do not require surgical closure of their defect, but they are at risk for infective endocarditis and should therefore receive antibiotic prophylaxis.
- Patients with large ventricular septal defects who survive to adulthood usually have left ventricular failure or pulmonary hypertension with associated right ventricular failure. Surgical closure of such defects is recommended, if the magnitude of pulmonary vascular obstructive disease is not prohibitive. Once the ratio of pulmonary to systemic vascular resistance exceeds 0.7, the risk associated with surgery is excessive.

Which patients merit surgical attention?

Usually, in an adult, VSD is small enough to be safely ignored, or the patient has Eisenmenger syndrome. However, there are exceptions to this and patients with the following conditions may benefit from surgery:

- Recurrent endocarditis.
- Development of aortic regurgitation due to prolapse of the right coronary cusp through the septal defect.
- Progressive left ventricular dilatation due to volume overload imposed by the shunt (pulmonary to systemic ratio is 3:1).
- When the defect is due to an acute rupture of the ventricular septum.

Note. If the VSD is large enough to cause heart failure or pulmonary hypertension, it usually manifests in the first few years of life.

Henri Roger (1809–1891), a French paediatrician, described maladie de Roger in 1879 in a paper entitled *Clinical researches on the congenital communication of the two sides of the hearts, but failure of occlusion of the interventricular septum.*

Case 22

ATRIAL SEPTAL DEFECT

INSTRUCTION

Examine this patient's heart.
Listen to her heart.

SALIENT FEATURES

History

Ostium secundum defect (anatomically in the region of the fossa ovalis)

- Asymptomatic, particularly small defects with minimal left-to-right shunting. Moderate or large defects often have no symptoms until the third or fourth decades despite substantial left-to-right shunting (characterized by a ratio of pulmonary to systemic flow of 1.5 or more).
- Fatigue.
- Dyspnoea.
- Palpitations indicating atrial arrhythmias.
- Productive cough indicating recurrent pulmonary infections.
- Symptoms of paradoxical emboli.
- Right heart failure.

Ostium primum defect (in the lower part of the atrial septum)

Patients may develop symptoms and heart failure in childhood:

- Failure to thrive.
- Chest infections.
- Poor development.

   In adults, in addition to the same symptoms as for secundum defect, the following occur:

- Syncope: indicating heart block.
- Symptoms suggesting endocarditis.

Examination

- Diffuse or normal apical impulse.
- Left parasternal heave.
- Ejection systolic flow murmur in the left second and third intercostal space.
- Wide, fixed, split second heart sound (occasionally a slight movement of P2 occurs).
- Infrequently, a mid-diastolic murmur may be heard in the tricuspid area (indicating a large left-to-right shunt).

Look for signs of:

- Pulmonary hypertension (Eisenmenger syndrome).
- Congenital defects of the thumb (Holt–Oram syndrome).

Note. Atrial secundum defect is often confused with pulmonary stenosis (P2 is soft, delayed and moves with respiration).

DIAGNOSIS

This patient has an atrial septal defect (lesion) which is congenital in origin (aetiology); she is not in cardiac failure and there is no reversal of shunt (functional status).

ADVANCED-LEVEL QUESTIONS

What are the types of atrial septal defect (ASD)?

- Ostium secundum defect accounts for 70% of the cases. The defect is in the middle portion of the atrial septum and is usually 2–4 cm in diameter (incomplete right bundle branch block pattern, QRS axis rightward).
- Sinus venosus type is a defect in the septum just below the entrance of the superior vena cava into the right atrium (leftward P wave axis so that P waves are inverted in at least one inferior lead).
- Ostium primum type is a defect in the lower part of the septum, and clefts may occur in the mitral and tricuspid valves (QRS axis leftward). A junctional or low atrial rhythm (inverted P waves in the inferior leads) occurs with sinus venosus defects.

What do you understand by the term 'patent foramen ovale'?

In the fetus, the right and left atria communicate with each other through an oblique valvular opening, which is called the foramen ovale. The foramen ovale persists throughout fetal life. After birth, the left atrium receives blood from the lungs and the pressure in this chamber becomes greater than that in the right atrium; this causes the closure of the foramen ovale.

What is the importance of patent foramen ovale?

The prevalence of patent foramen ovale is significantly higher in patients with stroke (*N Engl J Med* 1988; **318:** 1148–52).

What is Holt–Oram syndrome?

There is an ostium secundum ASD with a hypoplastic thumb and an accessory phalanx. In addition, the thumb lies in the same plane as the other digits (*Br Heart J* 1960; **22:** 236). The inheritance is autosomal dominant and is associated with mutations to chromosome 12q2 (*N Engl J Med* 1994; **330:** 885–91).

At what age does reversal of the shunt occur?

Usually after the end of the second decade.

What is the mechanism of the fixed split second sound?

In normal individuals on inspiration there is a widening of the split between the two components of the second sound due to a delay in closure of the pulmonary valve. In ASD the effect of respiration is eliminated due to the communication between the left and right sides of the heart.

In which conditions is an abnormally widely split second sound present?

- ASD, VSD, pulmonary regurgitation (due to increased right ventricular volume).
- Pulmonary stenosis (due to increased right ventricular pressure).

- Right bundle branch block (due to right ventricular conduction delay).
- Mitral regurgitation, VSD (due to premature left ventricular emptying).

What do you know about the embryology of atrial septal defect?

There are seven septa involved in the partitioning of the heart. Three form passively (i.e. when an area of tissue forms a septum because of the rapid growth of contiguous tissue); these include the septum secundum at the atrial septum, the muscular portion of the ventricular septum and the aorticopulmonary septum. The actively formed portions of the septa of the heart include the septum of the atrioventricular canal, the conal septum and the truncal septum.

The atrial septum begins as a passively formed septum; however, active growth from the endocardial cushions completes the septum.

What is Lutembacher syndrome?

ASD with an acquired rheumatic mitral stenosis (*Arch Mal Coeur* 1916; **9:** 237).

What is Fallot's trilogy?

ASD, pulmonary stenosis and right ventricular enlargement.

How would you investigate a patient with atrial septal defect?

ECG
- Often has right axis deviation and incomplete right bundle branch block.
- In ostium primum defects left axis deviation also occurs, whereas a junctional or low atrial rhythm (inverted P waves in inferior leads) occurs in sinus venosus defects.

Chest radiography
- Prominent pulmonary arteries (large pulmonary conus).
- A peripheral pulmonary vascular pattern of 'shunt vascularity' (in which the small pulmonary arteries are especially well visualized in the periphery of both lungs).
- Small aortic knob.
- Enlarged right ventricle and right atrium.
- 'Hilar dance' on fluoroscopy.

Echocardiography
- Transthoracic echocardiography visualizes ostium secundum and primum defects but usually does not identify sinus venosus defects.
- Sensitivity can be enhanced by injecting microbubbles into a peripheral vein, after which the movement across the defect can be seen.
- Trans-oesophageal and Doppler colour-flow echocardiography is useful in detecting and determining the location of atrial septal defects and also in identifying anomalous venous drainage and sinus venosus defects.

Cardiac catheterization
Often unnecessary in diagnosis but is useful in determining the magnitude and direction of shunting and to determine the severity and reversibility of pulmonary hypertension.

What are the complications of ASD?
- Atrial arrhythmias: atrial fibrillation is most common. Atrial fibrillation is often accompanied by the appearance of tricuspid regurgitation. Patients are usually in normal sinus rhythm in the first three decades of life, after which atrial

arrhythmias including atrial fibrillation and supraventricular tachycardia may appear.
- Pulmonary hypertension with the development of right ventricular disease.
- Eisenmenger syndrome with reversal of shunt.
- Paradoxical embolus.
- Infective endocarditis in patients with ostium primum defects only.
- Recurrent pulmonary infections.

How is pregnancy tolerated in a woman with ASD?

Pregnancy is usually well tolerated in uncomplicated atrial septal defects; however, when the defect is complicated by significant pulmonary hypertension there is increased maternal and fetal morbidity and mortality and hence pregnancy should be avoided in Eisenmenger syndrome. Rapidly progressive pulmonary vascular disease may develop during pregnancy, therefore routine closure of atrial septal defect is recommended before pregnancy.

How would you manage an uncomplicated atrial septal defect?

Early childhood

If the defect is detected in early childhood, surgical closure is recommended between the ages of 5 and 10 years to prevent the late onset of either right ventricular failure, atrial arrhythmias or right heart failure.

In adults

- Small ASDs can be left alone, although many believe that all ASDs must be closed. Those operated on before the age of 25 years have an excellent prognosis and one may anticipate normal long-term survival, but older patients require regular supervision. In a recent study, surgical repair of atrial septal defects in middle-aged and elderly patients was found to improve longevity and reduce functional limitation due to heart failure, and is therefore superior to medical treatment. However, the risk of atrial arrhythmias, especially fibrillation and flutter, and the attendant risk of thromboembolic events was not reduced by closure of the defect.
- Left-to-right shunt saturations of 1.5:1 or more require surgical closure to prevent right ventricular dysfunction.
- Closure in adults results in a reduction in right ventricular size and improves symptoms.

More recently, ASDs are being occluded by transcatheter button or 'clam-shell devices'.

Is prophylaxis against infective endocarditis recommended in ASD?

Prophylaxis against infective endocarditis is not recommended for patients with atrial septal defects (repaired or unrepaired) unless a concomitant valvular abnormality (e.g. mitral valve cleft or prolapse) is present.

Leonardo da Vinci's description in 1513 of a 'perforating channel' in the atrial septum is believed to be the first recorded account of a congenital malformation of the human heart.

Rene Lutembacher, a French physician, described the Lutembacher syndrome in 1916.

Mary Holt, cardiologist, King's College Hospital, London.

Samuel Oram, cardiologist, King's College Hospital, London.

Case 23

HYPERTROPHIC CARDIOMYOPATHY

INSTRUCTION

Examine this patient's cardiovascular system.

SALIENT FEATURES

History

- Patients may be asymptomatic.
- Severe cardiac failure (in infants).
- Premature unexpected death: may be presenting symptom in children or young adults.
- Dyspnoea on exertion: (in ~50% of patients).
- Chest pain (in ~50%; may be exertional or occur at rest).
- Syncope (in 15–25%).
- Dizziness and palpitations.
- Obtain a family history of the following: (a) similar cardiomyopathy, (b) sudden death.

Examination

- Carotid pulse is bifid.
- 'a' wave in the JVP.
- *Double apical impulse* (left ventricular heave with a prominent presystolic pulse caused by atrial contraction).
- Pansystolic murmur at the apex due to mitral regurgitation.
- Ejection systolic murmur along the left sternal border (across the outflow tract obstruction); accentuated by standing and Valsalva manoeuvre and softer on squatting (squatting increases LV cavity size and reduces outflow tract obstruction).
- Fourth heart sound.

DIAGNOSIS

This patient has hypertrophic cardiomyopathy (aetiology) as evidenced by a double apical impulse and ejection systolic murmur along the left sternal border which is heard better on standing (lesion); the patient is in cardiac failure.

ADVANCED-LEVEL QUESTIONS

How would you investigate this patient?

- Echocardiogram is useful for assessing left ventricular structure and function, gradients, valvular regurgitation, and atrial dimensions. Characteristic findings include systolic anterior motion of mitral valve (SAM), asymmetric hypertrophy (ASH) and mitral regurgitation.

- ECG may be normal (in about 5% of patients) or show abnormalities including left ventricular hypertrophy, atrial fibrillation, left axis deviation, right bundle branch block and myocardial disarray (e.g. ST–T wave changes, intraventricular conduction defects, abnormal Q waves); bizarre or abnormal findings in young patients should raise suspicion of hypertrophic cardiomyopathy, especially if family members are also affected.
- Chest radiograph may be normal or show evidence of left or right atrial or left ventricular enlargement.
- Treadmill exercise test is performed when patients have angina (ST segment changes of >2 mm documented in 25% associated with symptoms of angina).
- 48-hour Holter monitoring identifies established atrial fibrillation (in about 10% of patients), paroxysmal supraventricular arrhythmias (in 30%), non-sustained ventricular tachycardia (in 25%), and ventricular tachycardia (in 25%). Ventricular tachycardia is invariably asymptomatic during Holter monitoring, but the most useful risk marker of sudden death in adults. Sustained supraventricular arrhythmias are often symptomatic and predispose to thromboembolic complications.
- Endomyocardial biopsy may be necessary to exclude specific heart muscle disorder (amyloid, sarcoid) but has no role in diagnosis because of the patchy nature of myofibrillar disarray.

What are the complications of hypertrophic cardiomyopathy?
- Sudden death.
- Atrial fibrillation.
- Infective endocarditis.
- Systemic embolization.

How would you manage such a patient?
- Relief of symptoms.
- Prevention of arrhythmias and sudden death by administration of amiodarone (*Br Heart J* 1985; **53**: 412–16).
- Improvement of ventricular function using a beta-blocker (propranolol up to 640 mg per day), verapamil, amiodarone and diuretics (*N Engl J Med* 1997; **336**: 775).
- Prevention of infective endocarditis.
- Dual-chamber pacing or DDD pacing (see p. 98) is considered by some to be the initial procedure in symptomatic patients resistant to treatment with drugs. DDD pacing causes depolarization from the right ventricular apex, resulting in altered motion of the interventricular septum and diminished subaortic gradient.
- Septal ablation with alcohol or surgery – such as myotomy or myectomy – relieves symptoms but does not alter the natural history of the disease. Mitral valve replacement may be done simultaneously for severe mitral regurgitation.
- Counselling of sufferers and relatives is essential and they should be encouraged to contact the Hypertrophic Cardiomyopathy Association.

What is the most characteristic pathophysiological abnormality in hypertrophic cardiomyopathy?
Diastolic dysfunction.

Which condition has the most common association with hypertrophic cardiomyopathy?

Friedreich's ataxia.

What do you know about the genetics of hypertrophic cardiomyopathy?

- Hypertrophic cardiomyopathy is an autosomal dominant heart muscle disorder.
- Mutations in the gene encoding contractile proteins cause disease in 50–60% of patients.
- There are mutations in the gene encoding for myofibrillary proteins; at least 9 individual genes have been identified. Beta heavy chain myosin gene mutations are associated with left ventricular outflow obstruction, whereas troponin T mutations are associated with rather modest left ventricular wall thickening, and mutations in myosin binding protein C are associated with onset in late adult life. Arginine gene mutations have a worse prognosis than leucine gene mutations.

What do you know about the Brockenbrough–Braunwald–Morrow sign?

Diminished pulse pressure in post-extrasystolic beat occurs in hypertrophic cardiomyopathy/aortic stenosis (*Circulation* 1961; **23**: 189–94).

What do you know about the epidemiology of this condition?

- The male to female ratio is equal, although the disease tends to affect younger men and older women.
- In children and adolescents, myocardial hypertrophy often occurs during growth spurts (a negative diagnosis made before adolescent growth does not exclude the condition, and reassessment at a later age is important).
- Myocardial hypertrophy does not ordinarily progress after adolescent growth is completed.
- Sudden death can occur at any age (from childhood to over 90 years) in subjects who have been asymptomatic all their life. The annual mortality from sudden death is 3–5% in adults and at least 6% in children and young adults.
- First-degree relatives of affected patients have a 50% chance of carrying the disease gene; they should be investigated by ECG and two-dimensional echocardiogram. Genetic counselling is therefore important.

The pathology of hypertrophic cardiomyopathy was first described by two French pathologists in the mid 19th century and by a German pathologist in the early 20th century. The simultaneous reports of Sir Russel Brock, thoracic surgeon at Guy's and Brompton Hospitals (*Guy's Hosp Rep* 1957; **106**: 221–38), and of Teare in 1958 brought the condition to modern medical attention (*Br Heart J* 1958; **20**: 1).

Case 24

PATENT DUCTUS ARTERIOSUS

INSTRUCTION

Examine this patient's heart.
Examine this patient's cardiovascular system.

SALIENT FEATURES

History

* Asymptomatic.
* Bronchitis or dyspnoea on exertion in severe cases.
* Take a maternal history of rubella, particularly in the first trimester.
* Determine whether the patient was a premature baby or had a low birth weight. Remember, the frequency of PDA in infants weighing 501–1500 g was 31% (*Pediatrics* 1993; **91:** 540–5).
* Determine whether the patient was born in a place at high altitude.

Examination

* Collapsing pulse (due to an aortic diastolic run-off).
* Heaving apex beat.
* Systolic and/or diastolic thrill in the left second interspace.
* Loud, continuous 'machinery' murmur, i.e. pansystolic and extending into early diastole – known as Gibson murmur – is heard along the left upper sternal border and outer border of the clavicle. The murmur begins after the first heart sound, peaks with the second sound, and trails off in diastole (*Edinb Med* 1890; **8:** 1).
* The second sound is not heard.

DIAGNOSIS

This patient has a patent ductus arteriosus (lesion) which is probably congenital in origin (aetiology); the patient is not in heart failure (functional status).

QUESTIONS

Mention a few causes of a collapsing pulse.

Hyperdynamic circulation due to:

* Aortic regurgitation.
* Thyrotoxicosis.
* Severe anaemia.
* Paget's disease.
* Complete heart block.

ADVANCED-LEVEL QUESTIONS

Mention a few causes of continuous murmurs.

- Venous hum.
- Mitral regurgitation murmur with aortic regurgitant murmur.
- VSD with aortic regurgitation.
- Pulmonary arteriovenous fistula.
- Rupture of the sinus of Valsalva.
- Coronary arteriovenous fistula.
- Arteriovenous anastomosis of intercostal vessels following a fractured rib.

What happens to the continuous murmur of patent ductus arteriosus (PDA) in pulmonary hypertension?

First the diastolic murmur, then the systolic murmur, becomes softer and shorter, and P2 increases in intensity.

How would you investigate this patient?

- ECG may be normal or shows left ventricular hypertrophy.
- Chest X-ray (CXR) may be normal, or there may be left ventricular and left atrial enlargement. The chest film shows pulmonary plethora, proximal pulmonary arterial dilatation, and a prominent ascending aorta. The ductus arteriosus may be visualized as an opacity at the confluence of the descending aorta and the aortic knob. If pulmonary hypertension develops, right ventricular hypertrophy is noted.
- Echocardiogram: the ductus arteriosus can usually be visualized, and Doppler studies demonstrate continuous flow in the pulmonary trunk.
- Cardiac catheterization is useful to determine the presence and severity of the shunt; it also determines pulmonary vascular resistance. Angiography defines the anatomy.

Mention a few associated lesions.

- Ventricular septal defect.
- Pulmonary stenosis.
- Coarctation of aorta.

What are the complications?

- Congestive cardiac failure is the commonest complication.
- Infective endocarditis or endarteritis (involves the pulmonary side of the ductus arteriosus or the pulmonary artery opposite the duct orifice, from which septic pulmonary emboli may arise).
- Pulmonary hypertension and reversal of shunt (causes differential cyanosis and clubbing, i.e. toes, *not* fingers, are clubbed and cyanosed).
- Substantial left-to-right shunting through the ductus in infants may increase the risk of intraventricular haemorrhage, necrotizing enterocolitis, bronchopulmonary dysplasia and death.
- The ductus may become aneurysmal and calcified, which may lead to its rupture.

Remember. One third of patients with a patent ductus arteriosus that is not surgically repaired die of heart failure, pulmonary hypertension, or endarteritis by the age of 40 years, and two thirds die by the age of 60 years.

How would you manage such patients?

- Within 1–3 weeks of birth: administer a prostaglandin E synthesis inhibitor such as indometacin or ibuprofen. Ibuprofen is as effective as indometacin but is associated with a lower incidence of renal toxic effects (*N Engl J Med* 2000; **343**: 674–81).
- A Rashkind PDA occluder can be inserted percutaneously without the need for a thoracotomy. It consists of a series of miniature back-to-back umbrellas which are positioned across the duct.
- In children or adults with large shunts: perform surgery, i.e. ligation or division of the PDA.

Note

- Because of the risk of endarteritis associated with unrepaired patent ductus arteriosus (estimated at 0.45% annually after the second decade of life) and the low risk associated with ligation (mortality of less than 0.5%), it is recommended that even a small patent ductus arteriosus be ligated surgically or occluded with a percutaneously placed closure device.
- Once severe pulmonary vascular obstructive disease develops, surgical ligation or percutaneous closure is contraindicated.

Which congenital cardiac lesions are dependent on a PDA?

Hypoplastic left heart syndrome, complex coarctations of aorta and critical congenital aortic stenosis.

> Collapsing pulse is also called Corrigan's pulse after Sir Dominic J. Corrigan (1802–1880), a Dublin-born physician who graduated from Edinburgh.
>
> R.E. Gross was the first to report surgical closure of the PDA in 1939.

Case 25

PULMONARY STENOSIS

INSTRUCTION

Examine this patient's heart.

SALIENT FEATURES

History

- Ask for a history of maternal rubella.
- Patients may be asymptomatic.
- Dyspnoea on exertion or fatigability may occur (when the stenosis is severe); less often, patients may have retrosternal chest pain or syncope with exertion. Eventually, right ventricular failure may develop, with resultant peripheral oedema and abdominal swelling.

- Cyanosis and clubbing (if the foramen ovale is patent, shunting of blood from the right to the left atrium may occur).

Remember. The presence or absence of symptoms, their severity, and the prognosis are influenced by the severity of stenosis, the right ventricular systolic function, and the competence of the tricuspid valve.

Examination

- Round plump facies.
- Normal pulse.
- Prominent 'a' wave in the JVP.
- Left parasternal heave.
- Ejection click (valvular stenosis) (*Br Heart J* 1951; **13:** 519).
- Soft P2, with a wide split second sound.
- Ejection systolic murmur in the left upper sternal border, best heard on inspiration. The murmur radiates to the left shoulder and left lung posteriorly. The more severe the stenosis, the longer the murmur, obscuring the second aortic sound A2.

Proceed as follows:
Look for central cyanosis and clubbing (Fallot's tetralogy).

DIAGNOSIS

This patient has pulmonary stenosis (lesion) which is a congenital anomaly (aetiology) and the patient is severely limited by her symptoms (functional status).

QUESTIONS

What is the underlying cause of pulmonary stenosis?
- Congenital (commonest cause).
- Carcinoid tumour of the small bowel.

ADVANCED-LEVEL QUESTIONS

What is the normal area of the pulmonary valve?
The area of the pulmonary valve orifice in a normal adult is about 2.0 cm^2 per square metre of body surface area, and there is no systolic pressure gradient across the valve.

How is the severity of pulmonary valve stenosis determined?
- Mild: if the valve area is larger than 1.0 cm^2 per square metre, the transvalvular gradient is less than 50 mmHg, or the peak right ventricular systolic pressure is less than 75 mmHg.
- Moderate: if the valve area is 0.5–1.0 cm^2 per square metre, the transvalvular gradient is 50–80 mmHg, or the right ventricular systolic pressure is 75–100 mmHg.
- Severe: if the valve area is less than 0.5 cm^2 per square metre, the transvalvular gradient is more than 80 mmHg, or the right ventricular systolic pressure is more than 100 mmHg.

How would you investigate this patient?

- Electrocardiogram: Right axis deviation and right ventricular hypertrophy.
- Chest radiograph: The aortic knuckle is normal whereas the pulmonary conus is either normal or enlarged (due to post-stenotic dilatation of the main pulmonary artery) and the pulmonary vascular markings are diminished. The cardiac silhouette is usually normal in size or may be enlarged (when the patient has right ventricular failure or tricuspid regurgitation).
- Echocardiogram: The site of obstruction can be visualized in most patients but right ventricular hypertrophy and paradoxical septal motion during systole are evident. Doppler flow studies accurately assess the severity of stenosis so that cardiac catheterization and angiography are usually unnecessary.

What are the complications of this condition?

- Cardiac failure.
- Infective endocarditis: blood cultures are rarely positive; the emboli are entirely in the pulmonary circulation and not systemic.

What are the types of pulmonary stenosis?

- Valvular.
- Subvalvular: infundibular and subinfundibular.
- Supravalvular.

Do you know of any eponymous syndromes linked to pulmonary stenosis?

- Noonan's syndrome: short stature, ptosis, downward slanting eyes, wide-spaced eyes (hypertelorism), low-set ears, webbed neck, mental retardation and low posterior hairline. About two thirds of patients with Noonan's syndrome have pulmonary stenosis due to valve dysplasia.
- Watson's syndrome: café-au-lait spots, mental retardation and pulmonary stenosis.
- Williams syndrome: infantile hypercalcaemia, elfin facies and mental retardation, in addition to supravalvular pulmonary stenosis. Subvalvular pulmonary stenosis, which is caused by the narrowing of the right ventricular infundibulum or subinfundibulum, usually occurs in association with a ventricular septal defect.

How would you manage a patient with pulmonary stenosis?

- Mild valvular pulmonary stenosis: these patients are usually asymptomatic. Survival among such patients is excellent (94% are still alive 20 years after diagnosis) and therefore they do not require surgical correction. It is important that patients with mild valvular stenosis who are undergoing elective dental or surgical procedures should receive antibiotic prophylaxis against infective endocarditis.
- Severe stenosis: the stenosis should be relieved, since only 40% of such patients do not require any intervention by 10 years after diagnosis.
- Moderate pulmonary stenosis has an excellent prognosis with either medical or interventional therapy. Interventional therapy is usually recommended, since most patients with moderate pulmonary stenosis eventually have symptoms requiring such therapy. Valve replacement is required if the leaflets are dysplastic or calcified or if marked regurgitation is present.

What is the role of balloon valvuloplasty in pulmonary stenosis?

Relief of valvular stenosis can be accomplished easily and safely with percutaneous balloon valvuloplasty (*Am J Cardiol* 1990; **65**: 775) and a delay in intervention offers no advantage. Balloon valvuloplasty, the procedure of choice, is usually successful, provided the valve is mobile and pliant; its long-term results are excellent. The secondary hypertrophic subpulmonary stenosis that may occur with valvular stenosis usually regresses after successful intervention. In a series of 100 patients, balloon dilatation resulted in a significant reduction in the transvalvular gradient, which was maintained at 12 months' follow-up (*Int J Cardiol* 1988; **21**: 335–42).

What is Erb's point?

The third left intercostal space adjacent to the sternum is Erb's point. The murmur of infundibular pulmonary stenosis is best heard in this space and in the left fourth intercostal space.

Case 26

DEXTROCARDIA

INSTRUCTION

Examine this patient's precordium.
Listen to this patient's heart.

SALIENT FEATURES

History

- Asymptomatic.
- Obtain history of cough with purulent expectoration (bronchiectasis) and sinusitis.

Examination

- Apex beat is absent on the left side and present on the right.
- Heart sounds are better heard on the right side of the chest.
- Ascertain whether the liver dullness is present on the right or left side.
- Examine the chest for bronchiectasis.

Proceed as follows:

Tell the examiner that you would like to perform the following checks:

- Obtain a CXR (look for right-sided gastric bubble).
- Obtain an ECG (inversion of all complexes in lead I).

Note. Dextrocardia without evidence of situs inversus is usually associated with cardiac malformation. It may occur with cardiac malformation in Turner's syndrome.

DIAGNOSIS

This patient has dextrocardia (lesion) of congenital aetiology.

ADVANCED-LEVEL QUESTIONS

What is Kartagener's syndrome?

A type of immotile cilia syndrome in which there is dextrocardia or situs inversus, bronchiectasis and dysplasia of the frontal sinuses (*Beitr Klin Tuberk* 1933; **83:** 489; *N Engl J Med* 1953; **248:** 730).

Which other abnormality has been associated with dextrocardia?

Asplenia (blood smear may show Heinz bodies, Howell–Jolly bodies) (*Br Heart J* 1975; **37:** 840).

What do you understand by the term 'situs inversus'?

Right-sided cardiac apex, right stomach, right-sided descending aorta. The right atrium is on the left. The left lung has three lobes and the right lung has two.

What do you understand by the term 'dextroversion'?

Right-sided cardiac apex, left-sided stomach and left-sided descending aorta.

What do you understand by the term 'levoversion'?

Left-sided apex, right-sided stomach and right descending aorta.

M. Kartagener (b. 1897), a Swiss physician, described this condition in 1933.

Case 27

COARCTATION OF AORTA

INSTRUCTION

Examine this patient's cardiovascular system.

SALIENT FEATURES

History

- Usually asymptomatic.
- Symptoms are usually those of hypertension: headache, epistaxis, dizziness, and palpitations.
- Claudication (due to diminished blood flow to the legs).
- Occasionally, diminished blood flow to the legs can cause leg fatigue.
- Patients sometimes seek medical attention because they have symptoms of heart failure or aortic dissection. Women with coarctation are at particularly high risk for aortic dissection during pregnancy.

Examination

- The upper torso is better developed than the lower part.
- The systolic arterial pressure is higher in the arms than in the legs, but the diastolic pressures are similar, therefore a widened pulse pressure is present in the arms. (**Note.** This condition results in hypertension in the arms. Less commonly, the coarctation is immediately proximal to the left subclavian artery, in which case a difference in arterial pressure is noted between the arms.)
- Radial pulse on the left side may be less prominent.
- The femoral arterial pulses are weak and delayed (simultaneous palpation of the brachial and femoral arteries using the thumbs is the most convenient method of comparing pulsations in the upper and lower limbs).
- A systolic thrill may be palpable in the suprasternal notch.
- Heaving apex due to left ventricular enlargement.
- A systolic ejection click (due to a bicuspid aortic valve which occurs in 50% of cases) is frequently present, and the second heart sound is accentuated.
- A harsh systolic ejection murmur may be identified along the left sternal border and in the back, particularly over the coarctation.
- Scapular collaterals are visible (listen over these collaterals for murmur).
- A systolic murmur, caused by flow through collateral vessels, may be heard in the back.
- In about 30% of patients with aortic coarctation, a systolic murmur indicating an associated bicuspid aortic valve is audible at the base.

Look for:
- Turner's syndrome (female, webbing of the neck, increased carrying angle).
- Berry aneurysms (extraocular movements impaired due to third cranial nerve involvement).

DIAGNOSIS

This patient has coarctation of the aorta (lesion) with left ventricular failure (functional status).

ADVANCED-LEVEL QUESTIONS

What are the types of aortic coarctation?

Common:
- Infantile or preductal where the aorta between the left subclavian artery and patent ductus arteriosus is narrowed. It manifests in infancy with heart failure. Associated lesions include patent ductus arteriosus, aortic arch anomalies, transposition of the great arteries, ventricular septal defect.
- Adult type: the coarctation in the descending aorta is juxtaductal or slightly postductal. It may be associated with biscuspid aortic valve or patent ductus arteriosus. It commonly presents between the ages of 15 and 30 years.

Rare:
- Localized juxtaductal coarctation.
- Coarctation of the ascending thoracic aorta.

- Coarctation of the distal descending thoracic aorta.
- Coarctation of the abdominal aorta.
- Pseudocoarctation is of no haemodynamic significance and is a 'kinked' appearance of the aorta in the juxtaductal region without stenosis.

Is aortic coarctation more common in men or women?

This condition is two to five times as frequent in men and boys as in women and girls.

What conditions are associated with coarctation of aorta?

It may occur in conjunction with gonadal dysgenesis (e.g. Turner's syndrome), bicuspid aortic valve, ventricular septal defect, patent ductus arteriosus, mitral stenosis or regurgitation, or aneurysms of the circle of Willis.

At what age does the condition manifest?

It is particularly likely to produce significant symptoms in early infancy (presenting as cardiac failure) or between the ages of 20 and 30 years.

How would you investigate this patient?

- Electrocardiogram: usually shows left ventricular hypertrophy.
- Chest radiograph: symmetric rib notching. The coarctation may be visualized as the characteristic '3' sign on a chest radiograph (or a reverse '3' sign on the barium swallow). The upper bulge is formed by dilatation of the left subclavian artery high on the left mediastinal border, the sharp indentation is the site of the coarctation, and the lower bulge is called the poststenotic dilatation of the aorta.
- Echocardiogram: the coarctation may be visualized echocardiographically, and Doppler examination makes possible an estimate of the transcoarctation pressure gradient.
- Computed tomography, magnetic resonance imaging and contrast aortography are useful to determine the precise anatomy regarding the location and length of the coarctation; in addition, aortography permits visualization of the collateral circulation.

What causes rib notching?

Collateral flow through dilated, tortuous and pulsatile posterior intercostal arteries typically causes notching on the undersurfaces of the posterior portions of the ribs. The anterior parts of the ribs are spared because the anterior intercostal arteries do not run in the costal grooves. Notching is seldom found above the third or below the ninth rib and rarely appears before the age of 6 years.

Mention a few conditions in which rib notching is seen.

- Coarctation of aorta.
- Pulmonary oligaemia.
- Blalock–Taussig shunt.
- Subclavian artery obstruction.
- Superior vena caval syndrome.
- Neurofibromatosis.
- Arteriovenous malformations of the lung or chest wall.

What are the complications of aortic coarctation?

- Severe hypertension and resulting complications:
  - Stroke.
  - Premature coronary artery disease.

- Left ventricular failure (two thirds of patients over the age of 40 years who have uncorrected aortic coarctation have symptoms of heart failure).
  - Rupture of aorta.
- Infective endocarditis endarteritis (at the site of the coarctation or on a congenitally bicuspid aortic valve).
- Intracranial haemorrhage (combination of hypertension and ruptured berry aneurysm).
- Three quarters die by the age of 50, and 90% by the age of 60 (*Br Heart J* 1970; **32:** 633–40).

What are the fundal findings in coarctation of aorta?

Hypertension due to coarctation of aorta causes retinal arteries to be tortuous with frequent 'U' turns; curiously, the classical signs of hypertensive retinopathy are rarely seen.

What is the treatment of such patients?

- Surgical repair should be considered for patients with a transcoarctation pressure gradient of more than 30 mmHg. Although balloon dilatation is a therapeutic alternative, the procedure is associated with a higher incidence of subsequent aortic aneurysm and recurrent coarctation than surgical repair (*Circulation* 1993; **87:** 793–9).
- Surgical resection and end-to-end anastomosis, although a tubular graft may be required if the narrowed segment is too long.

What are the postoperative complications?

Postoperative complications include recurrent coarctation, persistent hypertension and the possible sequelae of a bicuspid aortic valve.

What happens to the hypertension after surgery?

Despite surgery, some patients may continue to have residual or recurrent hypertension and will require monitoring for hypertension and premature coronary artery disease (*Circulation* 1989; **80:** 840–5). The incidence of persistent or recurrent hypertension is influenced by the patient's age at the time of surgery:

- Among patients who undergo surgery during childhood, 90% are normotensive 5 years later, 50% are normotensive 20 years later, and 25% are normotensive 25 years later.
- Among those who undergo surgery after the age of 40 years, half have persistent hypertension, and many of those with a normal resting blood pressure after successful repair have a hypertensive response to exercise.

Is survival improved by surgery?

Survival after repair of aortic coarctation is influenced by the age of the patient at the time of surgery:

- After surgical repair during childhood, 89% of patients are alive 15 years later and 83% are alive 25 years later.
- When repair of coarctation is performed when the patient is between the ages of 20 and 40 years, the 25-year survival is 75%.
- When repair is performed in patients more than 40 years old, the 15-year survival is only 50%.

Case 28

EISENMENGER SYNDROME

INSTRUCTION

Examine this patient's heart.
Examine this patient's cardiovascular system.

SALIENT FEATURES

History

- Symptoms may not appear until early late childhood or early adulthood.
- Cyanosis (appears as right-to-left shunting develops).
- Dyspnoea on exercise and impaired exercise tolerance.
- Palpitations (common and usually due to atrial fibrillation or flutter).
- Angina of effort.
- Haemoptysis (may occur as a result of pulmonary infarction, or rupture of dilated pulmonary arteries, or aorticopulmonary vessels).
- Syncope (owing to inadequate cardiac output or, less commonly, an arrhythmia).
- Symptoms of hyperviscosity including visual disturbances, fatigue, headache, dizziness, and paraesthesia.
- Symptoms of heart failure are uncommon until the disease is in its advanced stages.

Examination

- Clubbing of fingers and central cyanosis.
- 'a' waves in the JVP, 'v' wave if tricuspid regurgitation is also present.
- Left parasternal heave and palpable P2.
- Loud P2, pulmonary ejection click, early diastolic murmur of pulmonary regurgitation (Graham Steell murmur).
- Loud pansystolic murmur of tricuspid regurgitation.
- Listen carefully to the second sound. The clinical findings resulting from the underlying defect are as follows:
  - VSD: single second sound
  - ASD: fixed, wide split second sound
  - PDA: reverse split of second sound and differential cyanosis where lower-limb cyanosis is marked.

DIAGNOSIS

This patient has Eisenmenger syndrome with a shunt at the ventricular level (lesion) which is congenital in origin (aetiology), and severe pulmonary hypertension (functional status).

QUESTIONS

What do you understand by the term 'Eisenmenger syndrome'?

Pulmonary hypertension with a reversed or bidirectional shunt. It matters very little where the shunt happens to be (e.g. VSD, ASD, patent ductus arteriosus, persistent truncus arteriosus, single ventricle or common atrioventricular canal).

ADVANCED-LEVEL QUESTIONS

What do you understand by the term 'Eisenmenger complex'?

Eisenmenger complex is a VSD with a right-to-left shunt in the absence of pulmonary stenosis. The onset of Eisenmenger syndrome is often heralded by a softening of the murmur, a decrease in the left heart size and an increase in the second pulmonic sound.

Mention some cyanotic heart diseases of infancy.

- Tetralogy of Fallot.
- Transposition of the great vessels.
- Tricuspid regurgitation.
- Total anomalous pulmonary venous connection.

What is the age of onset of Eisenmenger syndrome?

In the case of patent ductus arteriosus and VSD, about 80% occur in infancy, whereas in the case of ASD over 90% occur in adult life.

What are the complications of Eisenmenger syndrome?

- Haemoptysis.
- Right ventricular failure.
- Cerebrovascular accidents (as a result of paradoxical embolization, venous thrombosis of cerebral vessels, or intracranial haemorrhage).
- Sudden death.
- Brain abscess.
- Bleeding and thrombosis (patients at increased risks for both as a consequence of an abnormal haemostasis secondary to chronic arterial desaturation).
- Paradoxical embolization.
- Infective endocarditis.
- Hyperuricaemia.
- Recurrent haemoptysis.

How would you investigate this patient?

Electrocardiogram
- Right ventricular hypertrophy.
- Atrial arrhythmias, particularly in those with underlying atrial septal defect.

Chest radiograph
- Conspicuous dilatation of the pulmonary artery with narrowed 'pruned' peripheral vessels (due to pulmonary hypertension).
- Slight to moderate enlargement of the heart (predominantly right ventricle) may be seen in atrial septal defect, whereas the size of the heart is normal in ventricular septal defect or patent ductus arteriosus.

Echocardiogram
- Evidence of right ventricular overload and pulmonary hypertension.
- The underlying cardiac defect can be visualized although shunting may be difficult to demonstrate by colour Doppler imaging because of low-velocity jet.
- Contrast echocardiography permits localization of shunt.

Cardiac catheterization
- To determine the extent and severity of pulmonary vascular disease and to quantify accurately the magnitude of intracardiac shunting.
- Assessment of reversibility of shunting is done using pulmonary vasodilators (e.g. oxygen, inhaled nitrous oxide, intravenous adenosine or epoprostenol).

What is the prognosis in these patients?
- Survival is 80% 10 years after diagnosis, 77% at 15 years, and 42% at 25 years.
- Death is usually sudden; other causes include heart failure, haemoptysis, brain abscess or stroke.
- Poor prognostic factors include syncope, clinically evident right ventricular systolic dysfunction, low cardiac output, and severe hypoxaemia.

Is pregnancy safe in this patient?
Pregnancy is associated with a high incidence of early spontaneous abortion and rarely results in the birth of a healthy child. Mortality of the mother is high (30–60%) in those with underlying VSD, particularly in late pregnancy and the postpartum period. Pregnancy is, therefore, contraindicated and if it occurs is best terminated at an early stage. If pregnancy proceeds to term, a vaginal delivery is the preferred route with careful management of hydration, arrhythmias and hypoxaemia. Epidural anaesthesia is preferred over general anaesthesia in complicated cases.

What treatment is available for Eisenmenger syndrome?
- Phlebotomy to avoid symptoms of polycythaemia.
- Long-term intravenous epoprostenol (*Circulation* 1999; **99(14)**: 1858–65; *Ann Intern Med* 1999; **130(9)**: 740–3).
- Combined heart–lung transplantation (limited success and hence patients should be carefully selected).

Victor Eisenmenger was a German physician who described this condition in an infant in 1897. His patient had cyanosis since infancy and a fairly good quality of life until he succumbed at the age of 32 years. The patient was active until the age of 29 years when he developed right heart failure and died three years later following a massive haemoptysis. Post-mortem revealed a large VSD (2.5 cm), both the left and right ventricles having equally thick walls. The pulmonary arteries revealed atheroma with multiple thrombi leading to pulmonary infarctions.

Paul Wood, at the Brompton Hospital, in 1958 published a study of 127 patients and was the first to suggest that Eisenmenger reaction occurred with defects other than at the ventricular level (*BMJ* 1958; **2**: 701, 709).

Case 29

FALLOT'S TETRALOGY

INSTRUCTION

Examine this patient's heart.

SALIENT FEATURES

History

- Syncope (in 20% of cases).
- Squatting.
- Shortness of breath.
- Growth retardation.

Examination

- Clubbing.
- Central cyanosis.
- Left parasternal heave with normal left ventricular impulse.
- Ejection systolic murmur heard in the pulmonary area.

Signs indicating Blalock–Taussig shunt:
- The left radial pulse is not as prominent as the right.
- The arm on the side of the anastomosis (usually the left) may be smaller than the other arm.
- Blood pressure is difficult to obtain because of the narrow pulse pressure in the arm supplied by the collateral vessels.
- Thoracotomy scar.

DIAGNOSIS

This patient has Fallot's tetralogy with a Blalock–Taussig shunt and is mildly cyanosed, indicating a right to left shunt (functional status).

Read: *N Engl J Med* 1993; **329**: 655–6.

QUESTIONS

What are the constituents of Fallot's tetralogy?
- VSD with a right-to-left shunt.
- Pulmonary stenosis (infundibular or valvular).
- Right ventricular hypertrophy.
- Dextroposition of the aorta with it overriding the ventricular septal defect.

What are the complications of Fallot's tetralogy?
- Cyanotic and syncopal spells.
- Cerebral abscess (in 10% of cases).
- Endocarditis (in 10% of cases).

- Strokes – thrombotic secondary to polycythaemia.
- Paradoxical emboli.

ADVANCED-LEVEL QUESTIONS

What do you understand by a Blalock–Taussig shunt?

It is the anastomosis of the left subclavian artery to the left pulmonary artery with the intention to increase pulmonary blood flow.

Why is it less frequently seen in adults in the recent past?

With ready availability of cardiopulmonary bypass, such patients have total correction of their anomalies at an early age.

What do you know about the embryological development of Fallot's tetralogy?

It arises from the anterior displacement of the conal septum, which leads to unequal partitioning of the conus at the expense of the right ventricular infundibulum and results in the obstruction of the right ventricular outflow tract and failure to close the intraventricular foramen.

What is the treatment for Fallot's tetralogy?

- Total correction under the age of 1 year when there is no need for an outflow transannular patch. A second-stage total correction can be performed when the child is over the age of 2 years.
- Blalock–Taussig shunting is performed nowadays only if the anatomy is unfavourable for a total correction.
- Modified Blalock–Taussig shunting is the interposition of a tubular graft between the subclavian and pulmonary arteries.
- The Waterston shunt involves anastomosis of the back of the ascending aorta to the pulmonary artery. A Waterston shunt is performed when surgery is required under the age of 3 months because the subclavian artery is too small for a good Blalock–Taussig shunt.
- The Potts shunt involves anastomosis of the descending aorta to the back of the pulmonary artery (*JAMA* 1946; **132:** 627).
- The Glenn operation involves anastomosis of the superior vena cava to the right pulmonary artery. The bidirectional Glenn procedure involves anastomosis of the superior vena cava to both pulmonary arteries.
- Pulmonary balloon valvuloplasty is sometimes used as an alternative to surgery.

Which cardiac lesions favour an initial shunt?

- Anomalous coronary artery.
- Single pulmonary artery.
- Hypoplastic pulmonary arteries.
- Single pulmonary artery.

What is Fallot's trilogy?

ASD, pulmonary stenosis and right ventricular hypertrophy.

What is Fallot's pentalogy?

Fallot's tetralogy with associated ASD is known as Fallot's pentalogy.

What conditions are associated with Fallot's tetralogy?

- Right-sided aortic arch (in 30% of cases).
- Double aortic arch.
- Left-sided superior vena cava (in 10% of cases).
- Hypoplasia of the pulmonary arteries.
- ASD.

Mention the common congenital heart diseases.

VSD, ASD of the secundum type, patent ductus arteriosus and Fallot's tetralogy are the common congenital heart diseases, in order of frequency.

What are the CXR findings?

- Boot-shaped heart.
- Enlarged right ventricle.
- Decreased pulmonary vasculature.
- Right-sided aortic arch (in 30% of cases).

What do you know about the Taussig–Bing syndrome?

In this condition the aorta arises from the right ventricle; the pulmonary trunk overrides both ventricles at the site of an interventricular septal defect.

Etienne-Louis Arthur Fallot (1850–1911), Professor of Hygiene and Legal Medicine in Marseilles, published his *Contribution to the pathologic anatomy of morbus coeruleus cardiac cyanosis* in 1888. The tetralogy was first described by N. Stensen, Professor of Anatomy in Copenhagen, in 1672 (Fallot A. Contribution à l'anatomie pathologique de la maladie bleue (cyanose cardiaque). *Marseille Médical* 1888; **25**: 418–20).

Helen Brook Taussig (1898–1986) is the founder of American paediatric cardiology. She collaborated with Alfred Blalock (1899–1964), a vascular surgeon, in the development of palliative surgery for Fallot's tetralogy (*JAMA* 1945; **128**: 189).

Case 30

ABSENT RADIAL PULSE

INSTRUCTION

Examine this patient's pulses.

SALIENT FEATURES

History

- Past history of insertion of an arterial line for blood gases or arterial pressure.
- Systemic symptoms in the past (Takayasu's arteritis).

- Past history of cardiac surgery (Blalock–Taussig shunt).
- Cervical rib.

Examination

- Left radial pulse is weaker than the right.
- Examine all other pulses (including carotid, brachial, femoral, popliteal, posterior tibial and dorsalis pedis pulses).
- Check the blood pressure in both the upper limbs (differences in blood pressure between both arms of more than 10 mmHg systolic or 5 mmHg diastolic are abnormal).

DIAGNOSIS

This patient has an absent radial pulse (lesion) which is due to a previous Blalock–Taussig shunt.

QUESTIONS

In which conditions may the pulse rate in one arm differ from that in the other?

Usually, slowing of the pulse on one side occurs distal to the aneurysmal sac. Thus, an aneurysm of the transverse or descending aortic arch causes a retardation of the left radial pulse. Also, the artery feels smaller and is more easily compressed than usual. An aneurysm of the ascending aorta or common carotid artery may result in similar changes in the right radial pulse.

What are the causes of absent radial pulse?

- Aberrant radial artery or congenital anomaly (check the brachials and blood pressure).
- Artery tied off at surgery or previous surgical cut-down.
- Catheterization of the brachial artery with poor technique.
- Following a radial artery line for monitoring of blood gases or arterial pressure.
- Subclavian artery stenosis.
- Blalock–Taussig shunt on that side (shunt from subclavian to pulmonary artery).
- Embolism into the radial artery (usually due to atrial fibrillation).
- Takayasu's arteritis (rare).

What are the causes of differences in blood pressure between arms or between the arms and legs?

- Occlusion or stenosis of the artery of any cause.
- Coarctation of the aorta.
- Dissecting aortic aneurysm.
- Patent ductus arteriosus.
- Supravalvular aortic stenosis.
- Thoracic outlet syndrome.

ADVANCED-LEVEL QUESTIONS

What do you know about Takayasu's arteritis?

It tends to affect young women and most of the cases have been from Japan. Prodromal systemic symptoms include fever, night sweats, anorexia, weight loss, malaise, fatigue, arthralgia and pleuritic pain. It predominantly involves the aorta and is of three types: Type I (Shimizu–Sano) which involves primarily the aortic arch and brachiocephalic vessels; Type II (Kimoto) which affects the thoraco-abdominal aorta and particularly the renal arteries; Type III (Inada) with features of Types I and II. Types I and III may be complicated by aortic regurgitation.

> M. Takayasu (1860–1938), Japanese ophthalmologist.

Case 31

CONSTRICTIVE PERICARDITIS

INSTRUCTION

Examine this patient's cardiovascular system.

SALIENT FEATURES

History

- Dyspnoea.
- Fatigue.
- Ankle or abdominal swelling.
- Nausea, vomiting, dizziness and cough.

Examination

- The patient may appear cachectic.
- Pulse may be regular or irregularly irregular (one third have atrial fibrillation).
- Prominent x and y descents in the jugular venous pulse, and the level of the JVP may rise with inspiration (Kussmaul's sign).
- Apex beat is not palpable.
- Early diastolic pericardial knock along the left sternal border, which may be accentuated by inspiration.
- Lungs are clear but there may be pleural effusion.
- Markedly distended abdomen with hepatomegaly and ascites.
- Pitting leg oedema.

DIAGNOSIS

This patient has constrictive pericarditis (lesion) caused by radiation therapy for previous Hodgkin's disease (aetiology) and is now limited by dyspnoea and marked ascites (functional status).

QUESTIONS

Mention some causes of constrictive pericarditis.
- Tuberculosis (<15% of patients).
- Connective tissue disorder.
- Neoplastic infiltration.
- Radiation therapy (often years earlier).
- Postpurulent pericariditis.
- Haemopericardium after surgery (rare).
- Chronic renal failure.

ADVANCED-LEVEL QUESTIONS

What is the mechanism for pericardial knock?
It is caused by the abrupt halting of rapid ventricular filling.

Mention the differential diagnosis of the early diastolic sound.
- Loud P2 (see p. 103).
- S3 gallop (see p. 39).
- Opening snap (mitral stenosis).
- Pericardial sound.
- Tumour plop (atrial myxoma).

What is Beck's triad?
The presence of low arterial blood pressure, high venous pressure and absent apex in cardiac tamponade is known as Beck's triad.

How would you investigate a patient with constrictive pericarditis?
- Chest radiograph typically shows normal heart size and pericardial calcification (**note**: the combination of pulsus paradoxus, pericardial knock and pericardial calcification favours the diagnosis of constrictive pericarditis).
- ECG shows low voltage complexes, non-specific T wave flattening or atrial fibrillation.
- Echocardiogram shows myocardial thickness is normal and may reveal thickened pericardium; normal ventricular dimensions with enlarged atria and good systolic and poor diastolic dysfunction. Doppler shows increased right ventricular systolic and decreased left ventricular systolic velocity with inspiration, expiratory augmentation of hepatic vein diastolic flow reversal.
- CT scan or MRI: shows normal myocardial thickness usually, and pericardial thickening and calcification.
- Cardiac catheterization typically shows identical left and right ventricular filling pressures and pulmonary artery systolic pressure usually <45 mmHg, with normal myocardial biopsy. Haemodynamic tracings show rapid 'y' descent in atrial pressure and early dip in diastolic pressure, with pressure rise to plateau in mid or late diastole.

How would you treat a patient with constrictive pericarditis?
- Surgery is the only satisfactory treatment: Complete surgical resection of the pericardium (myocardial inflammation or fibrosis may delay symptomatic response).

- Patients with tuberculous pericarditis should be pre-treated with antituberculosis therapy; if the diagnosis is confirmed after pericardial resection, full antituberculous therapy should be continued for 6–12 months after resection.

> C.S. Beck (1894–1971), surgeon, Peter Bent Brigham Hospital in Boston.
>
> W. Broadbent (1868–1951), English physician who qualified from St Mary's Hospital Medical School, London. He described the Broadbent sign in constrictive pericarditis, which is an indrawing of the 11th and 12th left ribs with a narrowing and retraction of the intercostal space posteriorly; this occurs as a result of pericardial adhesions to the diaphragm.

Case 32

PERMANENT CARDIAC PACEMAKER/IMPLANTABLE CARDIOVERTER-DEFIBRILLATOR

INSTRUCTION

Examine this patient's cardiovascular system.

SALIENT FEATURES

History
- Past history of syncope (Stokes–Adams attacks) and heart block.
- Dizziness (pacemaker syndrome).

Examination
- Dropped beats due to occasional ventricular ectopics.
- Infraclavicular scar indicating pacemaker insertion.
- Palpate the infraclavicular area gently to confirm the presence of a pacemaker.

Remember. Electromagnetic interference during magnetic resonance imaging or lithotripsy may transiently cause malfunction of pacemakers.

DIAGNOSIS

This patient has a permanent pacemaker (lesion) for previous heart block (aetiology) which is functioning adequately (functional status).

QUESTIONS

What are the indications for a permanent pacemaker?
- Symptomatic bradyarrhythmias (heart rate <40 beats/min or documented periods of asystole >30 seconds when awake). Symptoms include syncope, pre-syncope, confusion, seizures, or congestive heart failure and they must be clearly related to the bradycardia.

- Asymptomatic Mobitz type II atrioventricular block (*N Engl J Med* 1998; **338**: 1147–8).
- Complete heart block.

ADVANCED-LEVEL QUESTIONS

What do you know about permanent pacemakers?

- They are connected to the heart by one or two electrodes and are powered by long-lasting (5–10 years) solid-state lithium batteries. Most pacemakers are designed to pace and sense the ventricles – called the VVI pacemakers because they pace the ventricle (V), sense the ventricle (V) and are inhibited (I) by the ventricular signal. They are inserted under local anaesthesia and fluoroscopic guidance, subcutaneously under the pectoral muscles.
- In symptomatic sinus tachycardia, an atrial pacemaker may sometimes be implanted (AAI).
- In sick sinus syndrome, a dual-chamber pacemaker DDD (because it paces two or dual chambers, senses both (D) and reacts in two (D) ways, i.e. pacing in the same chamber is inhibited by spontaneous atrial and ventricular signals, and ventricular pacing is triggered by spontaneous atrial events) is implanted.
- Rate-responsive pacemakers measure activity, respiration, biochemical and electrical indicators, and change their pacing rate so that it is suitable for that level of exertion.

How soon after pacemaker insertion can a patient drive?

The patient may not drive until the pacemaker has been shown to be functioning correctly for at least 1 month after implantation. Patients must inform driving licensing authorities and the motor insurers.

Mention some expanded uses of cardiac pacing.

- Dual chamber pacing has been used to optimize cardiac output and minimize the outflow tract gradient in patients with hypertrophic obstructive cardiomyopathy.
- Dual chamber pacing is currently being investigated in dilated cardiomyopathy with heart failure and intraventricular conduction delay to optimize AV delay and improve cardiac output.
- Dual-site atrial pacing to prevent atrial fibrillation is being evaluated.

What are the complications of pacemakers?

- Erosion through the skin due to mechanical factors.
- Infection.
- Lead displacement or lead fracture (the most common site of pacing lead fracture is between the first rib and the clavicle).
- Pacemaker malfunction.
- Electromagnetic interference.
- Pain/ecchymoses at the site of insertion.
- Pneumothorax.

What are the potential sources of electromagnetic interference?

These include heavy electric motors and arc welding. Devices such as airport security devices and ham radios cause single-beat inhibition but they should not cause significant clinical interference. Microwave ovens do not interfere with pacemakers. Cellular phones and anti-theft devices or electronic article surveillance equipment can potentially interfere with pacemakers (*N Engl J Med* 1997; **336:** 1518–19; *N Engl J Med* 1997; **336:** 1473–9). Analogue phones are less likely to cause interference than phones based on digital technology. Patients should avoid carrying a cellular phone in a pocket directly over the pacemaker.

What is the pacemaker syndrome?

It is seen in individuals with a single-chamber pacemaker who experience symptoms of low cardiac output (dizziness, etc.) when erect; it is attributed to the lack of atrial kick. Pacemaker syndrome is caused by haemodynamic changes as a consequence of inappropriate use of ventricular pacing: it occurs when ventricular pacing is uncoupled from atrial contraction. It is most common when the VVI mode is used in patients with sinus rhythm but can occur in any pacing mode when atrioventricular synchrony is lost. Levels of atrial natriuretic factor are high in pacemaker syndrome.

If pacemaker syndrome occurs in a patient with a VVI pacemaker the only definitive treatment is to convert to a dual-chamber pacemaker. If the patient has occasional bradycardia then often symptoms may be ameliorated by programming the pacemaker to a lower limit and programming with hysteresis 'on'. This allows the patient to stay in normal sinus rhythm for longer periods by minimizing the pacing.

If a patient with an implantable defibrillator required a pacemaker, would you put in a separate device or replace it with an ICD with associated pacemaker function?

Placement of a separate pacemaker into a patient who has a defibrillator has the potential to cause serious pacemaker–defibrillator interactions. The most commonly implanted defibrillators have the additional ability to attempt termination of ventricular tachycardia with antitachycardia pacing. The obvious advantage of this feature is that an arrhythmia can be terminated painlessly without delivery of a shock. If antitachycardia pacing is unsuccessful then the device will administer a shock.

Mention some indications for implantable cardiac defibrillators.

*   Cardiac arrest resulting from ventricular tachyarrhythmia not due to a reversible or transient cause (**remember:** patients who have cardiac arrest unrelated to acute myocardial infarction have approximately a 35% chance of recurrent ventricular arrhythmias within the first year).
*   Spontaneous sustained ventricular tachycardia.
*   Syncope of undetermined origin with inducible sustained ventricular tachycardia on electrophysiological study and when drug therapy is not effective or tolerated.
*   Non-sustained ventricular tachycardia with coronary artery disease and inducible ventricular tachycardia on electrophysiological study that is not suppressible by a class I antiarrhythmic drug.

What techniques are contraindicated in patients with ICDs?

*   Magnetic resonance imaging.
*   Lithotripsy, if the pulse generator is in the field.

Case 33

PERICARDIAL RUB

INSTRUCTION

Listen to this patient's heart.

SALIENT FEATURES

History

Obtain a history of:

* Precordial pain changing with posture (worse on lying down and relieved by sitting forward).
* Myocardial infarction.
* Viral infection (Coxsackie A and B viruses).
* Chronic renal failure.
* Trauma.
* Tuberculosis.

Examination

* Scratching and grating sound heard best with the diaphragm at the left sternal border, with the patient leaning forward and the breath held in expiration. **Note.** A pericardial rub does not occur in acute pericarditis and it is common for the rub to disappear when a pericardial effusion develops.
* Tell the examiner that you would like to do an ECG (see below).

DIAGNOSIS

This patient has a pericardial rub (lesion) resulting from pericarditis secondary to uraemia (aetiology) and is not in pain (functional status).

QUESTIONS

What are the characteristic features of a pericardial friction rub?
It typically consists of three components: a presystolic rub (during atrial contraction), a ventricular systolic rub (which is almost always present and usually the loudest component) and a diastolic rub which follows the second heart sound (during rapid ventricular filling).

ADVANCED-LEVEL QUESTIONS

What are the characteristic electrocardiographic findings?
* ST elevation in most ECG leads with the concavity upwards.
* T-wave inversion occurs after the ST segment returns to baseline (unlike in acute myocardial infarction where the ST segment is concave downwards like a cat's

back and there is some amount of T-wave inversion accompanying the ST elevation).
- PR-segment depression (due to inflammation of the atrial wall).

How common is pericardial rub in constrictive pericarditis?
It is not heard in constrictive pericarditis.

What is the treatment for acute pericarditis?
- Pain relief (codeine) and anti-inflammatory agents (non-steroidal anti-inflammatory drugs (NSAIDs) such as indometacin).
- Steroids should be considered only when the pain does not respond to a combination of NSAIDs.
- Treatment of the underlying cause.
- Colchicine has been used to treat recurrent pain of pericarditis, and rarely pericardiectomy may be required for pain even in the setting of no haemodynamic impairment.

What do you know about the transient constrictive phase of acute pericarditis?
About 10% of the patients with acute pericarditis have a transient constrictive phase which may last 2–3 months before it gradually resolves, either spontaneously or with treatment with anti-inflammatory drugs. These patients usually have a moderate amount of pericardial effusion and, as the effusion resolves, the pericardium remains thickened, inflamed and non-compliant resulting in constrictive haemodynamics. Clinical features include shortness of breath, raised jugular venous pressure, peripheral oedema and ascites. Constrictive haemodynamics can be documented by Doppler echocardiography and resolution of constrictive physiology can be serially followed by this technique.

What is Dressler's syndrome?
Dressler's syndrome is characterized by persistent pyrexia, pericarditis and pleurisy. It was first described in 1956 when Dressler recognized that post-myocardial infarction chest pain is not caused by coronary artery insufficiency. It usually occurs 2–3 weeks after myocardial infarction and is considered to be of autoimmune aetiology; it responds to NSAIDs.

What do you know about postcardiotomy syndrome?
It occurs in about 5% of patients who have cardiac surgery, with symptoms of pericarditis from three weeks to six months after surgery. It is initially treated with NSAIDs and systemic steroids in refractory cases. Pericardiectomy is rarely required. It is said to result from an autoimmune response and is most likely to be related to surgical trauma and irritation of blood products in the mediastinum and pericardium.

What are the functions of pericardium?
- The pericardium protects and lubricates the heart.
- It contributes to the diastolic coupling of the left and right ventricles – an effect that is important in cardiac tamponade and constrictive pericarditis.

W. Dressler (1890–1969), US physician educated in Vienna. He worked at the Manimoides Hospital, Brooklyn, New York.

Case 34

PRIMARY PULMONARY HYPERTENSION

INSTRUCTION

Listen to this patient's heart.

SALIENT FEATURES

History

- Dyspnoea (60–89%).
- Fatigue (19–73%).
- Syncope, near syncope or dizziness (13–88%).
- Oedema (3–37%).
- Palpitations (5–33%).
- Determine whether the patient is on oral contraceptives, fenfluramine or aminorex (*N Engl J Med* 1996; **335:** 609–16).
- Determine whether the patient has habitually consumed plant products from *Crotalaria* species (particularly if from the Caribbean).
- Determine whether there is a family history: the chromosome locus 2q31–q32 has been identified in one familial cohort of primary pulmonary hypertension (*Circulation* 1997; **95:** 2603–6).
- Determine whether there is a history of HIV (HIV-associated pulmonary hypertension is associated with poor prognosis).

Examination

- Young woman.
- Loud pulmonary second sound.
- Early diastolic murmur of pulmonary regurgitation best heard on inspiration (Graham Steell murmur).
- Examine the chest for chronic lung disease.

Tell the examiner that you would like to:
- Investigate for a tight or occult mitral stenosis.
- Perform a ventilation–perfusion (V/Q) scan to exclude pulmonary emboli.

DIAGNOSIS

This patient has pulmonary hypertension (lesion) and should be investigated for an underlying cause; she is in cardiac failure (functional status).

QUESTIONS

What are the signs of pulmonary hypertension?
- Large 'a' waves in JVP.
- Left parasternal heave.

- Loud or palpable P2.
- Ejection click in the pulmonary area.
- Early diastolic murmur (Graham Steell murmur) due to pulmonary regurgitation.

ADVANCED-LEVEL QUESTIONS

How would you investigate such a patient?

- Chest radiograph: enlarged main pulmonary arteries with reduced peripheral branches, enlargement of the right ventricle.
- Pulmonary function testing, arterial blood-gas study.
- ECG: right ventricular and right atrial hypertrophy.
- V/Q scan to exclude pulmonary emboli.
- Echocardiogram, right heart catheterization and pulmonary angiography.

What are the pathological features of primary pulmonary hypertension?

They are those of plexogenic pulmonary arteriopathy (which also occurs in post-tricuspid left-to-right atrial shunts such as VSD or PDA, and collagen vascular diseases), characterized by medial hypertrophy and concentric intimal fibrosis of the pulmonary arteries with complex plexiform lesions. Others have no plexiform lesions or concentric intimal fibrosis, but rather have recanalized thrombotic small pulmonary arteries which are said to be the result of small thrombi or recurrent emboli. The least common histological pattern is veno-occlusive disease.

What are the theories for the cause of primary pulmonary hypertension?

- Excess endothelial production of the vasoconstrictor thromboxane relative to dilator prostaglandins such as prostacyclin.
- Excess endothelin-1 levels relative to nitric oxide. Inhaled nitric oxide and endothelin-1 antagonists reduce pulmonary hypertension.
- Excessive thrombosis *in situ* due to increased platelet activation, plasminogen activator inhibitor levels and decreased thrombomodulin.
- Increased serotonin levels.
- Inhibition or downregulation of potassium (Kv) channels in pulmonary artery smooth muscle cells and platelets.
- Activation of elastase and matrix metalloprotease enhances production of mitogens.
- Monoclonal proliferation of endothelial cells.

What is the prognosis in pulmonary hypertension?

The prognosis is poor: median survival is approximately 3 years from the time of diagnosis, with about one third of patients surviving for 5 years. Death usually occurs suddenly, presumably from arrhythmias or right ventricular infarction.

What are the predictors of survival?

These include indicators of severity of disease as assessed by measurement of haemodynamic characteristics (mean pulmonary artery pressure, right atrial pressure, cardiac index and mixed venous oxygen concentration), functional class, exercise tolerance (6-minute walk test), anticoagulant therapy and the response to vaso-dilators. Most patients succumb to progressive right-sided failure, but sudden death accounts for approximately 7% of deaths.

What treatment is available for primary pulmonary hypertension?

- Diuretics are useful in reducing excessive preload in patients with right heart failure, particularly when hepatic congestion and ascites are present.
- Oral anticoagulants: warfarin is the anticoagulant of choice, in doses adjusted to achieve an INR of approximately 2.0. Anticoagulants nearly double the 3-year survival rate (*Circulation* 1984; **70:** 580–7).
- Calcium channel blockers: nifedipine, diltiazem. Patients who respond to calcium channel blockers have a 5-year survival rate of 95% (*N Engl J Med* 1992; **327:** 76–81).
- Intravenous epoprostenol (formerly prostacyclin or prostaglandin I_2), which is a potent short-acting vasodilator and inhibitor of platelet aggregation that is produced by the vascular endothelium (*N Engl J Med* 1996; **334:** 296–301; *N Engl J Med* 1998; **338:** 273–7).
- Atrial septostomy: the creation of a right-to-left shunt by blade-balloon atrial septostomy has been reported to improve forward output and alleviate right-sided heart failure by providing blood with a low-resistance channel, thereby decompressing the right atrium and improving filling of the left side of the heart (*Circulation* 1995; **91:** 2028–35).
- Lung transplantation and combined heart–lung transplantation: survival rates after the two procedures are similar. Even markedly depressed right ventricular function improves considerably with single- or double-lung transplantation.
- Possible future drugs: (a) UT-15, a prostaglandin I_2 analogue, has been shown to have sustained and favourable effects in patients when administered sub-cutaneously (*Circulation* 2000; **102(18):** 11–101); (b) Sitaxsentan, an oral selective endothelin-A receptor blocker, has been shown to produce sustained improvements in pulmonary artery pressure (*Circulation* 2000; **101(25):** 2922–7).

Graham Steell (1851–1942), assistant physician to the Manchester Royal Infirmary, described the murmur in a paper titled *The murmur of high pressure in the pulmonary artery* (Med Chron (Manchester) 1888; **9:** 182–8).

Case 35

EBSTEIN'S ANOMALY

INSTRUCTION

Listen to this patient's heart. He was told he had an innocent murmur during a school medical examination many years ago but now has a large globular heart on chest radiography.

SALIENT FEATURES

History

- An incidental cardiac murmur.
- Ask the patient about palpitations (paroxysmal supraventricular tachycardia).

- Symptoms of right-sided heart failure.
- History of maternal lithium ingestion.

Examination

- Raised jugular venous pulse; a large 'v' of tricuspid regurgitation is absent because the giant right atrium absorbs most of the regurgitant volume.
- Left parasternal heave.
- Loud first heart sound produced by the sail-like anterior tricuspid leaflet.
- Pansystolic murmur which increases on inspiration.
- Hepatomegaly.

Proceed as follows:
- Ascertain whether the patient has exertional cyanosis or dyspnoea.
- Exclude an atrial septal defect.

DIAGNOSIS

This patient has isolated tricuspid regurgitation (lesion) which is probably of congenital aetiology as there is no pulmonary hypertension. He has Ebstein's anomaly with cardiomegaly and cardiac failure (functional status).
Read recent paper on this condition: *J Am Coll Cardiol* 1994; **23:** 170–6.

ADVANCED-LEVEL QUESTIONS

What is the pathology in Ebstein's anomaly?
The tricuspid leaflets are abnormal and are displaced into the body of the right ventricle. The septal leaflet is variably deficient or even absent. The posterior leaflet is also variably deficient and there is a large 'sail-like' anterior leaflet that is the hallmark of this condition. The abnormally located tricuspid orifice results in a part of the right ventricle lying between the atrioventricular ring and the origin of the valve, which is continuous with the right atrial chamber. This proximal segment is known as the 'atrialized' portion of the right ventricle.
About 50% of the patients have either a patent foramen ovale or a secundum ASD, and 25% have one or more accessory atrioventricular conduction pathways. The anomaly is said to be associated with maternal lithium ingestion.

What are the mechanisms of cyanosis in these patients?
Right-to-left shunting at the atrial level, i.e. through a patent foramen ovale or atrial septal defect.

What are the predictors of a poor outcome?
- The earlier the presentation, the higher the risk of mortality.
- A large right atrium or cardiothoracic ratio >60%.
- Severe right outflow tract abnormalities.

How would you investigate such a patient?
- CXR: large right atrium with oligaemic lung fields.
- ECG: RBBB (right bundle branch block), prolonged PR interval, P pulmonale (indicating right atrial enlargement), the P waves are large (Himalayan P waves),

type B Wolff–Parkinson–White syndrome (where the QRS complex is downward in lead V1).

- Echocardiogram: characteristic findings include the abnormal positional relationship between the tricuspid valve and mitral valve with septal displacement of the septal tricuspid leaflet.
- Cardiac catheterization: in classical cases there is no place for this investigation, which in the past has been associated with serious morbidity and mortality.

What are the indications for surgery?
- Severe functional limitation.
- A cardiothoracic ratio >60%.
- An atrial communication and if the patient has cyanosis (due to risk of stroke).
- Accessory pathway is present.
- Severe tricuspid regurgitation.

How are such patients treated?
- Tricuspid valve replacement plus closure of the atrial septal defect.
- Tricuspid annuloplasty with plication of the atrialized portion of the right ventricle.

W. Ebstein (1836–1912), German physician who also described Armanni–Ebstein nephropathy (where there is glycogen vacuolation in the proximal convoluted tubules); L. Armanni (1839–1903) was an Italian pathologist.

HISTORY

Note. Mnemonic: **SHOVE**.

- **S**yncope, **s**peech defect, **s**wallowing difficulty.
- **H**eadache.
- **O**cular disturbances: diplopia, field defects.
- **V**ertigo.
- **E**pilepsy: seizures.
- History pertaining to motor and sensory components of the cranial nerves and limbs, e.g. pain, paraesthesia, weakness, incoordination, etc.

EXAMINATION OF THE CRANIAL NERVES

First cranial nerve

1. Ask the patient, 'Have you noticed any change in your sense of smell recently?' 'Can you differentiate between the odour of tea, coffee and bananas?'.
2. If the examiner requires you to test the sense of smell, use an odour that can be readily identified, such as soap or clove oil. If the patient has frequent nasal trouble, the value of this examination is limited.

Second cranial nerve

1. First check visual acuity with a pocket Snellen's chart and finger counting.
2. Make sure that the patient wears her spectacles should she use them, as one is not concerned with refractive errors.
3. Check visual fields with a white hat pin (10 mm in diameter); your instructions to the patient should be clear and precise. Smaller hat pins (5 mm in diameter) are used for detecting small scotomata. Red hat pins, for reasons that are not clear, are useful in the detection of pregeniculate lesions and are therefore useful in compression of the optic nerve, optic chiasm or optic tract.
4. Comment on the pupils (size, shape or inequality) and test their reaction to light (direct and indirect reaction) and to accommodation. The popular acronym PERRLA (**p**upils **e**qual, **r**ound and **r**eactive to **l**ight and **a**ccommodation) is a convenient description of normal pupillomotor function.
5. Examine the fundus in a definite sequence: retina, retinal vessels, optic nerve and macula.

Third, fourth and sixth cranial nerves

1. Test eye movements:
   - Remember to ask the patient whether she sees a double image – this is the most sensitive sign of defective eye movement and may be present even when there is no apparent weakness of extraocular muscle or an abnormality of gaze.
   - *Saccadic movements* are tested by asking the patient to look voluntarily to the right and left and up and down. Note whether these movements are carried out rapidly to the extremes of gaze.

- *Pursuit movements* are examined by asking the patient to follow an object moved to the right and left and up and down.

Note whether these movements are carried out smoothly without interruption.

- Remember to comment on nystagmus. Nystagmus is a repetitive drift of the eyeball away from the point of fixation, followed by a fast corrective movement towards it.
- Comment on ptosis if present (seen in third nerve palsy).

Fifth cranial nerve

1. Test the masseters – 'Clench your teeth' – taking care to palpate the muscles.
2. Test the pterygoids – 'Open your mouth' – and note if the jaw deviates to the side of the lesion.
3. Test corneal (not conjunctival) sensation by touching a wisp of cotton wool to the cornea while the patient looks upward and away from the examiner.
4. Test facial sensation: keep in mind that this nerve supplies not only the face but also the anterior half of the scalp. Impairment of sensation limited to the face only is usually psychogenic in origin.
5. Test jaw jerk: with the mouth half open, place your thumb over the patient's chin and lightly tap on the thumb. A mild jaw jerk or absent jerk is seen in normal individuals. In upper motor neuron lesions above the cervical cord, the jaw will manifest a marked jerk with this procedure.

Seventh cranial nerve

Remember that the facial nerve is a motor nerve.

1. Test the lower half of the face:
   - Ask the patient, 'Show me your teeth'.
   - Note the nasolabial fold, which often disappears in mild facial palsy.
2. Test the upper half of the face:
   - Ask the patient, 'Screw your eyes tightly shut and don't let me open them'.
   - Have the patient wrinkle his or her forehead and note the movement of the muscles of the forehead.

Note. Taste may be lost on the anterior two thirds of the tongue, but this is not usually tested.

Eighth cranial nerve

1. Test by bringing a watch from beyond auditory acuity into the zone of hearing.
2. Occlude each external auditory meatus with your finger and whisper short phrases, asking the patient to repeat them.
3. Perform Rinne's and Weber's tests (use a tuning fork with a frequency of 256 or 512 cycles per second). Normally air conduction is better than bone conduction.
4. Rinne's test: in obstructive deafness, bone conduction is better. In nerve deafness the normal relations are kept, i.e. air conduction is greater than bone conduction in the deaf ear.
5. Weber's test: if the base of the tuning fork is placed on the middle of the forehead of a person with an obstructive deafness, he or she will hear it better in the deaf ear; with a nerve deafness, the fork will be heard better in the normal ear.

Ninth and tenth cranial nerves

1. Ask the patient 'Open your mouth and say "aah" '; observe the soft palate with a torch (the soft palate is pulled to the normal side on saying 'aah').
2. Tell the examiner that you would like to check gag reflex. An absence of gag reflex is significant only if it is unilateral.

Eleventh cranial nerves

1. Ask the patient, 'Shrug your shoulders', and try to push them down simultaneously (this tests the trapezii muscles).
2. Test the sternomastoids by the patient's ability to resist lateral movement of the neck. Keep in mind that one rotates the head to the *right* by use of the *left* sternomastoid muscle.

Twelfth cranial nerve

1. Ask the patient, 'Open your mouth'; comment on fasciculations of the tongue while in the mouth. Comment on wasting.
2. Ask the patient, 'Stick your tongue out' (it deviates to the side of the lesion). Slight deviation of the tongue can be disregarded.

> H.A. Rinne (1819–1868), German ear, nose and throat physician.
>
> F.E. Weber-Liel (1832–1891), a German otologist.

NEUROLOGICAL EXAMINATION OF THE PATIENT'S UPPER LIMBS

1. *Introduce* yourself to the patient and ask him to take his top off so that both his arms are well exposed. If the patient is female, cover her breasts with suitable clothing so that she is decent.

2. Comment on wasting, tremor (see pp 161–4), fasciculations.

3. *Assess tone*: 'Let your arms go loose and let me move them for you'.
   - Flex and extend wrists passively – cogwheel rigidity is elicited by this method.
   - Flex and extend at the elbows, pronate and supinate at the forearm – lead-pipe rigidity and clasp-knife spasticity is elicited by these methods.

4. *Test power*: 'I am going to test the strength of the muscles of your arms'.
   - Tell the patient, 'Hold your arms stretched out in front of you and then close your eyes'. Observe for drift, action tremor.
   - Shoulder abduction: 'Hold your arms outwards at your sides (like this) and keep them up; don't let me stop you'. Chief movers are the deltoids, C5. (**Note.** Supraspinatus is responsible for the initiation of abduction and for the first 60 degrees of this movement. However, this method of testing only assesses the power of the deltoids.)
   - Shoulder adduction: 'Push your arms in towards you and don't let me stop you'. Chief movers are the pectoral muscles, C6–8.
   - Elbow flexion: 'Bend your elbows and pull me towards you; don't let me stop you'. Chief mover is the biceps, C5.
   - Elbow extension: 'Straighten your elbows and push me away; don't let me stop you'. Chief mover is the triceps, C7.

- Wrist extension: 'Clench your fist and cock your wrists up; don't let me stop you'. Chief mover is C7.
- Wrist flexion: 'Now push the other way'. Chief mover is C7.
- Finger abduction: 'Spread your fingers wide apart and don't let me push them together'. Chief movers are the dorsal interossei, T1 (ulnar nerve). **Note.** **D**orsal interossei **ab**duct: mnemonic, DAB.
- Finger adduction: 'Hold this piece of paper between your fingers and don't let me snatch it away'. Chief movers are the palmar interossei, T1 (ulnar nerve). **Note. P**almar interossei **ad**duct: mnemonic, PAD.
- Thumb abduction: 'Hold your palms facing the ceiling and now point your thumb towards the ceiling; don't let me stop you'. Chief mover is the abductor pollicis brevis, C8, T1 (median nerve).
- Flexion of fingers: 'Grip these two fingers of mine tightly and don't let them go'. Chief movers are the long and short flexors of the fingers, C8.

Note.

- The median nerve supplies the lateral two **l**umbricals, **o**pponens pollicis, **a**bductor pollicis brevis, **f**lexor pollicis brevis: mnemonic, LOAF.
- The ulnar nerve supplies all other small muscles of the hand.
- The lumbricals are responsible for flexion at the metacarpophalangeal joint when the interphalangeal joints are in extension.
- Power is graded from 0 to 5:
  0: Absence of movement.
  1: Flicker of movement on voluntary contraction.
  2: Movement present when gravity is eliminated.
  3: Movement against gravity but not against resistance.
  4: Movement against resistance but not full strength.
  5: Normal power.

5. *Test deep tendon reflexes*:
   - Biceps jerk, C5, C6.
   - Triceps, C7.
   - Supinator, C5, C6.

Note.

- If the reflexes are absent, test after reinforcement – ask the patient to clench his or her teeth.
- *Inversion of the supinator reflex.* When the supinator jerk is elicited the normal response is a slight flexion of the fingers, contraction of the brachioradialis and flexion at the elbow joint. The jerk is said to be 'inverted' when finger flexion is the sole response, with contraction of the brachioradialis and elbow flexion being absent. There is associated absence of the biceps jerk and exaggeration of the triceps jerk.

The inverted jerk indicates a lower motor neuron lesion at the fifth cervical level and an upper motor neuron lesion below this level. It could be caused by cervical spondylosis, trauma to the cervical cord, spinal cord tumours at this level and syringomyelia.

6. *Finger reflexes*
   - *Hoffmann's sign.* The examiner holds the patient's wrist in the horizontal pronated position with the fingers and wrists relaxed. Then the distal phalanx of the patient's middle finger is forcibly flexed. Normally no reflex occurs unless the patient is under emotional tension.
   - In upper motor neuron lesions, the patient's thumb undergoes a quick flexion–adduction–opposition movement while the other fingers move in flexion–adduction. This response is labelled as a 'positive' Hoffmann's sign.
   - *Wartenberg's sign.* The patient places his or her hand in partial supination resting on a table with the fingers slightly flexed. Then the examiner places his/her middle and index fingers on the volar surface of the patient's four fingers and taps his/her own fingers briskly with the tendon hammer. The response is one of flexion of the patient's four fingers and the distal phalanx of the thumb.
   - *Mayer's sign.* With the patient's thumb abducted and the hand relaxed, the proximal phalanx of the middle finger is forcibly flexed towards the palm. Normally the thumb adducts. In upper motor neuron lesions the thumb usually remains in the position of abduction.

7. *Test coordination*
   - Finger–nose–finger test: 'Touch your nose with your index finger and now touch my finger'.
   - Rapid alternating movement of one hand over the other.

8. *Test sensation*
   - Light touch: use cotton wool and check each dermatome.
   - Pinprick: demonstrate first the sharp end and then the blunt end on the sternum; then check each dermatome for sharp or blunt sensation with the eyes closed.
   - Joint position sense: check in the distal interphalangeal joint of the thumb.
   - Vibration sense: use a tuning fork of 128 c.p.s. (although some authorities believe that a fork of 64 c.p.s. is more accurate). First test on the sternum so that the patient can recognize the vibration and then check over the fingers, moving proximally if the vibration sense is absent distally. Pallaesthesia is the ability to perceive the presence of vibration when an oscillating tuning fork is placed over certain bony prominences. Loss of vibratory perception is referred to as pallanaesthesia.

Remember:
- Joint sense and vibration sense are carried in the dorsal columns.
- Pain and temperature are carried in the lateral spinothalamic tracts.
- Light touch is carried in both the above tracts.

NEUROLOGICAL EXAMINATION OF THE PATIENT'S LOWER LIMBS

1. *Introduce* yourself and then ensure that the lower limbs are well exposed. It is important to ensure that the patient is decent – cover the genital area with a towel or any suitable clothing.

2. *Inspect for wasting, fasciculations* (tap the muscles of the leg and thigh to elicit fasciculations if not seen).

3. *Assess tone:*
   - Ask the patient, 'Let your leg go loose and lax, and let me move it for you'; then passively flex and extend the leg at the knee and hip.
   - Roll the extended leg, feeling for resistance.
   - Put your hand behind the knee and pull it upwards, observing the foot to check whether or not it flops.
   - If there is spasticity or increased tone, then test for ankle clonus and patellar clonus.
     - *Patellar clonus*: With the patient in the supine position, grasp the upper edge of the patella between the thumb and index finger and apply a quick constant pressure in a downward direction. Avoid prolonging this manoeuvre as it is often painful to the patient. In upper motor neuron lesions the patella may manifest a few jerks (unsustained clonus) or a constant jerking as long as the pressure is applied (sustained clonus).
     - *Ankle clonus*: Ensure that the patient's knee is semi-flexed and the foot relaxed. The foot is suddenly pushed dorsally with moderate force and held there. In upper motor neuron lesions the posterior muscles of the leg will enter into a persistent contraction.

4. *Test power* (begin at the hips): 'I am going to test the strength of the muscles of your legs'.
   - Hip flexion: 'Lift your leg straight up and keep it there; don't let me stop you'. Chief mover is iliopsoas L1, L2.
   - Hip extension: 'Push your leg downwards into your bed and don't let me stop you'. Chief movers are glutei, L4, L5.
   - Hip adduction: 'Push your thigh inwards against my hand'. Chief movers are adductors of the thigh, L2–4.
   - Knee flexion: 'Bend your knee and pull your heel towards you; don't let me stop you'. Chief movers are the hamstrings, L5, S1.
   - Knee extension: 'Straighten your knee and don't let me stop you'. Chief movers are quadriceps, L3, L4.
   - Plantar flexion of the ankle: 'Push your foot downwards against my hand'. Chief mover is the gastrocnemius, S1.
   - Dorsiflexion of the ankle: 'Move your foot up and don't let me stop you'. Chief movers are the tibialis anterior and long extensors, L4, L5.
   - Inversion of the foot: 'Push your foot inwards against my hand'. Chief movers are tibialis anterior and posterior, L4.
   - Eversion of the foot: 'Push your foot outwards against my hand'. Chief movers are the peronei, S1.
   - Extension of the great toe: 'Pull your toe upwards and don't let me stop you'. Chief mover is the extensor hallucis longus, L5.

5. *Test the plantar response*: 'I am going to tickle the bottom of your foot'; use an orange stick to stimulate the outer portion of the sole and then across the ball to the base of the big toe. Always describe the response as either downgoing or upgoing. Normally the response is downgoing, i.e. all the toes flex towards the

plantar surface. Upgoing plantars or the Babinski response is a feature of upper motor neuron lesions where the four small toes fan and turn towards the sole while the big toe extends dorsally. There is associated slight flexion of the hip and knee. The contraction of the tensor fasciae lata is referred to as Brissaud's reflex and is a part of the spinal defence reflex mechanism. Other responses to plantar stimulation include: (a) quick avoidance response; (b) the grasp reflex; and (c) the support reaction. Remember that if the feet are cold (when outside the bedclothes for long) the response may be equivocal.

6. *Test deep tendon reflexes*
- Knee jerk, L4.
- Ankle jerk, S1. In the elderly, the plantar strike technique is said to be more reliable than the tendon-striking method for eliciting ankle jerks. The plantar strike technique of eliciting ankle jerks is as follows: the patient's legs are side by side and the foot is passively dorsiflexed; the reflex hammer strikes the examiner's own fingers, which are placed over the plantar surface.
- When the reflexes are absent, reinforce by asking the patient to pull outwards his or her clasped hands (Jendrassik manoeuvre). Do not tie your hands into a knot while testing the left ankle jerk from the patient's right-hand side. Avoid jabbing the patient while eliciting reflexes.

Note. By convention, deep tendon reflexes are graded as follows:

0 no response, abnormal.
1+ slight but definitely present response which may be normal or abnormal.
2+ brisk response, normal.
3+ very brisk response which may be normal or abnormal.
4+ a tap elicits clonus, abnormal.
Asymmetry of reflexes suggests abnormality.

7. *Test coordination*
Heel–shin test: Have the patient place the heel of one foot upon the knee of the opposite leg, and then move the heel downwards along the tibia. In a positive test, the patient has difficulty placing or holding the heel on the opposite knee or cannot keep the heel firmly on the tibia as the heel is moved downwards.

8. *Test sensation*
Avoid testing in a given rhythm where the patient can expect to be stimulated at a given time. Always compare sensory responses in different areas of the same side of the body, as well as the two sides of the body.

- Light touch.
- Pinprick: test irregularly with the pin-point and pin-head, asking the patient whether the perceived sensation is sharp or blunt.
- Joint position sense: hold the lateral aspect of the patient's big toe (not the dorsum of the toe) while eliciting this and move the toe gently up and down. The examiner's fingers should not rub against the skin of the adjoining toe during this test. Also, the joint should not be put in the extreme position of flexion during the test.
- Vibration sense.

Note. When there is weakness of the limbs, tell the examiner that you would like to check sensation in the sacral area.

9. *Romberg's test:* 'Please stand up with your legs together and now close your eyes'. Take care to protect the patient if he or she sways or tends to fall. A positive test result is shown by pronounced swaying of the trunk. Sometimes functional cases will sway without having a true Romberg. This may be proved by diverting the attention of the patient by instituting the finger–nose test at the same time as Romberg is being tested. In functional cases the 'rombergism' will usually disappear.

10. *Check gait* and, if the heel–shin test is affected, then test tandem walking (asking the patient to walk along a straight line with one heel in front of the other foot). *Candidates frequently forget to check the gait when asked to examine the legs.*

Special manoeuvres in suspected upper motor neuron lesions

* Rossolimo's sign: The undersurfaces of the patient's toes are tapped with the examiner's fingers to produce abrupt extension (dorsiflexion) of the toes. In normal individuals there is no response, whereas in patients with upper motor neuron lesions all the toes respond with a quick plantar flexion.

In upper motor neuron lesions, the big toe will often dorsiflex (i.e. upgoing toe) when any of the following manoeuvres is conducted:

* Gordon reflex: on applying pressure to the muscle of the calf.
* Oppenheim sign: on applying heavy pressure with the thumb and index finger to the shin, stroking downwards from below the knee down to the ankle.
* Bing reflex: when the dorsum of the toe is pricked with a pin.
* Schaefer reflex: pinching the Achilles tendon sufficiently to cause pain.
* Chaddock reflex: on stroking the lateral side of the foot, beginning below the malleolus and extending anteriorly along the dorsum of the foot to the base of the big toe.
* Gonda reflex: grasping the small toes between the fingers, slowly and forcibly flexing the toe and then suddenly releasing the toe.

J.J. Babinski (1857–1932), of Polish origin, graduated from the University of Paris with a thesis on multiple sclerosis. The Babinski response refers to upgoing plantars in upper motor neuron lesions. He described adiposogenitalis a year before Frolich.

Case 36

BILATERAL SPASTIC PARALYSIS (SPASTIC PARAPLEGIA)

INSTRUCTION

Carry out a neurological examination of this patient's lower limbs.

SALIENT FEATURES

History

- Ask about onset, duration and course of symptoms.
- Back pain – is it localized?
- Ask about radicular pain.
- Numbness and paraesthesia, particularly below the level of the lesion.
- Weakness: gradual or sudden?
- Sphincter control and bladder sensation.
- Functional status: wheel chair transfers, walking aids, orthotic shoes, has house been modified for the patient's disability?
- Take a family history (hereditary spastic paraplegia).
- Take a history of birth anoxia (cerebral palsy).
- History of urinary infections, pressure sores and deep venous thromboses.

Examination

- Increased tone in both lower limbs.
- Hyper-reflexia.
- Ankle clonus.
- Weakness in both lower limbs.
- Wasting.

Proceed as follows:
- Check the sensory level and examine the spine (spinal tenderness or deformity).
- Tell the examiner that you would like to do the following:
  - check sacral sensation
  - examine the hands to rule out involvement of upper limbs
  - check for cerebellar signs (multiple sclerosis, Friedreich's ataxia).
- Try to localize the level of lesion using the following:
  - spasticity of the lower limb alone: lesion of thoracic cord (T2–L1)
  - irregular spasticity of lower limbs with flaccid weakness of scattered muscles of lower limbs: lesion of lumbosacral enlargement (L2–S2)
  - radicular pain: useful early in the disease, with time becomes diffuse and ceases to have localizing value
  - superficial sensation: not good for localizing as the level of sensory loss may vary greatly in different individuals and in different types of lesions.

DIAGNOSIS

This patient has bilateral spastic paraparesis (lesion) at L1 spinal level due to trauma (aetiology); it is complicated by bladder involvement (functional status).

QUESTIONS

What are the causes of spastic paraparesis?

Youth:
- Trauma.
- Multiple sclerosis.
- Friedreich's ataxia.
- HIV.

Adults:
- Multiple sclerosis.
- HIV (*Neurology* 1989; **39:** 892).
- Trauma (motor vehicle or diving accident).
- Spinal cord tumour (meningioma, neuroma).
- Motor neuron disease.
- Syringomyelia.
- Subacute combined degeneration of the cord (associated peripheral neuropathy).
- Tabes dorsalis.
- Transverse myelitis.
- Familial spastic paraplegia.

Elderly:
- Osteoarthritis of the cervical spine.
- Vitamin deficiency.
- Metastatic carcinoma.
- Anterior spinal artery thrombosis.
- Atherosclerosis of spinal cord vasculature.

ADVANCED-LEVEL QUESTIONS

What intracranial cause for spastic paraparesis do you know of?
Parasagittal falx meningioma.

What do you know about paraplegia-in-flexion?
Paraplegia-in-flexion is seen in partial transection of the cord where the limbs are involuntarily flexed at the hips and knees because the extensors are more paralysed than the flexors. In complete transection of the spinal cord, the extrapyramidal tracts are also affected and hence no voluntary movement of the limb is possible, resulting in paraplegia-in-extension.

What do you know about transverse myelitic syndrome?
- Causes include: trauma, compression by bony changes or tumour, vascular disease.
- All the tracts of the spinal cord are involved.
- The chief clinical manifestation is spastic or flaccid paralysis.
- The lesion can be incomplete cord compression or total cord transection:

	Total cord transection	Incomplete cord compression
Paraplegia in flexion	+	+
Paralysis	Symmetrical	Asymmetrical
Flexor–withdrawal reflex	+ without return (withdrawal phase only)	Associated with return to original position
Other	Vasomotor and sphincter changes	Variable area of anaesthesia which is not consistent with motor loss

What investigations would you perform?

- Complete blood count (CBC) for anaemia; erythrocyte sedimentation rate (ESR) for infection.
- Serology: syphilis, vitamin B_{12}, prostate-specific antigen (PSA) and serum acid phosphatase, and serum protein electrophoresis.
- Magnetic resonance imaging (MRI) of the spine.
- Computed tomography (CT) of the head to exclude parasagittal meningiomas.
- CT myelography, or plain CT.
- Check cerebrospinal fluid (CSF) for oligoclonal bands.
- Serum vitamin B_{12} levels.

Where is the lesion in patients with spastic weakness of one leg?

The lesion may be localized to the spinal cord or the brain. Progression to involve the arm does not help to differentiate between the spinal cord or the brain. Similarly, spread to the opposite leg does not necessarily indicate that the lesion is the spinal cord. Full investigation would include radiography of the spine and CT, but if the latter is normal then myelography may be required.

What do you know about hereditary spastic paraplegia?

This is an autosomal dominant condition, first described by Seeligmuller and Strumpell, in which spasticity is more striking than muscular weakness. The age of onset is variable and the condition has a relatively benign course. When the onset is in childhood, there may be shortening of the Achilles tendon, often requiring surgical lengthening. There is usually no sensory disturbance.

What do you know about tropical spastic paraplegia?

This is seen in Japan, the Caribbean and parts of western Africa and South America where women, more often than men, in their third and fourth decades have spastic paraparesis with neurogenic bladder. Viral infection with human T-lymphotrophic virus 1 has been implicated as a cause of this disorder.

How do you localize the lesion to the 2nd and 3rd lumbar root level?

- Muscular weakness: hip flexors and quadriceps.
- Deep tendon reflexes affected: knee jerk.
- Radicular pain/paraesthesia: anterior aspect of thigh, groin and testicle.
- Superficial sensory deficit: anterior thigh.

How do you localize the lesion to the 4th lumbar root level?

- Muscular weakness: quadriceps, tibialis anterior and posterior.
- Deep tendon reflexes affected: knee jerk.

- Radicular pain/paraesthesia: anteromedial aspect of the leg.
- Superficial sensory deficit: anteromedial aspect of the leg.

How do you localize the lesion to the 5th lumbar root level?
- Muscular weakness: hamstrings, peroneus longus, extensors of all the toes.
- Deep tendon reflexes affected: none.
- Radicular pain/paraesthesia: buttock, posterolateral thigh, anterolateral leg, dorsum of foot.
- Superficial sensory deficit: dorsum of the foot and anterolateral aspect of the leg.

How do you localize the lesion to the 1st sacral root level?
- Muscular weakness: plantar flexors, extensor digitorum brevis, peroneus longus, hamstrings.
- Deep tendon reflexes affected: ankle jerk.
- Radicular pain/paraesthesia: buttock, back of thigh, calf and lateral border of the foot.
- Superficial sensory deficit: lateral border of the foot.

How do you localize the lesion to the lower sacral root level?
- Muscular weakness: none
- Deep tendon reflexes affected: none (but anal reflex impaired).
- Radicular pain/paraesthesia: buttock and back of thigh.
- Superficial sensory deficit: saddle and perianal areas.

What is the characteristic type of diplegia in cerebral palsy?
Diplegia associated with prematurity is a striking clinical entity – striking for the symmetry of neurological signs, for their distribution, for the relatively good intelligence of the patients, and for the comparative absence of seizures, the disability often being purely motor without sensory deficits.

What surgical treatment is available for the management of spastic diplegia in cerebral palsy?
Dorsal rhizotomy may be beneficial in selected patients.

What are the clinical features of spinal cord compression from epidural metastasis?
The initial symptom is progressive axial pain, referred or radicular, which may last for days to months. Recumbency frequently aggravates the pain, unlike the pain of degenerative joint disease where it is relieved. Weakness, sensory loss and incontinence typically develop after the pain. Once a neurological deficit appears, it can evolve rapidly to paraplegia over a period of hours to days. In suspected cases MRI of the spine must be done by the next day. About 50% of cases in adults arise from breast, lung or prostate cancer. Compression usually occurs in the setting of disseminated disease. It is at the thoracic level in 70% of cases, lumbar in 20% and cervical in 10%, and occurs at multiple, non-contiguous levels in less than half of the cases. The tumour usually occupies the anterior or anterolateral spinal canal. CSF findings are non-specific in metastatic epidural compression. The cell count is usually normal, but protein levels may be raised because the flow of CSF is impeded. Lumbar puncture has been known to worsen the neurological deficit, presumably due to impaction of the cord.

Case 37

HEMIPLEGIA

INSTRUCTION

Carry out a neurological examination of this patient.

SALIENT FEATURES

History
- Obtain history of headache, seizures and loss of consciousness (more common in subarachnoid haemorrhage or intracerebral bleeds than in cerebral infarction).
- History of speech defects, sensory loss and weakness of face and limbs.
- Risk factors: hypertension, smoking, diabetes mellitus.
- History of functional status: swallowing, mobility, pressure sores, independence in activities of daily living, visual difficulties (for visual field defects).

Examination
- Unilateral upper motor neuron seventh nerve palsy.
- The arm is held to the side, the elbow is flexed, and the fingers and wrist are flexed on to the chest.
- The leg is extended at both the hip and knee, while the foot is plantar flexed and inverted.
- Weakness of the upper and lower limbs on the same side with upper motor neuron signs – increased tone, hyper-reflexia and upgoing plantar response.
  - Hemiplegic weakness of the upper limbs affects the shoulder abductor, elbow extensors, wrist and finger extensors, and small hand muscles.
  - Hemiplegic weakness of the lower limbs affects hip flexors, knee flexors and dorsiflexors and evertors of the foot.
- Do not forget sensory signs, in particular joint sensation which is important in rehabilitation.

Proceed as follows:
- Examine:
  - For homonymous hemianopia and sensory inattention.
  - For carotid bruits.
  - For speech defects.
  - The pulse for atrial fibrillation.
  - The heart for murmurs.
- Tell the examiner that you would like to check the blood pressure and check the urine for sugar.

DIAGNOSIS

This patient has had a stroke causing a right or left hemiplegia (lesion) which can be caused either by a vascular event such as thrombosis, embolism or haemorrhage, or by a neoplasm of the brain (aetiology). This patient is limited by hemiplegia and hemianopia (functional status).

QUESTIONS

What are the causes of hemiplegia?

About 80% of all strokes are due to cerebral infarction resulting from thrombotic or embolic occlusion of a cerebral artery (*J Neurol Neurosurg Psych* 1990; **53:** 16–22). The remaining 20% are caused by either intracerebral or subarachnoid haemorrhage.

Elderly:
- Vascular event (thrombosis, embolism or haemorrhage).
- Tumour.
- Subdural haematoma.
- Syphilis.

Youth:
- Multiple sclerosis.
- Tumour.
- Trauma.
- Embolism (look for underlying valvular heart disease, atrial fibrillation).
- Connective tissue disorder.
- Neurosyphilis.
- Intracranial infection: look for underlying acquired immune deficiency syndrome (AIDS), otitis media, cyanotic heart disease.

How would you manage such a patient?

- Early hospital admission, preferably to a dedicated stroke unit, which has been shown to produce long-term reductions in death, dependency and need for institutional care (*BMJ* 1997; **314:** 1151–9).
- Aspirin given within 48 hours of ischaemic stroke reduces the risk of death and recurrent stroke. The international stroke trial (*Lancet* 1997; **349:** 1569–81) and the Chinese stroke trial (*Lancet* 1997; **349:** 1641–9), each concerning 20 000 patients, found that aspirin was associated with about 10 fewer deaths or recurrent strokes, but with slightly more haemorrhagic strokes. The international stroke trial reported no benefit from subcutaneous heparin given with or without aspirin.
- FBC, ESR.
- Urine sugar.
- ECG.
- Chest radiography.
- Echocardiography (looking for source of emboli), computed tomography (CT), carotid digital subtraction angiography (DSA) in selected patients.
- Physiotherapy, speech therapy and occupational therapy.
- Control of risk factors – stop smoking, hypertension, hyperlipidaemia, diabetes, stop oral contraceptives.

Discuss the importance of blood pressure reduction in a patient with acute ischaemic stroke

Randomized clinical trials suggest that acute ischaemic stroke patients treated with antihypertensive agents may have an adverse clinical outcome and increased mortality (*BMJ* 1988; **296:** 737–41; *Cerebrovasc Dis* 1994; **4:** 204–10).

ADVANCED-LEVEL QUESTIONS

What are the measures used to determine the outcome after an acute stroke?

Some of the standard measures include:

- Barthel index is a reliable and valid measure of the ability to perform activities of daily living such as eating, bathing, walking and using the toilet.
- Modified Rankin Scale is a simplified overall assessment of function in which a score of 0 indicates the absence of symptoms and a score of 5 shows severe disability.
- Glasgow Outcome Scale is a global assessment of function in which a score of 1 indicates good recovery, a score of 2 moderate disability, a score of 3 severe disability, a score of 4 survival but in a vegetative state, and a score of 5 death.
- NIH Stroke Scale, a serial measure of neurological deficit, is a 42-point scale that quantifies neurological deficits in 11 categories. For example, a mild facial paralysis is given a score of 1 and complete right hemiplegia with aphasia, gaze deviation, visual field deficit, dysarthria and sensory loss is given a score of 25. Normal function without neurological deficit is scored as zero.

What is the role of thrombolysis in acute stroke?

Treatment with intravenous tissue plasminogen activator (tPA) when administered within 3 hours after onset of the ischaemic event (and in the absence of any sign of brain injury on CT) improves clinical outcome at 3 months (*N Engl J Med* 1995; **333:** 1581–7). The CT scan in these patients must be examined very carefully for evidence of hemispheric brain ischaemia, which may increase the risk of deterioration, with or without cerebral haemorrhage, after thrombolytic treatment. An overview of previous trials found significant excesses of early and total deaths, and of symptomatic and fatal intracranial haemorrhages, after acute thrombolysis, but a significant reduction in death or dependency in patients randomized to treatment within 3 hours of stroke onset (*Lancet* 1997; **350:** 607–14). It remains unclear which patients are most likely to benefit or be harmed.

What is the role of anticoagulants in the immediate treatment of acute ischaemic stroke?

Anticoagulants (including unfractionated heparin, low molecular weight heparin or specific thrombin inhibitors) offer no short- or long-term benefits in the immediate treatment of acute ischaemic stroke. Although the risks of deep venous thrombosis or pulmonary embolus are significantly reduced, these benefits are offset by a dose-dependent increased risk of intracranial or extracranial bleeding.

What is the prognosis in a patient with acute ischaemic stroke?

About 10% of these patients will die within a month from the onset of the stroke (*J Neurol Neurosurg Psych* 1990; **53:** 824–9). Of those who survive the acute event, about half will experience some disability after 6 months (*J Neurol Neurosurg Psych* 1987; **50:** 177–82).

What is the significance of carotid artery stenosis?

- Carotid artery stenosis is an important predisposing factor for cerebrovascular ischaemic events, the risk increasing with the severity of the stenosis and the presence of symptoms.
- For severe (>70% narrowing) symptomatic stenosis, carotid endarterectomy is recommended.
- For severe symptom-free stenosis, optimal management has yet to be defined: one meta-analysis of trials showed only a small absolute benefit from surgery in reducing the odds of ipsilateral stroke (*BMJ* 1998; **317:** 1477–80). Also, 45% of strokes in patients with asymptomatic stenosis with 60–99% narrrowing are attributable to lacunae or cardioembolism (*N Engl J Med* 2000; **342:** 1693–700). Carotid endarterectomy can not, therefore, be routinely recommended.
- For mild to moderate symptomatic stenosis (<70% narrowing), antiplatelet agents such as aspirin are recommended. Persistent symptoms may necessitate use of other agents such as ticlopidine, or clopidogrel, which reduces the relative risk for further ischaemic events slightly more than aspirin (CAPRIE trial, *Lancet* 1996; **348:** 1329–39).

How would you manage a patient with a transient ischaemic attack (TIA)?

- Give advice on stopping smoking.
- Aspirin.
- Duplex ultrasonography of the carotid vessels.
- Carotid artery DSA.

What do you understand by the term 'TIA'?

An acute loss of focal cerebral or ocular function with symptoms lasting less than 24 hours.

Why is it important to differentiate a carotid TIA from a vertebrobasilar TIA?

Carotid TIAs may be amenable to surgery. Furthermore, a TIA in the anterior circulation is generally of more serious prognostic significance than a TIA in the posterior circulation.

What are the features of a carotid TIA?

Hemiparesis, aphasia or transient loss of vision in one eye only (amaurosis fugax).

What are the features of a vertebrobasilar TIA?

- Vertigo, dysphagia, ataxia and drop attacks (at least two of these should occur together).
- Bilateral or alternating weakness or sensory symptoms.
- Sudden bilateral blindness in patients aged over 40 years.

What are the clinical features that would interest you for the rehabilitation of a stroke patient?

- Independence in activities of daily living – bathing, dressing, toileting, transferring, continence and feeding.
- Independence in more complex activities such as meal preparation, shopping, financial management, housekeeping, transportation, medication-taking and laundering.

What are the risk factors for stroke?

Hypertension, ischaemic heart disease, atrial fibrillation, peripheral vascular disease, diabetes, smoking, previous TIA, cervical bruit, hyperlipidaemia, raised haematocrit, oral contraceptive pill, cardiomyopathy.

Why is it important to treat TIAs?

Prospective studies have shown that within 5 years of a TIA:

- One out of six patients will have suffered a stroke.
- One out of four patients will have died (due either to stroke or heart disease).

What is the role of carotid endarterectomy in patients with a carotid TIA?

- For patients with severe stenosis (70–99%) the risks of surgery are significantly outweighed by the later benefits.
- For patients with mild stenosis (0–50% of cases) there is little 3-year risk of ipsilateral ischaemic stroke, even in the absence of surgery, so that any 3-year benefits of surgery are small and outweighed by its early risks (*N Engl J Med* 2000; **342:** 1743–5).
- For patients with moderate stenosis (50–69% of cases) the balance of surgical risk and eventual benefit is still being evaluated.

What is the role of carotid angioplasties in patients with recent carotid artery TIAs who have severe stenosis of the ipsilateral carotid artery?

This procedure has not been adequately assessed in patients with recent carotid artery TIAs or those with non-disabling ischaemic stroke who have severe stenosis of the ipsilateral carotid artery, and hence is not recommended. However, registry data suggest that carotid artery stenting may be useful in carefully selected patients. The CREST trial – a randomized trial funded by the NIH to examine the role of carotid stenting – is currently ongoing.

What do you understand by the term 'RIND'?

Reversible ischaemic neurological disease, in which symptoms and signs reverse within 1 week but not within 24 hours.

What are lacunar infarcts?

Lacunar infarcts are seen in hypertensive patients and consist of small infarcts in the region of the internal capsule (causing partial hemiparesis or hemisensory impairment), pons (ataxia of cerebellar type, partial hemiparesis), basal ganglia or thalamus. They are often multiple. Lacunae are thought to be caused by occlusion of small branch arteries or by rupture of Charcot–Bouchard microaneurysms producing a small haematoma which resolves, leaving an area of infarction.

What areas of the brain are supplied by the anterior carotid artery?

The anterior carotid artery supplies the frontal lobes and the medial cerebral hemispheres with the exception of the visual cortex of the occipital lobes. Cortical areas supplied by this artery include the motor and sensory areas of the lower limbs, a 'micturition centre' and the supplementary motor cortex. Ischaemia in the territory of one anterior carotid artery produces weakness and mild sensory deficits in the opposite lower limb. Some patients with left anterior carotid artery ischaemia have a mild transient aphasia.

What do you understand by the term 'stroke'?

Stroke is characterized by rapidly progressive clinical symptoms and signs of focal, and at times global, loss of cerebral function lasting more than 24 hours or leading to death, with no apparent cause other than that of vascular origin (*Bull World Health Organ* 1976; **54:** 541–53).

How do you classify stroke?

Using the **Bamford clinical classification of stroke**:

Total anterior circulation syndrome

- Unilateral motor deficit of face, arm and leg.
- Homonymous hemianopia.
- Higher cerebral dysfunction (e.g. aphasia, neglect).

Parietal anterior circulation syndrome

Any two of the following features:

- Unilateral motor and/or sensory deficit.
- Ipsilateral hemianopia or higher cerebral dysfunction.
- Higher cerebral dysfunction alone or isolated motor and/or sensory deficit restricted to one limb or the face.

Posterior circulation syndrome

One or more of the following features:

- Bilateral motor or sensory signs not secondary to brainstem compression by a large supratentorial lesion.
- Cerebellar signs, unless accompanied by ipsilateral motor deficit (see ataxic hemiparesis).
- Unequivocal diplopia with or without external ocular muscle palsy.
- Crossed signs, for example left facial and right limb weakness.
- Hemianopia alone or with any of the four items above.

Lacunar syndromes

- *Pure motor stroke:*
  - unilateral, pure motor deficit
  - clearly involving two of three areas (face, arm and leg)
  - with the whole of any limb being involved.
- *Pure sensory stroke:*
  - unilateral pure sensory symptoms (with or without signs)
  - involving at least two of three areas (face, arm and leg)
  - with the whole of any limb being involved.
- *Ataxic hemiparesis:*
  - ipsilateral cerebellar and corticospinal tract signs
  - with or without dysarthria
  - in the absence of higher cerebral dysfunction or a visual field defect.
- *Sensorimotor stroke:*
  - pure motor and pure sensory stroke combined (i.e. unilateral motor or sensory signs and symptoms)
  - in the absence of higher cerebral dysfunction or a visual field defect.

M. Fischer wrote one of the earliest descriptions of the effect of 'occlusion of the internal carotid artery' including transient cerebral ischaemia and ischaemic stroke (*Arch Neurol Psychiatry* 1951; **65**: 346–77).

Charles Warlow, contemporary Professor of Neurosciences, Edinburgh.

Peter Sandercock, contemporary Professor of Neurology, Edinburgh.

NASCET = North American Symptomatic Carotid Endarterectomy Trial.

Case 38

PTOSIS AND HORNER'S SYNDROME

INSTRUCTION

Examine this patient's face.

SALIENT FEATURES

History

- Ask the patient whether or not there is absence of sweating on one side of the face.
- History of lung cancer.
- History of cervical sympathectomy.
- Migraine.

Examination

If you notice ptosis during the examination, then you must answer the following questions:

- Is ptosis complete or incomplete?
- Is it unilateral or bilateral?
- Is the pupil constricted (Horner's syndrome) or dilated (third nerve palsy)?
- Are extraocular movements involved (third nerve palsy or myasthenia gravis)?
- Is the eyeball sunken or not (enophthalmos)?
- Is the light reflex intact (intact light reflex in Horner's syndrome)?

If the patient has Horner's syndrome then quickly proceed as follows:

- Examine the supraclavicular area:
  Percuss the supraclavicular area, looking for dullness of Pancoast's tumour.
  - Look for scar of cervical sympathectomy (be prepared with indications for cervical sympathectomy).
  - Look for enlarged lymph nodes.

- Examine the neck:
  - For carotid and aortic aneurysms.
  - For tracheal deviation (Pancoast's tumour).
- Examine the hands:
  - For small muscle wasting.
  - For pain sensation with a pin.
  - For clubbing.
    (These should help in making a diagnosis of syringomyelia or Pancoast's tumour.)
- If there is no clue so far about the cause, tell the examiner that you would like to examine for nystagmus, cerebellar signs, cranial nerves and pale optic discs, and pyramidal signs to ascertain brainstem vascular disease or demyelination.

DIAGNOSIS

This patient has Horner's syndrome (lesion) associated with dullness in the supra-clavicular area indicating a Pancoast's tumour (aetiology).

QUESTIONS

What causes Horner's syndrome?

The syndrome results from the involvement of the sympathetic pathway which starts in the sympathetic nucleus and travels through the brainstem and spinal cord to the level of C8/T1/T2 to the sympathetic chain, stellate ganglion and carotid sympathetic plexus (*Am J Ophthalmol* 1958; **46:** 289–96: Horner's syndrome: an analysis of 216 cases).

What are the features of Horner's syndrome?

It is characterized by:

- Miosis (resulting from paralysis of the dilator of the pupil).
- Partial ptosis or pseudoptosis (due to paralysis of the upper tarsal muscle).
- Enophthalmos (due to paralysis of the muscle of Müller).
- Often, slight elevation of the lower lid (because of paralysis of lower tarsal muscles).

What additional feature would you see in congenital Horner's syndrome?

There would be heterochromia of the iris, i.e. the iris remains grey-blue.

How would you determine the level of the lesion using only the history?

The level of the lesion is determined by the distribution of the loss of sweating:

- Central lesion – sweating over the entire half of the head, arm and upper trunk is lost.
- Lesions of the neck:
  - Proximal to the superior cervical ganglion – diminished sweating on the face.
  - Distal to the superior cervical ganglion – sweating is not affected.

ADVANCED-LEVEL QUESTIONS

How would you differentiate whether the lesion is above the superior ganglion (peripheral) or below the superior cervical ganglion (central)?

Test	Above	Below
Sweating	Such lesions may not affect sweating at all as the main outflow to the facial blood vessels is below the superior cervical ganglion	Such lesions affect sweating over the entire head, neck, arm, and upper trunk. Lesions in the lower neck affect sweating over the entire face
Cocaine 4% in both eyes	Dilates the normal pupil No effect on the affected side	Dilates both pupils
Adrenaline 1:1000 in both eyes	Dilates affected eye No effect on normal side	No effect on both sides

Note. In peripheral lesions there is depletion of amine oxidase due to postganglionic denervation. As a result this sensitizes the pupil to 1:1000 adrenaline, whereas it has no effect on the normal pupil or in central lesions (where the presence of the enzyme rapidly destroys the adrenaline).

Mention one cause of intermittent Horner's syndrome.

Migraine.

What are the causes of ptosis?

Unilateral:
- Third nerve palsy.
- Horner's syndrome.
- Myasthenia gravis.
- Congenital or idiopathic.

Bilateral:
- Myasthenia gravis.
- Dystrophia myotonica.
- Ocular myopathy or oculopharyngeal dystrophy.
- Mitochondrial dystrophy.
- Tabes dorsalis.
- Congenital.
- Bilateral Horner's syndrome (as in syringomyelia).

If the patient has Pancoast's tumour, what is the most likely underlying pathology?

Squamous cell carcinoma.

> J.F. Horner (1831–1886), Professor of Ophthalmology in Zurich, conceded that Claude Bernard had recognized the syndrome before him.
>
> Henry K. Pancoast (1875–1939) was the first Professor of Radiology in the USA at the University of Pennsylvania.

Case 39

ARGYLL ROBERTSON PUPIL

INSTRUCTION

Examine this patient's eyes.

SALIENT FEATURES

History

- Ask the patient about lancinating pains.
- History of multiple sclerosis, sarcoidosis, syphilis.
- Difficulty in walking (remember the gait in tabes dorsalis).

Examination

- The pupils are small and irregular.
- Light reflex is absent.
- Accommodation reflex is intact.
- There may be depigmentation of the iris.
- Bilateral ptosis and marked overcompensation by frontalis muscle (in tabes dorsalis).

Proceed as follows:
Tell the examiner that you would like to do the following:

- Examine for vibration and position sense.
- Test for Romberg's sign and deep tendon reflexes (decreased).
- Check syphilitic serology.
- Check urine sugar.

Remember that these pupils show little response to atropine, physostigmine or methacholine.

DIAGNOSIS

This patient has Argyll Robertson pupil (lesion) and you would like to investigate for underlying neurosyphilis or leutic infection (aetiology).

QUESTIONS

What are the causes of Argyll Robertson pupil?
- Neurosyphilis – tabes dorsalis.
- Diabetes mellitus and other conditions with autonomic neuropathy.
- Pinealoma.
- Brainstem encephalitis.
- Multiple sclerosis.
- Lyme disease.

- Sarcoidosis (*BMJ* 1984; **289**: 356).
- Syringobulbia.
- Tumours of the posterior portion of the third ventricle.

ADVANCED-LEVEL QUESTIONS

What do you know about the nerve pathways of the light reflex?

- The afferent is through the optic nerve and the efferent limb is through the third cranial nerve. The relevant optic nerve fibres responsible for the light reaction leave those responsible for the perception of light to terminate in the pretectal region of the midbrain, from whence a further relay passes to the Edinger–Westphal nucleus.
- Disturbances of the pupillary light reflex occur when there is involvement of the following:
  - Superior colliculus.
  - Decussation of Meynert.
  - Edinger–Westphal nucleus (supplies the constrictor muscles of the iris).

Where is the lesion in Argyll Robertson pupil?

Damage to the pretectal region of the midbrain is believed to be responsible for the Argyll Robertson pupil of neurosyphilis (*Am J Ophthalmol* 1956; **42**: 105). This, however, does not explain the small irregular pupils and it has been suggested that local involvement of the iris is a separate lesion.

Which muscle in the eye is responsible for the accommodation reflex?

Paralysis of accommodation occurs when the ciliary muscle is involved. Remember that accommodation is a much more potent stimulus for constriction of the pupils than light, as there are more nerve fibres mediating the accommodation reflex than the light reflex.

Mention a few causes of a small pupil.

- Senile miosis.
- Pilocarpine drops in the treatment of glaucoma.

What is 'reversed' Argyll Robertson pupil?

The pupils react to light but not to accommodation – seen in parkinsonism caused by encephalitis lethargica.

What do you understand by the term 'anisocoria'?

Anisocoria is gross inequality of the pupils. Causes include:

- About 20% of normal individuals.
- Third nerve palsy.
- Iritis.
- Blindness or amblyopia in one eye (pupil larger in the affected eye).
- Cerebrovascular accidents.
- Severe head trauma.
- Hemianopia due to optic tract involvement.

Note. Eccentric pupil occurs when the pupil is not in the centre of the iris. It may result from trauma or iritis and need not be pathognomonic of neurological disease.

> Douglas M.C.L. Argyll Robertson (1837–1909) of Edinburgh described these pupils in 1869 with neurosyphilis (*Edinb Med J* 1869; **15**: 487). His studies on the effects of the extracts of the Calabar bean (*Physostigma venenosum*) on the pupil were widely acclaimed. He was the President of the Royal College of Surgeons of Edinburgh.

Case 40

HOLMES–ADIE SYNDROME

INSTRUCTION

Examine this patient's eyes.

SALIENT FEATURES

History

- The patient is usually a young woman.
- Impaired sweating.
- Onset may be acute.

Examination

- The pupil is large, regular, irregular, oval, or circular.
- The pupil will react sluggishly or fail to react to light. However, if a strong and persistent stimulus is used it can be shown that the pupil contracts excessively to a very small size and when the stimulus is removed it returns to its former size gradually – this is known as the 'myotonic' pupil.
- Delayed constriction in response to near vision.
- Delayed re-dilatation after near vision.
- Accommodation impaired.
- There is segmental palsy and segmental spontaneous movement of iris (*Lancet* 2000; **356**: 1760–1).

Proceed as follows:
Check the ankle jerks and tell the examiner that you expect them to be absent.

DIAGNOSIS

This woman has a sluggishly reacting pupil with absent ankle jerks (lesion) due to Holmes–Adie syndrome (aetiology), which is a benign disorder (functional status).

QUESTIONS

What is the significance of this condition?

It is benign and must not be mistaken for Argyll Robertson pupil.

What are the causes of a dilated pupil?

- Mydriatic eye drops.
- Third nerve lesion.
- Holmes–Adie syndrome (degeneration of the nerve to the ciliary ganglion).
- Lens implant, iridectomy.
- Blunt trauma to the iris (pupil may be irregularly dilated and reacts sluggishly to light – post-traumatic iridoplegia).
- Drug overdose, e.g. cocaine, amphetamine.
- Poisoning, e.g. belladonna.
- Deep coma, death.

What are the causes of a small pupil?

- Old age.
- Pilocarpine eye drops.
- Horner's syndrome.
- Argyll Robertson pupil.
- Pontine lesion.
- Narcotics.

ADVANCED-LEVEL QUESTIONS

What do you know about the factors that control the size of the pupil?

The sphincter muscle of the pupil (causing miosis) is supplied by the cholinergic parasympathetic nerves, whereas the dilator of the pupil (causing mydriasis) is supplied by noradrenergic sympathetic fibres. The parasympathetic fibres arise from the Edinger–Westphal nucleus. They travel by the third cranial nerve to the ciliary ganglion. Postganglionic fibres arise from the ciliary ganglion and are distributed by the ciliary nerve.

Where is the lesion in Adie's tonic pupil?

There is damage to the parasympathetic fibres within the ciliary ganglion.

What is the difference between Adie's tonic pupil and Holmes–Adie syndrome?

Adie's tonic pupil with absent deep tendon jerks is called Holmes–Adie syndrome.

How does the Holmes–Adie pupil react to weak pilocarpine (0.125%) or 2.5% methacholine?

It usually constricts, indicating a supersensitivity to acetylcholine secondary to parasympathetic denervation resulting from degeneration of postganglionic neurons and neurons in the ciliary ganglion. There is no effect on a normal pupil.

Which conditions may accompany this syndrome?

Dysautonomias such as:

- Ross's syndrome (segmental loss of sweating).
- Cardiac arrhythmias.

Sir Gordon M. Holmes (1876–1965) and William J. Adie (1886–1935) were London neurologists who described the condition independently in 1931 (Holmes: *Trans Ophthalmol Soc UK* 1931; **41**: 209; Adie: *Brain* 1932; **55**: 98; *Br J Ophthalmol* 1932; **16**: 449). The name Holmes–Adie syndrome was coined by Bramwell in 1936. Saenger and Strasburger indepedently described the syndrome in 1902; it was first recorded in the English literature by Markus in 1905.

Case 41

HOMONYMOUS HEMIANOPIA

INSTRUCTION

Examine this patient's eyes.
Examine this patient's visual fields.

SALIENT FEATURES

History

- The patient bumps into things on one side and may have a history of traffic accidents where one side of the car is damaged without the patient realizing.
- The patient may insist that he/she has one 'bad' eye (remember, blindness in one eye causes impairment in perceiving distances but the normal eye will provide a full field of vision on both sides and hence the patient will not bump into objects).
- Reading difficulty (suggests that the visual defect splits the midline: if the defect is on the right side, the patient is unable to scan along the line to the next word and hence reading is almost impossible, whereas when the defect is on the left side the patient cannot find the beginning of the next line).
- Determine whether the patient is aware of his/her defect (if the patient is aware of the visual defect it is likely that the defect 'splits' the macula and bisects the central field, whereas if the patient is unaware and bumps into things, then the defect is either macular sparing or an attention hemianopia).

Examination

Testing for homonymous hemianopia includes:

- Testing for an attention field defect using both hands of the examiner and asking the patient to determine which finger is moving.
- Testing of the whole field in each eye using a white hat pin.
- Re-evaluation of the field in each eye to determine whether there is macular sparing or macular splitting using a hat pin.

If you are unable to determine, then tell the patient that you would like to do formal field testing with a tangent screen or using a perimeter.

Proceed as follows:
- Check the visual acuity; examine the fundus.
- Tell the examiner that you would like to do a full neurological examination to look for an underlying cause:
  - Stroke.
  - Intracranial tumour.

DIAGNOSIS

This patient has a homonymous hemianopia (lesion) for which I would like to determine the aetiology, such as a stroke or tumour.

ADVANCED-LEVEL QUESTIONS

Where is the lesion?

The lesion is in the optic tract and beyond (visual acuity is intact when the macula is spared):

Site of lesion	Type of homonymous hemianopia
Optic tract and first part of radiations	Incongruous
Optic radiations	Generally congruous
Temporal lobe	Superior quadrantic defect in each eye
Posterior parietal lobe	Inferior quadrantic defect in each eye

What further investigations would you do?

- Formal field testing: perimetry is particularly important if the patient holds a driver's licence.
- CT head scan.

Case 42

BITEMPORAL HEMIANOPIA

INSTRUCTION

Examine this patient's eyes.
Examine this patient's visual fields.

SALIENT FEATURES

History

- Insidious onset of defects in visual field. Involvement of the macula is late and is associated with abrupt visual failure as the presenting feature.
- Hypogonadism (may precede the visual failure by many years): males have impotence and females have amenorrhoea.

Examination

- Bitemporal hemianopia, which is caused by a median lesion of the optic chiasma.

Proceed as follows:

- Examine the hands and face for acromegaly.
- Tell the examiner that you would like to look for signs of hypopituitarism (see pp 375–7). The probable causes are as follows:
  - Pituitary tumour (endocrine symptoms precede the visual symptoms; the upper temporal fields are affected first and then the defect spreads down).

– Craniopharyngioma (bitemporal hemianopia is initially worse in the lower quadrants).
– Suprasellar meningioma.
– Aneurysms.
– Metastases.
– Glioma.

DIAGNOSIS

This patient has bitemporal hemianopia (lesion) and I would like to investigate for a median mass lesion compressing the optic chiasma.

QUESTIONS

How would you investigate this patient?

- Formal field testing – perimetry.
- Serum prolactin.
- Skull radiography (calcification of craniopharyngioma and size of the pituitary fossa which is best seen in the lateral skull radiograph).
- CT head scan.

Case 43

CENTRAL SCOTOMA

INSTRUCTION

Examine this patient's visual fields.

SALIENT FEATURES

History

- Sudden onset usually.
- Patient notices a 'hole' in the vision while reading a poster or looking at a clock.

Examination

- Central scotoma (allow the patient to find the defect himself by moving the white hat pin in his own visual field). Then determine:
  1. The size and shape of the defect by moving the pin in and out of the blind area.
  2. Whether the defect crosses the horizontal midline (vascular defects of retina do not do so).
  3. Whether the defect crosses the vertical midline (defects due to pathway damage have a sharp vertical edge at the midline).

4. Whether the defect extends to the blind spot – so-called 'caecocentral scotoma' (seen in glaucoma, vitamin B_{12} deficiency).
5. Whether there is a similar defect in the other eye (to exclude homonymous hemianopic scotomas).
- Examine the fundus. Remember that the optic discs may be:
  - Pale (optic atrophy).
  - Normal (retrobulbar neuritis).
  - Swollen and pink (papillitis).

DIAGNOSIS

This patient has a central scotoma (lesion) due to optic atrophy (aetiology).

ADVANCED-LEVEL QUESTIONS

What do you understand by the term 'scotoma'?
It is a small patch of visual loss within the visual field.

Mention a few underlying causes for central scotoma.
- Demyelinating disorders (multiple sclerosis).
- Optic nerve compression by tumour, aneurysm.
- Glaucoma.
- Toxins – methanol, tobacco, lead, arsenical poisoning.
- Ischaemia – including central retinal artery occlusion due to thromboembolism, temporal arteritis, syphilis, idiopathic acute ischaemic neuropathy.
- Hereditary disorders – Friedreich's ataxia, Leber's optic atrophy.
- Paget's disease.
- Vitamin B_{12} deficiency.
- Secondary to retinitis pigmentosa.

Case 44

TUNNEL VISION

INSTRUCTION

Examine this patient's eyes.
Examine this patient's visual fields.

SALIENT FEATURES

History

See optic atrophy (pp 529–31), retinitis pigmentosa (pp 535–7).

Examination

Intact central vision with constriction of the peripheral fields.

Proceed as follows:
Examine for the following:

- Optic atrophy (primary and secondary).
- Retinitis pigmentosa (see pp 535–7).
- Choroidoretinitis (see p. 538).
- Glaucoma.

DIAGNOSIS

This patient has tunnel vision (lesion) due to retinitis pigmentosa (aetiology).

ADVANCED-LEVEL QUESTIONS

What are the other causes of tunnel vision?
- Hysteria.
- Slight contraction of field occurs when there is a significant refractive error.

Note. Before making a diagnosis of hysteria, it is essential to exclude contraction of the visual fields due to extreme fatigue, poor attention, inadequate vision, diminished visual acuity or delayed reaction time.

How would you differentiate hysteria from an organic cause of tubular vision?

In organic causes the field of vision widens progressively as the test objects are held further away from the eye, but in the hysterical person this widening is not seen and the entire width of the field is as great at 1 foot from the eye as it is at 5, 10 or 15 feet.

Case 45

PARKINSON'S DISEASE

INSTRUCTION

Examine this patient.

SALIENT FEATURES

History

- Tremor: usually unilateral at onset; usually starts in upper limbs. Also seen in the legs and jaws.

- Rigidity: ask about history of falls, poor balance, pain and muscle stiffness.
- Poverty of movement: ask about drooling of saliva, difficulty in writing (micrographia), difficulty in turning in bed and change in voice (softness of voice).
- Family history of disease.
- History of encephalitis.
- History of exposure to manganese dust, carbon disulphide, or carbon monoxide.
- Use of MTP for recreational purposes.
- Elicit a drug history, particularly regarding neuroleptics (reserpine, metoclopramide).

Examination

Usually florid cases are seen in the examination and the striking abnormalities are:

- An expressionless or 'mask-like' face (fixed stare, infrequent blinking and ironed-out wrinkles).
- Drooling of saliva.
- Resting or pill-rolling movement (most common in the distal extremities).

Proceed as follows:
- Comment on the expressionless face, pill-rolling movement and drooling of saliva so that the examiner knows that you have observed these abnormalities. Elicit bradykinesia by asking the patient to touch her thumb with each finger in turn.
- Examine the tone, in particular at the wrist for cog-wheel rigidity.
- Proceed to do the glabellar tap. Tap the forehead just above the bridge of the nose repeatedly (about twice per second): in normal subjects the blinking will stop whereas the patient with Parkinson's disease continues to blink – referred to as Myerson's sign. It must be remembered that this sign is unreliable.
- Ask the patient to walk, and comment on the paucity of movement including the absence of arm swing and festinating gait (the patient walks with a stooped posture as if trying to catch up with her centre of gravity). The feet may scrape the floor in taking steps so the patient trips easily (be prepared to prevent the patient from falling when examining the gait).
- Tell the examiner that you would like to:
  – Ask the patient a few questions with a view to assessing her speech.
  – Assess handwriting (tremulous and small, micrographia).
- Tell the examiner that you would like to look for:
  – Postural hypotension (Shy–Drager syndrome, L-dopa treatment).
  – Impaired vertical gaze (Steele–Richardson–Olzewski syndrome).
- Seborrhoea.

Note. The diagnosis of Parkinson's disease is entirely clinical but the results of certain investigations may help in recognizing alternative causes for parkinsonism.

DIAGNOSIS

This patient has features of Parkinson's disease (lesion) which is due to long-standing use of phenothiazines (aetiology). The patient is severely disabled by the bradykinesia (functional status).

QUESTIONS

What comprises Parkinson's disease?

Upper body dyskinesia

This must be present – it is a symptom complex containing many of the following features:

- Slowness of movement (bradykinesia).
- Poverty of movement (mask-like facies, diminished arm swing).
- Difficulty in initiating movement.
- Diminished amplitude of repetitive alternative movement.
- Inordinate difficulty in accomplishing some simultaneous or sequential motor acts.

Rigidity

This is usually but not always present:

- Leadpipe rigidity, where the increase in tone is equal in flexors and extensors of all four limbs but slightly more in flexors, resulting in a part flexed 'simian' posture.
- Cog-wheel rigidity is due to superimposed or underlying tremor.

Postural instability

Usually a late feature.

Tremor

Absent in about one third of patients with Parkinson's disease at presentation and throughout its course in some.

- Resting, 3–5 Hz pill, pronation and supination rolling tremor of the upper limb.
- Tremor is intermittent (can usually be brought about by getting the subject to count backwards with the eyes closed and hands dangling over the armrests of the seat).
- The tremor is intensified by emotion or stress and disappears during sleep.
- The legs, head and jaw may shake as well. Jaw tremor is rare but is most distressing; the teeth may pound together until they become unbearably painful.

ADVANCED-LEVEL QUESTIONS

What are the causes of Parkinson's disease?

- *True parkinsonism:*
  - Idiopathic (due to degeneration of the substantia nigra) – also known as Parkinson's disease.
  - Drug-induced (chlorpromazine, metaclopramide, prochlorperazine).
  - Anoxic brain damage such as cardiac arrest, exposure to manganese and carbon monoxide.
  - Postencephalitic – as a result of encephalitis lethargica or von Economo's disease.
  - 1-Methyl-4-phenyl-1,2,3,6-tetrahydropyridine toxicity – seen in drug abusers.
  - Multiple system atrophy.
  - Progressive supranuclear atrophy.

   – Familial.

   – Mutation of the α-synuclein gene or linkage to a region on chromosome 2.

- *Pseudoparkinsonism:*
  - Essential tremor.
  - Atherosclerotic (vascular) pseudoparkinsonism (mention that in the past atherosclerosis was thought to be a cause of Parkinson's disease but this is no longer accepted as a cause).
- *Hemiparkinsonism* (presenting feature of a progressive space-occupying lesion).

What are the pathological changes in Parkinson's disease?

The most typical pathological hallmarks of Parkinson's disease are:

- Neuronal loss with depigmentation of the substantia nigra.
- Lewy bodies, which are eosinophilic cytoplasmic inclusions in neurons consisting of aggregates of normal filaments.

The following associations have been made with clinical features and pathological changes:

Clinical deficit	Pathology
Motor symptoms	Degeneration of dopaminergic nigrostriatal pathway
Cognitive defects	Degeneration of dopaminergic mesocortical and mesolimbic pathways
Autonomic dysfunction	Dopamine depletion in the hypothalamus
'Freezing phenomenon'	Degeneration of the noradrenergic locus ceruleus
Dementia	Degeneration of the cholinergic nucleus

What is the mental status of patients with Parkinson's disease?

- In the initial stages, intellect and senses are usually preserved. Many patients have some intellectual deterioration – a slowness of thought and of memory retrieval (bradyphrenia), and subtle personality changes.
- Global dementia may develop in one fifth of patients.
- Depression occurs in one third of patients.
- Acute confusion can be precipitated by drug therapy.

Note. Parkinson's disease must be kept in mind in elderly patients presenting with a history of frequent falls.

What is the difference between rigidity, spasticity and gegenhalten?

- *Rigidity* indicates increased tone affecting opposing muscle groups equally and is present throughout the range of passive movement. When smooth it is called 'leadpipe' rigidity, and when intermittent is termed 'cog-wheel' rigidity. It is common in extrapyramidal syndromes, Wilson's disease and Creutzfeld–Jakob disease.
- *Spasticity* of the clasp-knife type is characterized by increased tone which is maximal at the beginning of movement and suddenly decreases as passive movement is continued. It occurs chiefly in the flexors of the upper limb and extensors of the lower limb (antigravity muscles).
- *Gegenhalten*, or paratonia, is where the increased muscle tone varies and becomes worse the more the patient tries to relax.

What do you understand by the 'wheelchair sign' in Parkinson's disease?

Patients with advanced disease and 'on–off' motor fluctuations require a wheelchair when 'off' and when 'on' are seen to walk about (sometimes pushing the chair!). These patients are rarely permanently wheelchair-bound; in contrast, those who never leave their wheelchair usually do not have Parkinson's disease.

What is the role of protein diets in patients who have episodes of sudden and substantial loss of mobility?

High-protein diets should be avoided in these patients, because a large influx of dietary amino acids can interfere with the transport of L-dopa into the brain (*N Engl J Med* 1967; **276:** 374–9).

How is the severity of Parkinson's disease graded?

The Hoehn–Yahr staging grades Parkinson's disease into five stages:

- Newly diagnosed disease – Stage I.
- Moderately severe disease – Stages II and III.
- Advanced disease – Stages IV and V.

How would you manage a patient with Parkinson's disease?

Symptomatic therapy:

- When *tremor* is the main problem – anticholinergic drugs such as trihexyphenidyl, benzatropine, biperiden, cycrimine, procyclidine, phenoxene, orphenadrine.
- When *bradykinesia* is the main problem – L-dopa with a decarboxylase inhibitor such as carbidopa or benserazide. Other drugs include amantadine and synthetic dopamine agonists (bromocriptine, pergolide). In early Parkinson's disease levodopa-sparing agents may be desirable to prevent dyskinesia. Bromocriptine alone improves about 50% of patients during the first year of treatment but there is a gradual loss thereafter with only 10% responding at 5 years; other dopamine agonists have similar effects. Ropinirole and pramipexole are dopamine agonists that are not derived from ergot and are more selective, have fewer adverse effects and tend to produce greater therapeutic response which is longer-lasting than that of the older ergot derivatives. In the elderly, L-dopa is the first line of treatment as it has the best therapeutic index.

Protective therapy:

Selegiline, a monoamine oxidase B inhibitor, is said to retard the progression of early Parkinson's disease (*N Engl J Med* 1993; **328:** 176–83); it delays the need for levodopa by a mean of 8 months. One study found increased mortality in patients taking levodopa in combination with selegiline (*BMJ* 1995; **311:** 1602–7) but a subsequent study has refuted this finding.

What is the role of ropinirole in early Parkinson's disease?

A 5-year study shows that the early use of the dopamine D_2 receptor agonist ropinirole significantly reduces the risk of dyskinesia in patients with Parkinson's disease. When all patients randomly assigned to ropinirole were compared with those randomly assigned to levodopa, the risk of dyskinesia was lower by a factor of almost three in the ropinirole group. The overall incidence of dyskinesia at

5 years was 20% in the ropinirole group compared to 45% in the levodopa group. This difference was even more striking among patients who did not require supplementary levodopa (rates of dyskinesia: ropinirole group, 5%; levodopa group, 36%). The reason why the early use of ropinirole reduced the risk of dyskinesia remains unclear. The early use of ropinirole did not reduce the occurrence of wearing-off and freezing during walking to the same extent as it did the occurrence of dyskinesia. However, delaying treatment with levodopa to prevent dyskinesia can be justified only if the underlying symptoms of Parkinson's disease are sufficiently controlled (*N Engl J Med* 2000; **342**: 1484–91).

In which condition is L-dopa absolutely contraindicated?

Melanoma.

What do you know about 'drug holidays' in levodopa therapy?

Drug holidays (i.e. discontinuation of therapy) were previously claimed to enhance the efficacy of treatment when it was resumed; this is now known to be dangerous (deaths have occurred) and of doubtful value.

What do you know about dopamine receptors?

At least four types of receptors have been reported: D_1 and D_2 are the two major families of dopamine receptors. For neurotransmission to occur, a complex consisting of a dopamine receptor and G protein (guanine nucleotide-binding protein) must be formed. This complex then usually couples to the enzyme adenylate cyclase which controls the formation of the second messenger, cyclic AMP. Alteration of the second messenger leads to a cascade of events that ultimately determines the transfer of information between nerve cells. The D_{2A} receptor is involved in the therapeutic response elicited by dopaminergic agonists in parkinsonism, although the mechanism at the physiological level is not clear. The role of the D_1 family is unclear; it is not certain whether the activation of these receptors leads to useful effects (i.e. reduction of parkinsonian deficits), undesirable effects (e.g. dyskinesia), or both. Bromocriptine, pergolide and lisuride all stimulate D_2 receptors, whereas bromocriptine and lisuride are D_1 receptor antagonists and pergolide is a D_1 receptor agonist.

Mention some newer drugs used in the treatment of Parkinson's disease.

- Dopamine antagonists: cabergoline, ropinirole, pramipexole.
- Inhibitors of catechol *O*-methyltransferase (COMT): entacapone, tolcapone. COMT inhibitors increase 'on' time and reduce the duration of the 'off' time and thus allow reduction of the daily dose of L-dopa.
- Inhibitors of glutamate receptors: CPP (3-(2-carboxy-piprazin-4-yl)propyl-l-phosphonate), lamotrigine.
- GM-1 ganglioside: when monkeys were treated with this drug from cow's brain their motor function was returned to normal.

What is the role of fetal tissue in Parkinson's disease?

Parkinson's disease is characterized by loss of midbrain dopamine neurons that innervate the caudate and putamen. Patients tend to have a reduced response to levodopa after 5–20 years of therapy, with 'on–off' fluctuations consisting of dyskinesia alternating with immobility. Animal experiments have suggested that fetal dopaminergic neurons can survive transplantation and restore neurological function. Trials are underway to determine whether fetal grafts can improve motor function in patients with Parkinson's disease. Fetal ventral mesencephalic tissue is implanted in the patient's postcommissural putamen (*N Engl J Med* 1995; **332:** 1118–24).

What is the role of thalamotomy in Parkinson's disease?

Thalamotomy used to be the main treatment until 1950, but with the introduction of levodopa it became less popular. However, there has been a revival of stereotactic surgery prompted by the failure of levodopa in four main aspects: in severe tremor, levodopa-induced dyskinesia, advanced Parkinson's disease and akinetic–rigid syndromes (*BMJ* 1998; **316:** 1259–60). Four types of stereotactic surgery are practised:

- Thalamotomy for intractable tremor, where a radiofrequency lesion is placed in the venterointermediate nucleus (VIM) of the thalamus. It is unsuitable for bilateral tremor as bilateral thalamotomy tends to cause impairment of speech.
- Thalamic stimulation with a fine electrode in the VIM nucleus and a pacemaker inserted under the skin on the chest. This relieves tremor and can be performed bilaterally. Neither procedure improves akinesia, the most disabling aspect of Parkinson's disease.
- Deep-brain stimulation of the globus pallidus and subthalamic nucleus may result in striking improvements in parkinsonism and dyskinesia, resulting in large reductions of levodopa dose and thus improvements in levodopa-induced dyskinesias (*Lancet* 1995; **345:** 91–5).
- Unilateral posteroventral medial pallidotomy – ameliorates contralateral parkinsonian symptoms and medication-related dyskinesia and is sustained for up to $5\frac{1}{2}$ years. Improvements in ipsilateral and axial symptoms are not sustained and many patients undergo a second contralateral procedure (*N Engl J Med* 2000; **342:** 1708–14).

Note. Patients with dementia and hallucinations tolerate all surgical procedures poorly and any benefit in patients with rapidly progressive parkinsonism is likely to be short lived.

What are Parkinson plus syndromes?

Some patients have other neurological deficits in addition to Parkinson's disease. Examples of these so-called 'Parkinson plus syndromes' are:

- Steele–Richardson–Olszewski disease (akinesia, axial rigidity of the neck, bradyphrenia, supranuclear palsy).
- Multiple system atrophy.
  Olivopontocerebellar degeneration.
  Strionigral degeneration.
  Progressive autonomic failure (Shy–Drager syndrome).
- Basal ganglia calcification.

What is tardive dyskinesia?

Tardive dyskinesia is seen in patients taking neuroleptics. Its manifestations are orofacial dyskinesia such as smacking, chewing lip movements, discrete dystonia or choreiform movements and, rarely, rocking movements. Withdrawal of the offending drug will improve these symptoms over a period of 3–4 years, except in a small minority of patients.

What is the drug of choice when these patients develop psychosis and delusions?

Clozapine.

Mention some heredo-degenerative parkinsonian disorders.

- Hallervorden–Spatz disease: autosomal recessive; patients also have dementia, dystonia, choreoathetosis, retinitis pigmentosa. There is increased iron deposition and increased cysteine in the globus pallidus.
- Fahr's disease or familial basal ganglia calcification: patients also have chorea, dementia and palilalia.
- Olivopontocerebellar and spinocerebellar degenerations: autosomal dominant, associated cerebellar ataxia and retinitis pigmentosa.

James Parkinson (1755–1824) first reported six cases of this syndrome in 1817 (at the age of 62 years).

J.C. Steele, J.C. Richardson and J. Olszewski were all US neurologists.

K. von Economo (1876–1931), an Australian neurologist, also wrote on Wilson's disease.

C.D. Marsden, contemporary Professor of Neurology, National Hospital, Queen's Square, London; his chief interest is Parkinson's disease and movement disorders.

Case 46

CEREBELLAR SYNDROME

INSTRUCTION

Examine this patient, who presented with a history of falling to one side. Demonstrate the cerebellar signs.

SALIENT FEATURES

History

- History of falls, wide-based gait, clumsiness and difficulty with fine coordinated movements.
- Tremor.
- Waxing and waning of symptoms (multiple sclerosis).
- Stroke (brainstem vascular lesion).
- Drug toxicity: phenytoin, alcohol abuse, lead poisoning and solvent abuse.
- History of intracranial tumours (posterior fossa including cerebellopontine angle tumour).
- History of hypothyroidism (a reversible cause).
- Family history (Friedreich's ataxia and other hereditary ataxias).
- Birth defects (congenital malformations at the level of the foramen magnum).

Examination

- Ask the patient a few questions to assess his speech.
- Ask the patient to keep his arms outstretched; then give them a small push downward and look for rebound phenomenon.
- Examine for rapid alternating movements with the hand.
- Do the finger–nose test: look for past-pointing and intention tremor.
- Do the heel–shin test.
- Examine the gait, in particular tandem walking. If ataxia is not marked, the patient's gait may be tested with eyes closed; he often progresses to the side of the lesion.
- Tell the examiner that you would like to examine the fundus for optic atrophy as demyelination is the commonest cause of cerebellar signs.

DIAGNOSIS

This patient has a cerebellar syndrome with optic atrophy (lesion) due to multiple sclerosis (aetiology) and is markedly ataxic (functional status).

QUESTIONS

How may cerebellar signs manifest?

- Disorders of movement:
  - Nystagmus: coarse horizontal nystagmus with lateral cerebellar lesions; its direction is towards the side of the lesion.
  - Scanning dysarthria: a halting, jerking dysarthria which is usually a feature of bilateral lesions.
  - Lack of finger–nose coordination (past-pointing): movement is imprecise in force, direction and distance – dysmetria.
  - Rebound phenomenon – inability to arrest strong contraction on sudden removal of resistance. This is known as Holmes' rebound phenomenon.
  - Intention tremor.
  - Dysdiadochokinesia – impairment of rapid alternating movements (clumsy).
  - Dyssynergia – movements involving more than one joint are broken into parts.
- Hypotonia.
- Absent reflexes or pendular reflexes.
- Lack of co-ordination of gait – patient tends to fall towards the side of the lesion.

Note.

1. The classical clinical triad of cerebellar disease is **A**taxia, **A**tonia, **A**sthenia.
2. The cerebellum is not primarily a motor organ. It is developed phylogenetically from a primary vestibular area and is involved in modulation of motor activity. It receives afferents from the vestibular nuclei, spinal cord and cerebral cortex via the pontine nuclei.

What are the causes of cerebellar syndrome?

- Demyelination (multiple sclerosis).
- Brainstem vascular lesion.
- Phenytoin toxicity.

- Alcoholic cerebellar degeneration (there is atrophy of the anterior vermis of the cerebellum).
- Space-occupying lesion in the posterior fossa including cerebellopontine angle tumour.
- Hypothyroidism (a reversible cause).
- Paraneoplastic manifestation of bronchogenic carcinoma.
- Friedreich's ataxia and other hereditary ataxias.
- Congenital malformations at the level of the foramen magnum.

ADVANCED-LEVEL QUESTIONS

How are cerebellar signs localized?
- Gait ataxia (inability to do tandem walking): anterior lobe (palaeocerebellum).
- Truncal ataxia (drunken gait, titubation): flocculonodular or posterior lobe (archicerebellum).
- Limb ataxia, especially upper limbs and hypotonia: lateral lobes (neocerebellum).

What is the difference between sensory ataxia and cerebellar ataxia?

	Cerebellar ataxia	Sensory ataxia
Site of lesion	Cerebellum	Posterior column or peripheral nerves
Deep tendon	Unchanged or pendular reflexes	Lost or diminished
Deep sensation	Normal	Decreased or lost
Sphincter disturbances	None	Decreased when posterior column involved, causing overflow incontinence

If you were allowed to perform one investigation, which one would you choose in a patient with a suspected cerebellar lesion?
Magnetic resonance imaging (MRI).

Sir Gordon M. Holmes (1876–1965), consultant neurologist, National Hospital for Nervous Diseases, Queen Square, London, whose observations on wartime gunshot wounds allowed him to study cerebellar disease (*Lancet* 1922; **ii**: 59, 111; *Brain* 1939; **62**: 1–30). He was the editor of the journal *Brain*.

Case 47

JERKY NYSTAGMUS

INSTRUCTION

Examine this patient's eyes.
Test the patient's eye movements.

SALIENT FEATURES

History

- Obtain history regarding cerebellar syndrome: multiple sclerosis, alcohol, etc. (p. 143).
- Ear infections (vestibular involvement).
- Horizontal nystagmus with fast components to right or left side (when eliciting nystagmus take care to keep your finger at least 2 feet away from the patient and avoid going laterally beyond the extent of binocular vision).

Proceed as follows:
- Look for other cerebellar signs (see p. 144).
- Tell the examiner that you would like to do the following:
  - Examine the fundus for optic atrophy (multiple sclerosis).
  - Take a history of vertigo (vestibular nystagmus).

Note. Remember that if the patient has vertical nystagmus in addition to horizontal nystagmus it is more likely to be vestibular nystagmus or brainstem disease.

DIAGNOSIS

This patient has a jerky nystagmus with optic atrophy (lesion) due to multiple sclerosis (aetiology). I would like to examine her neurological system to evaluate the disability (functional status).

QUESTIONS

What do you understand by the term 'nystagmus'?

Nystagmus is a series of involuntary, rhythmic oscillations of one or both eyes. It may be horizontal, vertical or rotatory.

ADVANCED-LEVEL QUESTIONS

What is pendular nystagmus?

In pendular nystagmus, the oscillations are equal in speed and amplitude in both directions of movement. It may be seen on central gaze when the vision is poor, as in severe refractive error or macular disease.

What do you understand by the term 'jerky' nystagmus?

Jerky or phasic nystagmus is a condition in which eye movement in one direction is faster than that in the other. This is usually seen in the horizontal plane and is brought out by lateral gaze to one or both sides. It is seen with lesions of the cerebellum, vestibular apparatus or their connections in the brainstem.

What is dissociated nystagmus?

Dissociated or ataxic nystagmus is irregular nystagmus in the abducting eye. It is bilateral in multiple sclerosis, brainstem tumour or Wernicke's encephalopathy. It is unilateral in vascular disease of the brainstem. It is due to a lesion in the medial longitudinal fasciculus (which links the sixth nerve nucleus on one side to the medial rectus portion of the third nerve on the other).

Where is the lesion in vestibular nystagmus?

It may be in one of two locations:

- Peripheral (labyrinth or vestibular nerve), as in labyrinthitis, Ménière's syndrome, acoustic neuroma, otitis media, head injury.
- Central (affecting vestibular nuclei), as in stroke, multiple sclerosis, tumours, alcoholism.

What do you know about 'downbeat' and 'upbeat' nystagmus?

Downbeat nystagmus is associated with brainstem lesions, meningoencephalitis and hypomagnesaemia. Upbeat nystagmus is caused by lesions of the anterior vermis of the cerebellum.

K. Wernicke (1848–1904) graduated from Poland; although aware that a toxic factor was important in the aetiology, he did not realize that this syndrome was due to a nutritional deficiency.

P. Ménière (1799–1862), French ear, nose and throat specialist.

Case 48

SPEECH

INSTRUCTION

Ask this patient some questions.

SALIENT FEATURES

Proceed as follows:

Ask the patient simple questions

Personal details such as name, age, occupation, address and handedness (remember that over 90% of left-handed people have a dominant left hemisphere).

Test the following:
Comprehension:

- Put your tongue out.
- Shut your eyes.
- Touch your nose.
- Smile.
- Two-step commands, such as touch your left ear with your right hand.

Orientation:

- Time–date.
- Place.
- Name familiar objects:
  - Pen.
  - Coin.
  - Watch.

Articulation. Ask the patient to repeat the following:

- British constitution.
- West Register Street.
- Baby hippopotamus.
- Biblical criticism.
- Artillery.

Abbreviated mental test:

- Address to recall: 42 West Street.
- Age.
- Date of birth.
- Time.
- Year.
- Recognition of two persons such as doctor and nurse.
- Name of this place.
- Name of the monarch or prime minister.
- Year of World War I or World War II.
- Count backwards from 20 to 1.
- Serially subtract 7 from 200.

Tell the examiner that you would like to check the 'primitive' reflexes:

- *Snout reflex*: brought about by tapping the upper lip slightly. There is puckering or protrusion of the lips with percussion. The muscles around the mouth and the base of the nose contract.
- *Palmomental reflex*: occurs when a disagreeable stimulus is drawn from the thenar eminence at the wrist to the base of the thumb (*Arch Neurol* 1988; **45**: 425–7). There is ipsilateral contraction of the orbicularis oris and mentalis muscles. The corner of the mouth elevates slightly and the skin over the chin wrinkles.
- *Sucking reflex*: elicited by tapping or lightly touching the lips with a tongue blade or the examiner's finger. Sucking movements of the lips occur when they are stroked or touched.

Note. The above three reflexes are normal in infants, may be present in normal individuals and are said to be present in a larger number of patients with neurological disease. They are most often seen in those with diffuse cerebral conditions that affect the frontal lobes and pyramidal tracts. The occurrence of more than one reflex is more suggestive of disease than normality.

- *Grasp reflex*: obtained when the examiner's hand is gently inserted into the palm of the patient's hand (when the patient is distracted, usually by engaging him in conversation). With a positive response the patient grasps the examiner's hand and continues to grasp it as it is moved. The presence of the grasp reflex indicates disease of the supplementary motor area of the frontal cortex.
- *Jaw jerk* (see p. 108).

DIAGNOSIS

This patient has expressive dysphasia (lesion) due to a stroke (aetiology) and is unable to express himself (functional status).

Read review on aphasia: *N Engl J Med* 1992; **326:** 531–9.

QUESTIONS

What do you understand by the term 'dysphasia'?

Dysphasia is a disorder of the content of speech and usually follows a lesion of the dominant cortex:

- When the *speech defect* is expressive dysphasia or nominal dysphasia or motor dysphasia, the *site of the lesion in the cortex* is the posterior inferior part of the dominant frontal lobe, i.e. *Broca's area.*
- When the *speech defect* is sensory dysphasia or receptive dysphasia, the *site of the lesion* is the superior temporal lobe or *Wernicke's area.*

What do you understand by the term 'dysarthria'?

Dysarthria is an inability to articulate properly because of local lesions in the mouth or disorders of speech muscles or their connections. There is no disorder of the content of speech. The causes of dysarthria are:

- Stutter.
- Paralysis of cranial nerves – Bell's palsy, ninth, tenth and eleventh nerves.
- Cerebellar disease – staccato, scanning speech.
- Parkinson's speech – slow, quiet, slurred, monotonous.
- Pseudobulbar palsy – monotonous, high-pitched 'hot potato' speech.
- Progressive bulbar palsy – nasal.

ADVANCED-LEVEL QUESTIONS

What are the components of speech?

- Phonation: abnormality is called dysphonia.
- Articulation: abnormality is called dysarthria.
- Language: abnormality is called dysphasia.

What are the other dominant hemisphere functions?
- Right–left orientation.
- Finger identification.
- Calculation.

What are the non-dominant hemisphere functions?
- Drawing ability.
- Topographic ability.
- Construction.
- Dressing.
- Facial recognition.
- Awareness of body and space.
- Motor persistence.

What are the parietal lobe signs?
- Loss of accurate localization of touch, position, joint sense and temperature appreciation.
- Loss of two-point discrimination.
- Astereognosis.
- Dysgraphaesthesia.
- Sensory inattention.
- Attention hemianopia, homonymous hemianopia, or lower quadrantic hemianopia.

What do you understand by the term 'agnosia'?
Agnosia is a failure to recognize objects despite the fact that the sensory pathways for sight, sound or touch are intact. This is tested by asking the patient to feel, name and describe the use of certain objects.

What are the different types of agnosia?
Different types of agnosia include:

- Tactile agnosia and astereognosis: where the patient is unable to recognize objects placed in his hands despite the fact that the sensory system of the hands and fingers is intact and there is adequate motor function to allow him to examine the object. The lesion is in the parietal lobe.
- Prosopagnosia: inability to recognize a familiar face. The lesion is in the parieto-occipital lobe.
- Visual agnosia: inability to recognize objects despite the fact that the main visual pathways to the occipital cortex are preserved. The lesion is in the parieto-occipital lobe.
- Anosognosia: the lack of awareness or realization that the limbs are paralysed, weak or have impaired sensation. The lesion is usually in the non-dominant parietal lobe.

What do you understand by the term 'apraxia'?
Apraxia is the inability to perform purposeful volitional movements in the absence of motor weakness, sensory deficits or severe incoordination. Usually the defect is in the dominant parietal lobe, with disruption of connections to the motor cortex and to the opposite hemisphere.

What are the different types of apraxia?
Different types of apraxia include:

- Dressing apraxias: the patient is unable to put on his clothes correctly.
- Gait apraxia: difficulty in walking, although patients may show intact leg movements when examined in bed.
- Ideomotor apraxia: patients are unable to perform movements on command, although they may do this automatically, e.g. lick their lips.
- Ideational apraxias: difficulty in carrying out a complex series of movements, e.g. to take a match from a box to light a cigarette.
- Constructional apraxia: the patient has difficulty in arranging patterns of blocks or copying designs.

What do you know about dyslexia?

Reading difficulties, including dyslexia, occur as a part of a continuum that also includes normal reading ability. It is not an all-or-none phenomenon but, like hypertension, occurs in degrees. It has been defined as a disorder that is manifested by difficulty in learning to read despite conventional instruction, adequate intelligence and sociocultural opportunity.

> Sir Charles Sherrington (1857–1952), Oxford University, and Lord Edgar Douglas Adrian (1889–1977), Cambridge University, were awarded the Nobel Prize in 1932 for their discoveries regarding the functions of neurons.

Case 49

EXPRESSIVE DYSPHASIA

INSTRUCTION

Ask this patient a few questions.

SALIENT FEATURES

History

See Case 48 (pp 147–8).

Examination

Patient has difficulty in finding the appropriate words, comprehension is intact and repetition may or may not be intact.

Proceed as follows:

Tell the examiner that you would like to carry out a neurological examination of the patient for a right-sided stroke.

DIAGNOSIS

This patient has expressive dysphasia (lesion) due to a right-sided stroke (aetiology).

QUESTIONS

Where is the lesion?

In Broca's area, which is located in the posterior portion of the third left frontal gyrus. It is the motor association cortex for face, tongue, lips and palate. It contains the motor patterns necessary to produce speech.

How would you manage this patient?

• CT head scan to localize the affected area.
• Aspirin.
• Referral to the speech therapist.
• General rehabilitation of a patient with stroke.

Pierre Paul Broca (1824–1880) was Professor of Surgery in Paris. His notable achievements were in anthropology and his suggestion of cerebral localization of speech was first made at a French Anthropological Society meeting in 1861. He is reported to have described muscular dystrophy (before Duchenne), venous spread of cancer (before Rokitansky) and rickets as a nutritional disorder (before Virchow).

Case 50

CEREBELLAR DYSARTHRIA

INSTRUCTION

Ask this patient a few questions.

SALIENT FEATURES

History

See Case 48 (pp 147–8).

Examination

• The speech may be scanning (enunciation is difficult, words are produced slowly and in a measured fashion) or staccato (in bursts). Scanning speech is more common in multiple sclerosis, whereas staccato speech is more common in Friedreich's ataxia.
• Articulation is uneven, words are slurred and variations in pitch and loudness occur.

Proceed as follows:

Tell the examiner that you would like to carry out a neurological examination of the patient for cerebellar signs.

See *Cerebellar syndrome* (pp 143–5) for discussion.

DIAGNOSIS

This patient has scanning speech (lesion) due to cerebellar involvement secondary to chronic alcohol abuse (aetiology).

QUESTIONS

What do you understand by the term 'dysarthria'?

Dysarthria is impaired articulation of speech. It may result from lesions of muscles, myoneural junctions or motor neurons of lips, tongue, palate and pharynx. Common causes include mechanical defects such as ill-fitting dentures or cleft palate. Dysarthria may also result from impaired hearing which begins in early childhood.

ADVANCED-LEVEL QUESTIONS

How would you test the different structures responsible for articulation?

- Lips: ask the patient to say, 'me, me, me'.
- Tongue: ask the patient to say, 'la, la, la'.
- Pharynx: ask the patient to say, 'kuh, gut'.
- Palate, larynx and expiratory muscles: ask the patient to say, 'ah'. In palatal paralysis the patient's speech is worse when the head is bent forwards.

Articulation can also be tested by asking the patient to repeat the following:

- British constitution.
- Hippopotamus.
- Methodist Episcopal.
- Constantinople is the capital of Turkey.

Case 51

THIRD CRANIAL NERVE PALSY

INSTRUCTION

Examine this patient's eyes.

SALIENT FEATURES

History

- Diplopia in all directions except on lateral gaze to the side of the third nerve lesion (because the lateral rectus muscle supplied by the sixth cranial nerve is intact).
- Painful onset (berry aneurysm or aneurysmal dilatation of the intracavernous part of the carotid artery causing third nerve palsy).
- Headaches (migraine, cranial arteritis).
- Obtain history of diabetes or hypertension.

Examination

- Unilateral ptosis (from paralysis of the levator palpebrae superioris).
- Dilated pupil reacting slowly or incompletely to light (paralysis of the constrictor of the pupil).
- Paralysis of accommodation (from involvement of ciliary muscle).
- Squint and diplopia resulting from weakness of muscles supplied by the third cranial nerve (superior, inferior, medial recti and inferior oblique). The eye will be in the position of abduction, i.e. down and out (if the fourth and sixth nerves are intact).
- Diplopia may not be obvious until the affected eyelid is elevated manually.

Proceed as follows:

- Exclude associated fourth cranial nerve lesion (supplies the superior oblique) by tilting the head of the patient to the same side – the affected eye will intort if the fourth cranial nerve is intact. Remember, superior oblique **in**torts the eye (SIN); inferior oblique externally rotates the eye.
- Tell the examiner that you would like to check:
  - The urine for sugar (diabetes mellitus).
  - The blood pressure (hypertension).

Note. Vascular lesions (such as those associated with diabetes and arteritis) which infarct the third nerve may produce a complete oculomotor palsy with pupillary sparing. The pupillomotor fibres are around the periphery of the third nerve. Compression of the mass or aneurysm often involves the pupil.

DIAGNOSIS

This patient has a R/L third nerve palsy (lesion) due to diabetes mellitus (aetiology).

QUESTIONS

What are the common causes of a third nerve palsy?

- Hypertension and diabetes are the most common causes of pupil-sparing third nerve palsy. (**Note.** The presence of pain is not a good discriminating feature between diabetes and aneurysm, as pain is present in both.) Diabetic third nerve palsy usually recovers within 3 months.
- Multiple sclerosis.
- Aneurysms of posterior communicating artery (painful ophthalmoplegia).
- Trauma.
- Tumours, collagen, vascular disorder, syphilis.
- Ophthalmoplegic migraine.
- Encephalitis.
- Parasellar neoplasms.
- Meningioma at the wing of sphenoid.
- Basal meningitis.
- Carcinoma at the base of the skull.

How would you investigate such a patient?

- Test blood pressure and urine for sugar.

- ESR to exclude temporal arteritis (in the elderly).
- Edrophonium test to exclude myasthenia if the pupil is not involved.
- Thyroid function tests and orbital ultrasonography to exclude thyroid disease.
- CT scan of the head.
- Arteriography, especially when the pupil is involved and there is severe pain.

ADVANCED-LEVEL QUESTIONS

When would you suspect a lesion of the third nerve nucleus?
In the following instances:

- Unilateral third nerve palsy with contralateral superior rectus palsy and bilateral partial ptosis.
- Bilateral third nerve palsy (with or without internal ophthalmoplegia associated with spared levator function).

What do you know about the muscles of extraocular movement?
Each eye is moved by three pairs of muscles, and the precise action of these muscles depends on the position of the eye; the actions are as follows:

- Medial and lateral recti (first pair of muscles): adduct and abduct the eye respectively.
- Superior and inferior recti: elevate and depress the abducted eye.
- Superior and inferior obliques: depress and elevate the adducted eye.

Note. Superior and inferior recti act in the abducted position (mnemonic RAB).

Do you know of any eponymous syndromes in which the third cranial nerve is involved?

- Weber's syndrome: ipsilateral third nerve palsy with contralateral hemiplegia. The lesion is in the midbrain.
- Benedikt's syndrome: ipsilateral third nerve palsy with contralateral involuntary movements such as tremor, chorea and athetosis. It is due to a lesion of the red nucleus in the midbrain.
- Claude's syndrome: ipsilateral oculomotor paresis with contralateral ataxia and tremor. It is due to a lesion of the third nerve and red nucleus.
- Nothnagel's syndrome: unilateral oculomotor paralysis combined with ipsilateral cerebellar ataxia.

M. Benedikt (1835–1920), an Austrian physician, described this syndrome in 1889.

Sir H.D. Weber (1823–1918) qualified in Bonn and worked at Guy's Hospital, London.

Henri Claude (1869–1945), a French psychiatrist.

Carl Wilhelm Nothnagel (1841–1905), an Austrian physician.

Case 52

SIXTH CRANIAL NERVE PALSY

INSTRUCTION

Examine this patient's eyes.

SALIENT FEATURES

History

- Diplopia in all directions of gaze except away from the affected side.
- Patient may rotate the head towards the weak side to produce a single image.
- Patient may intentionally close the affected eye to prevent diplopia (pseudoptosis).
- Hearing loss (acoustic neuroma).
- Diabetes or hypertension.

Examination

- The eye is deviated medially and there is failure of lateral movement.
- The diplopia is maximal when looking towards the affected side. The two images are parallel and separated in the horizontal plane. The outer image comes from the affected eye and disappears when the eye is covered.

Proceed as follows:
Tell the examiner that you would like to check the following:

- Blood pressure and urine sugar.
- Hearing and corneal sensation (early signs of acoustic neuroma).

DIAGNOSIS

This patient has a sixth nerve palsy (lesion) due to diabetes mellitus (aetiology) and is experiencing severe diplopia (functional status).

QUESTIONS

What are the causes of sixth nerve palsy?
- Hypertension.
- Diabetes.
- Raised intracranial pressure (false localizing signs).
- Multiple sclerosis.
- Basal meningitis.
- Encephalitis.
- Acoustic neuroma, nasopharyngeal carcinoma.

ADVANCED-LEVEL QUESTIONS

Where is the nucleus of the sixth nerve located?

In the pons. (**Note.** The nuclei of the first four cranial nerves are situated above the pons and those of the last four cranial nerves are situated below the pons.)

What are the structures in close proximity to the sixth nerve nucleus and fascicles?

These include:

- Facial and trigeminal nerves.
- Corticospinal tract.
- Median longitudinal fasciculus.
- Parapontine reticular formation.

A combination of clinical findings pointing to the involvement of these structures indicates the presence of an intrapontine lesion.

What do you know about the peripheral course of the abducens nerve?

It is a lengthy one from the brainstem and base of the skull, through the petrous tip and cavernous sinus, to the superior orbital fissure and orbit. Lesions at any of these sites may affect the nerve.

Have you heard of Gradenigo's syndrome?

Inflammation of the tip of the temporal bone may involve the fifth and sixth cranial nerves as well as the greater superficial petrosal nerve, resulting in unilateral paralysis of the lateral rectus nerve, pain in the distribution of the trigeminal nerve (particularly its first division) and excessive lacrimation.

Do you know of any eponymous syndromes in which the pons is infarcted and consequently the sixth cranial nerve is involved?

- Raymond's syndrome: ipsilateral sixth nerve paralysis and contralateral paresis of the extremities.
- Millard–Gubler syndrome, in which there is ipsilateral sixth and seventh nerve palsy with contralateral hemiplegia.
- Foville's syndrome has all the features of Millard–Gubler paralysis with lateral conjugate gaze palsy.

Mention other syndromes with sixth nerve involvement.

- Duane's syndrome: widening of the palpebral fissure on abduction and narrowing on adduction.
- Gerhardt's syndrome: bilateral abducens palsy.
- Möbius syndrome: paralysis of extraocular muscles, especially abducens, with paresis of facial muscles.

What do you know about Tolosa–Hunt syndrome?

It is a syndrome characterized by unilateral recurrent pain in the retro-orbital region with palsy of the extraocular muscles resulting from involvement of the third, fourth, fifth and sixth cranial nerves. It has been attributed to inflammation of the cavernous sinus.

C. Gradenigo (1859–1926), an Italian otolaryngologist, described this syndrome in 1904.

E. Tolosa, a Spanish neurosurgeon.

W.E. Hunt, an American neurosurgeon.

A.L.J. Millard (1830–1915), a French physician.

A.M. Gubler (1821–1915), Professor of Therapeutics in France.

A.L.F. Foville (1799–1878), Professor of Physiology at Rouen, described his syndrome in 1848.

Case 53

SEVENTH CRANIAL NERVE PALSY – LOWER MOTOR NEURON TYPE

INSTRUCTION

Look at this patient's face.
Examine the cranial nerves.

SALIENT FEATURES

History

- Onset: whether abrupt followed by worsening over the following day (Bell's palsy).
- Pain preceding or accompanying the weakness (Bell's palsy).
- The face itself feels stiff and pulled to one side.
- Ipsilateral restriction of eye closure.
- Difficulty with eating.
- Disturbance of taste (due to chorda tympani fibres).
- Hyperacusis (involvement of stapedius muscle in the inner ear).

Examination

- Weakness of muscles of one half of the face – patient is unable to screw her eyes tightly shut or move the angle of the mouth on the affected side.
- Loss of facial expression.
- Widened palpebral fissure.

Proceed as follows:
- Look for the following when the patient is unaware of being observed:
  – Flatter nasolabial folds on the affected side.
  – Mouth on the affected side droops and participates manifestly less while talking.
  – The eyelid on the affected side closes just after the opposite eyelid.
- Look at the external auditory meatus for herpes zoster (Ramsay Hunt syndrome).
- Look for parotid gland enlargement.
- Examine for taste (loss of taste with the involvement of chorda tympani).
- Check for hearing (for hyperacusis resulting from involvement of the nerve to stapedius muscle).

- Examine the tympanic membrane for otitis media.
- Tell the examiner that you would like to do the following:
  – Test the urine for sugar (diabetes).

DIAGNOSIS

The patient has lower motor neuron seventh cranial nerve palsy (lesion) which is idiopathic (aetiology). She is distressed because the condition causes severe disfigurement while talking (functional status).

QUESTIONS

How would you differentiate between upper and lower motor neuron palsy?

In lower motor neuron palsy the whole half of the face on the affected side is involved. In upper motor neuron palsy the upper half of the face (the forehead) is spared.

ADVANCED-LEVEL QUESTIONS

What are the causes of bilateral facial nerve palsy?

- Guillain–Barré syndrome (see pp 243–4).
- Sarcoidosis in the form of uveoparotid fever (Heerfordt's disease).
- Melkersson–Rosenthal syndrome, which is a triad of facial palsy, recurrent facial oedema and plication of the tongue (*Hygiea* (Stockholm) 1928; **90:** 737–41; *Z Neurol Psychiatr* 1931; **131:** 475–501).

Note. Myasthenia may mimic bilateral facial nerve palsy.

What are the causes of unilateral facial nerve palsy?

Lower motor neuron (all the muscles of one half of the face are affected):

- Bell's palsy (idiopathic). Recent studies using a polymerase chain reaction have implicated herpes simplex viral infection in Bell's palsy. The incidence of Bell's palsy is 23 per 100 000 individuals per year or about 1 in 60–70 individuals per year. Men and women are equally affected and the peak incidence is between the ages of 10 and 40. Both the right and left sides are affected with equal frequency.
- Herpes zoster.
- Cerebellopontine angle tumours.
- Parotid tumours.
- Old polio.
- Otitis media.
- Skull fracture.

Upper motor neuron (forehead spared):

- Stroke (hemiplegia).

Is the facial nerve a motor nerve or a sensory nerve?

The facial nerve is predominantly a motor nerve and supplies all muscles concerned with facial expression and the stapedius muscle. Uncommonly, it may have a sensory component which is small – the nervus intermedius of Wrisberg. It conveys taste sensation from the anterior two thirds of the tongue and, probably, cutaneous impulses from the anterior wall of the external auditory canal.

What do you know of nervus intermedius?

The nervus intermedius or pars intermedia of Wrisberg is the sensory or the parasympathetic root of the facial nerve, and is lateral and inferior to the motor root. Inside the internal auditory meatus it lies between the motor root and the eighth cranial nerve. The sensory cells are located in the geniculate ganglion (at the bend of the facial nerve in the facial canal) and their nerve fibres enter the pons with the motor root. The geniculate ganglion is continued distally as the chorda tympani, which carries taste and preganglionic parasympathetic fibres. This nerve consists of contributions from three areas:

- Superior salivary nucleus (in the pons) supplies secretory fibres to the glands.
- Gustatory or solitary nucleus (in the medulla) receives taste fibres via the chorda tympani.
- Dorsal part of the trigeminal nerve receives cutaneous sensation from the external auditory meatus and the skin behind the ear (distributed with the facial nerve proper).

How would you manage Bell's palsy?

About 50–60% of patients recover spontaneously without deficits, others have considerable improvement and about 10% have permanent residual deficits. Therefore many physicians tend to initiate treatment with steroids only in those with clinically complete deficit or when there is severe pain. Treatment includes:

- Physiotherapy: massage, electrical stimulation, splint to prevent drooping of the lower part of the face.
- Protection of the eye with lubricating eye drops and a patch during sleep.
- A short course of dexamethasone 2 mg three times a day for 5 days and tapered over the next 5 days (should be given within 48 hours of onset).
- Aciclovir–prednisone is more effective in improving volitional muscle activity and in preventing partial nerve degeneration as compared to placebo–prednisone treatment (*Ann Otol Rhinol Laryngol* 1996; **105:** 371).

What are the branches of the facial nerve?

- Greater superficial petrosal nerve (supplies lacrimal, nasal and palatine glands).
- Nerve to stapedius muscle.
- Chorda tympani (supplies taste to anterior two thirds of tongue, submaxillary and sublingual glands).
- Motor branches (exit from the stylomastoid foramen).

How would you localize facial nerve palsy?

- Involvement of the nuclei in the pons – associated ipsilateral sixth nerve palsy.
- Cerebellopontine angle lesion – associated fifth and eighth nerve involvement.
- Lesion in the bony canal – loss of taste (carried by the lingual nerve) and hyperacusis (due to involvement of the nerve to stapedius).

Mention reflexes involving the facial nerve.

- Corneal reflex (see p. 108).
- Palmomental reflex (see p. 148).
- Suck reflex.

- Snout reflex (see p. 148).
- Orbicularis oculi reflex or glabellar reflex (see p. 137).
- Palpebral–oculogyric reflex.
- Orbicularis oris reflex.

Mention a few examples of facial synkinesis.

Facial synkinesis means that attempts to move one group of facial muscles result in contraction of associated muscles. It may be seen during anomalous regeneration of the facial nerve. For example:

- If fibres originally connected with muscles of the face later innervate the lacrimal gland, anomalous secretion of tears (crocodile tears) may occur while eating.
- If fibres originally connected with the orbicularis oculi innervate the orbicularis oris, closure of the eyelids causes retraction of the mouth.
- Opening of the jaw may cause closure of the eyelids on the corresponding side (jaw-winking).

Have you heard of Möbius' syndrome?

Congenital facial diplegia, congenital oculofacial paralysis and infantile nuclear aplasia. It consists of congenital bilateral facial palsy associated with third and sixth nerve palsies.

What is the relationship between diabetes and Bell's palsy?

Diabetes is said to be an important cause in about 10% of cases of Bell's palsy. In one study Bell's palsy was associated with abnormal glucose tolerance in two thirds of patients (*Lancet* 1971; **i:** 108; *Arch Otolaryngol* 1974; **99:** 114).

> Sir Charles Bell (1774–1842) was Professor of Surgery in Edinburgh and a founder member of the Middlesex Hospital in London. He discovered that the anterior and posterior spinal nerve roots were motor and sensory respectively.
>
> James Ramsay Hunt (1874–1937), Professor of Neurology in New York.
>
> P.J. Möbius (1853–1907), a German neurologist.

Case 54

TREMORS

INSTRUCTION

Look at this patient's hands.
Demonstrate tremors.

SALIENT FEATURES

Patient 1

- Coarse resting tremor which is slow (4–6 per second).

- Adduction–abduction of the thumb with flexion–extension of fingers (pill-rolling movement).
- The tremor is halted by purposive movements of the hands. The upper limb tremor often increases as the patient walks.

Proceed as follows:
Tell the examiner that you would like to do the following:

- Look for cog-wheel rigidity.
- Comment on mask-like facies.
- Check gait for festinant gait.
- Ask the patient's relatives whether sleep relieves the tremor and whether emotion makes it worse.

Diagnosis
This patient with resting tremor and mask-like facies (lesion) has Parkinson's disease (aetiology) and is severely disabled by the tremor (functional status).

Patient 2

There is a 10-second physiological tremor which is brought on when the arms are outstretched. It can be amplified by laying a sheet of paper on the hands.

Proceed as follows:
Tell the examiner that you would like to do the following:

- Check for thyrotoxicosis.
- Take a history for alcoholism.
- Take a drug history (salbutamol, terbutaline, lithium).
- Occupational history to mercury ('hatter's shakes').
- Know whether tremor runs in the family and is relieved by alcohol (benign essential tremor).

Diagnosis
This patient has fine tremor with an enlarged thyroid gland (lesion), which could be due to hyperthyroidism (aetiology).

Patient 3

The patient does not have a resting tremor or a tremor with outstretched hands.

Proceed as follows:
- Check for past-pointing – the intention tremor of cerebellar disease.
- Tell the examiner that you would like to check for other cerebellar signs (see p. 144).

Diagnosis
This patient has an intention tremor (lesion) due to cerebellar syndrome (aetiology).

Patient 4

- Unsteadiness when standing still; by contrast patient has little or no difficulty while walking, which relieves the symptoms.
- Fine rippling of the muscles of the legs may be seen or felt when the patient attempts to stand still; after a short interval the patient becomes increasingly unsteady and is forced to take a step to regain balance.

Diagnosis
This patient has primary orthostatic tremor (lesion).
    Read this review on tremors: *Med Clin North Am* 1972; **56:** 1363–75.

QUESTIONS

What are the tremors?
Involuntary movements that result from alternating contraction and relaxation of groups of muscles, producing rhythmic oscillations about a joint or a group of joints.

How would you classify tremors?
* Resting tremor, as in Parkinson's disease.
* Postural tremor (brought on when the arms are outstretched) due to the following:
  – exaggerated physiological tremor, caused by anxiety, thyrotoxicosis, alcohol, drugs
  – brain damage seen in Wilson's disease, syphilis.
* Intention tremor (aggravated by voluntary movements) in cerebellar disease.
* Tremor due to neuropathy (postural tremor; arms more than legs).

Mention a few involuntary movements.
* Chorea.
* Athetosis.
* Hemiballismus.
* Fasciculation.
* Torticollis.
* Clonus.

What are the causes of drug-associated tremors?
* Drug-induced tremors: beta-2 agonists (e.g. salbutamol), caffeine, theophylline, lithium, tricyclic antidepressants, 5-HT reuptake inhibitors, neuroleptics, sodium valproate, corticosteroids.
* Tremors associated with drug withdrawal: alcohol (delirium tremens), benzodiazepines, barbiturates, opiates.

ADVANCED-LEVEL QUESTIONS

What do you know about the investigation and management of primary orthostatic tremor?
In primary orthostatic tremor:

* EMG shows rhythmic activation of lower limb muscles at a frequency of 4–18 Hz.
* Positron emission tomography shows increased activity in the cerebellum.
* Treatment is supportive; the patient is often relieved to know the diagnosis, especially when a psychiatric cause has been suspected previously.

What is the treatment for tremor?
* Tremor due to Parkinson's disease: Levodopa, anticholinergic agents, dopamine agonists, or budipine. When all other types of medication are not effective,

clozapine is often beneficial. More than 50% of patients respond to this treatment (*N Engl J Med* 2000; **342:** 505).

- Essential tremor: Beta-blockers, primidone or both; 40–70% of these patients have some improvement with this treatment.
- Cerebellar tremor: No standard treatment; clonazepam is sometimes effective, as is treatment with levodopa, anticholinergic agents or clozapine.
- Drug-resistant tremor: Thalamic stimulation (continuous deep-brain stimulation) and thalamotomy are equally effective, but thalamic stimulation has fewer adverse effects and results in a greater improvement of function (*N Engl J Med* 2000; **342:** 461–8).

Mercury poisoning was known as 'hatter's shakes' because workers involved in the manufacture of felt hats were exposed to mercury.

Case 55

PERIPHERAL NEUROPATHY

INSTRUCTION

Examine this patient's legs.
Carry out a neurological examination of this patient's legs.

SALIENT FEATURES

History

- Progressive and symmetrical numbness in the hands and feet which spreads proximally in a glove and stocking distribution.
- Distal weakness, which also ascends.
- History of diabetes, alcohol, connective tissue disorder, malignancy.

Examination

Bilateral symmetrical sensory loss for all modalities with or without motor weakness.

Proceed as follows:
- Look for evidence of the following:
  - **D**iabetes mellitus (diabetic chart, insulin injection sites, insulin pump).
  - **A**lcoholic liver disease (palmar erythema, spider naevi, tender liver).
  - **D**rug history.
  - **R**heumatoid arthritis.
  - **U**raemia.
  - **M**alignancy. (Mnemonic: **DAD, RUM**).
- Palpate for thickened nerves and look for Charcot's joints.

- Tell the examiner that you would like to do the following:
  - Look for anaemia and jaundice (vitamin B_{12} deficiency).
  - Check urine for sugar.
  - Take a history of alcohol consumption and a drug history.

DIAGNOSIS

This patient has symmetrical, bilateral sensory loss for touch and pain (lesion) due to diabetes mellitus (aetiology).

QUESTIONS

Mention a few causes of thickened nerves.
- Amyloidosis.
- Charcot–Marie–Tooth disease.
- Leprosy.
- Refsum's disease (retinitis pigmentosa, deafness and cerebellar damage).
- Déjérine–Sottas disease (hypertrophic peripheral neuropathy).

What are the causes of motor neuropathy?
- Guillain–Barré syndrome.
- Peroneal muscular atrophy.
- Lead toxicity.
- Porphyria.
- Dapsone toxicity.
- Organophosphorous poisoning.

What are the causes of mononeuritis multiplex?
Mononeuritis multiplex is a neuropathy affecting several nerves; causes include:

- **W**egener's granulomatosis.
- **A**myloidosis.
- **R**heumatoid arthritis.
- **D**iabetes mellitus.
- **S**LE.
- **P**olyarteritis nodosa.
- **L**eprosy.
- **C**arcinomatosis, Churg–Strauss syndrome. (Mnemonic: **WARDS, PLC**).

Mention a few causes of predominantly sensory neuropathy.
- Diabetes mellitus.
- Alcoholism.
- Deficiency of vitamins B_{12} and B_1.
- Chronic renal failure.
- Leprosy.

What are the types of neuropathy described in diabetes mellitus?
- Symmetrical, mainly sensory, polyneuropathy.
- Asymmetrical, mainly motor, polyneuropathy (diabetic amyotrophy).
- Mononeuropathy.
- Autonomic neuropathy.

What drugs are used for painful peripheral neuropathy of diabetes?
Tricyclic antidepressants, phenytoin, carbamazepine and topical capsaicin.

ADVANCED-LEVEL QUESTIONS

What are the other effects of alcohol on the central nervous system?
- Wernicke's encephalopathy (ophthalmoplegia, nystagmus, confusion and neuropathy).
- Korsakoff's psychosis (recent memory loss and confabulation).
- Cerebellar degeneration.
- Marchiafava–Bignami disease (symmetrical demyelination of corpus callosum).
- Central pontine myelinolysis.
- Amblyopia.
- Epilepsy.
- Myopathy and rhabdomyolysis.

K. Wernicke (1848–1904) worked in Poland.

S.S. Korsakoff (1853–1900), a Russian neuropsychiatrist.

J. Churg (b. 1910) qualified in Poland and was Professor of Pathology in New York.

L. Strauss, a pathologist in New York.

Case 56

CHARCOT–MARIE–TOOTH DISEASE (PERONEAL MUSCULAR ATROPHY)

INSTRUCTION

Examine this patient's legs.

SALIENT FEATURES

History
- See Case 55 (p. 164).
- Ask about a family history of similar weakness.

Examination
- Wasting of muscles of calves and thighs which stops abruptly, usually in the lower third of the thigh, and is described as 'stork' or 'spindle' legs, 'fat bottle' calves and 'inverted champagne bottles'.
- Pes cavus, clawing of toes, contractures of the Achilles tendon.
- Weakness of dorsiflexion.
- Absent ankle jerks, plantars are downgoing or equivocal.
- Mild sensory impairment or no sensory loss. Some patients have decreased responses to pain in the stocking distribution.

Proceed as follows:
- Feel for lateral popliteal nerve thickening (seen in some cases only).
- Look at the hands for small muscle wasting and clawing.
- Tell the examiner that you would like to: + hx of associated pain
  - Know whether there is a family history of disease.
  - Look for enlarged greater auricular nerves.
  - Examine the spine for scoliosis.
  - Examine the gait (high-stepping gait of foot-drop).

Note. There are two distinctive clinical features of this disease:

1. The muscular atrophy begins in the distal portions of the affected muscles in the lower and upper limbs, unlike the global atrophy of motor neuron disease or muscular dystrophy. The atrophy then creeps upwards, involving all muscles.
2. Second, the degree of disability is minimal in spite of marked deformity.

DIAGNOSIS

This patient has 'inverted champagne bottle' legs with sensory neuropathy (lesion) which is due to hereditary Charcot–Marie–Tooth disease (aetiology). She has severe foot-drop and requires calipers (functional status).

ADVANCED-LEVEL QUESTIONS

What is the mode of inheritance?
Both autosomal dominant and recessive inheritances are seen in different families. The responsible gene is usually located on the short arm of chromosome 17 (*Ann Neurol* 1992; **31**: 570; *N Engl J Med* 1993; **329**: 96–101) and less often shows linkage to chromosomes 1 or X. In hereditary motor sensory neuropathy (HMSN) type I with dominant inheritance, the locus is on the long arm of chromosome 1.

What are the three recognized forms?
- HMSN type I – a demyelinating neuropathy (marked slowing of conduction in motor nerves; absent deep tendon reflexes).
- HMSN type II – an axonal neuropathy (little or no slowing of nerve conduction; normal deep tendon reflexes).
- Distal spinal muscular atrophy.

What other uncommon features may these patients have?
Optic atrophy, retinitis pigmentosa, spastic paraparesis.

In which other condition is pes cavus seen?
Friedreich's ataxia.

What is the natural history of the disease?
The disease usually arrests in middle life.

How does the forme fruste of the disease manifest?
The forme fruste may be seen in family members of patients with Charcot–Marie–Tooth disease and manifests as pes cavus and absent ankle jerks.

Mention other hereditary neuropathies.

- Roussy–Lévy syndrome (where features of progressive muscular atrophy may be combined with tremor and ataxia).
- Hereditary amyloidosis.
- Refsum's disease (phytanic acid accumulates in the central and peripheral nervous systems).
- Fabry's disease (where there is a deficiency of α-galactosidase).
- Tangier disease.
- Bassen–Kornzweig disease (abetalipoproteinaemia, absence of low density lipoproteins and vitamin E deficiency).
- Metachromatic leukodystrophy (where galactosyl sulphatide accumulates in the central and peripheral nervous systems).

Mention a few conditions that Charcot is credited with having described for the first time.

- Ankle clonus.
- Tabes dorsalis and Charcot's joints.
- Multiple sclerosis.
- Peroneal muscular atrophy.
- Multiple cerebral aneurysms, called Charcot–Bouchard aneurysms.
- Hysteria.

> The syndrome was originally described by J.M. Charcot (1825–1923) and P. Marie (1853–1940) in 1886 at the Saltpêtrière in Paris, and independently by H.H. Tooth at St Bartholomew's Hospital and the National Hospital for Nervous Diseases, Queen Square, London, at the same time. P. Marie was a world-famed neurologist. He published extensively on aphasia. He succeeded Charcot's lineage of Raymond, Brissaud and Déjérine at the Saltpêtrière in 1918.

Case 57

DYSTROPHIA MYOTONICA

INSTRUCTION

Look at this patient's face.
Examine this patient's cranial nerves.

SALIENT FEATURES

History

- Onset usually in the third and fourth decade. However, if the mother is the carrier then the disease may manifest in infancy and undergo rapid deterioration at the usual age of onset.
- Onset dominated by weakness or myotonia or both.
- Difficulty in releasing grip.

- Leg weakness (difficulty in kicking a ball).
- 'Pseudo-drop attacks' (due to weakness of quadriceps muscle).
- Ask the patient whether or not he has dysphagia (oesophageal involvement).
- Impotence (due to gonadal atrophy).
- Recurrent respiratory infections (due to weakness of muscles of bronchioles).

Examination

- While shaking hands with the patient, note the myotonia.
- Frontal baldness. (**Note.** The patient may be wearing a wig and it is important to mention that he is wearing one.)
- Ptosis (bilateral or unilateral) with a *smooth* forehead.
- Cataracts (posterior capsular cataracts) or evidence of surgery for cataracts.
- Difficulty in opening the eyes after firm closure.
- Expressionless face ('hatchet face') with wasting of temporalis, masseters and *sternomastoids* and 'swan neck' due to thinning of the neck.

Proceed as follows:
- Test:
  – Sternomastoids.
  – Distal muscles of the upper limbs, wasting, percussion myotonia over thenar muscles and weakness.
  – Deep tendon jerks (depressed).
- Tell the examiner that you would like to do the following:
  – Check the urine for sugar (diabetes mellitus).
  – Test higher intellectual function (low IQ).
  – Examine for gynaecomastia and testicular atrophy.

DIAGNOSIS

This patient has frontal balding, myotonia, cataracts and wasting of the sternomastoids (lesion) due to dystrophia myotonica (aetiology). He has dysphagia and severe muscular weakness (functional status).

ADVANCED-LEVEL QUESTIONS

What is the inheritance of this condition?

Autosomal dominant; the gene is located on chromosome 19q13.3. The condition usually presents in the third and fourth decades. The disease tends to be worse in successive generations (known as anticipation). As a result the grandparent may merely have cataracts while the grandchild develops a severe progressive form of the disease. Positional cloning has helped to identify the myotonic dystrophy gene and localized a dynamic mutation with an increase in the number of trinucleotide repeats (AGC repeat). The repeat size typically increases from generation to generation, providing a molecular basis for the clinical phenomenon of anticipation (*Science* 1992; **255**: 1253–5; *Nature* 1992; **355**: 545–6; *N Engl J Med* 1993; **328**: 471).

What are the other features of this condition?

- Cardiomyopathy and cardiac conduction defects.
- Respiratory infection (low serum immunoglobulin G levels).

- Somnolence.
- External ophthalmoplegia (occasionally).

What do you understand by myotonia?

It is continued contraction of the muscle after voluntary contraction ceases, followed by impaired relaxation.

What therapeutic modalities are available?

Procainamide or phenytoin has been used in *disabling* myotonia. No treatment has altered the course of progressive weakness.

What other forms of myotonia do you know?

Myotonia congenita or Oppenheim's disease, an autosomal dominant condition which presents at birth with feeding difficulties. The myotonia improves with age and there is no dystrophy. Although this is considered to be a myopathy, changes have been reported in the motor nuclei of the spinal cord and motor cortex.

In which myopathies is distal weakness prominent?

- Myotonic dystrophy.
- Welander's distal myopathy.

If this patient requires major surgery, what fact would you keep in mind?

Patients with dystrophia myotonica tend to do poorly after the administration of general anaesthetic (due to impaired cardiorespiratory malfunction) and will require intensive postoperative observation.

Mention some causes of bilateral ptosis.

- Myasthenia gravis.
- Congenital muscular dystrophies.
- Ocular myopathy.
- Syphilis.

What is the pathognomonic pattern of cataract in dystrophia myotonica?

Stellate cataract.

The patient's sister is worried about risks to her offspring. What tests would you perform?

- Clinical examination.
- Electromyography (EMG).
- Slit-lamp examination for cataracts.

Is prenatal diagnosis available?

Yes – in some families. The myotonic dystrophy gene is linked to the ABH secretor gene. However, not all families are informative.

What is the characteristic EMG finding?

Waxing and waning of the potentials, known as the dive-bomber effect. EMG changes are found in almost any muscle.

How would you manage such patients?

- Foot-drop is controlled by calipers or moulded-foot orthoses.
- Myotonia, when disabling, may respond to phenytoin (avoid quinidine and procainamide as they can worsen cardiac conduction).

- Advanced heart block with or without syncope should be considered for pacemaker insertion.

Délége, in 1890, first described the association of myotonia with muscular atrophy.

Batten and Gibb (*Brain* 1909; **32**: 187), and Steinert (*Dtsch Z Nervenheilk* 1909; **37**: 58), in 1909 independently described the clinical features of the symptom complex.

Curschmann in 1912 emphasized the dystrophic symptoms and applied the term 'dystrophia myotonica'.

Case 58

PROXIMAL MYOPATHY

INSTRUCTION

Perform a neurological examination of this patient's arms or legs.

SALIENT FEATURES

History
- Weakness of proximal muscles.
- Patient has difficulty in standing from the sitting position (getting up from chairs, getting off the commode) or difficulty in combing her hair – elicit this history.

Examination
- Check the gait, looking for waddling gait (see p. 181).
- Look for an underlying cause:
  - Diabetic amyotrophy (asymmetrical, usually in the lower limbs in non-insulin-dependent diabetes mellitus).
  - Cushing's syndrome (characteristic facies, history of steroid ingestion; see p. 385).
  - Thyrotoxicosis (look for eye signs, goitre, rapid pulse, tremor).
  - Polymyositis (heliotropic rash, tender muscles).
  - Drug history (alcohol, steroids, chloroquine).
  - Carcinomatous neuropathy.
  - Osteomalacia (bone pain).
  - Hereditary muscular dystrophy.

DIAGNOSIS

This patient has weakness of the proximal muscles of the lower limbs (lesion) due to Cushing's syndrome (aetiology) and is severely limited by the weakness (functional status).

QUESTIONS.

What is Gowers' sign?

In severe proximal myopathy of the lower limbs, the patient on rising from the floor uses her hands to climb up herself. It has been classically described in Duchenne muscular dystrophy.

What do you know about diabetic amyotrophy?

It is an asymmetrical motor polyneuropathy which presents with asymmetrical weakness and wasting of the proximal muscles of the lower limbs and sometimes upper limbs, diminished or absent knee jerk and sensory loss in the thigh. It is usually accompanied by severe pain in the thigh, often awakening the patient at night. The prognosis is good and most patients recover over months or years with diabetic control.

ADVANCED-LEVEL QUESTIONS

What is the difference between type 1 and type 2 muscle fibres?

- Type 1 muscle fibres are high in myoglobin and oxidative enzymes and have many mitochondria. They perform tonic contraction and are involved in weight-bearing and movements requiring sustained force. Chloroquine causes vacuolation of myocytes, predominantly type 1 fibres.
- Type 2 muscle fibres are rich in glycolytic enzymes; they perform rapid phasic contractions and are involved in sudden movements and in purposeful motion. In steroid myopathy the muscle fibre atrophy predominantly affects these fibres.

Sir W.R. Gowers (1845–1915), Professor of Medicine at University College Hospital, London, invented a haemoglobinometer, personally illustrated an atlas of ophthalmology, and wrote a book on spinal cord diseases and a manual on the nervous system. He also founded a society of medical stenographers.

Guillaume-Benjamin-Amand Duchenne (1806–1875) was first to describe Duchenne muscular dystrophy in 1868, when he described 13 cases of the disease; by 1870 he had seen about 40 cases.

Case 59

DEFORMITY OF A LOWER LIMB

INSTRUCTION

Examine the lower limbs of this patient who has had this abnormality since childhood.

SALIENT FEATURES

History

- History of trauma to the spine and/or leg.

- History of poliomyelitis.
- History of weakness and fasciculations.
- Bladder and bowel symptoms.

Examination

- Wasting and deformity of one lower limb (or both, with one side being more affected than the other).
- Fasciculations.
- Normal tone in both lower limbs.
- Check the sensory system (L5 and/or S1 sensory loss in spina bifida).
- Examine the spine:
  – Kyphoscoliosis (seen in poliomyelitis, indicating involvement of trunk muscles).
  – Tuft of hair in the lower lumbosacral spine (closed spina bifida).
- Comment on bony deformity in the affected leg.

Note. Always check the gait and test for Romberg's sign.

DIAGNOSIS

This patient has unilateral wasting and deformity of the R/L leg (lesion) due to poliomyelitis in childhood (aetiology) and wears calipers on that leg (functional status).

QUESTIONS

What is the differential diagnosis?
- Old poliomyelitis.
- Spina bifida.

What are the causes of lower motor neuron signs in the legs?
- Peripheral neuropathy.
- Prolapsed intervertebral disc.
- Diabetic amyotrophy.
- Poliomyelitis.
- Cauda equina lesions.
- Motor neuron disease.

ADVANCED-LEVEL QUESTIONS

What is the cause of polio?
Polio is caused by a picornavirus of the genus Enterovirus; there are three antigenic types – type I (Brunhilde), type II (Lansing) and type III (Leon).

Is the muscular involvement of polio in childhood progressive?
Paralytic polio usually remains stable after the initial attack. However, in some patients new muscle weakness and atrophy involving previously affected muscles or even unaffected muscles occurs and this deterioration can occur as long as 30 years after the first attack – known as postpoliomyelitis muscular atrophy (PPMA). The

progression of this involvement is slow and is said to be distinct from motor neuron disease. It is not entirely clear why only some patients are affected but it has been reported that it is more likely to occur in those with widespread paralysis and poor immune status (*N Engl J Med* 1986; **314:** 959).

Is poliomyelitis preventable?

Yes, three types of polio vaccine are available (each containing all three strains of the virus):

* Oral polio vaccine of Sabin consists of live attenuated virus.
* Killed or inactivated vaccine of Salk.
* Enhanced potency vaccine of van Wezel.

With which vaccine is paralytic poliomyelitis associated?

Vaccine-associated paralytic poliomyelitis (VAPP) is associated with oral polio vaccine, particularly in immunodeficient individuals (*N Engl J Med* 1995; **332:** 500–6). Such individuals and their household contacts should be given inactivated vaccine.

What do you know about 'provocation poliomyelitis'?

Provocation poliomyelitis is caused by the administration of intramuscular injections during the incubation period of wild-type poliovirus or shortly after exposure to oral polio vaccine (either as a vaccine recipient or through contact with a recent recipient).

What do you understand by the term 'spina bifida'?

Spina bifida means an incomplete closure of the bony vertebral canal and is commonly associated with a similar anomaly of the spinal cord. The commonest site is the lumbosacral region but the cervical spine can be involved. It may be associated with hydrocephalus.

What are the features of closed spina bifida?

* Cutaneous: lumbosacral lipoma, hypertrichosis, sinus or dimple above the sacrum, naevus or scarring.
* Unilateral shortening of one leg and foot with a deficiency of the muscles below the knee. There may be calcaneovalgus or equinovarus deformity. Sensory loss in the fifth lumbar and first sacral dermatome is common.
* Neuropathic bladder, enuresis.
* Bony changes on radiography: sacral dysgenesis, scoliosis, laminar fusion of vertebral body, pedicle erosion and bony spurs.

Is the neurological deficit in closed spina bifida progressive?

This issue is contentious as much of the deficit is fixed antenatally and any progression occurs as a result of growth and posture. In some patients, however, the late appearance of bladder dysfunction indicates that the neurological deficit is progressive in these individuals.

Mention some teratogenic factors responsible for neural canal defects.

* Maternal diabetes and sacral dysgenesis.
* Sodium valproate in pregnancy and neural tube defects (*Lancet* 1982; **ii:** 1282).

Mention some prenatal screening tests for spina bifida.
- Amniotic α-fetoprotein levels.
- Amniotic acetylcholinesterase estimation.
- High-resolution diagnostic ultrasonography.

M.H. Romberg (1795–1873), German neurologist and Professor of Medicine in Berlin.

The 1952 Nobel Prize was jointly awarded to John F. Enders (1897–1985), Thomas H. Weller (1915–) both of Children's Medical Center and Harvard Medical School, Boston, and Frederick C. Robbins (1916–) of Western Reserve University, Cleveland, Ohio, for their discovery of the ability of poliomyelitis viruses to grow in cultures of various types of tissue.

Case 60

MULTIPLE SCLEROSIS

PATIENT 1

Instruction

Examine this patient's eyes.

Salient features

History
Remissions and relapses: visual loss, diplopia.

Examination
- Optic atrophy.
- Nystagmus.
- Internuclear ophthalmoplegia.
- Look for features of cerebellar syndrome (see pp 143–4).

Proceed as follows:
Tell the examiner that you would like to do a full neurological examination.

PATIENT 2

Instruction

Examine this patient's legs.

Salient features

History
Remissions and relapses: weakness, incoordination, pain, paraesthesias, urinary urgency, impotence. Steinberg's triad is history of incontinence of bladder, impotence and constipation.

Examination

- Spastic paraparesis (increased tone, upgoing plantars, weakness, brisk reflexes and ankle or patellar clonus). Spasticity is quantified using the Ashworth Scale, which scores muscle tone on a scale of 0–4 with 0 representing normal tone and 4 severe spasticity.
- Impaired coordination on heel–shin test (if there is marked weakness, this test may be unreliable).

Proceed as follows:

- Check abdominal reflexes (absent or diminished in over 80% of cases).
- Tell the examiner that you would like to do the following:
  - Look for optic atrophy and cerebellar signs.

In such patients, remember that spinal cord compression should be ruled out before making a diagnosis of multiple sclerosis.

Some examiners may consider it insensitive to use the term 'multiple sclerosis' in front of the patient and may prefer that the candidate uses the term 'demyelinating disorder' instead.

DIAGNOSIS

This patient has optic atrophy and spastic paraparesis (lesion) due to multiple sclerosis, and is wheelchair bound (functional status).

QUESTIONS

What investigations would you consider?

- Spinal radiography, including both cervical and thoracic regions.
- Lumbar puncture: total protein concentration may be raised (in 60% of cases), with an increase in the level of immunoglobulin G (in 40%) and oligoclonal bands (in 80%) on electrophoresis.
- Visual evoked potentials: despite normal visual function there may be prolonged latency in cortical response to a pattern stimulus. This indicates a delay in conduction in the visual pathways.
- MRI scan of the brain: about 50% of patients with early multiple sclerosis in the spinal cord show abnormal areas in the periventricular white matter.
- Serum vitamin B_{12} – to exclude subacute degeneration of the spinal cord.

Mention a few causes of bilateral pyramidal lesions affecting the lower limbs.

- Cord compression.
- Multiple sclerosis.
- Cervical spondylosis.
- Transverse myelitis.
- Motor neuron disease.
- Vitamin B_{12} deficiency.
- Cerebrovascular disease.

ADVANCED-LEVEL QUESTIONS

How common is multiple sclerosis?
The prevalence is about 1 in 800 people, with an annual incidence of 2–10 per 100 000. The age of onset varies but peaks between 20 and 40 years of age (*Brain* 1980; **112:** 133–46).

What are the main ways in which multiple sclerosis can present?
- Optic neuritis (in 40% of cases) resulting in partial loss of vision.
- Weakness of one or more limbs.
- Tingling in the extremities due to posterior column involvement.
- Diplopia.
- Nystagmus, cerebellar ataxia.
- Vertigo.

What is the natural history of multiple sclerosis?
The course of the disease is extremely variable and patients with multiple sclerosis face enormous prognostic uncertainty. The onset may be acute, subacute or insidious. The course may be rapidly downhill, or may spontaneously remit for periods lasting from days to years before a second exacerbation (*N Engl J Med* 2000; **343:** 938–52).

What are the clinical categories of multiple sclerosis?
- Relapsing-remitting: episodes of acute worsening with recovery and a stable course between relapses.
- Secondary progressive: gradual neurological deterioration with or without super-imposed acute relapses in a patient who previously had relapsing-remitting multiple sclerosis.
- Primary progressive: gradual, almost continuous neurological deterioration from the onset of symptoms.
- Progressive relapsing: gradual neurological deterioration from the onset of symptoms but with subsequent superimposed relapses.

What is Lhermitte's sign?
A tingling or electric shock-like sensation which radiates to the arms, down the back or into the legs on flexion of the patient's neck. It has also been called the barber's chair sign. It indicates disease near the dorsal column nuclei of the higher cervical cord. Causes include multiple sclerosis, cervical stenosis, subacute combined degeneration of the cord.

What is Uhthoff's symptom?
The exacerbation of symptoms of multiple sclerosis during a hot bath.

Do you know of any criteria for the diagnosis of multiple sclerosis?
Poser's criteria: a history of two episodes of neurological deficit and objective clinical signs of lesions at more than one site within the central nervous system establishes the diagnosis of definite multiple sclerosis. In the presence of only one clinical sign, the demonstration of an additional lesion by laboratory tests – such as evoked potentials, MRI, CT or urological studies – also fulfils the criteria.

A diagnosis of probable multiple sclerosis is defined as either two attacks with clinical evidence of one lesion, or one attack with clinical evidence of two lesions.

Which conditions may be considered formes fruste of multiple sclerosis?
• Optic neuritis.
• Single episode of transverse myelitis with optic neuritis.

What is the role of steroids in acute optic neuritis and the development of multiple sclerosis?
In acute optic neuritis, treatment with a 3-day course of high-dose intravenous methylprednisolone (followed by a short course of prednisone) reduces the rate of development of multiple sclerosis over a 2-year period (*N Engl J Med* 1993; **326:** 581–8; *N Engl J Med* 1993; **329:** 1764–9).

Does pregnancy affect the clinical features of multiple sclerosis?
Pregnancy itself may have a mildly protective effect but there is an increased risk of relapse during the puerperium; overall, the effect on the course of the disease is probably negligible.

What is the role of exercise in the treatment of such patients?
Patients should be encouraged to keep active during remission and to avoid excessive physical exercise during relapses.

What is the role of MRI in multiple sclerosis?
MRI can identify up to 80% of patients with multiple sclerosis. T2-weighted images show hyperintense focal periventricular lesions. Although periventricular white matter lesions are typical of multiple sclerosis, they are not pathognomonic. Small infarcts, disseminated metastases, moya-moya disease and inflammatory diseases can produce a similar picture. High-resolution MRI may provide useful prognostic information in patients who present with an acute, clinically isolated syndrome suggestive of multiple sclerosis. On 5-year follow-up, over half the patients who had asymptomatic white matter lesions at presentation had developed clinically definite multiple sclerosis, compared with 3% of patients who had normal results at presentation. The disease progressed rapidly if the scan showed four or more lesions at presentation, and a greater number of lesions also correlated with the development of moderate or severe disability (*N Engl J Med* 1993; **116:** 135–46; *Brain* 1998; **121:** 495–503).

Mention some other demyelinating disorders.
• Devic's disease: myelitis with optic neuritis. There has been debate as to whether this is a form of multiple sclerosis or a monophasic illness.
• Leukodystrophies.
• Tuberous sclerosis (patchy demyelination; see pp 511–13).
• Schilder's disease (diffuse cerebral sclerosis; may present with cortical blindness when the occipital cortex is involved).

What are the prognostic markers that predict more severe multiple sclerosis?
• Progressive disease from the onset of symptoms.
• Frequent relapses in the first two years.
• Motor and cerebellar signs at presentation to neurologist.
• Short interval between the first two relapses.
• Male gender.
• Poor recovery from relapse.
• Multiple cranial lesions on T2-weighted MRI at presentation.

Note. Women and patients with predominantly sensory symptoms and optic neuritis have a more favourable prognosis.

Is there any treatment for multiple sclerosis?

- Two forms of interferon β (i.e. 1b, Betaferon, and 1a, Avonex, Rebif) have been shown to reduce the relapse rate in relapsing-remitting (non-progressive) neurological deficit by one third (*Neurology* 1993; **43**: 655–67; *Lancet* 1998; **352**: 1491–7). Whether reduction in relapse rate reduces or prevents later disability is not known; some evidence has been presented in favour. The Association of British Neurologists recommends interferon β be prescribed for ambulant patients with at least two definite relapses in the previous two years followed by recovery, which may or may not be complete.

- Interferon β-1b has been reported to delay progression (for 9–12 months) in a study period of 2–3 years) in secondary progressive multiple sclerosis of moderate severity (minimum walking distance of 20 metres with assistance) and has been licensed for this indication. However, the SPECTRIMS study, which was a large trial, showed no significant benefit of interferon β-1b therapy in delaying disability in secondary progressive multiple sclerosis. Mitoxantrone hydrochloride has been shown to reduce the rate of clinical relapse and delay progression of disability in secondary progressive multiple sclerosis.

- Copolymer-1 (*Neurology* 1995; **45**: 1268–76), glatiramer acetate (Copaxone) and pulsed intravenous immunoglobulin (*Lancet* 1997; **349**: 589–93), like the interferon betas, reduce the relapse rate. However, the role of immunomodulatory agents needs to be defined.

- Intravenous methylprednisolone may hasten recovery from acute relapses but has no effect in the long term. A recent trial suggested that intravenous methylprednisolone is no better than equivalent oral doses of methylprednisolone for acute relapses (*Lancet* 1997; **349**: 902–6).

- Plasma exchange enhances recovery of relapse-related neurological deficits in patients with no response to high-dose corticosteroids.

- Fatigue is modestly reduced by amantadine (*Neurology* 1995; **45**: 1956–61).

- Bladder dysfunction usually consists of combined detrusor hyper-reflexia and incomplete emptying. Volumes of less than 100 ml of urine remaining in the bladder after micturition are managed with oxybutinin or detrusitol; volumes greater than 100 ml require clean, intermittent self-catheterization (*J Neurol Neurosurg Psychiatry* 1996; **60**: 6–13).

- Sexual dysfunction (erectile failure) may be helped with the phosphodiesterase inhibitor sildenafil citrate (Viagra), or yohimbine or other alpha-adrenergic blockers.

- Limb spasticity requires a multidisciplinary approach to ensure correct posture, prevention of skin ulceration from pressure, and management of bladder and bowel dysfunction as well as medications such as tizanidine (an alpha2-adrenoreceptor antagonist), an antispastic agent (*Neurology* 1994; **44** (suppl 9): 70–78S). Tizanidine reduces spasticity but there is no beneficial effect on mobility.

Remember that there is no evidence to suggest that any treatment alters the long-term outcome in multiple sclerosis.

J.L. Lhermitte (1877–1959), a French neurologist and neuropsychiatrist, wrote on spinal injuries, myoclonus, internuclear ophthalmoplegia and chorea.

Case 61

ABNORMAL GAIT

INSTRUCTION

Look at this patient while he walks.
Test this patient's gait.

SALIENT FEATURES

1. Cerebellar gait

The patient has a broad-based gait, reeling and lurching to one side.

Proceed as follows:

Tell the examiner that you would like to examine the patient for other cerebellar signs (see p. 144).

2. Parkinsonian gait

The steps are small and shuffling, and the patient walks in haste (festinates). The entire body stoops forwards, knees bent, head hunched forward, and the feet must hurry to keep up with it as if trying to catch up with the centre of gravity. There is associated loss of arm swing and mask-like facies.

Proceed as follows:

Tell the examiner that you would like to look for other signs of Parkinson's disease (see pp 136–7).

3. Hemiplegic gait

The gait is slow, spastic and shuffling. With each step the pelvis is tilted upwards on the involved side to aid in lifting the foot off the ground, and the entire affected limb is circumducted, rotated in a semicircle at the pelvis. The upper limb is flexed, adducted and does not swing, and the lower limb is extended.

4. Sensory ataxia

The feet stamp, the movement of the legs bearing no relation to the position of the legs in space since proprioception is impaired or absent. The patient has to look down at the ground to compensate for the loss of proprioception. The patient walks on a wide base; the feet are lifted too high off the ground and are brought down too vigorously.

Proceed as follows:

- Check for Romberg's sign, vibration and position sense.
- Sensory ataxic gait may be due to the following:
  - Tabes dorsalis.
  - Subacute combined degeneration of the cord.
- Tell the examiner that you would like to look for Argyll Robertson pupils and anaemia.

5. High-stepping gait
This is usually unilateral and results from foot-drop. The patient has to lift the foot high in order to avoid dragging the forefoot.

It may be due to the following:

- Lateral popliteal nerve palsy.
- Poliomyelitis.
- Charcot–Marie–Tooth disease.
- Lead or arsenic poisoning.

6. Scissor gait
This is seen in spastic paraplegia. The adductor spasm may be so severe as to lead to the legs crossing in front of one another. Short steps with the front of the feet clinging to the ground result in a wearing out of the toes of shoes.

Proceed as follows:
Tell the examiner that the underlying aetiology would probably be cord compression, multiple sclerosis or cerebral palsy.

7. Waddling gait
The legs are held wide apart and the patient shifts weight from one side to the other as he walks. Comment on the lumbar lordosis. It is seen in advanced pregnancy and proximal weakness (Cushing's syndrome, osteomalacia, thyrotoxicosis, polymyositis, diabetes, hereditary muscular dystrophies).

ADVANCED-LEVEL QUESTIONS

What do you understand by the term 'astasia abasia'?
This is seen in psychogenic disturbances in which the patient is unable to walk or cannot stand. The patient falls far to the side on walking but usually regains balance before hitting the ground. The legs may be thrown out wildly or the patient may kneel with each step.

What do you understand by the term 'marche à petits pas'?
This describes a gait in which the movement is slow and the patient walks with very short, shuffling and irregular steps with loss of associated movements. It is seen in normal-pressure hydrocephalus. This gait bears some resemblance to that seen in Parkinson's disease.

Case 62

WASTING OF THE SMALL MUSCLES OF THE HAND

INSTRUCTION

Examine this patient's hands.
Ask the patient whether her hands are painful.

SALIENT FEATURES

History

- Rheumatoid arthritis.
- Painful neck movements (cervical spondylosis).
- Fasciculations, weakness (motor neuron disease).
- Associated sensory loss (syringomyelia).
- Family history (Charcot–Marie–Tooth disease).
- Ascending muscle weakness (Guillain–Barré syndrome).
- Trauma to upper limbs (bilateral median and ulnar nerve lesions).

Examination

Wasting of thenar and hypothenar eminences and dorsal interossei.

Proceed as follows:
- Look for deformity and swelling.
- Look for fasciculations.
- Check sensation over the hand, especially index and little fingers.
- Test grip and pincer movements.
- Test for median and ulnar nerve compression.
- Ask the patient to unbutton clothes or to write.
- Palpate for cervical ribs and compare radial pulses.
- Look for Horner's syndrome.
- Examine the neck and test neck movements.

DIAGNOSIS

This patient has bilateral wasted hands (lesions) due to cervical myelopathy (aetiology) and is unable to button her clothes (functional status).

Remember that the causes of bilateral wasted hands are as follows:

- Rheumatoid arthritis.
- Old age.
- Cervical spondylosis.
- Bilateral cervical ribs.
- Motor neuron disease.
- Syringomyelia.
- Charcot–Marie–Tooth disease.

- Guillain–Barré syndrome.
- Bilateral median and ulnar nerve lesions.

If the wasting is seen in only one hand, then in addition to the above causes consider the following:

- Brachial plexus trauma.
- Pancoast's tumour.
- Cervical cord lesions.
- Malignant infiltration of the brachial plexus.

QUESTIONS

In unilateral wasting, what is the level of the lesion?

C8, T1. These muscles are predominantly supplied by the ulnar nerve (the median nerve supplies the thenar eminence), the inner cord of the brachial plexus, the T1 spinal root and the anterior horn cells. Thus lesions of these structures may all produce wasting of the small muscles of the hand:

1. Lesions of the radial, median and ulnar nerves (trauma).
2. Brachial plexus (trauma, cervical lymph nodes, cervical ribs, tumour of superior sulcus of lung).
3. Anterior root (cervical spondylosis).
4. Anterior horn cell (motor neuron disease, tumours of spinal cord, syringomyelia, poliomyelitis).

Case 63

FACIOSCAPULOHUMERAL DYSTROPHY (LANDOUZY–DÉJÉRINE SYNDROME)

INSTRUCTION

Perform a neurological examination of this patient's cranial nerves and upper limbs.

SALIENT FEATURES

History

- Age of onset (usually between 10 and 40 years of age).
- Family history (parents or siblings may only have facial weakness).
- Weakness begins in the face and subsequently affects the shoulder girdle (particularly the lower trapezii, pectoralis, triceps and biceps).

Examination

Face
- Prominent ptosis.
- Difficulty in closing the eyes.
- Marked facial weakness, resulting in a dull expressionless face with lips open and slack, and inability to whistle or puff the cheeks.
- Speech is impaired owing to difficulty in articulation of labial consonants.

Neck
Wasted sternomastoids and marked weakness of neck muscles.

Shoulder girdle
- Winging of the scapula.
- Lower pectorals and lower trapezii severely affected.
- Weakness of triceps and biceps.
- True hypertrophy of deltoids to compensate for other muscles.
- Absent biceps and triceps jerk.

Uncommon features
Congenital absence of pectoralis, biceps or brachioradialis.
Tibialis anterior may be the only muscle involved outside the shoulder girdle.

DIAGNOSIS

This patient has weakness of the muscles of the face, neck and shoulder girdle (lesion) due to inherited facioscapulohumeral dystrophy (aetiology).

QUESTIONS

What is the mode of inheritance?
Autosomal dominant; both sexes are equally affected. The gene has been recently localized to the long arm of chromosome 4 (*Nat Genet* 1992; **2:** 26).

Are higher mental functions affected in this condition?
The IQ is normal in such patients.

What is the lifespan in such a patient?
Normal.

What is the age of onset of this disorder?
Between 10 and 40 years.

Are levels of muscle enzymes raised in this condition?
The enzyme levels usually remain normal. About half the cases show a very slight increase.

L.T.J. Landouzy (1845–1917), Professor of Therapeutics in Paris; although he is remembered for his description of the syndrome which bears his name, his major research interest was tuberculosis.

J.J. Déjérine (1849–1917), a French neurologist, was a pioneer in the localization of function in the brain. This syndrome was described in 1885.

Case 64

LIMB GIRDLE DYSTROPHY

INSTRUCTION

Perform a neurological examination of this patient's upper and lower limbs.

SALIENT FEATURES

History
- Age of onset (between 10 and 30 years of age).
- Onset may be either in the pelvic or shoulder girdle.
- It may remain confined to the pelvic or shoulder girdle and may be static for years before peripheral weakness and wasting occur.

Examination

Upper limbs
- Biceps and brachioradialis are involved late; wrist extensors are first involved when it extends to the wrist.
- Deltoids may show pseudohypertrophy and are spared until late.

Lower limbs
- In the early stages of the disease, hip flexors and glutei are weak.
- There is early wasting of medial quadriceps and tibialis anterior.
- Lateral quadriceps and calves may show hypertrophy.

Note. The face is never affected.

DIAGNOSIS

This patient has weakness of the proximal muscles of the arms and legs (lesion) due to limb girdle dystrophy (aetiology).

ADVANCED-LEVEL QUESTIONS

What is the mode of inheritance?
Autosomal recessive; males and females are equally affected.

What is the age of onset?
Between 10 and 30 years, causing disability 10–20 years after onset.

How is the intelligence affected?
It is unaffected and IQ is normal.

Is the lifespan affected?
No.

What happens to the serum enzymes?

Levels of serum enzymes are slightly affected or normal.

John Walton, Professor of Neurology at Oxford and Newcastle, was made a peer following his retirement and carries the title of Lord Walton of Detchant. His chief interest was muscular diseases.

Sir Roger Bannister, Master of Pembroke College at Oxford, worked at the National Hospital for Nervous Diseases, Queen Square, and St Mary's Hospital, London. His main interest was chronic autonomic failure. He was the first person to run the 4-minute mile.

Case 65

MYASTHENIA GRAVIS

INSTRUCTION

This patient complains of drooping of the eyelids in the evenings; examine this patient.

SALIENT FEATURES

History

- Weakness in muscles is more marked in the evening.
- Muscle weakness which increases with exercise (remember that *fatigability* is the hallmark of myasthenia gravis) and is painless.
- Muscle weakness affects smiling, chewing, speaking, muscles of the neck, walking, breathing, movements at the elbow and hand movements.
- Obtain history of thyrotoxicosis, diabetes mellitus, rheumatoid arthritis, SLE and thymoma.
- D-Penicillamine treatment for rheumatoid arthritis (myasthenia gravis is sometimes caused by D-penicillamine).

Examination

- The patient may have obvious ptosis.
- Check for worsening of ptosis after sustained upward gaze for at least 45 seconds.
- Check extraocular movements for diplopia and variable squint.
- Comment on snarling face when the patient attempts to smile.
- Weakness without loss of reflexes, or alteration of sensation or coordination. The weakness may be generalized; it may affect the limb muscles, often proximal in distribution, as well as the diaphragm and neck extensors.
- Speech is nasal.
- Muscle wasting is rare and presents late in the disease.

Proceed as follows:
Tell the examiner that myasthenia is associated with thyrotoxicosis, diabetes mellitus, rheumatoid arthritis, SLE and thymoma.

DIAGNOSIS

This patient has diplopia at the end of each day with ptosis; the weakness is marked on repeated exertion of the muscle (lesion) and is due to myasthenia gravis (aetiology).

Read classic review: *N Engl J Med* 1994; **330:** 1797–810.

QUESTIONS

At what age is myasthenia common?
The incidence has two age peaks: one peak in the second and third decades affecting mostly women and a peak in the sixth and seventh decades affecting mostly men.

What groups of muscles are commonly involved?
The muscles affected are as follows, in order of likelihood: extraocular, bulbar, neck, limb girdle, distal limbs and trunk.

What investigations would you like to perform in this patient?
- Edrophonium (Tensilon) test.
- Vital capacity.
- Imaging of the mediastinum: chest radiography, CT or MRI of the chest.
- Serum acetylcholine receptor antibodies (present in more than 80% of cases) (*J Neurol Neurosurg Psychiatry* 1985; **48:** 1246–52). Remember, the basic deficit is a deficiency of acetylcholine receptors at the neuromuscular junction (*Science* 1973; **182:** 293–5).
- Plasma thyroxine (to rule out an associated thyroid disorder).
- Anti-striated muscle antibody (seen in association with thymoma).
- Antinuclear antibody, rheumatoid factor, antithyroid antibodies may be positive.
- Tuberculin test if immunosuppressive therapy is contemplated.
- EMG abnormalities include a decremental response to tetanic train stimulation at 5–10 Hz (*Bull Johns Hopkins Hospital* 1941; **68:** 81–93; *Ann N Y Acad Sci* 1976; **274:** 203–22), and evidence of neuromuscular blockade is seen on single-fibre EMG in the form of jitter and blocking of motor action potentials (*Muscle Nerve* 1992; **15:** 720–4).

What is the differential diagnosis?
- Botulism.
- Eaton–Lambert syndrome.

What are the treatment modalities available?
- Symptomatic treatment entails administration of an anticholinesterase drug, e.g. pyridostigmine given up to five times per day.
- Definitive treatment entails immunosuppression, e.g. steroids, azathioprine, ciclosporin, plasmapheresis, thymectomy.

Mention a drug that can cause myasthenia.

D-Penicillamine therapy given for rheumatoid arthritis.

Why may a 'gin and tonic' exacerbate myasthenia?

The quinine in tonic water causes muscle weakness.

If this patient develops an infection, which group of antibiotics would you avoid?

Aminoglycosides.

Mention a few exacerbating features.

Fatigue, exercise, infection, emotion, change of climate, pregnancy, magnesium enemas, drugs (aminoglycosides, propranolol, morphine, barbiturates, procainamide, quinidine).

ADVANCED-LEVEL QUESTIONS

What do you know about Eaton–Lambert syndrome?

Eaton–Lambert syndrome (*JAMA* 1957; **163:** 1117) is a myasthenic disorder associated with malignancy (*Brain* 1988; **111:** 577; a review of 50 cases). It is associated with small cell carcinoma of the bronchus. Weakness of the truncal and proximal limb muscles is common. The pelvic girdle and thighs are almost invariably involved. Transient improvement in muscle strength and deep tendon reflexes may follow brief exercise. Unlike myasthenia, bulbar symptoms are rare. Antibodies to calcium channels may be detected. EMG is diagnostic. In the rested muscle there is marked depression of neuromuscular transmission after a single submaximal stimulus and marked facilitation of response during repetitive stimulation at rates greater than 10 per second.

What is myasthenic crisis?

Exacerbation of myasthenia. The need for artificial ventilation occurs in about 10% of patients with myasthenia. Those with bulbar and respiratory involvement are prone to respiratory infection. The crisis can be precipitated by respiratory infection and surgery. Such patients should be closely monitored for pulmonary function. Those with artificial ventilation are not given cholinergics as this avoids stimulation of pulmonary secretions and uncertainties about overdosage.

How does a cholinergic crisis manifest?

Excessive salivation, confusion, lacrimation, miosis, pallor and collapse. It is important to avoid edrophonium in such patients.

Mention a few associated disorders.

Thyroid disorders (thyrotoxicosis, hypothyroidism), rheumatoid arthritis, diabetes mellitus, dermatomyositis, pernicious anaemia, SLE, Sjögren's disease, sarcoidosis, pemphigus.

What is the role of thymectomy in such patients?

In the case of thymoma, thymectomy is necessary to prevent tumour spread, although most thymomas are benign. In the absence of a tumour, thymectomy has been found to be beneficial in 85% of patients, and 35% go into drug-free remission. The improvement is noticed 1–10 years after surgery (*Neurology* 1990; **40:**

1828–9). The role of thymectomy in ocular myasthenia, in adults over 55 years of age (*Acta Neurol Scand* 1994; **12:** 343–68) and in children is still under debate.

How is myasthenia graded clinically?

Osserman's grading of severity:
- Grade I: ocular myasthenia.
- Grade IIA: mild generalized myasthenia with slow progression; no crises; drug responsive.
- Grade IIB: moderate generalized myasthenia; severe skeletal and bulbar involvement, but no crises; drug response is less satisfactory.
- Grade III: acute fulminating myasthenia: rapid progression of severe symptoms of respiratory crises and poor drug response; high incidence of thymoma; high mortality rate.
- Grade IV: late severe myasthenia; same as grade III but takes two years to progress from Class I to II; crises; high mortality rate.

Newsom-Davies clinical subgroups include:
1. Patients with thymoma, equal sex incidence, peak age of onset 30–50 years, no HLA association and poor response to thymectomy.
2. Young onset (<40 years), typically female, thymic medullary germinal centres present, strong association with HLA-B8 and -DR3, and usually a good response to thymectomy.
3. Older onset (>40 years), more common in males, thymic involution, an association with HLA-B7 and -DR9, and doubtful response to thymectomy.

What is the role of immunomodulation in myasthenia gravis?
Intravenous immunoglobulin seems as efficacious as plasma exchange (*Ann Neurol* 1997; **41:** 789–96).

L.M. Eaton (1905–1958), Professor of Neurology at the Mayo Clinic, Rochester, Minnesota.

E.H. Lambert (b. 1915), Professor of Physiology, University of Minnesota.

Sir Samuel Wilks (1824–1911), physician, Guy's Hospital, London. Myasthenia gravis was known as Wilks' syndrome.

Myasthenia gravis was first described by the physiologist Thomas Willis in 1672 and by Erb in 1878. It was also known as Hoppe–Goldflam disease after H.H. Hoppe (1867–1919), a US neurologist (*Berl Klin Wochenschr* 1892; **29:** 332–6) and S.V. Goldflam (1852–1932), a Polish neurologist. In 1895 F. Jolly named the disease myasthenia gravis pseudoparalytica (*Berl Klin Wochenschr* 1895; **32:** 1–7).

John Newsom-Davies, FRS, contemporary Professor of Clinical Neurology, Oxford.

Alastair Composton, PhD, FRCP, contemporary Professor of Neurology, Cambridge.

Case 66

THOMSEN'S DISEASE (MYOTONIA CONGENITA)

INSTRUCTION

Look at this patient.

SALIENT FEATURES

History

- Ask the patient whether or not there is any seasonal variation in symptoms – myotonia is worse in winter because of the cold.
- Take a family history (inheritance is usually autosomal dominant; gene on long arm of chromosome 7).

Examination

- Diffuse muscle hypertrophy.
- Myotonia – may be apparent while shaking hands with the person.

DIAGNOSIS

This patient has diffuse muscular hypertrophy with myotonia (lesion) due to Thomsen's disease (aetiology).

ADVANCED-LEVEL QUESTIONS

How is the disease recognized in infancy?

Myotonia is present from birth and may be recognized by the child's peculiar cry. Also noticed in early infancy are difficulty in feeding and inability to reopen the eyes while having the face washed.

When does muscle hypertrophy manifest?

It is usually apparent in the second decade.

What is the cause of muscle hypertrophy?

It is caused by almost continual involuntary isometric exercise.

What is the life expectancy in such patients?

These patients have a normal life expectancy.

What drugs would you use to ameliorate the myotonia?

Procainamide, quinidine.

In which other conditions is myotonia seen?

- Myotonia dystrophica.
- Paramyotonia congenita (episodic myotonia after exposure to the cold).
- Following the administration of drugs such as clofibrate.

A.J.T. Thomsen (1815–1896) was a Danish physician who described this condition in his family and himself in 1876.

Case 67

FRIEDREICH'S ATAXIA

INSTRUCTION

Perform a neurological examination of this patient's legs.

SALIENT FEATURES

History
- Age of onset (usually the same in each family and ranges from 8 to 16 years of age).
- High-arched foot in childhood in the family (Friedreich's foot).
- Scoliosis developing in childhood.
- Cerebellar dysarthria (pp 152–3) and ataxia (p. 180).

Examination
- Pes cavus.
- Pyramidal weakness in legs.
- Cerebellar signs, ataxia being a constant sign.
- Impaired vibration and joint sense.
- Romberg's sign positive.
- Absence of deep tendon reflexes (due to degeneration of peripheral nerves)
- Distal muscle wasting (in 50% of cases), especially in the hands.

Proceed as follows:
- Check for nystagmus (present in 25% of the cases), scanning speech, intention tremor.
- Examine the heart for hypertrophic cardiomyopathy.
- Check the eyes for optic atrophy (present in 30% of cases).
- Check the spine for kyphoscoliosis.
- Check the urine for sugar (10% of patients have diabetes).
- Check IQ, looking for intellectual deterioration.

DIAGNOSIS

This patient has kyphoscoliosis, pes cavus and a combination of pyramidal, cerebellar and sensory deficits (lesions) in the lower limbs due to Friedreich's ataxia (aetiology); he is severely disabled by his deformity.

ADVANCED-LEVEL QUESTIONS

What is the mode of inheritance?
Autosomal recessive or, rarely, sex linked.

Why are the deep tendon reflexes absent even though plantars are upgoing?
This is due to a combination of pyramidal weakness with peripheral neuropathy.

In which other condition is there a mixture of cerebellar, pyramidal and dorsal column signs?
Multiple sclerosis.

Mention a few conditions with absent knee jerks and upgoing plantars.
- Peripheral neuropathy in a stroke patient.
- Motor neuron disease.
- Conus medullaris – cauda equina lesion.
- Tabes dorsalis.
- Subacute combined degeneration of the spinal cord.

What is the forme fruste of this condition?
Pes cavus or hammer toes, without any other signs, are seen in family members of such patients.

On which chromosome is the gene for this disorder localized?
Chromosome 9.

What are the clinical criteria for diagnosis of Friedreich's ataxia?
Harding's criteria (*Brain* 1981; **104:** 589):

- Essential criteria are onset before the age of 25 years, ataxia of limbs and gait, absent knee and ankle jerks, extensor plantars, autosomal recessive inheritance, motor conduction velocity greater than 40 ms, small or absent sensory nerve action potentials, dysarthria within 5 years of onset.
- Additional criteria (present in two thirds) are scoliosis, pyramidal weakness of lower limbs, absent upper limb reflexes, loss of vibration and joint position sense in the legs, abnormal ECG, pes cavus.
- Other features (present in less than 50% of cases) are nystagmus, optic atrophy, deafness, distal muscle wasting and diabetes.

What is the prognosis of Friedreich's ataxia?
Friedreich's ataxia usually progresses slowly and few patients live for more than 20 years after the onset of symptoms. Occasionally it may appear to be arrested, and abortive cases may be encountered in apparently healthy relatives of affected patients.

What are the pathological changes in Friedreich's ataxia?
- Marked loss of cells in the posterior root ganglia.
- Degeneration of peripheral sensory fibres.
- Involvement of the posterior and lateral columns of the cord.

Name a few syndromes with spinocerebellar degeneration (*N Engl J Med* 1995; **333:** 1351–3).
- Roussy–Lévy disease: hereditary spinocerebellar degeneration with atrophy of lower limb muscles and loss of deep tendon reflexes.
- Refsum's disease (see p. 537).
- Bassen–Kornzweig syndrome (see p. 537): caused by cellular deficiency of vitamin E (α-tocopherol) resulting from a defect in the α-tocopherol-transfer protein and abetalipoproteinaemia associated with a defect of very low density lipoproteins.
- Olivopontocerebellar degeneration: first described in 1882; autosomal dominant inheritance and has been mapped to HLA loci on the short arm of chromosome 6;

a highly polymorphic CAG repeat sequence has been found in this region. The CAG repeat sequence is longer than normal and unstable in affected patients.

- Machado–Joseph disease: dominant inheritance, first described in families of Portuguese origin. Clinical features include progressive ataxia, ophthalmoparesis, spasticity, dystonia, amyotrophy and parkinsonism. This disorder has been linked to chromosome 14 and is caused by the expansion of unstable CAG repeat sequences.
- Dentatorubral pallidoluysian atrophy is similar to Machado–Joseph disease but maps on the short arm of chromosome 12. The abnormally expanded CAG repeat sequences identified in the gene for olivopontocerebellar degeneration, Machado–Joseph disease and dentatorubral pallidoluysian atrophy each result in the expression of a specific ataxin.

Nikolaus Friedreich (1825–1882), Professor of Pathology and neurologist in Heidelberg, described this condition in a series of papers from 1861 to 1876.

Anita Harding (1953–1995) Professor of Neurology at the National Hospital, Queen Square, London, died at the age of 42 years from colonic cancer.

G. Roussy (1874–1948), a French neuropathologist.

G. Lévy (b. 1881), a French neurologist.

Sigvald Refsum (1907–1991), a Norwegian neurologist, was successively Professor of Neurology at Bergen University and at the National Hospital in Oslo (*BMJ* 1991; **303:** 919).

Case 68

MOTOR NEURON DISEASE

INSTRUCTION

Examine this patient's cranial nerves.
Examine this patient's upper limbs.
Examine this patient's lower limbs.

SALIENT FEATURES

History

- Fasciculations and cramps: these may precede other symptoms by months.
- Painless, asymmetrical weakness of muscles of the upper limb or lower limb.
- Dysarthria and dysphagia.
- Emotional lability if there is bulbar involvement.

Examination

- Fasciculations, absent reflexes and weakness in the upper limbs.
- Spasticity, exaggerated reflexes and upgoing plantars in lower limbs.
- Sluggish palatal movements, absent gag reflex, brisk jaw jerk.

A combination of the above signs may be seen.

DIAGNOSIS

This patient has a combination of upper and lower motor neuron signs (lesions) due to motor neuron disease (aetiology), although I would like to exclude cervical cord compression. The patient is wheelchair bound as a result of the disease (functional status).

QUESTIONS

What important cause should be ruled out before making a firm diagnosis of motor neuron disease?

Cord compression may produce a similar clinical picture and hence it is important to do an MRI scan of the spine and/or a myelogram to exclude it.

ADVANCED-LEVEL QUESTIONS

What are the characteristic features of this disease?

- It rarely begins before the age of 40 years.
- Presence of upper and lower motor neuron involvement of a single spinal segment, and motor dysfunction involving at least two limbs or one limb and bulbar muscles.
- Sensory symptoms or signs are not seen.
- Ocular movements are not affected.
- There are never cerebellar or extrapyramidal signs.
- Sphincters are involved late, if at all.
- Remission is unknown and the disease is fatal within 5–7 years (due to bronchopneumonia).

What are the clinical patterns of motor neuron disease?

- Bulbar: bulbar or pseudobulbar palsy (25% of cases).
- Amyotrophic lateral sclerosis (50% of cases): flaccid arms and spastic legs.
- Progressive muscular atrophy (25% of cases): a lesion in the anterior horn cells affecting distal muscles. Characteristically there is retention of deep tendon reflexes in the presence of severe muscular atrophy.
- Primary lateral sclerosis (rare): signs progress from an upper motor neuron to a lower motor neuron type.

Others affect lower motor neurons and include:

- Werdnig–Hoffman disease: presents in the neonatal period as a 'floppy infant' and is known as infantile progressive spinal muscular atrophy.
- X-linked spinal muscular atrophy: the patient has associated testicular atrophy resulting in oligospermia and gynaecomastia. It is associated with the amplification of a trinucleotide repeat in the coding sequence of the androgen receptor gene; the severity of the disease is directly related to the number of repeats present.
- Spinal muscular atrophy linked to locus on the large arm of chromosome 5.

What are the other types of motor neuron disease?

- Madras motor neuron disease is common in southern India. The onset is early (before the age of 30); asymmetrical limb weakness and wasting, bulbar and facial involvement occur along with sensorineural deafness. The course is more benign than the disorder observed in Europe and America (Srinivas K, Jagannathan K, Valmikinathan K 1984 The spectrum of motor neuron disease in Madras. In: Rose FC, ed. *Research Progress in Motor Neuron Disease*, p. 142. London: Pitman).

- Amyotrophic lateral sclerosis associated with a parkinsonism–dementia complex in Guam (*Science* 1987; **237**: 517). It also tends to have an earlier onset and a more protracted course than the sporadic cases seen in Europe and America.

What is the pathology of motor neuron disease?

The clinical manifestations are a result of degeneration of Betz cells, pyramidal tracts, cranial nerve nuclei and anterior horn cells. Both upper and lower motor neurons may be involved, but sensory involvement is not seen.

What is the explanation of fasciculation?

It results from spontaneous firing of large motor units formed by branching fibres of surviving axons that are striving to innervate muscle fibres that have lost their nerve supply.

What are the cerebrospinal fluid (CSF) changes in the disease?

The CSF is usually normal (the protein level may be slightly raised).

What do you know about the heredity of amyotrophic lateral sclerosis?

Most cases are sporadic. Five to ten per cent of cases are familial, and familial amyotrophic lateral sclerosis is linked to a gene on the long arm of chromosome 21 (*N Engl J Med* 1991; **324**: 1381). This genetic locus appears to be the copper–zinc-binding superoxide dismutase gene, with various missense mutations identified in different families.

Is there any treatment for motor neuron disease?

No treatment has been shown to influence the course of the disease. Riluzole, a glutamate antagonist, is being used in limb or bulbar palsy (*N Engl J Med* 1994; **330**: 585–91). Patients often require treatment for painful muscle cramps, constant drooling, severe fatigability, sleep problems, incipient contractures, subluxation of the shoulder joint, dysphagia and neuralgia – all of which can be ameliorated. Patients often have extreme lability of emotion, particularly in the early stages of amyotrophic lateral sclerosis. In order to alleviate distress before or during respiratory failure, which is usually the terminal event, narcotic drugs should not be withheld.

What is the rationale for using riluzole?

The suggestion that accumulation of toxic levels of glutamate at synapses may cause neuronal death through a calcium-dependent pathway. Riluzole has been shown to be useful in patients with disease of bulbar onset but not in those with disease of spinal onset. The risk of death or tracheostomy is lower with 100 mg riluzole than placebo in limb or bulbar onset disease (*Lancet* 1996; **347**: 1425–31), but it is debatable whether this translates into an improved quality of life.

Is there any test to monitor the rate of disease progression?

Antibodies to L-type voltage-gated calcium channels are present in the serum of patients with sporadic amyotrophic lateral sclerosis, and antibody titres correlate with the rate of disease progression (*N Engl J Med* 1992; **327**: 1721–8).

What is the role of magnetic cortical stimulation in amyotrophic lateral sclerosis?

Magnetic cortical stimulation uses time-varying magnetic fields to induce electrical currents within the brain painlessly. It is said to activate cortical motor neurons trans-synaptically through thalamocortical and corticocortical afferents, and allows detection of degeneration of cortical Betz cells. In patients with amyotrophic lateral sclerosis the sensitivity of this technique to detect upper motor neuron involvement in those with clinical signs is high, but the sensitivity of the technique in those without clinical signs is unknown.

Is there any animal model for amyotrophic lateral sclerosis?

A transgenic mouse model possesses mutations in the gene encoding the cytosolic form of the enzyme copper–zinc superoxide dismutase (*Nature* 1993; **362:** 59).

Lou Gehrig, the American baseball player, died from amyotrophic lateral sclerosis 50 years ago.

Charcot gave a detailed clinical and pathological description of amyotrophic lateral sclerosis in 1865.

Professor Stephen Hawking, the Cambridge theoretical physicist, is the most famous sufferer of motor neuron disease. It claimed the lives of the actor David Niven, the football manager Don Revie and the wartime pilot Sir Leonard Cheshire, VC.

Case 69

NEUROFIBROMATOSIS

INSTRUCTION

Examine this patient.

SALIENT FEATURES

History

- Presents in childhood with cutaneous features including café-au-lait spots, axillary freckles and neurofibromas.
- Obtain history of learning disabilities (about half the patients with neurofibroma 1 are affected; *Nature* 2000; **403:** 846–7).
- Childhood leukaemia. (The risk of malignant myeloid disorders, particularly juvenile myelomonocytic leukaemia and the monosomy 7 syndrome, a childhood variant of myeloid dysplasia, is 200–500 times normal; *N Engl J Med* 1997; **336:** 1713–20.)

Examination

- Multiple neurofibromas and café-au-lait spots (brown macules, >2.5 cm diameter, and more than 5 lesions).
- Examine the axilla for freckles.

- Visual acuity and fundus for optic glioma.
- Hearing and corneal sensation for acoustic neuroma.
- The iris for Lisch nodules (often apparent only by slit-lamp examination) – present in over 90% of patients.
- The spine for kyphoscoliosis.
- Tell the examiner that you would like to check the blood pressure (for renal artery stenosis or phaeochromocytoma).

Remember. The triad for neurofibromatosis – neurofibromas, café-au-lait spots and Lisch nodules – allows identification of virtually all patients with neurofibromatosis type 1.

DIAGNOSIS

This patient has multiple café-au-lait spots and neurofibromas (lesion) due to von Recklinghausen's disease (aetiology) which are cosmetically disfiguring (functional status).

ADVANCED-LEVEL QUESTIONS

What are the criteria for neurofibromatosis type 1 (von Recklinghausen's disease)?
Neurofibromatosis type 1 may be diagnosed when two or more of the following are present:

- Six or more café-au-lait spots, the greatest diameter of which is more than 5 mm in prepubertal patients and more than 15 mm in postpubertal patients.
- Two or more neurofibromas or one plexiform neurofibroma. Plexiform neurofibroma is considered by some to be a defining lesion of neurofibromatosis type 1.
- Freckling in the axilla or inguinal region (Crowe's sign).
- Optic glioma.
- Two or more Lisch nodules (iris hamartoma).
- A distinctive osseous lesion such as sphenoid dysplasia or thinning of long bone cortex with or without pseudoarthroses.
- A parent, sibling or child with neurofibromatosis according to the above criteria.

What are the criteria for neurofibromatosis type 2?
- Bilateral eighth nerve palsy confirmed by CT or MRI.
- A parent, sibling or child with neurofibromatosis type 2 and either unilateral eighth nerve mass or any two of the following: neurofibroma, meningioma, glioma, schwannoma or juvenile posterior subcapsular lenticular opacity (*N Engl J Med* 1988; **318:** 685).

What is the significance of the Lisch nodules?
Lisch nodules are melanocytic hamartomas that appear as well-defined, dome-shaped elevations projecting from the surface of the iris and are clear to yellow and brown. The incidence increases with age: at the age of 5 years only 22% have Lisch nodules whereas, at the age of 20 years, 100% have them. Older patients who do not have Lisch nodules are also, therefore, unlikely to have neurofibromatosis 1. Lisch

nodules are an important tool in establishing the diagnosis of neurofibromatosis type 1 and in providing accurate genetic screening (*N Engl J Med* 1991; **324:** 1264).

What is the histology of the skin tumours?
The peripheral nerve tumours are of two types:

- Schwannomas: arise in cranial and spinal nerve roots and also in peripheral nerve trunks.
- Neurofibromas: composed of a proliferation of all elements of the peripheral nerve including nerve trunks, Schwann cells and fibroblasts. In sensory nerve twigs they appear as subcutaneous nodules, while in peripheral nerve trunks they may appear as a fusiform enlargement or a plexiform neurofibroma.

Is biopsy of the neurofibromas required to make a diagnosis?
No, as the diagnosis is usually evident on clinical grounds.

What are the associated abnormalities of neurofibroma?
- Lung cysts.
- Retinal hamartomas.
- Skeletal lesions: rib notching and other erosive bony defects, intraosseous cystic lesions, subperiosteal bony cysts, dysplasia of the skull, bowed legs and pseudo-arthrosis of the tibia.
- Intellectual disability.
- Aqueductal stenosis.
- Epilepsy.
- Sarcomatous change.

What do you know about the inheritance of these two disorders?
Both are autosomal dominant syndromes, type 1 being carried on chromosome 17q11.2 and type 2 on chromosome 22 (*Science* 1987; **236:** 110; *Nature* 1993; **363:** 515). The gene for neurofibromatosis type 1 encodes a protein called neurofibromin which downregulates the function of the p21 ras oncoprotein (*Neuron* 1993; **10:** 335). Learning disabilities have been ascribed to abnormal brain development as a result of deficiency in neurofibromin signalling (*Nature* 2000; **403:** 895–8). The gene for type 2 neurofibromatosis is also a tumour suppressor gene which encodes a protein that links integral membrane proteins of the cytoskeleton. How this protein is involved in tumorigenesis is not clear. Family members at risk for type 2 neurofibromatosis should be screened regularly with hearing tests and brainstem auditory evoked responses.

How would you manage these patients?
- Most are asymptomatic and require no treatment.
- Large plexiform neurofibromas should be usually left alone.
- Small neurofibromas can be removed if painful.
- Optic gliomas are treated with radiation.

When one child is affected with neurofibromatosis 1, what is the risk of another child being affected when one parent is affected and when neither parent is affected?
If one parent is affected then there is a 50% chance that another child will be affected, whereas when neither parent is affected the risk of another child being affected is no more than the standard risk in the normal population.

> Friedreich Daniel von Recklinghausen (1833–1910) was Professor of Pathology successively at Königsberg, Würzburg and Strasbourg. He also described another disease, arthritis deformans neoplastica, to which his name is attached.
>
> The elephant man, John Merrick, is commonly believed to have suffered from neurofibromatosis, but according to *Science* (1994; **264:** 188) a rare condition, Proteus syndrome, is the more likely diagnosis.
>
> Professor Lisch first described the association of the Lisch nodule with neurofibromatosis in 1937 (*Z Augenheilkd* 1937; **93:** 137–43). These nodules were first described by Waardenburg in 1918 but he did not appreciate the association with neurofibromatosis.

Case 70

SYRINGOMYELIA

INSTRUCTION

Examine this patient's arms.

SALIENT FEATURES

History

- Classically patient has a history of painless trauma or burns with cigarettes, hot water.
- Patient may have cuts that never seem to hurt.
- Patient may have a long history of poorly localized unpleasant pain (although pain sensation is impaired, these patients have severe pain).
- Patient may notice scoliosis during childhood.

Examination

- Wasting and weakness of the small muscles of the hands and forearm (if fasciculation is seen, then the other diagnosis that comes to mind at this stage is motor neuron disease).
- Rarely patients may have hypertrophy in limbs, hand and feet (*Lancet* 1996; **347:** 1593–5).
- Tone and deep tendon reflexes are diminished.
- Loss of pain and temperature sensation with intact vibration, light touch and joint position sense – this deficit is the underlying cause for any burns present.
- There may be Charcot's joints of the shoulder and elbow.

Proceed as follows:
- Examine vibration sense over the fingers, lower end of radius, elbow and clavicles (note that vibration sense is impaired only at a later stage).
- Look for Horner's syndrome.
- Examine the neck posteriorly for scar of previous surgery.

- Ask whether you may examine the following:
  - The lower limbs for pyramidal signs.
  - The face for loss of temperature and pain sensation (starting from the outer part of the face and progressing forward, looking for the 'onion-skin pattern' of sensory loss due to a lesion in the spinal nucleus of the fifth cranial nerve which extends from the pons down to the upper cervical cord).
  - For lower cranial nerve palsy.
  - For nystagmus and ataxia (due to involvement of the medial longitudinal bundle from C5 upwards).
  - For kyphoscoliosis (due to paravertebral muscle involvement).

DIAGNOSIS

This patient has dissociated sensory loss (lesion) due to syringomyelia (aetiology), and has had severe painless trauma or burns (functional status).

QUESTIONS

How common is syringomyelia?

It is a rare disorder affecting both sexes equally; the usual age of onset is the fourth or fifth decade.

How do you explain the clinical features?

At the level of the syrinx:
- Anterior horn cell involvement causing a lower motor neuron lesion.
- Involvement of the central decussating fibres of the spinothalamic tract producing dissociated sensory loss and late development of neuropathic arthropathy and other trophic changes.

Below the level of the syrinx:
Involvement of pyramidal corticospinal tracts resulting in spastic paraparesis (sphincter function is usually well preserved).

Involvement of cervical sympathetics:
Horner's syndrome (miosis, enophthalmos, ptosis).

ADVANCED-LEVEL QUESTIONS

What is la main succulente?

In some patients with syringomyelia the hands have an ugly appearance as a result of trophic and vasomotor disturbances; these commonly result in cold, cyanosed and swollen fingers and palms.

What are the other causes of dissociated sensory loss?

- Anterior spinal artery occlusion (affecting the dorsal horn and lateral spinothalamic tract).
- Diabetic small-fibre polyneuropathy.
- Hereditary amyloidotic polyneuropathy.
- Leprosy (the latter three conditions affect small peripheral nerve axons).

What investigations would you perform?

MRI scan (*J Neurosurg* 1988; **68:** 726). In the past, myelography was performed to confirm the diagnosis but was associated with deterioration of the condition in a large number of patients.

What associated abnormalities may be present?

Arnold–Chiari malformation, spina bifida, bony defects around the foramen magnum, hydrocephalus, spinal cord tumours.

What conditions may present with a similar picture?

- Intramedullary tumours of the spinal cord.
- Arachnoiditis around the foramen magnum obstructing the CSF pathway.
- Haematomyelia.
- Craniovertebral anomalies.
- Late sequelae of spinal cord injuries (manifest as a painful ascending myelopathy).

What is the difference between hydromyelia and syringomyelia?

Hydromyelia is the expansion of the ependyma-lined central canal of the spinal cord, whereas syringomyelia is the formation of a cleft-like cavity in the inner portion of the cord. Both these lesions are associated with destruction of the white and grey matter and an accompanying reactive gliosis. In syringomyelia the process generally begins in the cervical cord, and with expansion of the cavity the brainstem and distal cord also become affected.

What are the clinical features of syringobulbia?

- Dissociated sensory loss of the face of the 'onion-skin' pattern (extending from behind forwards, converging on the nose and upper lip).
- Vertigo (common symptom).
- Wasting of the small muscles of the tongue (important physical sign).
- The process may be limited to the medullary region.
- The main cranial nerve nuclei involved are those of the fifth, seventh, ninth and tenth cranial nerves.

What does the cavity of the syrinx contain?

It contains a fluid similar to CSF but with a higher protein content.

What treatment is available? (J Neurol Neurosurg Psychiatry *1981; 44: 273–84*)

- Syringoperitoneal shunting (particularly in patients with basal arachnoiditis and without tonsillar descent).
- Direct drainage of the syrinx into the subarachnoid space (in post-traumatic cavitation).
- When there is an association with Arnold–Chiari malformation, the pressure is relieved by removing the lower central portion of the occipital bone and cervical laminectomy to restore normal CSF dynamics.

What other causes of Charcot's joints do you know?

- Diabetes mellitus, especially when toes and ankles are affected.
- Tabes dorsalis, especially when knee and hip joints are affected.

What do you know about Morvan's syndrome?

The term was initially used to describe painless whitlows on the fingers but was subsequently applied to the progressive loss of pain sensation and its effects (such as ulceration, resorption of the phalanges and loss of soft tissue) in both hands and feet (*Gazette Hebdomadaire Medicine et de Chirurgie* 1883; **35:** 580). These changes are now more commonly seen in leprosy.

What do you know about the management of syringomyelia?

- Syringomyelia associated with Arnold–Chiari malformation: suboccipital craniectomy and upper cervical laminectomy to decompress the malformation at the foramen magnum.
- Intramedullary tumour: surgery, with or without radiation therapy.
- Post-traumatic syringomyelia: surgery when the neurological deficit or pain is intolerable.

The term 'syringomyelia' (from *syringx*, a pipe or tube) was first used by Ollivier in 1824, in his monograph on diseases of the spinal cord, to denote cavity formation. It denotes the presence of a large fluid-filled cavity in the grey matter of the spinal cord which is in communication with the central canal and contains CSF.

J. Arnold (1835–1915), Professor of Pathology at Heidelberg.

H. Chiari (1851–1916), an Austrian pathologist.

Case 71

SUBACUTE COMBINED DEGENERATION OF THE SPINAL CORD

INSTRUCTION

Carry out a neurological examination of the patient's legs.

SALIENT FEATURES

History

- Family history of pernicious anaemia.
- History of alcohol consumption and previous gastrectomy.
- History of chronic diarrhoea (Crohn's disease, etc.).
- Tingling distal paraesthesia (common presenting symptom).
- Whether the patient is a vegan.

Examination

- Absent ankle jerks (due to peripheral neuropathy and motor involvement).
- Brisk knee jerks.
- Upgoing plantars (usually first evidence of spinal cord lesion).
- Diminished light touch, vibration and posterior column signs.
- Romberg's sign positive.

Proceed as follows:

- Examine the following:
  - Mucous membranes for anaemia (pernicious anaemia).

– Abdomen for scars of previous gastrectomy (carcinoma of the stomach).
– Pupils (Argyll Robertson pupil because tabes is a differential diagnosis).
– Fundus for optic atrophy, seen in this condition.
- Tell the examiner that you would like to perform the following investigations:
  – A mini-mental status examination for dementia.

DIAGNOSIS

This patient has absent ankle jerks, brisk knee jerks and upgoing plantars with posterior column signs (lesion) due to subacute combined degeneration of the spinal cord (aetiology) and paralysis (functional status).

QUESTIONS

Mention a few causes of vitamin B_{12} deficiency.

- Vegan diet.
- Impaired absorption:
  – From the stomach (pernicious anaemia, gastrectomy).
  – From the small bowel (ileal disease, bacterial overgrowth, coeliac disease).
  – From the pancreas (chronic pancreatic disease).
  – As a result of fish tapeworm (rare).

ADVANCED-LEVEL QUESTIONS

What is the pathology of this condition?

There is degeneration of the axons in both the ascending tracts of the posterior columns and the descending pyramidal tracts (hence combined degeneration).

How would you investigate such a patient?

- FBC and reticulocyte count.
- Vitamin B_{12} and folate concentrations.
- Serum ferritin levels (since associated iron deficiency is common).
- Bone marrow examination.
- Parietal cell and intrinsic factor antibodies.
- Schilling test.
- MRI findings are diverse but vitamin B_{12} deficiency should be considered in differential diagnosis of all spinal cord, peripheral nerve and neuropsychiatric disorders (*J Neurol Neurosurg Psychiatry* 1998; **65:** 822–7).

If this patient had a haemoglobin level of 6 g/dl, how would you treat it?

I would avoid giving packed cells before replacing vitamin B_{12} as this may irreversibly exacerbate the neurological manifestations. Furthermore, blood transfusion is reported to precipitate incipient heart failure and death.

What type of anaemia may be seen in such patients?

Macrocytic anaemia.

Mention a few other causes of macrocytic anaemia.

- With megaloblastic bone marrow: vitamin B_{12} deficiency, folate deficiency.

- With normoblastic marrow: haemolytic anaemias, post-haemorrhagic anaemia, severe hypoxia, myxoedema, hypopituitarism, bone marrow infiltration, acute leukaemia and aplastic anaemia.

What do you know about intrinsic factor antibodies?

Intrinsic factor antibodies are seen in about 50% of patients with pernicious anaemia. About 45% of the patients have no antibody to intrinsic factor. There are two types of antibody:

- Type 1 – the blocking antibody which prevents vitamin B_{12} from binding to intrinsic factor and occurs in 55% of patients.
- Type 2 – the binding or precipitating antibody, which reacts with intrinsic factor or with vitamin B_{12}–intrinsic factor complex and is seen in 35% of patients.

What is the relationship between pernicious anaemia and gastric carcinoma?

The incidence of gastric carcinoma in patients with pernicious anaemia is increased three-fold compared with that in the general population.

What gastrointestinal investigations would you perform in an asymptomatic patient with pernicious anaemia?

In the absence of gastrointestinal symptoms, gastroscopy or barium meal is not indicated, although many physicians tend to perform one of these investigations.

What do you understand by the term 'combined' degeneration of the cord?

This refers to the combined demyelination of both pyramids (or lateral columns) and posterior columns of the spinal cord.

What is the response of the neurological lesions to treatment with vitamin B_{12}?

The response to vitamin B_{12} therapy is variable: the lesions may improve, remain unchanged or even deteriorate. Sensory abnormalities improve more than motor abnormalities, and peripheral neuropathy responds better to treatment than myelopathy.

Subacute combined degeneration is also known as Putnam–Dana syndrome or Lichtheim's disease. James Jackson Putnam (1846–1918) and Charles Loomis Dana (1852–1935) were both US neurologists.

Ludwig Lichtheim (1845–1928), a German physician.

Pernicious anaemia was usually fatal until 1926, when Whipple, Minot and Murphy described the beneficial effects of feeding liver. The 1934 Nobel Prize in Medicine was awarded jointly to George Whipple (1878–1976) of University of Rochester, New York, and to George Minot (1885–1950) and William P. Murphy (1892–1987) of Harvard Medical School and Peter Brent Brigham Hospital, Boston, for their discoveries concerning liver therapy in cases of anaemia.

William B. Castle first found that oral administration of gastric juice (intrinsic factor) or beef (extrinsic factor, i.e. vitamin B_{12}) alone was not effective in the treatment of pernicious anaemia but that a mixture of both these factors rendered the patient erythropoietically active. Castle worked with Francis Peabody at the Harvard Medical School Unit at Boston City Hospital before he became Professor of Medicine at Harvard.

Case 72

TABES DORSALIS

INSTRUCTION

Examine this patient with lightning pains (lightning denotes that the pains are fleeting and does not necessarily mean they are excruciating).

SALIENT FEATURES

History

- 'Lightning pains' – sensation like an electric shock in the limbs, throat, stomach or rectum.
- High-stepping gait – patient may only hear his or her feet slapping the ground and feels as if walking on cotton-wool (due to loss of joint position sense).
- Constipation (this is present as a rule).
  - Ask the patient about bladder sensation (lost), overflow incontinence and impotence (if male).

Examination

- Examine the eyes:
  - Bilateral ptosis with frontalis overaction.
  - Argyll Robertson pupil (irregular, small pupil which reacts sluggishly to light as compared with accommodation).
  - Optic atrophy (primary).
- Examine the sensory system:
  - Posterior column signs.
  - Look for loss of pain sensation but with normal touch and temperature sensation over the nose, cheeks, inner aspects of the arms and legs, a band across the nipple and in the anal area.
  - Squeeze calf muscles and the Achilles tendon (evokes no pain as deep sensation is lost).
- Examine:
  - The ankle jerks (absent) and plantar response (normal).
  - The gait for ataxia (high-stepping gait) and Romberg's sign.
  - The knees and hips for Charcot's joints.
  - The feet for trophic ulcers.
- Tell the examiner that you would like to:
  - Check testicular sensation (usually lost early).

Note. Remember that, as a rule, the lower limbs are affected before the upper limbs. Very rarely, the upper limbs may be affected first – called 'cervical tabes'.

DIAGNOSIS

This patient has posterior column signs and Argyll Robertson pupil (lesion) due to tabes dorsalis (aetiology), and has severe ataxia (functional status).

ADVANCED-LEVEL QUESTIONS

What do you know about neurosyphilis?

There are five clinical patterns of neurosyphilis:

- Meningovascular disease, which occurs 3–4 years after primary infection.
- Tabes dorsalis, which occurs 10–35 years after primary infection.
- Generalized paralysis of the insane (GPI), which occurs 10–15 years after primary infection.
- Taboparesis (a combination of the latter two).
- Localized gummata.

Tertiary syphilis of the nervous system never develops in those who have received appropriate therapy in the early stages.

What is the underlying pathology?

A combination of neuronal degeneration and/or arterial lesions.

How would you confirm the diagnosis?

The Wassermann reaction, Venereal Disease Reference Laboratory (VDRL) or *Treponema pallidum* haemagglutination assay (TPHA):

- Meningovascular syphilis – 70% positive, whereas CSF shows 90% positive.
- Tabes dorsalis – 75% positive.
- GPI – nearly 100% positive.

Mention a few conditions in which the Wassermann reaction may be falsely positive.

Rheumatoid arthritis, SLE, chronic active hepatitis, infectious mononucleosis.

How would you treat the active syphilitic infection?

A course of parenteral penicillin.

How would you manage other symptoms of tabes?

- Lightning pains: simple analgesics, carbamazepine.
- Sensory ataxia: re-educational exercises to improve limb coordination.
- Bladder symptoms: avoid anticholinergics, employ urodynamic studies and intermittent self-catheterization.
- Visceral crises: opiate analgesics; in recurrent cases, section of lower thoracic spinal dorsal roots.
- Perforating ulcer: well-fitting shoes and regular foot care.
- Charcot's arthropathy: symptomatic treatment; avoid insertion of prostheses as results are poor.

In which group of patients is syphilis now common?

Those with underlying human immunodeficiency virus (HIV) infection.

What is the Jarisch–Herxheimer reaction?

An acute hypersensitivity reaction seen when a patient with syphilis is treated with penicillin. Toxins from the killed spirochaetes cause this reaction, which can be fatal. Steroids are often given during the first few days of penicillin therapy.

How may this patient present to the surgeons?

With acute abdominal pain (lancinating pains).

What are the methods of eliciting deep pain?

- Abadie's sign – the loss of pain sense in the Achilles tendon.
- Biernacki's sign – the absence of pain on pressure on the ulnar nerve.
- Pitres' sign – loss of pain on pressure on the testes.
- Haenel's sign – analgesia to pressure on the eyeballs.

Tabes was first recognized by Romberg and Duchenne. Fournier was the first to suspect that it was caused by syphilis.

A.P. Wassermann (1866–1925), a German physician.

A. Jarisch (1850–1902), Professor of Dermatology in Austria.

K. Herxheimer (1861–1944), a Jewish German dermatologist who died in a concentration camp.

In the first half of the 19th century, three European physicians – namely Mortiz Romberg, Marshall Hall and Bernadus Brach – described the loss of postural control in darkness of patients with severely impaired proprioceptive sensation (*Neurology* 2000; **55**: 1201–6). Romberg and Brach showed the relationship between this sign and tabes dorsalis.

Case 73

ULNAR NERVE PALSY

INSTRUCTION

Carry out a neurological examination of this patient's upper limbs.

SALIENT FEATURES

History

- Repeated trivial trauma to the elbow – the patient feels the 'funny bone'.
- Patient may be immobilized in the orthopaedic ward and use elbows to shuffle in bed.
- History of fracture of the upper arm in childhood (supracondylar fracture of humerus in childhood has an insidious course and can result in acute ulnar nerve palsy 20–30 years later – tardy ulnar palsy).

Examination

- Generalized wasting of the small muscles of the hand.
- There may be features of ulnar claw hand, i.e. hyperextension at the metacarpophalangeal joints and flexion at the interphalangeal joints of the fourth and fifth fingers.
- There is weakness of movement of the fingers, except that of the thenar eminence.
- There is sensory loss over the medial one and half fingers.

Proceed as follows:
- Examine the elbow for scars and signs of osteoarthrosis.
- Comment on the large carrying angle at the elbow, particularly in women (repeated extension and flexion of the arm can result in damage to the olecranon and consequently the ulnar nerve).

DIAGNOSIS

This patient has wasting of the small muscles of the hand and claw hand with sensory loss over the medial one and half fingers (lesion) due to ulnar nerve palsy caused by trauma (aetiology). She is unable to button her clothes (functional status).

ADVANCED-LEVEL QUESTIONS

What are the muscles supplied by the ulnar nerve?

The ulnar nerve is derived from the eighth cervical and first thoracic spinal nerves. It gives no branches above the elbow and supplies:

In the forearm:
- Flexor carpi ulnaris.
- Medial half of the flexor digitorum profundus.

In the hand:
- Movers of the little finger – abductor digiti minimi, flexor digiti minimi and opponens digiti minimi.
- Adductor pollicis (oblique and transverse heads).
- Dorsal and palmar interossei.
- Third and fourth lumbricals.
- Palmaris brevis.
- Inner head of flexor pollicis brevis.

How would you differentiate between a lesion above the cubital fossa and a lesion at the wrist?

- In lesions above the cubital fossa the flexor carpi ulnaris is involved.
- In lesions at the wrist, the adductor pollicis is involved.

How would you test the flexor carpi ulnaris?

- Ask the patient to keep her hand flat on a table with the palm facing upwards and then ask her to perform flexion and ulnar deviation at the wrist.

How would you test the adductor pollicis?

Ask the patient to grip a folded newspaper between the thumb and index finger of each hand so that the thumbs are uppermost – this causes the adductor to contract. When the muscle is paralysed, the thumb is incapable of adequate adduction and becomes flexed at the interphalangeal joint due to contraction of the flexor pollicis longus (innervated by the median nerve). This is known as Froment's sign.

What is ulnar paradox?

The higher the lesion in the upper limb, the lesser is the deformity. A lesion at or above the elbow causes paralysis of the ulnar half of the flexor digitorum profundus, interossei and lumbricals. Thus, the action of the paralysed profundus is not unopposed by the interossei and lumbricals; as a result the ring and little fingers are not flexed and hence there is no claw, whereas a lesion at the wrist causes an ulnar claw hand.

What causes the ulnar claw hand?

A lesion of the ulnar nerve at the wrist. The little and ring fingers are flexed at the interphalangeal joints and hyperextended at the metacarpophalangeal joints. The index and middle fingers are less affected as the first and second lumbricals are supplied by the median nerve.

What are the causes of claw hand?

True claw hand is seen in the following conditions:

- Advanced rheumatoid arthritis.
- Lesions of both the median and ulnar nerves, as in leprosy.
- Lesions of the medial cord of the brachial plexus.
- Anterior poliomyelitis.
- Syringomyelia.
- Polyneuritis.
- Amyotrophic lateral sclerosis.
- Klumpke's paralysis (lower brachial plexus, C7–8 involvement).
- Severe Volkmann's ischaemic contracture.

How is the ulnar nerve affected at the wrist?

The deep branch of the ulnar nerve is motor and may be compressed in Guyon's canal, which runs between the pisiform and hook of the hamate. This results in wasting and weakness of the interossei, particularly the first and the adductor pollicis, but sensation is spared. Also the hypothenar muscles are usually spared, although the third and fourth lumbricals may be affected. The nerve may be compressed in Guyon's canal by a ganglion, neuroma or repeated trauma. Surgical exposure of the nerve may be necessary when there is no history of trauma.

What is the most common cause of an ulnar nerve lesion at the elbow?

It is due to compression of the nerve by the fibrous arch of the flexor carpi ulnaris (the cubital tunnel) which arises as two heads from the medial epicondyle and the olecranon.

What do you understand by the term 'tardy ulnar nerve palsy'?

This occurs as a result of injuries or arthritic changes at the elbow causing a delayed or slowly progressive involvement of the ulnar nerve.

How would you rapidly exclude an injury to a major nerve in the arm?

- Radial nerve: test for wrist-drop.
- Ulnar nerve: test for Froment's sign (see above).
- Median nerve: Ochsner's clasping test.

Jules Froment (1876–1946), Professor of Clinical Medicine, Lyons, France.

A.J. Ochsner (b. 1896), a US surgeon, also investigated the role of tobacco in lung cancer.

Augusta Déjérine-Klumpke (1859–1927), a French neurologist, was the first woman to receive the title 'Internes des Hôpitaux' in 1877.

R. von Volkmann (1830–1889), Professor of Surgery in Halle, Germany.

Case 74

LATERAL POPLITEAL NERVE PALSY, L4, L5 (COMMON PERONEAL NERVE PALSY)

INSTRUCTION

Examine this patient's legs.
Test this patient's gait.

SALIENT FEATURES

History

- History of trauma to the nerve, particularly where it winds around the neck of the fibula where it is protected by only skin and fascia.
- Whether the symptoms occur after sitting cross-legged for prolonged periods.
- Recent weight loss, particularly in those who have been confined to bed (nerve more vulnerable because the protective fat and muscle is lost).
- Plaster around the knee.
- History of diabetes, polyarteritis nodosa, collagen vascular diseases (all causes of mononeuritis multiplex, p. 165).

Examination

- Wasting of the muscles on the lateral aspect of the leg, namely the peronei and tibialis anterior muscle.
- Weakness of dorsiflexion and eversion of the foot.
- Foot-drop.
- High-stepping gait.
- Loss of sensation on the lateral aspect of the leg and dorsum of the foot. If the deep peroneal branch is affected, the sensory loss may be limited to the dorsum of the web between the first and second toes.

Proceed as follows:
- Test the ankle jerk:
  - Absent ankle jerk: suspect an S1 lesion.
  - Normal jerk: common peroneal nerve palsy.
  - Brisk jerk: suspect an upper motor neuron lesion.
- Comment on calliper shoes by the bedside (if any).

DIAGNOSIS

This patient has wasting of the lateral aspect of the leg and sensory loss (lesion) due to common nerve palsy caused by trauma to the head of the fibula (aetiology), and has to wear callipers (functional status).

QUESTIONS

Mention a few causes.

- Compression resulting from application of a tourniquet or plaster of Paris cast. The nerve is vulnerable at the head of the fibula, where it lies on the surface of the hard bone and is covered only by skin.
- Direct trauma to the nerve.
- Leprosy (commonest cause worldwide).
- Ganglion arising from the superior tibiofibular joint may compress the nerve.
- Compression of the nerve by the tendinous edge of the peroneus longus.

ADVANCED-LEVEL QUESTIONS

How would you manage such a patient?

- Nerve conduction studies: there may be a local conduction block or slowing in the region of the head of the fibula. There may be denervation in the tibialis anterior and extensor digitorum profundus.
- If the intact nerve is severed: surgery.
- If the nerve is intact and concussed: 90 degree splint at night, calliper shoes with a 90 degree stop, and galvanic or faradic stimulation to maintain the bulk of the muscle until the nerve recovers.

What other types of nerve injury do you know?

- Neurapraxia, i.e. concussion of the nerve after which a complete recovery occurs.
- Axonotmesis, in which the axon is severed but the myelin sheath is intact; recovery may occur.
- Neurotmesis, in which the nerve is completely severed and the prognosis for recovery is poor.

What are the other causes of foot-drop?

- Peripheral neuropathy (see pp 164–6).
- L4, L5 root lesion.
- Motor neuron disease
- Sciatic nerve palsy.
- Lumbosacral plexus lesion.

Case 75

CARPAL TUNNEL SYNDROME

INSTRUCTION

Examine this patient's hands.

SALIENT FEATURES

History

- Ask the patient about nocturnal pain (commonest cause of hand pain at night).
- History of oral contraceptives, rheumatoid arthritis, myxoedema, acromegaly, chronic renal failure, sarcoidosis.
- Take a family history (abnormally small size of carpal tunnel runs in families).

Examination

- Wasting of the thenar eminence.
- Weakness of flexion, abduction and opposition of thumb.
- Diminished sensation over lateral three and half fingers.

Proceed as follows:

- Look carefully for scar of previous surgery (hidden by the crease of the wrist).
- Percuss over the course of the median nerve in the forearm: patient may experience tingling – this is Tinel's sign.
- Ask the patient to hyperextend the wrist maximally for 1 minute; this may bring on symptoms (dysaesthesia over the thumb and lateral two and half fingers).
- Tell the examiner that you would like to:
  - Examine for underlying causes such as myxoedema, acromegaly and rheumatoid arthritis.
  - Look for cervical spondylosis, frozen shoulder and tennis elbow (these may be associated).
  - Look for the Cimino–Brescia fistula for haemodialysis (*J Neurol Neurosurg Psychiatry* 1997; **40:** 511).

DIAGNOSIS

This patient has median nerve involvement of the hand with Tinel's sign (lesion) due to carpal tunnel syndrome as a complication of chronic haemodialysis (aetiology). The patient has disabling tingling and pain at night (functional status).

QUESTIONS

Mention a few causes of carpal tunnel syndrome.

- Pregnancy.
- Oral contraceptives.
- Rheumatoid arthritis.

- Myxoedema.
- Acromegaly.
- In chronic renal failure patients on long-term dialysis it is due to β_2-microglobulin as amyloid deposition.
- Sarcoidosis.
- Hyperparathyroidism.
- Amyloidosis (e.g. due to multiple myeloma).

How would you treat this condition?
- Diuretics.
- Wrist splint and ultrasound treatment (*BMJ* 1998; **316**: 731–5).
- Local steroid injection should be given proximal to the carpal tunnel (not into the tunnel because it may damage the nerve) (*BMJ* 1999; **319**: 884–6).
- Surgical decompression.

ADVANCED-LEVEL QUESTIONS

How would you confirm the diagnosis?
Nerve conduction studies (increased latency at the wrist on stimulation of the median nerve; the muscle action potential from abductor pollicis brevis is a valuable diagnostic sign). Rarely, the proximal latency may be normal with a prolonged distal latency due to an anastomosis between the ulnar and median nerves in the forearm. A negative test thus does not rule the syndrome out absolutely but calls it into question (*J Neurol Neurosurg Psychiatry* 1976; **39**: 449).

Mention a few clinical diagnostic tests (Lancet 1990; 335: 393).
- Wrist extension test: the patient is asked to extend his wrists for 1 minute; this should produce numbness or tingling in the distribution of the median nerve.
- Phalen's test: the patient is asked to keep both hands with the wrist in complete palmar flexion for 1 minute; this produces numbness or tingling in the distribution of the median nerve.
- Tourniquet test: the symptoms are produced when the blood pressure cuff is inflated above the systolic pressure.
- Pressure test: if pressure is placed where the median nerve leaves the carpal tunnel, it causes pain.
- Luthy's sign: if the skinfold between the thumb and index finger does not close tightly around a bottle or cup because of thumb abduction paresis, this test is regarded as positive.
- Durkan's test: direct pressure over the carpal tunnel – the carpal compression test – is more sensitive and specific than the Tinel and Phalen sign.

Mention other entrapment neuropathies.
- Meralgia paraesthetica (lateral cutaneous nerve of the thigh trapped under the inguinal ligament).
- Elbow tunnel syndrome (ulnar nerve trapped in the cubital tunnel; see p.207).
- Common peroneal nerve trapped at the head of the fibula (see p. 211).
- Morton's metatarsalgia (trapped medial and lateral plantar nerves causing pain between third and fourth toes).
- Tarsal tunnel syndrome (posterior tibial nerve is trapped).

- Suprascapular nerve trapped in the spinoglenoid notch.
- Radial nerve trapped in the humeral groove.
- Anterior interosseous nerve trapped between the heads of the pronator muscle.

> Jules Tinel (1879–1952), a French neurologist, described it as the 'sign of formication' in his book on nerve wounds. He took an active part in the French resistance.
>
> T.G. Morton (1835–1903), a US surgeon, described this syndrome in 1876.

Case 76

RADIAL NERVE PALSY

INSTRUCTION

Perform a neurological examination of this patient's arms.

SALIENT FEATURES

History

- An intoxicated person sleeping with the head resting in the upper arm, causing compression of the nerve over the middle third of the humerus; this is known as Saturday night palsy.
- Trauma to the nerve while it courses through the axilla, e.g. crutch palsy, shoulder dislocation, fractures of humerus or radius.
- History of exposure to lead (lead neuropathy).

Examination

- There is weakness of extension of the wrist and elbow (wrist flexion is normal).
- The patient is unable to straighten her fingers.
- If the wrist is passively extended, however, the patient is able to straighten her fingers at the interphalangeal joints (due to the action of interossei and lumbricals) but is unable to extend the metacarpophalangeal joint.
- There appears to be a weakness in abduction and adduction of the fingers, but this is not present when the hand is kept flat on a table and the fingers are extended.

Proceed as follows:

- Test the brachioradialis, looking for weakened elbow flexion. When the patient attempts to flex the elbow against resistance, the brachioradialis no longer springs up.
- Test the triceps.
- Check sensation over the first dorsal interosseous.

Note.

1. The radial nerve gives off two branches at the elbow:
   – Superficial radial (entirely sensory).
   – Posterior interosseous (entirely muscular).

2. If the injury is situated above the junction of the upper and middle thirds of the humerus, the action of triceps is lost.
3. If the lesion is situated in the middle third of the humerus (frequent site of fracture of the humerus), the brachioradialis is spared.

DIAGNOSIS

This patient has features of radial nerve palsy with the brachioradialis remaining unaffected (lesion) resulting from a fracture located in the middle third of the humerus (aetiology); she is disabled by the deficits (functional status).

ADVANCED-LEVEL QUESTIONS

What is the cutaneous supply of the radial nerve?
Overlap in the areas supplied by the median and ulnar nerves means that only a small area of skin over the first dorsal interosseous is exclusively supplied by the radial nerve.

What do you know about the origin of the radial nerve?
The radial nerve is the termination of the posterior cord of the brachial plexus and is derived from the fifth, sixth, seventh and eighth cervical spinal nerves.

What are the branches of the radial nerve in the forearm?
The radial nerve enters the forearm and passes between the two heads of the supinator muscle to become the posterior interosseous nerve.

What muscles are supplied by the radial nerve?
The radial nerve supplies the triceps, anconeus, brachioradialis, extensor carpi radialis longus and, through the posterior interosseous nerve, extensor carpi radialis brevis, supinator, extensor digitorum, extensor digiti minimi, extensor ulnaris, the three extensors of the thumb and extensor indicis.

Case 77

CHOREA

PATIENT 1: SYDENHAM'S CHOREA

Instruction
Look at this patient.

Salient features

History
- Ask about sore throats if the patient is an adolescent, particularly if female; suspect Sydenham's chorea (St Vitus' dance) in rheumatic fever.

- Take a family history (especially in the middle-aged adult) for Huntington's disease.
- Take a history of oral contraceptive use in a young woman or recent pregnancy (chorea gravidorum).

Examination

- Irregular, jerking, ill-sustained, unpredictable, quasipurposive movements of the upper limbs.
- The patient is clumsy and keeps dropping objects. Patients with mild disease may show increased fidgeting or restlessness.

Proceed as follows:

- Check the grip of the hands – ask the patient to squeeze your fingers. A squeezing and relaxing motion occurs which has been described as a 'milkmaid's grip'.
- Look at the tongue for any involuntary movements – known as 'jack-in-the box' tongue or 'bag of worms'.
- Test deep tendon reflexes ('pendular' or 'hung-up' reflexes).
- Tell the examiner that you would like to assess mental status (to exclude premature dementia seen in Huntington's disease).

Diagnosis

This young patient has Sydenham's chorea (lesion) secondary to streptococcal sore throat (aetiology); this condition is usually self-limiting.

ADVANCED-LEVEL QUESTIONS

Mention a few more causes of chorea.

- SLE.
- Polycythaemia vera.
- Chorea gravidorum, seen in pregnancy.
- Idiopathic hypoparathyroidism.
- Following a stroke.
- Kernicterus.

What is the prognosis of patients with Sydenham's chorea?

Most patients recover within 1 month; a few may have relapses. A small proportion may develop valvular heart disease and hence should receive penicillin prophylaxis to prevent recurrence of rheumatic fever.

Is there any haematological disorder associated with chorea?

- Polycythaemia vera.
- Neuroacanthocytosis or 'chorea–acanthocystosis' where more than 15% of the red blood cells are acanthocytes (*Brain* 1991; **114:** 13).

Thomas Sydenham (1624–1689) was a Puritan from Dorset, and in 1666 published his first work on fevers which he dedicated to Robert Boyle.

Chorea in Greek means 'dance'.

PATIENT 2: HUNTINGTON'S DISEASE

Instruction

Look at this patient and ask him a few questions.

Salient features

History

Tell the examiner that you would like to take a family history of dementia and chorea.

Examination

- Young adult (aged 30–50 years).
- Chorea.
- Patient has dementia.

Diagnosis

This patient has chorea (lesion) due to Huntington's disease, and is severely limited by the disease and chorea.

ADVANCED-LEVEL QUESTIONS

What do you know about Huntington's disease?

It is an autosomal dominant disorder with full penetrance characterized by progressive chorea and dementia in middle life. These characteristic findings result from severe neuronal loss, initially in the neostriatum and later in the cerebral cortex. The defect is on the small arm of chromosome 4. There is associated random repetition of a sequence of trinucleotides (viz. CAG; normal chromosomes contain about 11–34 copies of this repeat). In Huntington's disease, the greater the number of CAG repeats, the earlier the onset of disease (*Cell* 1993; **72:** 971). The protein product for the gene has been termed 'huntingtin'. It has been proposed that the huntingtin protein is cleaved to fragments which are conjugated with ubiquitin and carried to the proteasome complex. Components of both huntingtin and the proteasome then translocate to the nucleus to form intranuclear inclusions, and over time this process leads to cell death.

There is a marked reduction in acetylcholine, substance P and γ-aminobutyric acid (GABA) activity in the corpus striatum, whereas dopamine activity is normal and somatostatin is increased (*Ann Neurol* 1990; **27:** 357).

Using neuropeptide immunochemistry, the chorea has been shown to be associated with damage to the lateral globus pallidus, whereas the parkinsonian signs result from additional damage in projections of the medial globus pallidus.

What is the advantage of assessing CAG expansion in persons at risk for Huntington's disease?

It is a direct test that allows more accurate assessment of genetic risk without the need to obtain DNA from family members. This also allows privacy and confidentiality to be maintained because of the reduced need for blood samples from relatives. However, since the misdiagnosis of other illnesses as Huntington's disease may occur, the testing of DNA from at least one affected relative is recommended to confirm that CAG expansion is present in other affected persons in the family. This finding will allow the correct interpretation of a normal number of CAG repeats in a person at risk.

Are any other diseases known to be associated with increased numbers of triplet repeats?

Yes; these include myotonic muscular dystrophy, spinocerebellar ataxia type 1, FRAXE mental retardation (a variant of fragile X syndrome) and hereditary dentatorubral pallidoluysian atrophy (DRPLA).

How would you manage this patient?

A combination of valproate and olanzapine may help in relieving the psychosis and movement disorders associated with Huntington's disease (*N Engl J Med* 2000; **343**: 973).

George Summer Huntington (1851–1916) first documented (in 1909) the clinical and hereditary features of this condition in a family from Suffolk settled in Long Island in New York.

Case 78

HEMIBALLISMUS

INSTRUCTION

Look at this patient.

SALIENT FEATURES

History

- Sudden onset.
- Cardiovascular disease for source of emboli – atrial fibrillation, valvular heart disease or severe left ventricular dysfunction.

Examination

Unilateral, involuntary, flinging movements of the proximal upper limbs.

DIAGNOSIS

This patient has hemiballismus (lesion) due to a stroke (aetiology), and has severe exhaustion (functional status).

ADVANCED-LEVEL QUESTIONS

Where is the lesion?

In the ipsilateral subthalamic nucleus of Luys.

What is the underlying cause?

- Vascular event, usually an infarct.

- Rarely tumour, abscess, multiple sclerosis, arteriovenous malformation, cerebral trauma.

What investigations would you perform?
- ECG for atrial fibrillation.
- Echocardiogram to rule out source of emboli.
- CT scan, but this is usually unhelpful because the lesion is small.

What is the prognosis?
The prognosis for recovery is usually good and most patients recover within 1 month. Hemiballismus may occasionally prevent the patient from eating and can be exhausting or even life threatening.

Which drug is usually used to ameliorate this condition?
Tetrabenazine or haloperidol is usually effective. Prolonged and medically intractable hemiballismus can be treated with contralateral thalamotomy or pallidectomy.

> J.B. Luys (1828–1897), a French neurologist who also studied insanity, hysteria and hypnotism.

Case 79

OROFACIAL DYSKINESIA

INSTRUCTION

Look at this patient.

SALIENT FEATURES

History
- Ask the patient about removal of teeth and how long he/she has been edentulous.
- Date of onset and duration.
- Drug history (phenothiazines, L-dopa and related drugs).

Examination

Smacking, chewing or chomping movement of the lips, seen particularly in elderly patients; it usually involves the masticatory, lower facial and tongue muscles.

Proceed as follows:
Comment if the patient is edentulous (*Ann Neurol* 1983; **13:** 97).

DIAGNOSIS

This patient has orofacial dyskinesia (lesion) due to phenothiazines (aetiology) and is in considerable distress (functional status).

ADVANCED-LEVEL QUESTIONS

What is Meige's syndrome?
A combination of blepharospasm, oromandibular dystonia and cranial dystonia. There is spastic dysarthria when the throat and respiratory muscles are affected. The neck muscles are invariably involved.

What do you understand by tardive dyskinesia?
It is a drug-induced dyskinesia which may appear long after drug therapy has been discontinued. It is troublesome and may resist all forms of treatment.

How would you manage such patients?
Anticholinergic drugs, baclofen, benzodiazepines and tetrabenazine, but pharmaco-therapy is usually ineffective. Injection of botulinum toxin into the masseter, temporalis and internal pterygoid muscles results in improvement in chewing and speech in approximately 80% of patients with jaw closure due to oromandibular dystonia (*Ophthalmology* 1987; **2**: 237–54).

Mention a few other dystonias.
Blepharospasm, spasmodic torticollis, laryngeal dystonias, writer's cramp.

> H. Meige (1866–1940), a French physician, also wrote on ancient Egyptian diseases.

Case 80

INTERNUCLEAR OPHTHALMOPLEGIA

INSTRUCTION
Examine this patient's eyes.

SALIENT FEATURES

History
- Diplopia.
- History of multiple sclerosis.
- Neurofibroma (causing pontine gliomas).
- Drugs (phenytoin, carbamazepine).

Examination
- Nystagmus is more prominent in the abducting eye (Harris' sign).
- Diverging squint.
- Abduction in either eye is normal, whereas adduction is impaired, i.e. there is dissociation of eye movements. On covering the abducting eye, the adduction in the other eye is normal.

Proceed as follows:
Tell the examiner that you would like to look for other signs of demyelination: optic atrophy, pale discs, pyramidal signs.

DIAGNOSIS

This patient has internuclear ophthalmoplegia (lesion) which is probably due to multiple sclerosis (aetiology).

ADVANCED-LEVEL QUESTIONS

Where is the lesion?
In the medial longitudinal bundle which connects the sixth nerve nucleus on one side to the third nerve nucleus on the opposite side of the brainstem. The eye will not adduct because the third nerve and, therefore, the medial rectus have been disconnected from the lateral gaze centre and sixth nucleus of the opposite side.

What are the causes?
- Multiple sclerosis.
- Vascular disease.
- Tumour (pontine glioma).
- Inflammatory lesions of the brainstem.
- Drugs (phenytoin, carbamazepine).

How would you investigate?
- MRI scan.
- Edrophonium (Tensilon) test to exclude myasthenia.

What are the mechanisms to elicit conjugate gaze?
There are four mechanisms for eliciting conjugate gaze in any direction:

1. The saccadic system involves voluntary gaze (even when the eyes are shut). Pathways mediating saccadic gaze arise in the frontal lobe and pass to the pontine gaze centre.
2. The pursuit system allows the subject to follow a moving object. Pathways mediating pursuit movements arise in the parieto-occipital lobe and pass to the pontine gaze centre.
3. The optokinetic system involves the restoration of gaze despite movements from the outside world, e.g. while a subject is sitting in a railway train and looking out of the window, the eyes move slowly as the train moves, to be followed by rapid corrective movement back to the initial position of gaze. This is tested with a hand-held drum bearing vertical black and white stripes. Optokinetic nystagmus is often disturbed even before damage to the pursuit system is apparent.
4. The vestibulo-ocular system involves correction of gaze for movements of the head. This is achieved by inputs from the labyrinths and neck proprioreceptors to the brainstem. The patient is asked to fixate to the examiner's face and the head is briskly rotated by the examiner from side to side or up and down (doll's head manoeuvre). In supranuclear gaze palsy, these vestibulo-ocular reflex eye movements are preserved, despite the absence of both saccadic and pursuit movements. Caloric tests are used to demonstrate the vestibulo-ocular reflex.

Note.
1. Diplopia is not a feature of defects in conjugate gaze.
2. The centres for saccadic and pursuit movements in the cerebral hemispheres control deviation of the eyes towards the opposite side of the body. These pathways descend towards the brainstem and cross before they reach the pons.
3. The centres for conjugate vertical gaze lie in the midbrain.
4. The centres for conjugate downward vertical gaze are not well localized, and lesions both in the midbrain and at the level of the foramen magnum can cause defects of voluntary downgaze.

What do you know about 'Fisher's one and a half syndrome'?

It is a syndrome in which horizontal eye movement is absent and the other eye is capable only of abduction – one and a half movements are paralysed. The vertical eye movements and the pupils are normal. The cause is a lesion in the pontine region involving the medial longitudinal fasciculus and the parapontine reticular formation on the same side. This results in failure of conjugate gaze to the same side, impairment of adduction of the eye, and nystagmus on abduction of the other eye.

Internuclear ophthalmoplegia was first reported by Bielschowsky (1902) and then subsequently by Lhermitte in 1922. Spiller in 1924 described the necropsy findings, implicated the median longitudinal fasciculus and suggested the name 'ophthalmoplegia internuclearis anterior'.

Case 81

CEREBELLOPONTINE ANGLE TUMOUR

INSTRUCTION

Examine this patient's cranial nerves.

SALIENT FEATURES

Damage to the seventh and eighth cranial nerves is the hallmark of this lesion in this region.

Proceed as follows:
- Check the corneal reflex and test the trigeminal nerve (see p. 108).
- Tell the examiner that you would like to look for the following:
  - Cerebellar signs (see pp 143–5).
  - Signs of neurofibroma type 2 (see p. 197).
  - Papilloedema (seen uncommonly as a result of raised intracranial pressure).

DIAGNOSIS

This patient has features of cerebellopontine angle tumour (lesion) usually due to an acoustic neuroma (aetiology), and has severe hearing loss (functional status).

ADVANCED-LEVEL QUESTIONS

Mention a few causes of cerebellopontine angle lesions.

- Acoustic neuroma.
- Meningioma, cholesteatoma, haemangioblastoma, aneurysm of the basilar artery.
- Pontine glioma.
- Medulloblastoma and astrocytoma of the cerebellum.
- Carcinoma of the nasopharynx.
- Local meningeal involvement by syphilis and tuberculosis.

What do you understand by the term 'cerebellopontine angle'?

It is the shallow triangular fossa lying between the cerebellum, lateral pons and the inner third of the petrous temporal bone. It extends from the trigeminal nerve (above) to the glossopharyngeal nerve (below). The abducens nerve runs along the medial edge, whereas the facial and auditory cranial nerves transverse the angle to enter the internal auditory meatus.

What is the histology of acoustic neurofibroma?

It consists of elongated cells similar to spindle fibroblasts with much collagen and reticulum. They are believed to arise from Schwann cells and are also known as schwannomas.

How would you investigate such patients?

- Skull radiography, tomography of the internal auditory meatus, and CT head scan.
- Serology for syphilis.
- Audiography.
- Caloric test (which will reveal that the labyrinth is destroyed).
- Vertebral angiography.
- CSF: may be abnormal or have raised protein concentration.
- MRI.

What is the treatment in this condition?

- Microsurgical resection.
- Stereotactic radiosurgery (*N Engl J Med* 1998; **339**: 1426–33).
- Conservative approach.

F.T. Schwann (1810–1882), a German anatomist, was Professor of Anatomy in the Louvain. He was one of the first to demonstrate that fermentation was associated with living organisms. Independently from Schleiden, he concluded that plants are formed of cells; this is known as the Schleiden–Schwann cellular theory. Schwann also discovered that the upper oesophagus contains striated muscle. He discovered pepsin and showed that bile was essential for digestion.

The first surgical removal of an acoustic neuroma was performed in 1894 (*N Engl J Med* 1998; **339**: 1471).

L. Leksell was the first to use radiosurgery – what he called the 'gamma knife' (*Acta Chir Scand* 1971; **137**: 763–5).

Case 82

JUGULAR FORAMEN SYNDROME

INSTRUCTION

Examine this patient's cranial nerves.

SALIENT FEATURES

History

The clinical presentation consists of symptoms of impaired function of the last four cranial nerves:

- Hoarseness of voice.
- Nasal quality to the speech.
- Nasal regurgitation and dysphagia.
- Aspiration of food with choking attacks.
- Weakness of the sternomastoids and trapezii.
- Wasting of the tongue (often noticed by the dentist).
- Pain in and around the ear (due to damage of the ninth and tenth cranial nerves which carry sensation to the external auditory meatus and behind the ear).
- Headache.
- Ptosis (due to Horner's syndrome).

Examination

- Sluggish movement of the palate when the patient says 'aah' on the affected side.
- Absent gag reflex on the same side.
- Flattening of the shoulder on the same side.
- Wasting of the sternomastoid.
- Weakness when the patient moves her chin to the opposite side.
- Difficulty in shrugging the shoulder on the same side.

Proceed as follows:
- Look for wasting and deviation of the tongue (twelfth cranial nerve palsy).
- Tell the examiner that you would like to check for two signs:
  - Bovine cough.
  - Husky voice.

DIAGNOSIS

This patient has features of jugular foramen syndrome (lesion) which could be due to several causes including pharyngeal neoplasm (aetiology); she has difficulty in swallowing and requires a nasogastric tube (functional status).

ADVANCED-LEVEL QUESTIONS

Where is the jugular foramen located?

Between the lateral part of the occipital bone and the petrous portion of the temporal bones.

Which cranial nerves leave the skull through the jugular foramen?

The ninth, tenth and eleventh cranial nerves.

Through which foramen does the twelfth cranial nerve leave the skull?

The anterior condylar foramen.

Mention a few causes of jugular foramen syndrome.

- Carcinoma of the pharynx is the commonest cause.
- Fractured base of the skull.
- Paget's disease.
- Basal meningitis.
- Neurofibroma or any tumour.
- Thrombosis of jugular vein.

Do you know of any eponymous syndromes of the lower cranial nerves?

- Vernet's syndrome: paresis of the ninth, tenth and eleventh cranial nerves due to extension of tumour into the jugular foramen.
- Collet–Sicard syndrome: fracture of the floor of the posterior cranial fossa, causing palsy of the last four cranial nerves.
- Villaret's syndrome: ipsilateral paralysis of the last four cranial nerves and cervical sympathetics.
- Syndrome of Schmidt: vagus and accessory nerve involvement.
- Syndrome of Hughlings Jackson: accessory and hypoglossal nerve involvement.

What is the cause of unilateral eleventh cranial nerve palsy?

- Trauma to the nerve in the neck.
- In hemiplegia.

How would you test for eleventh cranial nerve palsy?

- Sternocleidomastoids are tested by having the patient turn her head forcibly against the examiner's hand in a direction away from the muscle being tested while the muscle is observed and palpated.
- Upper portion of the trapezii is tested by having the patient forcibly elevate (shrug) her shoulder while the examiner attempts to depress the shoulder.

M. Vernet (b. 1887), a French neurologist, described this syndrome in 1916.

M. Villaret (1877–1946), Professor of Neurology in France, described this syndrome in 1918.

F.J. Collet (b. 1870), a French otolaryngologist, described his patient in 1915.

J.A. Sicard (1872–1929), a French physician and radiologist, was the first to perform myelography, use alcohol in trigeminal neuralgia and inject a sclerosing substance in varicose veins. He described his patient in 1917.

Case 83

PSEUDOBULBAR PALSY

INSTRUCTION

Examine this patient's cranial nerves.

SALIENT FEATURES

History

- Ask the patient whether he has difficulty in swallowing or nasal regurgitation.
- Any changes in speech.
- Emotional lability.
- History of stroke, multiple sclerosis or motor neuron disease.

Examination

- Spastic tongue.
- Donald Duck speech.
- Patient is emotionally labile (uncontrollable laughter or crying).
- Sluggish movements of the palate when the patient is asked to say 'aah'.

Proceed as follows:
- Check the jaw jerk.
- Tell the examiner that you would like to do the following:
  - Check the gag reflex.
  - Look for upper motor neuron signs in the limbs.

DIAGNOSIS

This patient has pseudobulbar palsy (lesion) due to a stroke (aetiology); he has difficulty in swallowing and emotional lability (functional status).

QUESTIONS

What could be the underlying cause?
- Bilateral stroke.
- Multiple sclerosis.
- Motor neuron disease.

ADVANCED-LEVEL QUESTIONS

How would you manage the swallowing and speech difficulties?
The patient would initially require assessment by a speech therapist for the difficulty in swallowing and speech deficits. Barium swallow with videofluoroscopy may be required to 'visualize' the swallowing.

How would you differentiate bulbar palsy from pseudobulbar palsy?

	Pseudobulbar palsy	Bulbar palsy
Prevalence	Common	Rare
Type of lesion	Upper motor neuron	Lower motor neuron, muscular
Site of lesion	Bilateral, usually in the internal capsule	Medulla oblongata
Tongue	Small, stiff and spastic	Flaccid, fasciculations
Speech	Slow, thick and indistinct	Nasal twang
Nasal regurgitation	Not prominent	Prominent
Jaw jerk	Brisk	Normal or absent
Other findings	Upper motor neuron lesions of the limbs	Lower motor neuron lesions of the limbs
Affect	Emotionally labile	Normal affect
Causes	Stroke, multiple sclerosis, motor neuron disease, Creutzfeld–Jakob disease	Motor neuron disease, poliomyelitis, Guillain–Barré syndrome, myasthenia gravis myopathy

Case 84

BULBAR PALSY

INSTRUCTION

Examine this patient's cranial nerves.
Ask the patient a few questions.
Test this patient's speech.

SALIENT FEATURES

History

- Ask the patient about nasal regurgitation, dysphagia.
- Slurring of speech (patient may sound intoxicated).
- Difficulty in chewing and swallowing.
- Choking on liquids.

Examination

- Nasal speech lacking in modulation, and great difficulty with all consonants.
- Wasting of the tongue with fasciculations.
- Weakness of the soft palate: ask the patient to say 'aah'.
- There may be accumulation of saliva.
- Fasciculation elsewhere (particularly trunk muscles).

Proceed as follows:
- Check the jaw jerk (normal or absent).
- Tell the examiner that you would like to do the following:
  - Check the gag reflex.
  - Examine the hands for fasciculations, dissociated sensory loss.

DIAGNOSIS

This patient has bulbar palsy (lesion) due to motor neuron disease (aetiology) and has difficulty in swallowing (functional status).

QUESTIONS

What may be the underlying cause?
- Motor neuron disease – after the age of 60, rapidly progressive bulbar palsy is the commonest presenting symptom (see pp 193–6).
- Guillain–Barré syndrome.
- Syringomyelia (see pp 199–202).
- Poliomyelitis.
- Nasopharyngeal tumour.
- Neurosyphilis.
- Neurosarcoid.

Case 85

WALLENBERG'S SYNDROME (LATERAL MEDULLARY SYNDROME)

INSTRUCTION

Examine this patient's cranial nerves.

SALIENT FEATURES

History

- Severe nausea, vomiting, nystagmus (involvement of the lower vestibular nuclei).
- Limb ataxia (involvement of the inferior cerebellar peduncle).
- Intractable hiccups, dysphagia (ninth and tenth cranial nerve involvement).

Examination

- Nystagmus.
- Ipsilateral involvement of fifth, sixth, seventh and eighth cranial nerves.
- Bulbar palsy: impaired gag, sluggish palatal movements.
- Horner's syndrome.

Proceed as follows:
Tell the examiner that you would like to check for the following:

- Cerebellar signs on the same side.
- Pain and temperature sensory loss on the opposite side (dissociated sensory loss).

Remember. The main features of this syndrome are *ipsilateral* Horner's syndrome and *contralateral* loss of pain and temperature sensation.

DIAGNOSIS

This patient has lateral medullary syndrome (lesion) due to a stroke (aetiology) and has dysphagia (functional status).

ADVANCED-LEVEL QUESTIONS

Which vessel is occluded?
Any of the following five vessels:

- Posterior inferior cerebellar artery.
- Vertebral artery.
- Superior, middle or inferior lateral medullary arteries.

How may these patients present?
With sudden onset of vertigo, vomiting and ipsilateral ataxia, with contralateral loss of pain and temperature sensations.

Where is the lesion in lateral medullary syndrome?
The syndrome results from infarction of a wedge-shaped area of the lateral aspect of the medulla and inferior surface of the cerebellum. The deficits are caused by involvement of one side of the nucleus ambiguus, trigeminal nucleus, vestibular nuclei, cerebellar peduncle, spinothalamic tract and autonomic fibres.

What is the medial medullary syndrome?
It is caused by occlusion of the lower basilar artery or vertebral artery. Ipsilateral lesions result in paralysis and wasting of the tongue. Contralateral lesions result in hemiplegia and loss of vibration and joint position sense.

Mention a few other eponymous syndromes with crossed hemiplegias.
- Weber's syndrome: contralateral hemiplegia with ipsilateral lower motor neuron lesion of the oculomotor nerve. The lesion is in the midbrain.
- Millard–Gubler syndrome: contralateral hemiplegia with lower motor neuron lesion of the abducens nerve. The lesion is in the pons.
- Foville's syndrome: as Millard–Gubler syndrome with gaze palsy.

What is Benedikt's syndrome?
It causes cerebellar signs on the side opposite the third nerve palsy (which is produced by damage to the nucleus itself or to the nerve fascicle). It is due to a midbrain vascular lesion causing damage to the red nucleus, interrupting the dentatorubrothalamic tract from the opposite cerebellum.

Auguste L.J. Millard (1830–1915) and Adolphe Marie Gubler (1821–1879), Parisian physicians.
Achille L.F. Foville (1799–1878), a Parisian neurologist.
A. Wallenburg (1862–1949), a German neurologist, described this syndrome in 1895.

Case 86

WINGING OF THE SCAPULA

INSTRUCTION

Look at this patient's back.

SALIENT FEATURES

History

• Difficulty in raising the arms above the level of the shoulders.
• Winging of the scapula.

Examination

• Winging of the scapula.
• Difficulty in raising the arms above the horizontal.

Proceed as follows:
• Check whether the winging is unilateral or bilateral.
• Ask the patient to push the outstretched arm firmly against your hand, and check whether or not the winging is more prominent.
• Tell the examiner that you would like to examine the muscles in the arm to rule out muscular dystrophy.

DIAGNOSIS

This patient has winging of the scapula (lesion) due to palsy of the long thoracic nerve of Bell (aetiology).

ADVANCED-LEVEL QUESTIONS

Which nerve lesion is responsible for these signs?
Long thoracic nerve of Bell arising from the anterior rami of C5, C6 and C7.

Which muscle is supplied by this nerve?
Serratus anterior.

What is the action of the serratus anterior?
It is responsible for the lateral and forward movement of the scapula, keeping it closely applied to the thorax.

Which other muscle palsy can cause winging of the scapula?
Paralysis of the trapezius.

How would you differentiate winging of the scapula caused by serratus anterior palsy from that of trapezius palsy?
In serratus anterior palsy, abduction of the arm laterally produces little winging of the scapula, whereas winging due to weakness of the trapezius is intensified by abduction of the arm against resistance.

What do you know about brachial neuritis?
Brachial neuritis (neuralgic amyotrophy, Parsonage–Turner syndrome) often follows an infection or surgery. Diagnosis may be difficult initially when the patient has only pain. Later the patient has muscular weakness, affecting particularly the deltoid and serratus anterior (winging of the scapula). Atrophy often becomes prominent. In this syndrome there is often more than one lesion. The white cell count in the cerebrospinal fluid is occasionally raised. Recovery occurs over the next year and may not be complete.

Case 87

BECKER MUSCULAR DYSTROPHY

INSTRUCTION
Examine this patient's muscles.

SALIENT FEATURES

History
- Is there is a family history of the condition?
- Age of onset.
- Ask about shortness of breath (heart failure due to cardiomyopathy).
- History of mental retardation.

Examination
- Young adult male (>15 years).
- Proximal weakness of the lower extremities (in later stages more generalized muscle involvement).
- Pseudohypertrophy of calves.
- Facial muscle weakness is characteristically absent or insignificant.
- Kyphoscoliosis in late stages.

Proceed as follows:

Tell the examiner that you would like to check the IQ (mental retardation may be seen).

DIAGNOSIS

This young patient has proximal muscle weakness and pseudohypertrophy (lesion) due to Becker's dystrophy (aetiology). The patient has mild disability and the condition is usually progressive (functional status).

QUESTIONS

What is the difference between Duchenne and Becker muscular dystrophy?

By definition, patients with Becker muscular dystrophy can ambulate beyond the age of 15 years. The onset in Becker is usually between the ages of 5 and 15 years, but onset can occur in the third or fourth decades or even later. The majority survive into the fourth or fifth decades.

Is there any difference between the genetics of Duchenne and Becker muscular dystrophy?

No; both Duchenne and Becker muscular dystrophy are caused by mutations in the same dystrophin gene, located at Xp21. Another protein, utrophin, closely related to dystrophin, is encoded by a second gene on chromosome 6. In normal muscle, utrophin is located predominantly in the neuromuscular junction, whereas dystrophin is found in the sarcolemmal surface.

How would you confirm the clinical diagnosis of Becker dystrophy?

It requires Western blot analysis of muscle biopsy samples, demonstrating abnormal or reduced dystrophin.

ADVANCED-LEVEL QUESTIONS

Mention other X-linked myopathies.

- X-linked tubular myopathy, linked to Xq28.
- McLeod syndrome, where the responsible gene has been localized to Xp21 and the phenotype is characterized by mild, even subclinical, myopathy, acanthocytosis and haemolytic anaemia. The definitive diagnosis rests on determination of the Kell red cell antigen phenotype.
- Emery–Dreifuss muscular dystrophy, first described in a large family in Virginia by Emery and Dreifuss in 1966. Known association with deutan colour blindness led to localization of the gene on Xq28. The weakness presents in early childhood and is slowly progressive. The distribution of weakness is unique: an early humeral–peroneal pattern eventually evolves into a scapulo-humero-pelvo-peroneal distribution. Marked focal atrophy of the humeral and peroneal muscles is a consistent feature. Pseudohypertrophy is absent, except in extensor digitorum brevis.

P.E. Becker, Professor of Human Genetics at the University of Göttingen, Germany. Edward Meryon described Duchenne muscular dystrophy in 1852, 10 years before the French neurologist Guillaume Benjamin Amand Duchenne, with remarkably prescient pathological observations: '... the sarcolemma or tunic of the elementary fibre was broken and destroyed' (Emery AEH, Emery MLH 1995 *The History of a Genetic Disease: Duchenne Muscular Dystrophy or Meryon's Disease*).

Duchenne is reported to have designed a version of the modern muscle biopsy needle which he kept in alcohol to prevent rusting. He could not have known that this also prevented sepsis.

Newton Morton, a geneticist, was the first to introduce discriminant and segregation analysis into modern human genetics as a part of a large population study of Duchenne muscular dystrophy. Tony Murphy used the disease to develop bayesian risk-analysis procedures.

Case 88

TETRAPLEGIA

INSTRUCTION

Carry out a neurological examination of this patient's lower limbs.

SALIENT FEATURES

History

- Ask about bladder symptoms and check sacral sensation.
- Ask about radicular pain.
- Ask whether the weakness was sudden or gradual.
- History of trauma, multiple sclerosis.

Examination

- Increased or decreased tone in both lower limbs.
- Hyper-reflexia.
- Ankle clonus.
- Weakness in all four limbs.
- Wasted hands (cervical spondylosis, motor neuron disease or syringomyelia).

Proceed as follows:
- Remember to check the sensory level and examine the spine.
- Tell the examiner that you would like to do the following:
  - Check for cerebellar signs (multiple sclerosis, Friedreich's ataxia).
  - Check blood pressure (postural hypotension, autonomic dysreflexia).
- Try to localize the level of lesion using the following:
  - Spasticity of all four limbs: lesion above the C4 spinal cord segment.
  - Spasticity of the lower limbs with flaccid weakness of some muscles of the upper limb: lesion of cervical cord enlargement (C5–T2).

- Deep tendon reflexes – an absent biceps jerk with a brisk supinator jerk (inversion of the supinator jerk) or an absent biceps and supinator with a brisk triceps jerk localizes the lesion to C5–6.
- Radicular pain – useful early in the disease; with time becomes diffuse and ceases to have localizing value.
- Superficial sensation – not good for localizing as the level of sensory loss may vary greatly in different individuals and in different types of lesion.

DIAGNOSIS

This patient has weakness in all four limbs (lesion) due to spinal trauma (aetiology), and is wheelchair bound (functional status).

ADVANCED-LEVEL QUESTIONS

What is autonomic dysreflexia?

It is bradycardia, sweating, rhinorrhoea, pounding headaches and severe paroxysmal hypertension which presents quickly and can rapidly precipitate seizures and death if not relieved. Precipitating factors include blockage of urinary catheter, visceral distension from full bowel, stimulation of the skin secondary to an irritative pressure sore, and vesicoureteric reflux. Labour in a high-tetraplegic female may also be complicated by it.

Does ingestion of food affect blood pressure in tetraplegics?

The ingestion of food causes a small fall in blood pressure and this exacerbates the postural hypotension in these patients.

How would you manage spasticity in these patients?

- Drugs: diazepam, baclofen.
- Surgery: dorsal rhizotomy, neurectomy, myelotomy, orthopaedic procedures that divide and lengthen tendons of spastic muscles.

How do you localize the lesion to the fifth cervical root level?

- Muscular weakness: deltoid, supraspinatus, brachioradialis.
- Deep tendon reflexes affected: biceps and supinator jerks.
- Radicular pain/paraesthesia: neck, top of shoulder, outer aspect of the arm, forearm.
- Superficial sensory deficit: outer aspect of the upper arm.

How do you localize the lesion to the sixth cervical root level?

- Muscular weakness: biceps, brachioradialis, extensor carpi radialis longus.
- Deep tendon reflexes affected: biceps and supinator jerks.
- Radicular pain/paraesthesia: neck, shoulder, outer arm, forearm, thumb and index finger.
- Superficial sensory deficit: thumb and index finger.

How do you localize the lesion to the seventh cervical root level?

- Muscular weakness: triceps and most of the muscles on the dorsum of the forearm.
- Deep tendon reflexes affected: triceps jerk.

- Radicular pain/paraesthesia: neck, shoulder, arm, forearm to index and middle finger.
- Superficial sensory deficit: mostly middle and index fingers.

How do you localize the lesion to the eighth cervical root level?
- Muscular weakness: flexors of the forearm.
- Deep tendon reflexes affected: finger jerk.
- Radicular pain/paraesthesia: neck, shoulder, arm, ring and little fingers.
- Superficial sensory deficit: ring and little fingers.

How do you localize the lesion to the first thoracic root level?
- Muscular weakness: small muscles of the hand.
- Deep tendon reflexes affected: finger jerk.
- Radicular pain/paraesthesia: neck, axilla, medial aspect of the arm and forearm, little and ring finger.
- Superficial sensory deficit: medial arm and little finger.

What precautions would you take when transporting patients with acute high spinal injuries by air?
- Lung function should be stable before transfer.
- Air humidifier and supplemental oxygen should be available.
- Patient should be accompanied by someone trained in manoeuvres to clear airway secretions. Tracheal suction should be done regularly; this may be complicated by reflex bradycardia and cardiac arrest, and so atropine and orciprenaline should be readily available (*BMJ* 1990; **300:** 1498).

What is the mode of onset in patients with the classical syndrome of foramen magnum?
First, there is weakness of the shoulder and arm, followed by weakness of the ipsilateral leg, then contralateral leg and, finally, contralateral arm. Neoplasms in this region can cause suboccipital pain spreading to the neck and shoulders.

What is Raymond–Cestan syndrome?
Raymond–Cestan syndrome results from the obstruction of twigs of the basilar artery causing lesions of the pontine region; it is characterized by tetraplegia, nystagmus and anaesthesia.

Sir Ludwig Guttman, FRS, fled from Nazi persecution and worked at the National Spinal Injuries Centre in Stoke Mandeville Hospital, Aylesbury. He was entrusted to look after the paraplegics and tetraplegics of the war. He was the first to show that pressure sores can be avoided by 2-hourly turning of patients.

Hans L. Frankel, OBE, contemporary Physician, National Hospital of Spinal Injuries, Stoke Mandeville Hospital, Aylesbury.

Case 89

BROWN-SÉQUARD SYNDROME

INSTRUCTION

Examine this patient's neurological system.

SALIENT FEATURES

History

- Weak leg which feels normal whereas the other leg is moving perfectly but the patient has no sensation for pain and temperature.
- Trauma to the spine, e.g. stab injury.
- Tell the examiner that you would like to take a history for bladder and bowel symptoms.
- History of degenerative spine disease or multiple sclerosis.

Examination

- Deficits below the level of the lesion include:
  - Ipsilateral monoplegia or hemiplegia.
  - Ipsilateral loss of joint position and vibration sense.
  - Contralateral loss of spinothalamic (pain and temperature) sensation. The latter is sometimes localized to one or two segments below the anatomical level of the lesion.
- Deficits in the segment of the lesion:
  - Ipsilateral lower motor neuron paralysis.
  - Ipsilateral zone of cutaneous anaesthesia and zone of hyperaesthesia just below the anaesthetic zone.
  - Segmental signs such as muscular atrophy, radicular pain or decreased tendon reflexes are usually unilateral.
- Tell the examiner you would like to examine the spine and exclude multiple sclerosis.

DIAGNOSIS

This patient has Brown-Séquard syndrome (or hemisection of the spinal cord) at the level of T8 (lesion), probably due to a compressive or destructive lesion of the spinal cord (aetiology). The patient is limited by the weakness in one limb (functional status).

ADVANCED-LEVEL QUESTIONS

What are the causes of hemisection of the spinal cord?

- Syringomyelia (see pp 199–202).
- Cord tumour.

- Haematomyelia.
- Bullet or stab wounds.
- Degenerative disease of spine.
- Multiple myeloma.

Charles-Edouard Brown-Séquard (1817–1894) was Professor of Physiology in Virginia, USA, at the National Hospital, Queen Square, London, at Harvard, and finally in Paris. He was the first physician-in-chief of the National Hospital in Queen Square which was founded in 1860. In 1889 he is said to have drawn much attention and criticism for injecting himself with a testicular extract (*BMJ* 1889; **1**: 1416). Several nations lay claim to Brown-Séquard: he was born in Mauritius, then a British colony, the son of a French woman and an American sea captain (*Lancet* 2000; **356**: 61–3).

Case 90

CAUDA EQUINA SYNDROME

INSTRUCTION

This patient has bowel and bladder dysfunction; examine the lower limbs.

SALIENT FEATURES

History

- Ask the patient whether there is pain, usually projected to the perineum and thighs (this is root pain in the dermatomes L2 or L3 or S2 or S3, whereas pain in L4, L5 or S1 distribution is commonly attributed to disc disease).
- Determine whether there is a history of trauma and 'neural claudication' (where the patient develops root pain and leg weakness, usually a foot-drop while walking; this rapidly recovers on resting).
- Pain in the anterior thigh, wasting of the quadriceps muscle, weakness of the foot invertors (due to L4 root lesion) and an absent knee jerk.
- Obtain history of leukaemia or prostatic carcinoma (primaries for bony metastases).

Examination

- Flaccid, asymmetrical paraparesis.
- Knee and ankle jerks are diminished or absent.
- Saddle distribution of sensory loss up to the L1 level.
- Downgoing plantars.

DIAGNOSIS

This patient has flaccid paraparesis with saddle anaesthesia due to cauda equina syndrome (lesion) caused by a compressive lesion (aetiology).

ADVANCED-LEVEL QUESTIONS

What is the relationship of the spinal cord to the vertebrae?

The spinal cord extends from the foramen magnum to the interspace between the 12th thoracic (dorsal) and first lumbar spines, although the thecal membranes may extend down the body of the second sacral vertebra. To determine the spinal segments in relation to the vertebral body: for cervical vertebrae add 1, for thoracic 1–6 add 2, for thoracic 7–9 add 3, and the lumbar segments lie opposite the 10th and 11th thoracic spines and the next interspinal space. The first lumbar arch overlies the sacral and coccygeal segments. (Remember that the sacral segments are compressed into the last inch of the cord known as the conus medullaris; the latter is located behind the ninth thoracic to the first lumbar vertebra.)

At which vertebral level is the lesion in cauda equina syndrome?

A lesion in the spinal canal at any level below the tenth thoracic (dorsal) vertebra can cause cauda equina syndrome.

How would you differentiate between cauda equina and conus medullaris syndrome?

The cauda equina consists of lower spinal roots (T12 to S5) and hence a lesion causes lower motor neuron signs, whereas the conus medullaris is the lowest part of the spinal cord and lesions result in upper motor neuron signs. Lesions involving both conus and cauda result in a mixed picture.

What are the causes of cauda equina syndrome?

- Centrally placed lumbosacral disc or spondylolisthesis at the lumbosacral junction.
- Tumours of the cauda equina (ependymoma, neurofibroma).

What are the types of cauda equina syndrome in adults?

- The lateral cauda equina syndrome: pain in the anterior thigh, wasting of the quadriceps muscle, weakness of the foot invertors (due to L4 root lesion) and an absent knee jerk. Causes include neurofibroma, a high disc lesion.
- The midline cauda equina syndrome: bilateral lumbar and sacral root lesions. Causes include disc lesion, primary sacral bone tumours (chordomas), metastatic bone disease (from prostate) and leukaemia.

Case 91

TORSION DYSTONIA (DYSTONIA MUSCULORUM DEFORMANS)

INSTRUCTION

Look at this patient.

SALIENT FEATURES

History

- Perinatal anoxia, birth trauma or kernicterus.
- Family history.
- Drug history (neuroleptics).
- The age of onset of clinical features (abnormal movements are usually present before the age of 5 years in birth anoxia).

Examination

- Dystonic movements of head and neck.
- Torticollis.
- Blepharospasm.
- Facial grimacing.
- Forced opening or closing of the mouth.
- Limbs may adopt abnormal but characteristic postures.

DIAGNOSIS

This patient has torsion dystonia (lesion) which may be due to birth anoxia (aetiology), and is confined to a wheelchair because of the disability (functional status).

QUESTIONS

What do you understand by the term 'dystonia'?
It implies a movement caused by a prolonged muscular contraction when a part of the body is thrown into spasm.

ADVANCED-LEVEL QUESTIONS

What is the inheritance of idiopathic torsion dystonia?
Idiopathic torsion dystonia can occur sporadically, or on a hereditary basis with autosomal dominant (where the gene is on chromosome 9q), X-linked recessive or autosomal recessive inheritance. The recessive variety has been described in Jewish families. There is a normal birth and developmental history in idiopathic torsion dystonia.

What are the other causes of dystonia?

- Birth anoxia (abnormal movements develop before the age of 5 years; often associated with a history of seizures and mental disability).
- Wilson's disease, Huntington's disease or parkinsonism.
- Drugs.

How would you treat such patients?

- Drugs: patients respond poorly to drugs. Occasionally helpful medications include diazepam, levodopa, amantadine, carbamazepine, tetrabenazine, phenothiazines and haloperidol.
- Stereotactic thalamotomy may be useful in predominantly unilateral dystonia.

Case 92

EPILEPSY

INSTRUCTION

This patient is suspected to have seizures; ask her a few questions. The eye-witness (usually the spouse) of the suspected event is next to the patient and you may ask him or her any relevant questions.

SALIENT FEATURES

Proceed as follows:

- Ask the patient about aura, whether she bit her tongue, whether she was incontinent during the attack, any hallucinations (*déjà vu* phenomenon). Ask the patient about triggering factors (including television, disco strobes, hypoglycaemia and alcohol ingestion) and whether they are recurrent. Take a family history (about 30% of patients with epilepsy have a history of seizures in relatives) and past history of head injury.
- Confirm this by asking the eye-witness for a description of the seizures (note whether they were tonic–clonic), frothing at the mouth, whether the patient was unconscious or incontinent, how long the whole 'episode' lasted and how long she was unconscious after the attack, and whether there was any weakness after the attack (Todd's paralysis).

DIAGNOSIS

This patient has recent-onset generalized tonic–clonic epilepsy (lesion) which could be due to an intracranial tumour (aetiology). The patient will have to give up her job as a truck-driver as a consequence of this (functional status).

QUESTIONS

How would you investigate the patient?

• Full blood count, urea and electrolytes, blood glucose, liver function tests.
• Chest radiography.
• EEG.
• CT scan.
• Magnetic resonance imaging and telemetry.

Mention some metabolic abnormalities found in these patients.

Hypoglycaemia, hyponatraemia (e.g. syndrome of inappropriate antidiuretic hormone secretion, SIADH), hypocalcaemia, hepatic failure, uraemia.

How would you classify seizures?

• Generalized seizures: generalized tonic–clonic seizures, petit mal and atypical absences, myoclonus, akinetic seizures. Petit mal describes only 3 Hz seizures, rather than clinically similar absence attacks which are partial seizures.
• Partial or focal seizures (a partial seizure is epileptic activity confined to one area of cortex with a recognizable clinical pattern): simple partial seizures (no impairment of consciousness), complex partial seizures, partial seizures evolving to tonic–clonic.

ADVANCED-LEVEL QUESTIONS

What is jacksonian epilepsy?

It is a simple partial seizure which usually originates in one portion of the prefrontal motor cortex so that fits begin in one part of the body (e.g. thumb) and then proceed to involve that side of the body and then the whole body. It suggests a space-occupying lesion.

What is Todd's paralysis?

Paresis of a limb or hemiplegia occurring after an epileptic attack, which may last up to 3 days.

How would you manage epilepsy?

• General advice: Avoid ladders, heights, unsupervised swimming and cycling for 2 years from the last episode.
• Antiepileptic drugs: The first line drugs for epilepsy monotherapy remain carbamazepine and sodium valproate; phenytoin is now less used, and although lamotrigine has a monotherapy licence its place has still to be defined. Several new 'add-on drugs' have been licensed in recent years including vigabatrin, gabapentin, lamotrigine, and topiramate. An overview of trials in patients with refractory partial seizures suggests no major differences between these agents in either efficacy or tolerability (*BMJ* 1996; **313:** 1169–74). Prolonged use of vigabatrin can result in severe visual field defects, prompting the development of guidelines for monitoring vision (*BMJ* 1998; **317:** 1322).
• Vagal stimulation remains an experimental approach in seizure control (*J Clin Neurophysiol* 1997; **14:** 358–68).
• Advice about driving: In the UK, those who have had more than one seizure are unable to hold a driving licence unless they have been free from any form of

epileptic attack whilst awake for a period of one year before the issue of a licence; in the case of attacks whilst asleep, these attacks must have occurred only during sleep over a period of 3 years and no awake attacks before the issue of a licence. Drivers of heavy goods vehicles and public service vehicles must have been free of epileptic attacks for at least the last 10 years and must not have taken anticonvulsant medications during this 10-year period.

What do you understand by the term 'status epilepticus'?

It is a medical emergency in which seizures follow each other without recovery of consciousness.

What is the prognosis in epilepsy?

- Most individuals with newly diagnosed epilepsy enter prolonged remission from seizures and have an excellent prognosis, but seizures remain refractory in 20–30%.

- Up to 75% of patients with refractory partial epilepsy show evidence of abnormalities on magnetic resonance imaging (*J Neurol Neurosurg Psych* 1995; **59**: 384–7), some of which are amenable to surgery.

- Population based studies show that patients with epilepsy have an increased risk of sudden death compared with age and sex matched controls (*J Neurol Neurosurg Psych* 1995; **58**: 462–4). Some of these deaths are related to epilepsy itself, for example as a consequence of accidents, but others are unexplained. This has been termed 'SUDEP' (sudden unexpected death in epilepsy) and is more common in refractory epilepsy (about 1 in 200 patients per year). Many of these deaths may be related to unwitnessed seizures, possibly associated with respiratory arrest, cardiac arrest or neurologically mediated pulmonary oedema; therefore a proportion of these deaths can potentially be prevented by better control of seizures.

Robert B. Todd (1809–1860), FRS, an Irish physician, graduated from Pembroke College, Oxford, and was Professor of Physiology at King's College, London (*J Neurol Neurosurg Psychiatry* 1994; **57**: 359). He was founder of King's College Hospital.

J. Hughlings Jackson (1835–1911), an English neurologist, worked at the National Hospital, Queen Square, London.

Case 93

GUILLAIN–BARRÉ SYNDROME

INSTRUCTION

Examine this patient's lower limbs, in which weakness began distally.

SALIENT FEATURES

History

- Weakness: difficulty in rising up from sitting position or climbing stairs; legs usually affected before upper limbs.
- Dyspnoea late in the course, suggesting diaphragmatic and intercostal muscle weakness.
- Cranial nerve involvement: diplopia, drooling of saliva, regurgitation of food.
- Paraesthesias.
- Urinary symptoms.
- Systemic symptoms: fatigue.
- Ascertain whether the onset was preceded by a trivial viral illness.

Examination

- Weakness of distal limb muscles.
- Distal numbness.
- Areflexia.

Proceed as follows:
Tell the examiner that you would like to:

- Assess respiratory function (forced vital capacity).
- Check blood pressure (for labile blood pressure).

DIAGNOSIS

This patient has Guillain–Barré syndrome (lesion) and is currently experiencing weakness of the distal limb muscles (functional status).

QUESTIONS

What is the pathology?

It is a demyelinating neuropathy.

ADVANCED-LEVEL QUESTIONS

How is the diagnosis confirmed?

- Nerve conduction studies demonstrate slowing of conduction or conduction block.

- CSF shows albumino-cytological dissociation, i.e. cell count is normal but the protein concentration is frequently raised.

What is Miller–Fisher syndrome?

A rare proximal variant of Guillain–Barré syndrome which initially affects the ocular muscles and in which ataxia is prominent.

What is the differential diagnosis?

Poliomyelitis, botulism, primary muscle disease or other neuropathy (porphyric, diphtheric, heavy metal or organophosphorus poisoning).

How would you treat such patients?

- High-dose intravenous γ-globulin during the acute phase to reduce the severity and duration of symptoms (*N Engl J Med* 1992; **326**: 1123–9). This is equivalent to plasma exchange in reducing disability, but the combination of intravenous immunoglobulin and plasma exchange offers no significant additional advantage (*Lancet* 1997; **349**: 225–30).
- Ventilatory support if respiratory muscles are affected.
- Physiotherapy and occupational therapy for muscle weakness.

C. Guillain (1876–1961), Professor of Medicine in Paris.

J.A. Barré (1880–1967), Professor of Neurology in Strasbourg, trained in Paris.

Case 94

MULTIPLE SYSTEM ATROPHY

INSTRUCTION

Perform a neurological examination on this patient.

SALIENT FEATURES

History

- Dizziness when standing up (due to postural hypotension).
- Dysphagia.
- Ataxia.
- Symptoms of Parkinson's disease (pp 136–8).
- Impotence, bladder disturbances (pp 246–7).
- Anhidrosis.

Examination

- Mask-like facies and other features of bradykinesia.
- Increased tone (rigidity).
- Cerebellar signs.

Proceed as follows:
Tell the examiner that you would like to look for:

- Postural hypotension, the hallmark of this condition (due to autonomic failure).
- Signs of autonomic dysfunction (pupillary asymmetry, Horner's syndrome).

DIAGNOSIS

This patient has cerebellar and Parkinson's signs (lesion) due to multiple system atrophy, a degenerative disorder (aetiology), and has marked disability including incontinence (functional status).

ADVANCED-LEVEL QUESTIONS

What are the types of multisystem atrophy?

- Striatonigral degeneration: clinical picture resembles Parkinson's disease but without tremor. These patients do not respond to anti-Parkinson medications and often develop adverse reactions to these agents.
- Shy–Drager syndrome: clinical picture consists of Parkinson's disease combined with severe autonomic neuropathy (particularly postural hypotension). Other important clinical features are impotence and bladder disturbances.
- Olivopontocerebellar atrophy: combination of extrapyramidal manifestations and cerebellar ataxia. Patients may also have autonomic neuropathy and anterior horn cell degeneration.
- Parkinsonism and motor neuron disease: rare.

What is the pathology in Shy–Drager syndrome?

In 1960, Shy and Drager described changes in the brainstem and ganglia; subsequently, loss of neurons has been shown in the autonomic nervous system and in the cells of the intermediolateral column of the spinal cord. Positron emission tomography shows decreased uptake of dopamine in the putamen and caudate lobe.

What factors can lower blood pressure in these patients?

Standing up (orthostatic hypotension, a hallmark of this condition), food and exercise. Food and exercise can produce hypotension even in the supine position (*J Neurol* 1990; **237**(suppl 1): S24; *J Am Coll Cardiol* 1993; **21**: 97A).

What is the morbidity of this condition?

It tends to disable most patients severely by the end of 5–7 years.

How would you treat these patients?

Treatment is symptomatic and supportive for hypotension and neurological deficits. Symptoms of postural hypotension may be ameliorated by antigravity stockings and fluorohydrocortisone.

G.M. Shy (1919–1967), a US neurologist who obtained his MRCP in London in 1947.

G.A. Drager (1917–1967), a US neurologist.

Bradbury and Eggleston in 1925 first described the combination of postural hypotension, incontinence, impotence and abnormality of sweating (anhidrosis). Neurological manifestations develop later.

Christopher J. Mathias, FRCP, DSc, contemporary Professor of Medicine, St Mary's Hospital Medical School and National Hospital, Queen Square, London, whose chief interest is the autonomic control of the cardiovascular system.

Case 95

NEUROLOGICAL BLADDER

INSTRUCTION

This patient is suspected to have difficulty in micturition accompanying paraparesis. Would you like to ask him a few questions?

SALIENT FEATURES

Proceed as follows:

Ask the patient the following questions:

- Do you get a sensation when the bladder is full?
- Do you feel the urine passing?
- Are you able to stop urine passing in midstream at your own will?
- Does the bladder leak continually?
- Do you suddenly pass large volumes?
- Is there any difficulty in defaecation?
- Is there any numbness in the perineal region?

Tell the examiner that in a male patient you would like to take a history of impotence and examine the neurological system and spine.

DIAGNOSIS

This patient has a spastic bladder (lesion) accompanying his paraparesis which occurred as a result of trauma (aetiology) and requires an indwelling urinary catheter (functional status).

ADVANCED-LEVEL QUESTIONS

What are the types of neurogenic bladder?

Spinal or spastic bladder

The bladder is small and spastic and holds less than 250 ml. It is seen in lesions of the spinal cord secondary to trauma, multiple sclerosis, and spinal cord tumour (upper motor neuron lesion). Bladder fullness is not appreciated and the bladder tends to empty reflexly and suddenly – the automatic bladder. Evacuation may be incomplete unless the bladder is massaged by pressure in the suprapubic region.

The autonomous bladder

This results from damage to the cauda equina, i.e. lower motor neuron lesion (see pp 237–8). The patient is incontinent with continual dribbling and there is no sensation of bladder fullness. Despite the dribbling there is considerable residual urine. There is loss of perineal sensation and sexual dysfunction. (In conus medullaris–cauda equina lesions, it is possible to have a flaccid lower motor neuron detrusor with a spastic sphincter. The reverse may also occur.)

The sensory bladder

This is similar to autonomous bladder and is seen in tabes dorsalis, subacute combined degeneration of the cord and multiple sclerosis. There is loss of awareness of bladder fullness with a loss of spinal reflex. This results in retention of large quantities of urine, incontinence with dribbling, and a high volume of residual urine which can be voided by considerable straining.

The uninhibited bladder

This occurs with lesions affecting the second gyrus of the frontal lobe, e.g. frontal lobe tumours, parasagittal meningiomas, aneurysms of the anterior communicating arteries and dementia. Patients have urgency despite low bladder volumes and have sudden uncontrolled evacuation. There is no residual urine. When there is deterioration of the intellect, the patient may pass urine at any time without concern.

What do you know about the neurological control of the bladder?

- Micturition follows activation of the parasympathetic pathways to the detrusor muscle and inhibition of the somatic input to the external urethral sphincter. The parasympathetic reflex is based in the S3 roots and S3 segments of the cord.
- The sympathetic system promotes urinary storage by increasing urethral resistance and depressing detrusor contractions. The sympathetic supply descends into the pelvis from the hypogastric reflex.
- A cortical representation of the bladder is present in the paracentral lobule, stimulation of which may evoke bladder contractions. It may play a part in initiating voluntary contractions and in stopping micturition by initiating contraction of the external sphincter.

What investigations are performed to evaluate bladder function?

Cystometry, sphincter electromyography, uroflowmetry with measurement and recording of urinary flow, urethral pressure profiles, and electrophysiological tests of bladder wall innervation.

What are the different types of urinary incontinence?

Urinary continence is dependent on a compliant reservoir (the bladder) and sphincteric efficiency which relies on its two components: the involuntary smooth muscle of the bladder neck and the voluntary skeletal muscle of the external sphincter. Urinary incontinence occurs when urine leaks involuntarily and is of five types:

- Total incontinence: the patient loses urine at all times and in all positions. It occurs when the sphincter is damaged (by surgery, cancerous infiltration and nerve damage) or when there is a fistula between the urinary tract and the skin, or ectopic ureters.
- Stress incontinence: occurs when there is an increase in intra-abdominal pressure (on coughing, sneezing, lifting, exercising). It is seen in patients with a lax pelvic floor (e.g. multiparous women, patients who have undergone pelvic surgery). Patients do not lose urine in the supine position.
- Urge incontinence: loss of urine preceded by a strong, unexpected urge to void urine. It occurs with inflammation or neurogenic disorders.
- Overflow incontinence occurs in chronic urinary retention from a chronically distended bladder.
- Enuresis: a form of involuntary nocturnal incontinence. It is usually seen in children.

HISTORY AND EXAMINATION OF THE CHEST

Introduce yourself to the patient.

HISTORY

1. Cough.
2. Sputum.
3. Haemoptysis (acute infection including in COPD, pulmonary infarction, bronchogenic carcinoma, bronchiectasis, TB, Goodpasture's syndrome, pulmonary haemosiderosis, mitral stenosis).
4. Dyspnoea
   - Intermittent (asthma, recurrent pulmonary oedema, exacerbations of COAD).
   - Over days (pleural fluid, carcinoma of bronchus, heart failure).
   - Over months to years (COAD, fibrosing alveolitis, anaemia, fibrotic lung disease).
   - Over a few hours (pulmonary oedema, bronchial asthma, pneumonia).
   - Acute or sudden (pneumothorax, pulmonary oedema, inhaled foreign body).
5. Wheezing (airways limitation including asthma, COAD).
6. Chest pain (pleurisy, tracheitis).
7. Smoking.
8. Family history.

EXAMINATION

1. Place the patient in a sitting position and ask whether he or she is comfortable.
2. Examine the sputum cup and comment on the sputum.
3. Examine the patient from the foot end of the bed and comment as follows:
   - Whether the patient is breathless at rest.
   - On wasting, if any, in the infraclavicular region.
   - On diminished movement on the right or left side.
   - Count the respiratory rate.
4. Examine the hands:
   - Clubbing.
   - Cyanosis.
   - Tar staining (the yellow 'nicotine' staining is actually due to tar).
   - Examine the pulse for bounding pulse and asterixis (signs of carbon monoxide narcosis).
5. Examine the face:
   - Comment on the tongue, looking for central cyanosis.
   - Comment on the eyes, looking for pallor and evidence of Horner's syndrome.
6. Examine the neck:
   - Comment on neck veins.
   - Check for cervical lymphadenopathy.
   - Comment on the trachea:
     - Whether or not it is deviated.
     - The distance between the cricoid cartilage and suprasternal notch.

7. Palpate:
   - Apex beat.
   - Movements on both sides with the fingers symmetrically placed in the intercostal spaces on both sides.
   - Vocal fremitus (tell the examiner that you would prefer to do vocal resonance because it gives the same information and is more reliable).
8. Percussion: percuss over supraclavicular areas, clavicles, upper, middle and lower chest on both sides.
9. Auscultation:
   - Over supraclavicular areas, upper, middle and lower chest on both sides – comment on breath sounds (whether vesicular or bronchial) and on adventitious sounds (wheeze, crackles or pleural rub). If crackles are heard, ask the patient to cough and then repeat auscultation. It is important to time the crackles to ascertain whether they occur in early, mid or late inspiration.
   - While auscultating the front of the chest, seize the opportunity to listen to the second pulmonary sound.
   - Check for vocal resonance by asking the patient to repeat 'one, one, one'.
   - Check for forced expiratory time (FET) if your diagnosis is chronic obstructive airways disease (COAD) by asking the patient to exhale forcefully after full inspiration while you are listening over the trachea: if the patient takes more than 6 seconds, airway disease is indicated.
10. Ask the patient to sit forward:
    - Palpate – assess expansion posteriorly.
    - Percuss – on both sides including axillae.
    - Auscultate – posteriorly including the axillae.
11. Remember to look for signs of middle lobe disease in the right axilla.

Case 96

PLEURAL EFFUSION

INSTRUCTION

Examine this patient's chest.
Examine this patient's chest from the back.
Examine this patient's chest from the front.

SALIENT FEATURES

History

- Fever.
- Pleuritic pain (made worse on coughing or deep breathing).
- Cough (pneumonia, TB).
- Haemoptysis (associated parenchymal involvement in bronchogenic carcinoma or TB).
- Shortness of breath (large effusions, cardiac failure).
- Exposure to asbestos (mesothelioma).
- Nephrotic syndrome.

Examination

- Decreased movement on the affected side.
- Tracheal deviation to the opposite side.
- Stony dull note on the affected side.
- Decreased vocal resonance and diminished breath sounds on the affected side.

Proceed as follows:
- Comment on aspiration marks.
- Percuss for the upper level of effusion in the axilla.
- Listen for bronchial breath sounds.
- Listen for aegophony at the upper level of the effusion.
- It is important to elicit any evidence of an underlying cause, such as clubbing, tar staining, lymph nodes, radiation burns and mastectomy, raised JVP, rheumatoid hands or butterfly rash.

Remember. 500 ml of pleural fluid should be present for clinical detection and there are 5 major types of pleural effusion: exudate, transudate, empyema, haemorrhagic pleural effusion or haemothorax, and chylous effusion.

DIAGNOSIS

This patient has a pleural effusion (lesion), probably due to bronchogenic carcinoma, and is short of breath at rest (functional status).

Read review: *Postgrad Med J* 1993; **69**: 12–18; *Thorax* 1979; **304**: 106.

QUESTIONS

How would you investigate this patient?

Chest radiography (CXR)

Standard posteroanterior and lateral chest radiographs detect pleural fluid in excess of 175 ml. Obliteration of costophrenic angle to hemithorax suggests fluid. Subpulmonic effusion can simulate an elevated diaphragm.

Pleural tap

- Pleural fluid for determination of the levels of protein, albumin, LDH, glucose, cholesterol and cytology. A simultaneous blood sample should be obtained for estimation of glucose, protein, albumin and LDH.
- When empyema is suspected or seen, pleural fluid pH should be obtained.
- When tuberculosis is suspected, pleural fluid adenosine deaminase or lysozyme levels should be determined and Ziehl–Neelsen staining and pleural fluid mycobacterial cultures should be done.
- Pleural fluid amylase levels should be estimated when malignancy, pancreatitis or oesophageal rupture is suspected.
- In autoimmune disorders, pleural fluid rheumatoid factor or antinuclear antibodies should be tested.

Pleural biopsy

The biopsy specimen is sent for histopathological examination and mycobacterial culture.

What are the causes of dullness at a lung base?

- Pleural effusion.
- Pleural thickening.
- Consolidation and collapse of the lung.
- Raised hemidiaphragm.

How would you differentiate between the above?

- Pleural effusion: stony dull note; trachea may be deviated to the opposite side in large effusions.
- Pleural thickening: trachea not deviated; breath sounds will be heard.
- Consolidation: vocal resonance increased; bronchial breath sounds and associated crackles.
- Collapse: trachea deviated to the affected side; absent breath sounds.

How would you differentiate between an exudate and a transudate?

- The protein content of an exudate is more than 3 g/l. However, if this criterion alone is applied, about 10% of the exudates and 15% of the transudates will be wrongly classified. A more accurate diagnosis is made when Light's criteria (*Ann Intern Med* 1972; **77**: 507–13) for an exudate are applied: (1) the ratio of the pleural fluid to serum protein is greater than 0.5; (2) the ratio of pleural fluid to serum lactic dehydrogenase (LDH) is greater than 0.6; (3) pleural fluid LDH is greater than two thirds the upper normal limit for blood LDH levels. Roth et al (1990) found that, although Light's criteria had a sensitivity of 100%, they had a low specificity of 72% (*Chest* 1990; **98**: 546–9). This was due to the fact that many patients with effusion due to chronic cardiac failure have protein values in

the exudate range, particularly when on chronic diuretic therapy. They found that the serum–effusion albumin gradient (i.e. serum albumin minus pleural fluid albumin) was 95% sensitive but a more specific (100%) marker of exudative effusion. A gradient of less than 1.2 g/dl indicates an exudative effusion whereas a gradient greater than 1.2 g/dl indicates a transudative effusion.
- The pleural fluid cholesterol level is below 60 mg/dl in transudates. All malignant effusions have a pleural cholesterol level greater than this value, and therefore this test is useful to separate these two categories of effusion (*Chest* 1987; **92:** 296–302; *Chest* 1991; **99:** 1097–102).

Mention a few causes for an exudate and a transudate.

Causes for an exudate:
- Bronchogenic carcinoma (presence of effusion is an ominous sign).
- Secondaries in the pleura (lung, breast, ovary and pancreas).
- Pneumonia.
- Pulmonary infarction.
- Tuberculosis.
- Rheumatoid arthritis.
- SLE.
- Lymphoma (in young individuals).
- Mesothelioma.

Causes of a transudate:
- Nephrotic syndrome.
- Cardiac failure.
- Liver cell failure.
- Hypothyroidism.

ADVANCED-LEVEL QUESTIONS

Mention a few conditions in which the pleural fluid pH and glucose levels are low with a raised LDH concentration.
Empyema, malignancy, tuberculosis, rheumatoid arthritis, systemic lupus erythematosus and oesophageal rupture.

What is the value of measuring pleural fluid pH and glucose concentrations in cases of malignant effusions?
This is of value in determining the prognosis (*Ann Intern Med* 1988; **108:** 345–9). Patients with a low pleural fluid pH (<7.3) or low glucose concentration (<60 mg/dl) have a shorter life expectancy than those with higher values: 2.1 months versus 9.8 months. The low pH group tends to have more extensive pleural involvement as determined by thoracoscopy and a higher failure rate for chemical pleurodesis.

What further investigation would you perform to determine the underlying cause of the pleural effusion?
- Pleural biopsy.
- CT chest scan.
- Magnetic resonance imaging of the chest: although this technique has limited value owing to motion artefacts caused by cardiac and respiratory movements,

radiologists were able to differentiate transudates, simple exudates and complex exudates.

What is the role of pleural fluid cytology in the diagnosis of pleural effusion?

- Pleural fluid usually contains about 1500 cells per μl (predominantly mono-nuclear cells). Counts above 50 000 are seen in parapneumonic effusions, whereas transudates usually have counts of less than 1000 cells per μl.
- Pleural fluid eosinophilia, i.e. greater than 10%, suggests a benign disease, including pneumothorax, asbestos-related effusions and post haemothorax, although malignancy cannot be excluded.
- Pleural fluid lymphocytosis is seen in about one third of transudates, in malignancy, tuberculosis, lymphoma, collagen vascular diseases and sarcoidosis.
- Computerized interactive morphometry (analyses the size and nuclei of cells in a stained centrifuged specimen) differentiates between malignant cells and reactive lymphocytosis. This method is particularly useful when differentiating between benign reactive mesothelial cells and malignancy.

What characteristics of the pleural fluid in a parapneumonic effusion indicate a need for closed-tube drainage?

A pleural fluid glucose concentration of less than 40 mg/dl or a pH less than 7.0 indicates the need for closed-tube drainage.

What does a pleural fluid total neutral fat level greater than 400 mg/dl suggest?

It suggests chylothorax and is seen most often in patients with lymphomas, solid tumours, nephrotic syndrome and cirrhosis, and occasionally in rheumatoid arthritis.

What is the significance of pleural fluid amylase levels?

A pleural fluid amylase level greater than the serum amylase concentration is seen in patients with pancreatitis, carcinoma, bacterial pneumonia and oesophageal rupture. In malignant effusions, when cytology cannot differentiate adenocarcinoma from mesothelioma, a raised amylase level suggests the presence of the former. Amylase-rich pleural effusions occur frequently, and pleural fluid isoamylase determination can be useful; the finding of a pleural effusion rich in salivary isoamylase should prompt an evaluation for carcinoma (particularly a lung primary), but may also be seen in other pleural inflammatory conditions (*Chest* 1992; **102:** 1455–9).

What are the causes of an exudate with negative cytology findings and pleural fluid lymphocytosis?

Possible causes include tuberculosis, collagen vascular diseases and tumours, including lymphoma.

In such patients, what other tests could you perform on the pleural fluid to determine the underlying cause?

- Pleural fluid adenosine deaminase concentration (an enzyme involved in purine metabolism and found in T lymphocytes) is markedly raised in tuberculous and rheumatoid effusions compared with malignant effusions.
- Increased pleural fluid lysozyme concentration (muramidase) is used to differ-entiate tuberculosis, rheumatoid arthritis and empyema from malignant effusions.

- Combined use of the latter two tests yields a sensitivity and specificity of 100% for tuberculous effusions if empyema is excluded.
- Gamma-interferon and soluble interleukin 2 receptor levels are also raised in tuberculous effusions compared with malignant effusions.
- Estimation of pleural fluid rheumatoid factor and antinuclear antibodies is useful in confirming the diagnosis of rheumatoid and lupus erythematosus respectively.

In which conditions is the pleural fluid bloody?
Haemorrhagic fluid is seen in malignancy, pulmonary embolus, tuberculosis and trauma to the chest.

What are the earliest radiological signs of pleural fluid?
The earliest radiological signs are blunting of the costophrenic angle on the anterior–posterior view or loss of clear definition of the diaphragm posteriorly on the lateral view.

How would you confirm your suspicions when in doubt of a small effusion?
Either by a lateral decubitus view (which shows a layering of the fluid along the dependent chest wall unless the fluid is loculated) or by ultrasonography.

What are the other uses of ultrasonography in the diagnosis of pleural effusion?
Ultrasonography is also useful for loculated effusions, for guided thoracocentesis, closed pleural biopsy or insertion of a chest drain, and to differentiate pleural fluid from pleural thickening.

What is a pseudotumour?
It is the accumulation of fluid between the major or minor fissure or along the lateral chest wall, and can be mistaken for a tumour on the radiograph. Such loculated effusions can be confirmed with ultrasonography.

What do you know about pleural disease in rheumatoid arthritis?
About 70% of patients with rheumatoid arthritis have pleural inflammation at autopsy and about 5% have radiological evidence of pleural inflammation at some time. Pleural involvement is associated with male sex, rheumatoid factor in serum, the presence of nodules and other systemic manifestations. The effusion is thought to develop as an inflammatory response to the presence of multiple subpleural nodules. For reasons that are entirely unclear, the left side is the more common site of unilateral rheumatoid pleural effusions. The pleural fluid glucose level is characteristically low and is said to be due to an 'entrance block' in which glucose is unable to enter the pleural space, unlike in empyema and malignant effusions where the low pleural fluid glucose concentration is attributed to the increased use of glucose by cells. Cytological appearances of slender and elongated macrophages, round giant multinucleated macrophages, presence of very few mesothelial cells and necrotic background material are thought to be pathognomonic of rheumatoid pleuritis.

What are the complications of thoracocentesis?
Pneumothorax, haemothorax, intravascular collapse and unilateral pulmonary oedema (the latter after withdrawal of large quantities of fluid).

What do you know about Meigs' syndrome?

Meigs' syndrome comprises pleural effusion (usually right-sided and a transudate) associated with ovarian tumours (usually benign ovarian fibroma).

Mention some causes of drug-induced pleural effusion.

Practolol, procarbazine, methysergide, bromocriptine, methotrexate and nitrofurantoin.

The patient used to be a shipbuilder: what diagnosis would you consider?

It is most likely that this patient has malignant mesothelioma. If the diagnosis is confirmed, I would advise him to apply for industrial injuries benefit.

What are the mechanisms for abnormal accumulation of pleural fluid?

There are three main mechanisms:

- An abnormality of the pleura itself, such as a neoplasm or inflammatory process, usually associated with increased permeability.
- Disruption of the integrity of a fluid-containing structure within the pleural cavity, such as the thoracic duct, oesophagus, major blood vessels or tracheobronchial tree, with leakage of the contents into the pleural space.
- Abnormal hydrostatic or osmotic forces operating on an otherwise normal pleural surface and producing a transudate.

Case 97

PLEURAL RUB

INSTRUCTION

This patient presented with sudden onset of lateral chest pain aggravated by deep inspiration and coughing. Listen to this patient's chest. Examine her chest.

SALIENT FEATURES

History

- Sharp localized pain worse on coughing or deep respiration.
- Nature of the sputum (purulent expectoration in a patient with chest infection, haemoptysis in pulmonary embolism).
- Drug history (oral contraceptives).

Examination

Pleural rub (superficial, scratchy, grating sound heard on deep inspiration).

Proceed as follows:
- Differentiate between pleural rub and crackles by asking the patient to cough and check whether or not there is any change in the nature. (**Note.** No change with the pleural rub.)
- Tell the examiner that you would like to listen for tachycardia and right ventricular gallop (pulmonary embolism).

DIAGNOSIS

This patient has a pleural rub (lesion) which is caused by either underlying infection or pulmonary embolism (aetiology). You would like to analyse blood gases to determine whether she is hypoxic (functional status).

QUESTIONS

How would you investigate this patient?
- Full blood count.
- Sputum cultures.
- Blood gases.
- ECG.
- CXR.
- Ventilation–perfusion scan.

ADVANCED-LEVEL QUESTIONS

What would you expect to see in the ventilation–perfusion scan in a patient with pulmonary embolism?
In acute pulmonary embolism the area of decreased perfusion usually has normal ventilation, whereas in pneumonia there are abnormalities in both the ventilation and perfusion scan.

How would you treat a patient with pulmonary embolism?
- Initially with heparin and then with oral anticoagulants for at least 3 months.
- Pain relief for pleurisy.

What are the ECG changes in pulmonary embolism?
These include:
- Sinus tachycardia.
- Tall R wave in lead VI.
- S1, S2, S3 syndrome (S waves in limb leads I, II and III).
- S1, Q3, T3 syndrome (S in limb lead 1 and Q wave and inverted T wave in limb lead III).

Case 98

ASTHMA

INSTRUCTION

Examine this patient's chest.

SALIENT FEATURES

History

- Determine whether there is a reversible airway obstruction by history. Are the wheezing and breathlessness reversible?
- Tightness in the chest.
- Recurrent cough.
- Exacerbation of the cough or wheeze at night or after exercise.
- Improvement of the cough or wheeze with bronchodilator therapy.
- Fever, yellowish sputum.
- History of atopy (eczema, hay fever).
- History of rhinitis, nasal polyps.

Examination

- Bilateral scattered wheeze.
- Examine the sputum cup.
- Comment on accessory muscles of respiration, tachycardia, pulsus paradoxus and whether the patient can utter sentences without stopping to take a breath.

DIAGNOSIS

This patient has a history of hay fever and bilateral scattered wheeze (lesion) due to bronchial asthma (aetiology), and is breathless at rest (functional status).

QUESTIONS

Mention a few trigger factors known to aggravate asthma.
- Infection.
- Emotion.
- Exercise.
- Drugs, e.g. beta-blockers.
- External allergens.

What do you understand by the term 'asthma'?
Asthma is an inflammatory disorder characterized by hyper-responsiveness of the airway to various stimuli, resulting in widespread narrowing of the airway. The changes are reversible, either spontaneously or as a result of therapy.

ADVANCED-LEVEL QUESTIONS

What do you understand by the term 'intrinsic asthma'?

Intrinsic asthma is of non-allergic aetiology and usually begins after the age of 30 years. It tends to be more continuous and more severe; status asthmaticus is common in this group.

What do you understand by the term 'extrinsic asthma'?

Extrinsic asthma has a clearly defined history of allergy to a variety of inhaled factors and is characterized by a childhood onset and seasonal variation.

What are the indications for steroids in chronic asthma?

- Sleep is disturbed by wheeze.
- Morning tightness persists until midday.
- Symptoms and peak expiratory flows progressively deteriorate each day.
- Maximum treatment with bronchodilators.
- Emergency nebulizers are needed.

What is the effect of reducing or discontinuing inhaled budesonide in patients with mild asthma?

Early treatment with inhaled budesonide results in long-lasting control of mild asthma (i.e. FEV_1 more than 85% of predicted value). Maintenance therapy can usually be given at a reduced dose, but discontinuation of treatment is often accompanied by exacerbation of the disease.

How would you manage a patient with acute asthma?

- Nebulized beta-agonists, e.g. terbutaline or salbutamol.
- Oxygen, using a high concentration.
- High-dose steroids: intravenous hydrocortisone or oral prednisolone or both.
- Blood gases.
- CXR to rule out pneumothorax.

When life-threatening features are present:

- Add ipratropium to nebulized beta-agonist.
- Intravenous aminophylline or salbutamol or terbutaline.

What do you know about the British Thoracic Society step care regimen for the management of chronic asthma in adults (Thorax 1997; 52: S1–24)?

- Step 1: Inhaled short-acting beta-agonists used as required for symptom relief. If required more than once, go to step 2.
- Step 2: Step 1 plus regular inhaled anti-inflammatory agents (such as beclomethasone, budesonide, cromoglicate or nedocromil sodium).
- Step 3: Step 1 plus high-dose inhaled steroids (using a large-volume spacer) or low-dose inhaled steroids plus a long-acting inhaled beta-agonist bronchodilator.
- Step 4: Step 1 plus high-dose inhaled steroids and regular bronchodilators (long-acting inhaled or oral beta-agonists, sustained-release theophylline, inhaled ipratropium).
- Step 5: Step 4 plus addition of oral steroids.

Patients should be started on treatment at the step most appropriate to the initial severity. A rescue course of prednisolone may be needed at any time and at any step. Stepwise reduction in treatment should be undertaken after the asthma has been stable over a 3–6-month period.

What are the features of acute severe asthma?

- Inability to complete a sentence in one breath.
- Respiration rate greater than 25 per minute.
- Pulse rate greater than 110 beats per minute.
- Peak expiratory flow rate less than 50% of predicted or best.

What are the life-threatening indicators in acute asthma?

- Peak expiratory flow rate less than 33% of predicted or best.
- Exhaustion, confusion, coma.
- Silent chest, cyanosis or feeble respiratory effort.
- Bradycardia or hypotension.

Note. Arterial blood gases should be measured if *any* of these features are present or if oxygen saturation is less than 92%.

What are the indicators of a very severe, life-threatening attack?

- Normal (5–6 kPa, 36–45 mmHg) or increased carbon dioxide tension.
- Severe hypoxia of less than 8 kPa (60 mmHg).
- Low pH.

What is the value of assessing pulsus paradoxus in a patient with acute severe asthma?

It is a poor guide to the severity of acute asthma as it compares poorly with the measurement of peak flow.

In which other conditions is wheeze a prominent sign?

Chronic obstructive airway disease, left ventricular failure (cardiac asthma), polyarteritis nodosa, eosinophilic lung disease, recurrent thromboembolism, tumour causing localized wheeze.

What are the indications for mechanical ventilation with intermittent positive pressure ventilation?

- Worsening hypoxia (Pao_2 <8 kPa) despite 60% inspired oxygen.
- Hypercapnia ($Paco_2$ >6 kPa).
- Drowsiness.
- Unconsciousness.

Professor Peter J. Barnes, contemporary chest physician, National Institute for Heart and Lung Diseases, London; his major interest is asthma.

Case 99

CHRONIC BRONCHITIS

INSTRUCTION

Examine this patient's chest.

SALIENT FEATURES

History

- Productive cough.
- Increasing dyspnoea.
- Weight loss.
- History of smoking.
- History of α_1-antitrypsin deficiency.

Examination

- Begin with examination of the *sputum pot.*
- Observe the patient from the end of the bed – for obvious breathlessness, pursed lip breathing and symmetrical chest movements – and count respiratory rate.
- Look for nail changes such as tar staining.
- Feel the palms for warmth and the pulse for rapid bounding pulse (signs of carbon dioxide retention).
- Look at the lips and tongue for central cyanosis.

Neck

- Comment on the active contractions of the accessory muscles of respiration such as sternocleidomastoids, scaleni and trapezii.
- Palpate for tracheal deviation and measure the distance between the cricoid cartilage and suprasternal notch (less than three fingers' breadth in emphysema).
- Comment on the raised JVP.

Chest

Comment on the barrel-shaped chest.

Palpate for:
- Apex beat.
- Chest expansion.
- Vocal fremitus.

Percussion:
Look for hyper-resonance and obliteration of cardiac and liver dullness.

Auscultate for:
- Breath sounds (diminished breath sounds).
- Vocal resonance.
- Forced expiratory time: normal individuals can empty their chest from full inspiration in 4 seconds or less. The end-point of FET is detected by auscultating

over the trachea in the suprasternal notch. Prolongation of the FET to more than 6 seconds indicates airflow obstruction.

- Loud pulmonary second heart sound.

Abdomen

Palpable liver due to hepatic displacement (comment on upper border of liver by percussion).

DIAGNOSIS

This patient has features of chronic obstructive airway disease (COAD) (lesion) due to cigarette smoking (aetiology) and is very cyanosed at rest (functional status).

QUESTIONS

What do you understand by the term 'chronic bronchitis'?

Chronic bronchitis is cough with mucoid expectoration for at least 3 months in a year for 2 successive years.

What is the definition of emphysema?

Emphysema is the abnormal permanent enlargement of the airway distal to the terminal respiratory bronchioles with destruction of their walls. Clinical, radiological and lung function tests give an imprecise picture in an individual case but a combination of all these features gives a reasonable picture.

What do you understand by the term 'COAD'?

The term COAD encompasses chronic obstructive bronchitis (with obstruction of small airways) and emphysema (with destruction of lung parenchyma, loss of lung elasticity, and closure of small airways). Most patients also have mucus plugging (*N Engl J Med* 2000; **343:** 269).

ADVANCED-LEVEL QUESTIONS

What is the mechanism of airflow limitation in COAD?

It is a variable mixture of loss of alveolar attachments, inflammatory obstruction of the airway and luminal obstruction with mucus.

What is the role of inflammatory mechanisms in COAD?

Macrophages and epithelial cells in airways are activated by cigarette smoke and other irritants and release neutrophil chemotactic factors including interleukin-8 and leukotriene B4. Neutrophils and macrophages then release proteases that break down connective tissue in the lung parenchyma, resulting in emphysema, and also stimulate hypersecretion of bronchial mucus. The chronic inflammatory process in COPD differs markedly from that seen in bronchial asthma, with different inflammatory cells, mediators, inflammatory effects and responses to treatment (*Thorax* 1998; **53:** 129–36; *Chest* 2000; **117** (suppl): 10S–14S).

What is the role of proteolysis in COAD?

In COAD the protease–antiprotease balance is tipped in favour of proteolysis because of either an increase in proteases (including neutrophil elastase, proteinase

3, cathepsins, matrix metalloproteases 1, 2, 9 and 12) or a deficiency of anti-proteases (including α_1-antitrypsin, elafin, secretory leukoprotease inhibitor and tissue inhibitors of matrix metalloproteases).

What is the role of high-resolution CT in the diagnosis of emphysema?

It is the most sensitive (but expensive) technique for the diagnosis of emphysema. It is useful in evaluating symptomatic patients with almost normal pulmonary function except for a low carbon monoxide diffusing capacity – a combination of findings that occurs in emphysema, interstitial lung disease and pulmonary vascular disease (*Radiology* 1992; **182**: 817–21).

How would you differentiate emphysema from chronic bronchitis?

	Emphysema	Chronic bronchitis
	Pink puffer	Blue bloater
Cyanosis	Absent	Prominent
Dyspnoea	++	+
Hyperinflation	++	+
Cor pulmonale	–	Common
Respiratory drive	High	Low

If the patient was between the ages of 30 and 45 years, what would you consider to be the underlying cause of the emphysema?

Smoking, α_1-antitrypsin (AAT) deficiency.

How would you treat an acute exacerbation?

- Nebulized bronchodilators (terbutaline, ipratropium bromide).
- Intravenous antibiotics (*BMJ* 1994; **308**: 871–2), initially amoxicillin and, if there is no clinical response, then a second-generation cephalosporin, quinoline or co-amoxiclav.
- Oxygen (24%).
- Intravenous hydrocortisone and oral steroids. (**Note.** Steroid therapy is useful only in acute exacerbations and, unlike in asthma, it does not influence the course of chronic bronchitis.)

What is the role of inhaled steroids in COPD?

Inhaled steroids are recommended for symptomatic patients with moderate to severe COAD and for patients with frequent exacerbations but not for patients with mild COAD (*N Engl J Med* 2000; **343**: 1960–1). Budenoside, fluticasone and triamcinolone were studied in long-term clinical trials (*N Engl J Med* 1999; **340**: 1948–53; *Lancet* 1999; **353**: 1819–23; *BMJ* 2000; **320**: 1297–303) and all were similar except that triamcinolone has deleterious effects on bone density (*N Engl J Med* 2000; **343**: 1902–9).

What are the organisms commonly associated with exacerbations of COAD?

Haemophilus influenzae and *Streptococcus pneumoniae* are the commonest organisms identified in the sputum during exacerbations of COAD, accounting for 43% and 25% respectively of positive cultures in one study. *Moraxella* (previously

Branhamella) *catarrhalis* is also frequently isolated from sputum during exacerbations. Less commonly, *Chlamydia pneumoniae* or *Pseudomonas aeruginosa* have been associated with some exacerbations.

What clinical features would suggest that this patient is suitable for long-term domiciliary oxygen therapy?

- COAD: forced expiratory volume in 1 second (FEV_1) less than 1.5 litres; forced vital capacity (FVC) less than 2 litres; stable chronic respiratory failure (Pao_2 <7.3 kPa, that is, 55 mmHg) in patients who have (1) had peripheral oedema or (2) not necessarily had hypercapnia or oedema (*N Engl J Med* 1995; **333:** 710–14); carboxyhaemoglobin of less than 3% (i.e. patients who have stopped smoking).
- Terminally ill patients of whatever cause with severe hypoxia (Pao_2 <7.3 kPa).

How can the sensation of breathlessness be reduced?

By the use of either promethazine or dihydrocodeine.

How would you treat acute respiratory failure?

If Pao_2 is less than 8 kPa, administer 24% oxygen. There is no need for oxygen when Pao_2 is greater than 8 kPa. Monitor blood gases after 30 minutes. If Pao_2 is rising (by 1 kPa), monitor blood gases hourly. If Pao_2 continues to rise, administer doxapram. If, in spite of this, the patient continues to deteriorate, artificial ventilation may be called for.

What do you know about non-invasive ventilation?

Non-invasive ventilation is an alternative approach to endotracheal intubation to treat hypercapnic ventilatory failure which occurs in COAD. It thus reduces the complications of endotracheal intubation such as infection and injury to the trachea. Non-invasive ventilation is pressure-support ventilation delivered with a face mask and a piece of white foam placed in the face mask to reduce the amount of internal dead space. In a recent randomized trial, non-invasive ventilation was shown to reduce the need for endotracheal intubation, length of hospital stay and in-hospital mortality rate in selected patients with acute exacerbations of COAD (*N Engl J Med* 1995; **333:** 817–22).

What do you know about the molecular genetics of COAD?

α₁-antitrypsin deficiency

- It was first described in Sweden. The patient is deficient in α_1-antitrypsin, with activity approximately 15% that of the normal value; concentrations of 40% or more are required for health. The patient is homozygous for the protease inhibitor (Pi) ZZ gene. Other genetic combinations and their percentage normal activity are PiMS (80%), PiMZ (60%), PiSS (60%), PiSZ (40%). Six per cent of the population is heterozygous for S(PiMS) and 4% for Z(PiMZ), making an overall frequency of 1 in 10 for the carriage of the defective gene. Liver transplantation results in conversion to the genotype of the donor.
- In the lung, α_1-antitrypsin inhibits the excessive actions of neutrophil and macrophage elastase, which cigarette smoke promotes. When the lung is heavily exposed to cigarette smoke, the protective effect of α_1-antitrypsin may be overwhelmed by the amount of elastase released or by a direct oxidative action of cigarette smoke on the α_1-antitrypsin molecule. The emphysema is panacinar and is seen in the lower lobes of the lungs. Smoking increases the severity and

decreases the age of onset of emphysema. Liver disease is a much less common complication. Human α_1-antitrypsin prepared from pooled plasma from normal donors is recommended for patients over 18 years with serum levels below 11 μmol/l and abnormal lung function.

- The siblings of an index case should be screened for this disorder. Their identification should be followed by counselling to avoid smoking and occupations with atmospheric pollution. Children of homozygotes will inherit at least one Z gene and hence will be heterozygotes. They should avoid pairing with another heterozygote if they wish to avoid the risk of producing an affected homozygote.

Tumour necrosis factor-alpha (TNF-α)

COAD is 10 times more common in Taiwanese with a polymorphism in the promoter region of the gene for TNF-α resulting in increased production of TNF-α (*Am J Respir Crit Care Med* 1997; **156:** 136–9). However, the same polymorphism in the UK population is not associated with increased risk of COAD (*Eur Respir J* 2000; **15:** 281–4).

Microsomal epoxide hydrolase

A polymorphism variant of microsomal epoxide hydrolase, an enzyme involved in the metabolism of epoxides that may be generated in tobacco smoke, has been associated with a quintupling of the risk of COAD (*Lancet* 1997; **350:** 663).

What is the role of surgery in COAD?

- Bullectomy may improve gas exchange and airflow, and reduce dyspnoea in selected patients with bullae larger than one third of the hemithorax and accompanying lung compression.
- Lung-volume reduction surgery (*N Engl J Med* 2000; **343:** 239–45) results in functional improvements including increased FEV_1, reduced total lung capacity, improved function of respiratory muscles, improved exercise capacity and improved quality of life (*J Thorac Cardiovasc Surg* 1999; **112:** 1319–29; *Am J Respir Crit Care Med* 1999; **160:** 2018–27). These benefits persist for at least a year but the long-term benefits are not known and are currently being investigated by the National Emphysema Treatment Trial Group (*Chest* 1999; **116:** 1750–61).
- Single lung transplantation: this has been successful for at least 3–4 years in patients with COAD. The criteria for selecting patients for transplantation have not been established. It does not improve survival but improves quality of life (*J Thorac Cardiovasc Surg* 1991; **101:** 623–32).

What are the general indications for lung transplantation?

The general indication is end-stage lung disease without alternative forms of therapy. Patients should be below 60 years of age and should have a life expectancy of less than 12 or 18 months; they should not have an underlying cancer or other serious systemic illness. The most common lung diseases are pulmonary fibrosis, emphysema (particularly α_1-antitrypsin deficiency), bronchiectasis, cystic fibrosis and primary pulmonary hypertension.

What is the role of nutrition in COAD?

Undernutrition is associated with reduced respiratory muscle function and an increased mortality rate. A high dietary intake of n-3 fatty acids may protect cigarette smokers against COAD.

Mention some newer treatments for COAD.

- Antagonists of inflammatory mediators: 5-lipoxygenase inhibitors, leukotriene B4 antagonists, interleukin-8 antagonists, tumour necrosis factor inhibitors and antioxidants.
- Protease inhibitors: neutrophil elastase inhibitors, cathepsin inhibitors, non-selective matrix metalloprotease inhibitors, elafin, secretory leukoprotease inhibitor, α_1-antitrypsin.
- New anti-inflammatory agents: phosphodiesterase-4 inhibitors, nuclear factor-kappaB inhibitors, adhesion molecule inhibitors and p38 mitogen-activated protein kinase inhibitors (*N Engl J Med* 2000; **343:** 1960–1).

Peter Howard, contemporary chest physician, Sheffield; his chief interest is long-term domiciliary oxygen therapy.

Peter Barnes, contemporary physician and professor, National Heart and Lung Institute London

---

Case 100

BRONCHIECTASIS

INSTRUCTION

Examine this patient's chest.
Listen to this patient's chest.

SALIENT FEATURES

History

- Cough with copious purulent sputum, recurrent haemoptysis.
- Intermittent fever and night sweats.
- History of recurrent chest infections.
- Weight loss.

Examination

- Copious purulent expectoration (remember to check the sputum cup in a chest case).
- Finger clubbing.
- Bilateral coarse, late, inspiratory crackles.

Proceed as follows:

- Comment on kyphoscoliosis if present.
- Tell the examiner that you would like to know whether the bronchiectasis is of long standing; if so, you would like to examine the abdomen for splenomegaly (amyloidosis).

In addition there may be signs of collapse, fibrosis or pneumonia.

DIAGNOSIS

This patient has bilateral, coarse, late inspiratory crackles with purulent sputum (lesion) due to bronchiectasis (aetiology), and is cyanosed.

QUESTIONS

What do you understand by the term 'bronchiectasis'?

It is a chronic necrotizing infection of the bronchi and bronchioles leading to abnormal, permanent dilatation of the airways.

Mention the causes of bronchiectasis.

- Postpneumonic, measles, pertussis, tuberculosis (TB).
- Mechanical bronchial obstruction, as in TB, carcinoma, nodal compression.
- Allergic bronchopulmonary aspergillosis.
- γ-Globulin deficiency – congenital, acquired.
- Immotile cilia syndrome (Kartagener's syndrome).
- Cystic fibrosis.
- Neuropathic disorders (namely Riley–Day syndrome, Chagas' disease).
- Idiopathic.

What investigations would you perform in such a patient?

FBC, sputum culture, CXR, bronchography, CT scan of the chest.

ADVANCED-LEVEL QUESTIONS

How can CT assess bronchiectasis?

High-resolution CT performed at the end of expiration suggests that small airways disease may be an early feature of bronchiectasis, which leads to more progressive injury and bronchiolar distortion. Larger studies with long-term follow-up are required to confirm this. Conventional CT has a sensitivity of 60–80% for detecting bronchiectasis, whereas high-resolution CT has a sensitivity of more than 90%, using bronchography as the 'gold standard'.

What is the difference between standard and high-resolution CT?

In standard CT the resolution is 10 mm thick whereas with high-resolution CT the slices are 1–2 mm thick and high spatial resolution algorithms are used to recon-struct images (*Radiology* 1994; **193**: 369–74).

What do you know about spiral CT?

This is a rapidly evolving technique to image the chest which has the advantage of truly contiguous sections; consequently completely seamless reconstructions are possible. This may allow virtual-reality bronchoscopy imaging (*Am J Roentgenol* 1994; **162**: 561–7).

What are the complications of bronchiectasis?

- Pneumonia, pleurisy, pleural effusion, pneumothorax.
- Sinusitis.
- Haemoptysis.
- Brain abscess.
- Amyloidosis.

What are the major respiratory pathogens in bronchiectasis?
Staphylococcus aureus, Haemophilus influenzae, Pseudomonas aeruginosa.

How would you treat such patients?
- Postural drainage.
- Antibiotics.
- Bronchodilators.
- Surgery in selected cases.

What abnormalities may be associated with bronchiectasis?
- Congenital absence of bronchial cartilage (Williams–Campbell syndrome).
- Tracheobronchomegaly (Mounier–Kuhn syndrome).
- Obstructive azoospermia and chronic sinopulmonary infection (Young's syndrome), said to be due to mercury intoxication. It was first described from the north of England by Young in 1970.
- Congenital kyphoscoliosis.
- Situs inversus and paranasal sinusitis (Kartagener's syndrome).
- Unilateral absence of pulmonary artery.

What is the indication for surgery in bronchiectasis?
Bronchiectasis localized to a single lobe or segment without clinical, bronchographic or CT evidence of bronchiectasis or bronchitis affecting other parts of the lung.

What are the common sites for localized disease?
Left lower lobe and lingula.

What do you understand by the term 'bronchiectasis sicca'?
Bronchiectasis or 'dry' bronchiectasis is that which presents with recurrent dry cough associated with intermittent episodes (months or years apart) of haemoptysis. The haemoptysis can be life threatening as bleeding is from bronchial vessels with systemic pressures. There is usually a past history of granulomatous infection, particularly tuberculosis. The upper lobes are often primarily affected, allowing good drainage.

What do you know about bronchiectasis in allergic bronchopulmonary aspergillosis?
The bronchial dilatation occurs in more proximal bronchi as a result of type III immune complex reactions.

What do you know about Reid's classification of bronchiectasis?
In 1950, Reid correlated pathological changes with bronchography and described three different appearances. All three types can be present in the same patient.

- Cylindrical bronchiectasis: refers to bronchi that are uniformly dilated and do not taper, but rather end abruptly. This is due to plugging of smaller bronchi by thick mucus and casts. The bronchi are dilated to greater than 2 mm but can be so large as to admit a finger.
- Varicose bronchiectasis: refers to dilated bronchi with irregular bulging contours similar to a varicose vein. They do not taper and terminations are bulbous. Bronchial subdivisions are reduced.

- Cystic or saccular bronchiectasis: the most severe form, characterized by sharply reduced bronchial subdivisions and dilated bronchi ending in cystic pus-filled cavities.

Laennec was the first to describe bronchiectasis in 1819.

M. Kartagener (b. 1897), a Swiss physician.

C.M. Riley and R.L. Day, both US paediatricians. Riley–Day syndrome consists of dysautonomia and lack of coordination in swallowing.

C.J.R. Chagas (1879–1934), a Brazilian physician.

Case 101

COR PULMONALE

INSTRUCTION

Examine this patient's chest.

SALIENT FEATURES

History
- Symptoms of COAD (see pp 261–6).
- Easy fatiguability, shortness of breath on exertion, weakness.
- Leg oedema, and right upper quadrant pain.

Examination
- Patient is short of breath at rest and is centrally cyanosed.
- Tar staining of the fingers.
- JVP is raised: both 'a' and 'v' waves are seen, 'v' waves being prominent if there is associated tricuspid regurgitation.
- On examination of the chest there is bilateral wheeze and other signs of chronic bronchitis (see pp 261–6).

Proceed as follows:
- Examine the cardiovascular system for signs of pulmonary hypertension:
  - Left parasternal heave (often absent when the chest is barrel shaped).
  - Right ventricular gallop rhythm.
  - Loud P_2 and a loud ejection click.
  - Pansystolic murmur of tricuspid regurgitation.
  - Early diastolic Graham Steell murmur in the pulmonary area.
- Look for signs of:
  - Hepatomegaly.
  - Pedal oedema.

DIAGNOSIS

This patient has chronic cor pulmonale (lesion) due to long-standing COAD (aetiology) and is in congestive cardiac failure (functional status).

QUESTIONS

What do you understand by the term 'cor pulmonale'?

Cor pulmonale is right ventricular enlargement due to the increase in afterload that occurs in diseases of the lung, chest wall or pulmonary circulation.

Mention a few causes of cor pulmonale.

Respiratory disorders:
- Obstructive:
  - COAD.
  - Chronic persistent asthma.
- Restrictive:
  - Intrinsic – interstitial fibrosis, lung resection.
  - Extrinsic – obesity, muscle weakness, kyphoscoliosis, high altitude.

Pulmonary vascular disorders:
- Pulmonary emboli.
- Vasculitis of the small pulmonary arteries.
- Adult respiratory distress syndrome.
- Primary pulmonary hypertension.

ADVANCED-LEVEL QUESTIONS

How would you manage a patient with cor pulmonale?

- Treat the underlying cause.
- Treat respiratory failure. If PaO_2 is less than 8 kPa, administer 24% oxygen. There is no need for oxygen if PaO_2 is more than 8 kPa. Monitor blood gases after 30 minutes. If PCO_2 is rising (by 1 kPa), monitor blood gases hourly. If PCO_2 continues to rise, administer doxapram. If, in spite of this, the deterioration continues, the patient may merit artificial ventilation.
- Treat cardiac failure with furosemide (frusemide).
- Consider venesection if the haematocrit is more than 55% (*Lancet* 1989; **ii:** 20–1).

What is the prognosis in cor pulmonale?

Approximately 50% of patients succumb within 5 years.

Case 102

CONSOLIDATION

INSTRUCTION

Examine this patient's chest.

SALIENT FEATURES

History

- Abrupt onset of symptoms.
- Cough with purulent sputum.
- Fever with sweating or rigors.
- Pleuritic chest pain (pp 251, 256).
- Shortness of breath.
- Haemoptysis.
- Nausea, vomiting, diarrhoea (consider *Legionella*).
- Mental status changes (esp. elderly).

Examination

- Purulent sputum (if bacterial in aetiology).
- Tachypnoea.
- Reduced movement of the affected side.
- Trachea central.
- Impaired percussion note.
- Bronchial breath sounds.
- Crackles.

DIAGNOSIS

This patient has left lower lobe consolidation with purulent sputum (lesion) indicating a bacterial pneumonia (aetiology).

Read *N Engl J Med* 1995; **333:** 1618–24; *Br J Hosp Med* 1993; **49:** 346–50.

QUESTIONS

What is the aetiology?

- Bacterial pneumonia.
- Bronchogenic carcinoma.
- Pulmonary infarct.

How would you investigate suspected bacterial pneumonia?

- Full blood count, serum urea, electrolytes and liver function tests.
- Sputum and blood cultures.
- Arterial blood gases.
- CXR.

- Test for *Legionella* (culture, direct fluorescent-antibody test, or urinary antigen assay), mycoplasma immunoglobulin M.
- Consider serological testing for human immunodeficiency virus (for patients 15–54 years old, particularly when there is lymphopenia or a low CD4 cell count).

ADVANCED-LEVEL QUESTIONS

What are the causes of a poorly resolving or recurrent pneumonia?
- Carcinoma of the lung.
- Aspiration of a foreign body.
- Inappropriate antibiotic.
- Sequestration (rare; suspect if left lower lobe is involved).

What do you know about atypical pneumonias?
Typical pneumonia is caused by pneumococcus (*Streptococcus pneumoniae*), whereas atypical pneumonia is that *not* due to pneumococcus; the latter may be caused by *Mycoplasma, Legionella, Chlamydia, Coxiella*, etc. The clinical picture in atypical pneumonia is dominated by constitutional symptoms, such as fever and headache, rather than respiratory symptoms.

What do you know about mycoplasma pneumonia?
Mycoplasma pneumoniae is an important cause of atypical pneumonia. It is an important community-acquired pneumonia and epidemics are seen every 4 years or so. Its incubation is 2–3 weeks and it is usually seen in children and young adults. Reinfection can occur in older patients with detectable *M. pneumoniae* antibody. Like all other pneumonias, mycoplasma pneumonia is common in winter months.

What are the extrapulmonary manifestations of mycoplasma pneumonia?
- Arthralgia and arthritis.
- Autoimmune haemolytic anaemia.
- Neurological manifestations involving both central and peripheral nervous systems.
- Pericarditis, myocarditis.
- Hepatitis, glomerulonephritis.
- Non-specific rash, erythema multiforme and Stevens–Johnson syndrome.
- Disseminated intravascular coagulation (DIC).

What are the complications of pneumonia?
- Septicaemia.
- Lung abscess.
- Empyema.
- Adult respiratory distress syndrome.
- Multiorgan failure, renal failure.
- Haemolytic syndrome.
- Death.

Which antibiotics would you use in a patient with community-acquired pneumonia where the pathogen is not known?
The British Thoracic Society recommends that empirical therapy 'should always cover' *Strep. pneumoniae*. The preferred regimen is amoxicillin or penicillin; when

Legionella or *M. pneumoniae* is specifically suspected, erythromycin should be given, and antibiotics directed against *Staphylococcus aureus* should be considered during epidemics of influenza.

What are the poor prognostic factors in patients with community-acquired pneumonia?

- Age over 65 years.
- Coexisting conditions such as cardiac failure, renal failure, chronic obstructive pulmonary disease, malignancy.
- Clinical features: respiratory rate >30 per min, hypotension (systolic blood pressure <90 mmHg or diastolic pressure <60 mmHg), temperature >38.3°C, impaired mental status (stupor, lethargy, disorientation or coma), extrapulmonary infection (e.g. septic arthritis, meningitis).
- Investigations: haematocrit <30%, white cell count <4000 or >30 000 per mm^3, azotaemia, arterial blood gas <60 mmHg while breathing room air, chest radiograph showing multiple lobe involvement, rapid spread or pleural effusion.
- Microbial pathogens: *Staph. aureus, Legionella, Strep. pneumoniae.*

What do you know about pulmonary eosinophilic disorders?

Crofton et al described five classes of pulmonary eosinophilic disorder (*Thorax* 1952; **7**: 1–35):

- Löffler's syndrome: characterized by transient pulmonary infiltrates and peripheral eosinophilia. It is associated with parasitic infections, drug allergies and exposure to inorganic chemicals such as nickel carbonyl. The course is benign and respiratory failure almost unknown.
- Eosinophilia in asthmatics: the most common cause is allergic bronchopulmonary aspergillosis. This condition is benign but chronic.
- Tropical eosinophilia which is secondary to filarial infection (*Wuchereria bancrofti* or *W. malayi Brug*).
- Churg–Strauss syndrome. Diagnosis requires four of the following features: asthma; eosinophilia greater than 10%; mononeuropathy or polyneuropathy; paranasal sinus abnormality; non-fixed pulmonary infiltrates visible on chest radiographs; blood vessels with extravascular eosinophils found on biopsy.
- Chronic eosinophilic pneumonia: chronic debilitating illness characterized by malaise, fever, weight loss and dyspnoea. The chest radiograph shows a peripheral alveolar filling infiltrate predominantly in the upper lobes (the 'photographic negative' of pulmonary oedema).

What do you know about bronchopulmonary sequestration?

It is an uncommon congenital lesion in which a portion of non-functioning lung tissue is detached from the normal lung and supplied by an anomalous systemic artery, usually arising from the aorta or one of its branches. The tissue has no communication with the bronchopulmonary tree. Two types of sequestration have been described: extralobar and intralobar. An extralobar sequestration has its own pleural lining, which separates it from the remaining lung tissue, and the intralobar type shares its pleura with the adjacent normal lung. Patients usually present in childhood with cough and recurrent pneumonia, and occasionally present with haemoptysis.

Case 103

BRONCHOGENIC CARCINOMA

INSTRUCTION

Examine this patient's chest.

SALIENT FEATURES

History

- Symptoms related to:
  - Primary tumour (cough, dyspnoea, haemoptysis, post-obstructive pneumonia).
  - Mediastinal spread (hoarseness with left-sided lesions due to recurrent laryngeal nerve palsy; obstruction of the superior vena cava with right-sided tumours or associated lymphadenopathy; elevation of the hemidiaphragm as result of phrenic nerve paralysis; dysphagia from oesophageal obstruction and pericardial tamponade).
  - Metastases (sites include liver, brain, pleural cavity, bone, adrenal glands, contralateral lung and skin). (Initial presentation with symptoms from a metastatic focus is particularly common with adenocarcinoma.)
  - Paraneoplastic syndrome (pain in arms or legs due to hypertrophic osteoarthropathy, symptoms of hypercalcaemia due to squamous cell carcinoma, neurological syndromes).
  - Systemic effects (anorexia, weight loss, weakness and profound fatigue).
- History of smoking.

Examination

- *Patient 1* has clubbing and tar staining of the fingers.
  - Dull percussion note at the apex with absent breath sounds.
  - Look for Horner's syndrome and wasting of the small muscles of the hand.
- *Patient 2* has signs of pleural effusion on one side.
- *Patient 3* shows signs of unilateral collapse or consolidation of the upper lobe on one side.

Note. If you suspect bronchogenic carcinoma, always look for clubbing, tar staining, cervical lymph nodes and radiation marks, and comment on cachexia.

DIAGNOSIS

This patient with marked clubbing and large pleural effusion (lesion) probably has bronchogenic carcinoma (aetiology) and is very short of breath due to the large effusion (functional status).

Read *BMJ* 1992; **304:** 1298; *BMJ* 1990; **301:** 1287.

QUESTIONS

How may patients with bronchogenic carcinoma present?

- Cough (in 80% of cases), haemoptysis (70%) and dyspnoea (60%); loss of weight, anorexia.
- Skeletal manifestations: clubbing (in 30% of cases).
- Local pressure effects: recurrent laryngeal nerve palsy, superior vena caval obstruction, Horner's syndrome.
- Endocrine manifestations: 12% of tumours – in particular small cell tumours – present with syndrome of inappropriate antidiuretic hormone (SIADH), hypercalcaemia, adrenocorticotrophic hormone (ACTH) secretion, gynaecomastia. SIADH does not usually cause symptoms. When Cushing's syndrome occurs the manifestations are primarily metabolic (hypokalaemic alkalosis).
- Neurological manifestations: Eaton–Lambert syndrome, cerebellar degeneration, polyneuropathy, dementia, proximal myopathy, encephalomyelitis, subacute sensory neuropathy, limbic encephalitis, opsoclonus and myoclonus.
- Cardiovascular: thrombophlebitis migrans, atrial fibrillation, pericarditis, non-bacterial thrombotic endocarditis.
- Cutaneous manifestations: dermatomyositis, acanthosis nigricans, herpes zoster.
- Anaemia, disseminated intravascular coagulation, thrombotic thrombocytopenic purpura. Hypercoagulopathy in the form of venous thromboembolism is seen, especially with adenocarcinoma.
- Membranous glomerulonephritis.

How would you investigate this patient?

- Sputum cytology: high yield for endobronchial tumours such as squamous cell and small cell carcinoma but poor yield for adenocarcinoma.
- CXR.
- Pleural fluid cytology.
- Bronchoscopy gives a high yield in excess of 90%, particularly when the tumour is viewed endobronchially. For tumours that are not visualized, the yield for washing and brushing is about 75% in central lesions and 55% in peripheral lesions. The yield in small-cell and squamous cell carcinomas is higher than in adenocarcinomas.
- CT scan of the chest and upper abdomen (to image the liver and adrenals).
- Bone scan for metastases (helpful in staging).
- PET scanning is highly sensitive and specific for mediastinal staging.
- Pulmonary function tests (most surgeons aim for a FEV_1 of about 1 litre after planned resection); a DLCO below 60% predicted is associated with a mortality rate as high as 25% due to respiratory complications.

ADVANCED-LEVEL QUESTIONS

What is the aim of staging?

The main aim of staging is to identify candidates for surgical resection, since this approach offers the highest potential cure for lung cancer. The staging assessment covers three major issues: distant metastases, the state of the chest and mediastinum, and the condition of the patient.

What is the role of surgery in lung carcinoma?

Surgery is beneficial in peripheral non-small cell carcinoma. Its role is limited in small cell carcinoma, as over 90% have metastasized by the time of diagnosis.

Which tumours respond well to chemotherapy?

Small cell carcinoma: cyclophosphamide, doxorubicin, cisplatin, etoposide and vincristine are some of the drugs used. The combination of etoposide and cisplatin appears to have the best therapeutic index of any regimen. A meta-analysis of the role of chemotherapy in non-small cell lung cancers suggested that the benefits are small.

What are the drugs used in non-small cell lung cancer?

- Old agents: cisplatin, carboplatin, etoposide, vinblastine, vindesine.
- Newer agents: docetaxel, paclitaxel, irinotecan, vinorelbine, gemcitabine.

What are the indications for radiotherapy?

- Pain – either local or metastatic.
- Breathlessness due to bronchial obstruction.
- Dysphagia.
- Haemoptysis.
- Superior venal caval obstruction.
- Pancoast's tumour.
- Before and after operation in selected patients.

What are the contraindications for surgery?

- Metastatic carcinoma.
- FEV_1 less than 1.5 litres.
- Transfer factor less than 50%.
- Severe pulmonary hypertension.
- Uncontrolled major cardiac arrhythmias.
- Carbon dioxide retention.
- Myocardial infarction in the past 3 months.

Is the progression of cancer associated with genetic change?

Yes: it is accompanied by a mutation in the p53 gene and loss of a portion of the short arm of chromosome 3 in small cell cancer; the functional significance of this is not clear.

Robert Souhami, Professor of Clinical Oncology, University College and Middlesex School of Medicine, London.

Case 104
CYSTIC FIBROSIS

INSTRUCTION

Examine the chest of this male patient who has had a good appetite, poor weight gain and foul fatty stool.

SALIENT FEATURES

History

- Cough with purulent and viscous expectoration.
- Diabetes mellitus.
- Gastrointestinal symptoms (steatorrhoea, failure to thrive in childhood, rectal prolapse, meconium ileus or distal intestinal obstruction).
- Heat stroke, salt depletion.
- Sterility in men and decreased fertility in women.

Examination

- Sputum is purulent.
- Patient is short of breath.
- Central cyanosis.
- Finger clubbing.
- Bilateral coarse crackles.

Proceed as follows:
Tell the examiner that you would like to check the following levels:

- Urine sugar.
- Faecal fat.
- Sweat sodium.

DIAGNOSIS

This patient has bilateral coarse crackles, asthenia and foul fatty stool (lesion) due to cystic fibrosis (aetiology) and requires continuous oxygen indicating respiratory failure (functional status).

QUESTIONS

What are the chances of this male patient having a child?

Males are sterile owing to the failure of development of the vas deferens and epididymis.

What are the clinical manifestations of this condition?

Neonates
Recurrent chest infections, failure to thrive, meconium ileus and rectal prolapse.

In childhood and young adults
- Respiratory: infection, bronchiectasis, pneumothorax, haemoptysis, nasal polyps, allergic bronchopulmonary aspergillosis, deterioration during and after pregnancy.
- Cardiovascular: cor pulmonale.
- Gastrointestinal: rectal prolapse, distal ileal obstruction (meconium ileus equivalent), cirrhosis, gallstones, intussusception.
- Miscellaneous: male infertility, diabetes mellitus, hypertrophic pulmonary osteoarthropathy.

How would you treat steatorrhoea?
- Low-fat diet.
- Pancreatic supplements.
- H_2-receptor antagonist.

How would you treat chest complications?
- Postural drainage.
- Antibiotics.
- Bronchodilators.
- Heart–lung transplantantion.

What is the role of physiotherapy?
Physiotherapy has been shown to be useful, but there remains considerable debate regarding the effectiveness of different techniques including traditional postural drainage and percussion, forced expiratory technique, positive expiratory pressure masks, autodrainage and flutter valves.

ADVANCED-LEVEL QUESTIONS

What is the inheritance in cystic fibrosis?
Autosomal recessive. On the long arm of chromosome 7 resides the gene coding for a 1480-amino-acid protein a cyclic AMP-regulated chloride channel, now called the cystic fibrosis transmembrane conductor regulator (CFTR). The CFTR gene is carried by 1 in 20 Caucasians and its incidence is about 1 in 2000 live births. There is a mutation on the long arm of chromosome 7 in 70% of patients. There is a deletion of the codon for phenylalanine at position 508 (Δ508; *N Engl J Med* 1990; **323**: 1517). This defect leads to a failure of the chloride channel to open in response to cyclic AMP (*Science* 1992; **256**: 774–9; *N Engl J Med* 1991; **325**: 575–7). More than 175 other types of lesion in the cystic fibrosis gene are responsible for the disease in the remaining 30% of patients.

How is this condition diagnosed in infancy?
Immunoreactive trypsin assay in dried blood.

What do you know about sweat testing?
A sweat sodium concentration over 60 mmol/l is indicative of cystic fibrosis. It identifies over 75% by the age of 2 years and about 95% by the age of 12 years. It is more difficult to interpret in older children and adults.

What is the basic defect in the airways of these patients?
The opening of chloride channels at the luminal surface of the airway epithelial cells in normal individuals allows the passive transport of chloride along an electro-chemical gradient from the cytoplasm to the lumen. In patients with cystic fibrosis

there is a defect in these channels which prevents the normal secretion of chloride into the airway lumen. Simultaneously, there is a three-fold increase in the reabsorption of sodium from the airway lumen into the cytoplasm of the epithelial cell. As the movement of water into airway secretions follows the movement of salt, it is believed that a decreased secretion of chloride into the airway lumen and the increased reabsorption of sodium from the airway lumen combine to reduce water content and increase the viscosity and tenacity of the airway secretions.

If the patient has persistent purulent cough, which organisms are usually responsible?

Staphylococcus aureus, Haemophilus influenzae, Burkholderia cepacia and *Pseudomonas aeruginosa*. The latter is associated with poor prognosis as this organism is almost impossible to eradicate.

Which antibiotics are usually used to treat pseudomonal infections?

Intravenous or aerosol carbenicillin and gentamicin in combination.

What is the risk of cancer in patients with cystic fibrosis?

The overall risk of cancer is similar to that of the general population, but there is an increased risk of digestive tract cancers (*N Engl J Med* 1995; **332:** 494–9). Persistent or unexplained gastrointestinal symptoms in these patients ought to be investigated carefully.

What is the lifespan in such patients?

The median age of survival is currently in the early 30s. It is estimated that at least half of those with cystic fibrosis will be adults by the year 2000.

What is the cause of death in cystic fibrosis?

Death occurs from pulmonary complications, such as pneumonia, pneumothorax or haemoptysis, or as a result of terminal chronic respiratory failure.

What parameters can predict death in cystic fibrosis?

Prediction of death within 2 years can be made for 50% of the patients whose forced expiratory volume in 1 second (FEV$_1$) is less than 30%. Thus the necessity for referral for transplantation can be anticipated about 1 year in advance of death (*N Engl J Med* 1992; **326:** 1187–91).

How would you manage a patient who has been accepted for transplantation?

The aim is to sustain life by aggressive therapy with nocturnal oxygen, continuous intravenous antibiotics, enteral feeding, respiratory stimulants and nasal intermittent positive pressure ventilation (*Eur Respir J* 1991; **4:** 524–7).

If this patient requires lung transplantation, which type of transplantation is the treatment of choice?

Bilateral lung transplantation is necessary for patients with chronic bronchial infection such as cystic fibrosis (or bronchiectasis) to avoid contamination of the donor lung by spill-over of infected material from the recipient's remaining lung (*J Thorac Cardiovasc Surg* 1992; **103:** 287–94).

What are the complications of lung transplantation?

Early post-transplantation lung oedema, infection and rejection (including obliterative bronchiolitis).

What are the indications for combined heart–lung transplantation?

Combined heart–lung transplantation has relatively few indications, the primary one being congenital heart disease with Eisenmenger syndrome.

What new methods of treatment are available?

- High-dose ibuprofen in patients with mild disease (FEV_1 of at least 60% of the predicted value), taken consistently for 4 years, significantly slows the progression of lung disease without serious adverse effects (*N Engl J Med* 1995; **332**: 848–54).
- Aerosolized recombinant human DNAse, which is capable of degrading DNA in the bronchial secretion, has been shown to improve forced expiratory flow rates when given by aerosol (*N Engl J Med* 1994; **331**: 637–42).
- Gene therapy: the gene is transferred in a 'carrier' (either in a cationic lipid envelope known as a liposome (*Nat Med* 1995; **1**: 39–46), or in an adenovirus). On transferring the gene for cystic fibrosis to the nasal epithelium using a cationic liposome, the deficit was partly restored without provoking a local inflammatory response.
- Improvement of the hydration of secretion:
  - By blocking the reabsorption of sodium from the airway lumen with amiloride.
  - By stimulating the secretion of chloride with triphosphate nucleotides (ATP or uridine triphosphate) through nucleotide receptors by a pathway independent of cylic AMP metabolism (*N Engl J Med* 1991; **322**: 1189–94).
- Immunization to various components of *Pseudomonas*.

What advice would you give a patient with cystic fibrosis who wishes to become pregnant?

- The couple will be offered genetic counselling and the man will be offered testing to determine his genetic status. If he is a carrier, chorionic villous sampling will be considered as the risk of the couple conceiving an infant with cystic fibrosis is 1 in 2 and they may wish to consider selective termination in the first trimester. The hazards of general anaesthesia (as lung function is impaired) for termination of pregnancy will be brought to their attention. Termination of pregnancy either with spinal anaesthesia or medications is an alternative.
- Women with severe disease will be informed that they may be unable to complete pregnancy and that their premature demise may leave a motherless child.
- In women with an FEV_1 less than 60% of the predicted value there is an increased risk of premature delivery, an increased rate of caesarean section, some loss of lung function and risk of respiratory complications, and early death of the mother (*BMJ* 1995; **311**: 822–3).
- Pregnancy after heart–lung transplantation offers better health and increased longevity in the mother, but the risk of organ rejection and exposure of the fetus to potentially teratogenic immunosuppressants means that pregnancy should not be attempted by women with transplants.

What is the 'forme fruste' of cystic fibrosis?

Increasingly, with the availability of neonatal screening with immunoreactive trypsin and thorough diagnosis by genetic studies, milder forms of disease have been recognized without the increase in sweat sodium. It is predicted that a considerable number of patients will present with a pattern of disease in adult life that has not been recognized in the past as being due to cystic fibrosis.

Sir Magdi H. Yacoub, contemporary Egyptian-born cardiothoracic surgeon at Harefield Hospital, London, popularized cardiac transplantation in the UK.

The first successful pregnancy in a woman with cystic fibrosis was reported in 1960.

Case 105

FIBROSING ALVEOLITIS

INSTRUCTION

Examine this patient's chest.
Examine the respiratory system from the back.

SALIENT FEATURES

History

- Progressive exertional dyspnoea (90%).
- Chronic cough (74%).
- Arthralgia/arthritis (19%).
- Obtain a drug history (amiodarone, nitrofurantoin and busulfan).

Examination

- Clubbing.
- Central cyanosis.
- Bilateral, basal, fine, end-inspiratory crackles which disappear or become quieter on leaning forwards. Furthermore, the crackles do not disappear on coughing (unlike those of pulmonary oedema). The crackles have been called 'Velcro' or 'Cellophane' crackles.
- Tachypnoea (in advanced cases).

Proceed as follows:
- Examine the following:
  - Hands (for rheumatoid arthritis, systemic sclerosis).
  - Face (for typical rash of SLE, heliotropic rash of dermatomyositis, typical facies of systemic sclerosis, lupus pernio of sarcoid).
  - Mouth (for aphthous ulcers of Crohn's disease, dry mouth of Sjögren's syndrome).
- Look for signs of pulmonary hypertension: 'a' wave in the JVP, left parasternal heave and P_2.

DIAGNOSIS

This patient has bilateral, basal, fine, end-inspiratory crackles (lesion) due to fibrosing alveolitis (aetiology) and is tachypnoeic at rest (functional status).

QUESTIONS

In which other conditions is clubbing associated with crackles?
- Bronchogenic carcinoma (crackles are localized).
- Bronchiectasis (coarse crackles).
- Asbestosis (history of exposure to asbestos).

ADVANCED-LEVEL QUESTIONS

Mention possible aetiological factors.
These include metal dust (steel, brass, lead); wood dust (pine); wood smoke and smoking.

Mention other conditions which have similar pulmonary changes.
- Rheumatoid arthritis, SLE, dermatomyositis, chronic active hepatitis, ulcerative colitis, systemic sclerosis.
- Pneumoconiosis.
- Granulomatous disease: sarcoid, TB.
- Chronic pulmonary oedema.
- Radiotherapy.
- Lymphangitis carcinomatosa.
- Extrinsic allergic alveolitis: farmer's lung, bird fancier's lung.

What is the pathology in fibrosing alveolitis?
Fibrosing alveolitis is characterized by the presence of connective tissue matrix proteins within the acinar regions of the lung in association with a variable cellular infiltrate within the alveoli and in the interstitium.

What are the types of interstitial pneumonitis?
Liebow and Carrington (Liebow AA, Carrington CB 1969 The interstitial pneumonias. In: Simon M, Potchen EJ, LeMay M (eds) *Frontiers of Pulmonary Radiology*. Grune & Stratton, New York, pp 102–141) initially described five subgroups, depending on histology, to which there has recently been an addition:

- Classical (usual) interstitial pneumonia (UIP), characterized by thickening of the alveolar interstitium by fibrous tissue and mononuclear cells; characteristically varying in severity from one focus to another. The mean survival is 2.8–5.6 years. Twelve per cent respond to steroids and spontaneous improvement does not occur.
- Desquamative interstitial pneumonia (DIP) where there is a marked accumulation of macrophages in the alveolar airspaces associated with a relatively mild but uniform thickening of the interstitial space caused by mononuclear inflammatory cells. The mean survival is 12.4–14 years. The response to steroids is 62% and spontaneous improvement is 22%.
- Non-specific interstitial pneumonia (NSIP). The survival is 14 years and therapeutic response is similar to DIP.
- A diffuse lesion similar to UIP but with superimposed bronchiolitis obliterans.
- Lymphoid interstitial pneumonia (LIP) in which there is marked infiltration of interstitium by lymphocytes that may be indistinguishable from lymphoma.
- Giant-cell interstitial pneumonia consisting of a mononuclear cell infiltrate in the interstitium associated with large numbers of multinucleated giant cells.

How would you investigate this patient?

- CXR typically shows bilateral basal reticulonodular shadows which advance upwards as the disease progresses. In advanced cases there is marked destruction of the parenchyma causing 'honeycombing' (due to groups of closely set ring shadows), and nodular shadows are not conspicuous. The mediastinum may appear broad as a result of a decrease in lung volume.
- Blood gases: arterial desaturation worsens while upright and improves on recumbency. There is arterial hypoxaemia and *hypocapnia*.
- Pulmonary function tests: in the early stages lung volumes may be normal, but there is arterial desaturation following exercise. Typically there is a restrictive defect with reduction of both the gas transfer factor and gas transfer coefficient.
- High ESR; raised immunoglobulins; raised antinuclear factor; rheumatoid factor is positive.
- Bronchial lavage: a large number of lymphocytes indicates a good response to steroids and a good prognosis. A large number of neutrophils and eosinophils indicates a poor prognosis (5-year survival rate of 60% for steroid responders versus 25% for non-responders). The patients are more likely to respond to cyclophosphamide if the number of neutrophils is increased (*Am Rev Respir Dis* 1987; **135**: 26).
- Lung biopsy: in early stages there is mononuclear cell infiltration in the alveolar walls, progressing to interstitial fibrosis – known as usual interstitial pneumonitis (UIP); in later stages fibrotic contraction of the lung, honeycombing, bronchial dilatation and cysts are seen. DIP – alveolar macrophages with little mononuclear infiltration or fibrosis – has a better prognosis than UIP as it responds to steroids.
- MRI is useful in determining disease activity without ionizing radiation but it is an expensive method.
- High-resolution CT (HRCT) is useful to assess the pattern and extent of disease. Patients with a predominantly ground-glass appearance are treated whereas those with a predominantly reticular appearance undergo technetium diethylenetriamine penta-acetate scanning (DPTA) to assess the probability of deterioration. HRCT may avoid the need for biopsy, especially if there is predominantly reticular shadowing. It acts as a guide for ideal biopsy site.
- Technetium-99m diethylenetriamine penta-acetate (DPTA) scanning in non-smokers is of value in identifying which patients are more likely to deteriorate. Therapy can be postponed when there is slow clearance, whereas those with fast clearance should receive treatment (*Eur Respir J* 1993; **6**: 797–802).

Mention prognostic factors.

Short duration of disease, young age of patient at onset, female, predominantly ground-glass shadowing on CXR and presence of little fibrosis on lung biopsies are good prognostic factors.

How would you manage this patient?

- All patients should receive a course of steroids (unless there are contraindications): prednisolone 40 mg per day for 6 weeks. Monitor symptoms, CXR, lung function tests. If response is good, continue; if no response then taper over 1 week.
- Steroid non-responders may benefit from a course of cyclophosphamide. Occasionally, patients who are unresponsive to prednisolone and cyclophosphamide will respond to prednisolone and azathioprine.
- Identify the underlying cause and manage accordingly.

What is the prognosis?

The 5-year overall survival rate is 50%, 65% in steroid responders and 25% in steroid non-responders.

What are the causes of death in such patients?

- Respiratory failure or cor pulmonale precipitated by chest infection.
- Ten-fold increase in bronchogenic carcinoma compared with normal controls.

What is the role for lung transplantation?

Single-lung transplantation is now an established and effective form of treatment for certain individuals. Current survival rate at 1 year is approximately 60% (*N Engl J Med* 1986; **314:** 1140–45).

What do you know about the Hamman–Rich syndrome?

The Hamman–Rich syndrome is a rapidly progressive and fatal variant of interstitial lung disease described by Hamman and Rich (*Bull Johns Hopkins Hosps* 1944; **74:** 177).

Mention indications for transbronchial and open lung biopsy.

- Transbronchial: sarcoidosis, tuberculosis, berylliosis, lymphangitis carcinomatosa, extrinsic allergic alveolitis.
- Open lung biopsy: fibrosing alveolitis, rheumatological disease, pulmonary vasculitis, lymphangioleiomyomatosis, Langerhans cell histiocytosis.

L.V. Hamman (1877–1946), physician, and A.R. Rich (1893–1968), pathologist, worked at the Johns Hopkins Hospitals, Baltimore (Hamman L, Rich AR 1944 Acute diffuse interstitial fibrosis of the lungs. *Bull Johns Hopkins Hosps* 1944; **74:** 177).

Dame Margaret Turner-Warwick, contemporary chest physician, was the first woman President of the Royal College of the Physicians of London; her chief interest is fibrotic lung disease.

Case 106

PULMONARY FIBROSIS

INSTRUCTION

Examine this patient's chest.

SALIENT FEATURES

History

- History of TB, ankylosing spondylitis, radiation.
- History of phrenic nerve crush, plombage, thoracotomy.

Examination

- The fibrosis is usually apical.
- Flattening of the chest on the affected side.
- Tracheal deviation to the affected side.
- Reduced expansion on the affected side.
- Dull percussion note.
- Presence of localized crackles; bronchial breathing may be present.

Proceed as follows:
Look for the following signs:

- Scars of phrenic nerve crush, plombage, thoracotomy.
- Radiation scars.

DIAGNOSIS

This patient has flattening of the R/L side of the chest with diminished movements on that side, tracheal deviation and localized crackles (lesion) due to pulmonary fibrosis secondary to tuberculosis (aetiology), and is comfortable at rest (functional status).

QUESTIONS

Mention a few causes of upper lobe fibrosis.

- Tuberculosis.
- Ankylosing spondylitis.
- Radiation-induced fibrosis.

ADVANCED-LEVEL QUESTIONS

Which is the best imaging procedure for the upper lobe lesions?
MRI is better for upper lobe lesions than CT of the chest.

What is the role of MRI of the thorax?
MRI of the thorax is less useful than CT scanning because of poorer imaging of the pulmonary parenchyma and inferior spatial resolution. However, MRI can provide images in multiple planes (e.g. sagittal, coronal as well as transverse) which CT can not. MRI is excellent for evaluating processes near the lung apex, spine and thoraco-abdominal junction.

On 8 November 1895 Röntgen discovered what he called X-rays. In the subsequent 7 weeks he meticulously performed experiments, and an X-ray picture of his wife's hand convinced him about the potential role of the new ray. In 1901 he was awarded the Nobel Prize for physics.

Hounsfield's work on CT in the EMI laboratories at Hounslow made it possible to obtain detailed cross-sectional views of the soft tissues, particularly the brain.
Sir Godfrey N. Hounsfield (1919–) and Alan M. Cormack (1924–), the latter of Tufts University, Boston, were jointly awarded the 1979 Nobel Prize for Medicine for the development of computer-assisted tomography.

Case 107

PNEUMOTHORAX

INSTRUCTION

Examine this patient's chest.

SALIENT FEATURES

History

- Sudden onset or rapidly progressive dyspnoea.
- Ipsilateral acute pleuritic pain – the pain is either sharp or a steady ache.
- A small pneumothorax may be asymptomatic.
- Obtain history of recent pleural aspiration or insertion of subclavian line (*J R Soc Med* 1997; **90:** 319–21), recent surgery to head and neck, abdominal procedures using bowel or peritoneal distension.
- History of asthma, COAD, ARDS, pneumonia, trauma to chest.
- History of Marfan's syndrome.
- History of HIV.
- History of positive pressure ventilation.

Examination

- Decreased movement of the affected side.
- Increased percussion note.
- Trachea may be central (small pneumothorax) or deviated to the affected side (underlying collapse of lung) or the opposite side (large pneumothorax).
- Increased vocal resonance with diminished breath sounds.

Proceed as follows:
- Look for clues regarding aetiology:
  - Pleural aspiration site.
  - Infraclavicular region for a bruise from the central line.
  - Comment if the patient is thin or has marfanoid features.
  - Inhaler or peak flow meter by the bedside (asthma, COAD).
- Tell the examiner that you would suspect tension pneumothorax when there is tachycardia (>135 beats/minute), hypotension and pulsus paradoxus.

DIAGNOSIS

This patient has diminished breath sounds and hyper-resonant note on R/L side of the chest (lesion) due to pneumothorax secondary to Marfan's syndrome (aetiology), and is not breathless at rest (functional status).

Read recent review: *N Engl J Med* 2000; **342:** 868–74.

QUESTIONS

What do you understand by the term 'pneumothorax'?
Air in the pleural cavity.

How would you investigate this patient?
- CXR, both inspiratory and expiratory phases. In critically ill patients pneumo-thorax is suspected when (a) the costophrenic angle extends more inferiorly than usual due to air – the 'deep sulcus sign' (*Radiology* 1980; **136:** 25–7), (b) liver appears more radiolucent due to air in the CP angle, or on the left side, when the air will outline the medial aspect of the hemidiaphragm under the heart.
- Blood gases if the patient is breathless: hypoxaemia depending on the shunting, whereas hypercapnia does not develop.

ADVANCED-LEVEL QUESTIONS

How would you grade the degree of collapse?
British Thoracic Society grading:

- Small: where there is a small rim of air around the lung.
- Moderate: when the lung is collapsed towards the heart border.
- Complete: airless lung, separate from the diaphragm (aspiration is necessary).
- Tension: any pneumothorax with cardiorespiratory distress (rare and requires immediate drainage).

How would you manage this patient?
- Small pneumothoraces (less than 20% in size) spontaneously resolve within weeks.
- Larger ones (irrespective of size) with normal lungs are managed by simple aspir-ation rather than an intercostal tube as the initial drainage procedure. Aspiration is less painful than intercostal drainage, leads to a shorter admission and reduces the need for pleurectomy with no increase in recurrence rate at 1 year.
- When there is rapid re-expansion following simple aspiration, an intercostal tube with underwater seal drainage is used. The tube should be left in for at least 24 hours. When the lung re-expands, clamp the tube for 24 hours. If repeat radio-graphy shows that the lung remains expanded, the tube can be removed. If not, suction should be applied to the tube. If it fails to resolve within 1 week, surgical pleurodesis should be considered. Video-assisted thoracoscopic surgery with several chest ports allows clear visualization of the pleural cavity for resection of bullae and pleurodesis.

What are the causes of pneumothorax?
- Spontaneous (usually in thin males).
- Trauma.
- Bronchial asthma.
- COAD – emphysematous bulla (*JAMA* 1975; **234:** 389–93).
- Carcinoma of the lung.
- Cystic fibrosis.
- TB (the original descriptions of pneumothorax were commonly associated with TB, *JAMA* 1931; **96:** 653–7).

- Mechanical ventilation.
- Marfan's syndrome, Ehlers–Danlos syndrome.
- Catamenial pneumothorax, i.e. pneumothorax that occurs in association with menstruation.

How would you perform a pleurodesis?
By injecting talc into the pleural cavity via the intercostal tube.

In which patients would you avoid doing a pleurodesis?
In patients with underlying cystic fibrosis. These patients may require lung transplantation in the future and pleurodesis may make this procedure technically not feasible.

When would you suspect a tension pneumothorax?
Tension pneumothorax should be suspected in the presence of any of the following:

- Severe progressive dyspnoea.
- Severe tachycardia.
- Hypotension.
- Marked mediastinal shift.

When should open thoracotomy be considered?
It should be considered if one of the following is present:

- A third episode of spontaneous pneumothorax.
- Any occurrence of bilateral pneumothorax.
- Failure of the lung to expand after tube thoracostomy for the first episode.

O.K. Williamson (1866–1941), an English physician, described the Williamson sign, i.e. blood pressure in the leg is lower than that in the upper limb on the affected side in pneumothorax.

The use of simple aspiration to manage pneumothorax was first reported by O.G. Raja in 1981 when he was a medical registrar (*Br J Dis Chest* 1981; 75: 207–8).

Case 108

OLD TUBERCULOSIS

INSTRUCTION

Examine this patient's chest.

SALIENT FEATURES

History
- Fever and night sweats.
- Malaise, fatigue, anorexia.
- Weight loss.
- Cough with sputum.

Examination

These patients tend to have signs of common chest diseases which are not cut and dried. There are several reasons for this, such as pleural thickening, thoracotomy and pneumonectomy, associated COAD, associated chest infection, plombage or phrenic nerve crush.

The following provide some examples:

Patient 1

The candidate was asked to examine the chest from the front, as a result of which the old thoracotomy scar was not seen. The patient was wheezy. The trachea was deviated to the right. Percussion note was stony dull from the right second intercostal space downwards. Wheeze was present on the left side. This patient had a right pneumonectomy with COAD in the left lung. The candidate's diagnosis of right-sided pleural effusion with underlying collapse and left-sided COAD was accepted.

Patient 2

The trachea was central. A phrenic nerve crush scar was seen. Percussion note was dull in the left infra-axillary region and there were associated crackles. The diagnosis of pleural thickening with associated chest infection was accepted; that of pleural effusion was not.

QUESTIONS

How would you manage a patient with old tuberculosis?

Old tuberculosis requires no antituberculosis treatment. However, the patient may require symptomatic treatment for wheeze and shortness of breath.

In which groups of people is the risk of tuberculosis high?

- Asian and Irish immigrants.
- The elderly.
- Immunocompromised individuals, particularly AIDS patients.
- Alcoholics.
- Occupations at risk: doctors, nurses, chest physiotherapists.

ADVANCED-LEVEL QUESTIONS

Would you isolate a patient with newly diagnosed, sputum-positive, pulmonary TB?

Yes. Segregation in a single room for 2 weeks is recommended for patients with smear-positive tuberculosis. Barrier nursing, however, is unnecessary. Adults with smear-negative or non-pulmonary disease may be in a general ward. A child with TB should be segregated until the source case is identified as this person may be visiting the child.

How are contacts investigated?

Contacts are investigated by inquiry into bacille Calmette–Guérin (BCG) vaccination site, Heaf testing and CXR examination.

To whom would you offer BCG vaccination?

BCG vaccination is offered to previously unvaccinated, persistently Heaf test-negative or grade 1 contacts aged under 35 years unless there is a special occupational, travel or ethnic risk. Patients with known or suspected HIV infection should not be offered the vaccination.

What are the indications for chemoprophylaxis?

- Chemoprophylaxis may be given to those with strongly positive Heaf test reactions but no clinical or radiological evidence of TB (*Thorax* 1994; **49:** 1193–200).
- Chemoprophylaxis should be given to children under 5 years who are close contacts of a smear-positive adult irrespective of their tuberculin test result.
- If chemoprophylaxis is not undertaken, follow-up with periodic CXR examinations for 2 years is recommended in all these groups.

Which rapid test allows early diagnosis of tuberculosis?

Polymerase chain reaction (PCR).

Robert Koch (1843–1910), Institute for Infectious Diseases, Berlin, was awarded the 1905 Nobel Prize for Medicine for his investigations and discoveries in relation to tuberculosis.

Kary Mullis of the USA was awarded the Nobel Prize for developing the technique of polymerase chain reaction.

Case 109

PICKWICKIAN SYNDROME

INSTRUCTION

Look at this patient.

SALIENT FEATURES

History

- Daytime somnolence.
- Unrefreshing sleep.
- Daytime fatigue.
- Snoring.
- Shortness of breath.
- Headache, particularly in the morning.
- Swelling of feet.
- Poor concentration.
- Systemic hypertension.
- Family history of obesity.
- Gastro-oesophageal reflux.
- Poor quality of life.

Examination

- Obese patient who is plethoric and cyanosed.
- Maxillary or mandibular hypoplasia.
- Shortness of breath at rest.
- May be nodding off to sleep.
- Systemic hypertension.
- Nocturnal angina.
- Look for signs of pulmonary hypertension and right heart failure.

Remember. Nearly 50% of patients with sleep apnoea syndrome are *not* obese.

DIAGNOSIS

This patient has marked obesity and hypersomnolence with signs of pulmonary hypertension (lesion) which indicate that she has pickwickian syndrome. The patient is in cardiac failure (functional status).

Read reviews: *J R Coll Phys (Lond)* 1993; **27**: 363–4; *J R Coll Phys (Lond)* 1993; **27**: 375.

ADVANCED-LEVEL QUESTIONS

What is the cause of cyanosis in such a patient?

A mixture of obstructive apnoea and sleep-induced hypoventilation. The blood gas picture is hypoxia and carbon dioxide retention.

Where is the obstruction?

It is caused by the apposition of the tongue and the palate on the posterior pharyngeal wall.

How would you treat such a patient?

- Weight reduction.
- Avoidance of smoking and alcohol.
- Progesterone (enhances respiratory drive).
- Continuous nasal positive airway pressure delivered by a nasal mask (*Lancet* 1999; **353**: 2100–5).
- Home oxygen.
- Surgery: tracheostomy, uvulopalatopharyngoplasty, linguoplasty, mandibular advancement, plastic remodelling of the uvula (laser-assisted or radiofrequency ablation).
- Drugs: serotonin receptor blockade, acetazolamide, methylxanthines, weight loss medications.

> Mr. Pickwick is a character in the novel *Pickwick Papers*, written by Charles Dickens; the term was applied by Sir William Osler.

Case 110

COLLAPSED LUNG

INSTRUCTION

Examine this patient's chest.

SALIENT FEATURES

History

- Sudden onset of breathlessness.
- History of cough.
- History of asthma, TB, lung cancer.

Examination

- Trachea deviated to the affected side.
- Movements decreased on the affected side.
- Percussion note dull on the affected side.
- Breath sounds diminished on the affected side.

Proceed as follows:

Tell the examiner that you would like to look for tar staining (tobacco smoking), clubbing and cachexia (bronchogenic carcinoma, see pp 274–6).

DIAGNOSIS

This patient has a collapsed lung (lesion); you would like to exclude malignancy (aetiology). He is breathless at rest (functional status).

QUESTIONS

What are the causes of lung collapse?

These include:

- Bronchogenic carcinoma.
- Mucus plugs (asthma, allergic bronchopulmonary aspergillosis; *BMJ* 1982; **285:** 552).
- Extrinsic compression from hilar adenopathy (e.g. primary TB).
- Tuberculosis (Brock's syndrome).
- Other intrabronchial tumours including bronchial adenoma.

What are the chest radiograph findings of collapse of the right middle lobe?

The loss of definition of the right heart border reflects collapse (or consolidation) affecting the right middle lobe.

What is Brock's syndrome?

It is collapse due to compression of the right middle lobe bronchus by an enlarged lymph node.

Sir Russell C. Brock (1903–1980) graduated from Guy's Hospital and was surgeon at Guy's and Brompton Hospitals. His interests included both thoracic and cardiac surgery. He was the President of the Royal College of Surgeons, 1963–1966.

HISTORY AND EXAMINATION OF THE ABDOMEN

HISTORY

- Fever, loss of weight, fatigue, lassitude.
- Gastrointestinal symptoms: dysphagia, nausea, vomiting, altered bowel movement, jaundice.
- Renal symptoms: oliguria, history of renal failure.
- History of diabetes, hypertension.
- History of ascites, swelling of feet, mass in the abdomen.

EXAMINATION OF THE ABDOMEN

1. Ensure the patient is lying flat (remove any extra pillows, if present, with the permission of the patient); the hands should lie by the patient's side with the abdomen exposed from the inframammary region to just above the genitalia. Do not expose the genitalia.
2. Begin with the hands, looking for the following signs:
   - Clubbing, leukonychia (white chalky nails).
   - Palmar erythema.
   - Dupuytren's contracture (feel for thickening of the fascia).
   - Hepatic flap.
3. Examine the arms: look for arteriovenous fistula, haemodialysis catheters, spider naevi.
4. Comment on the skin:
   - Pigmentation.
   - Scratch marks.
5. Examine the following:
   - Supraclavicular and cervical lymph nodes.
   - Tongue for pallor.
   - Eyes for anaemia, jaundice, xanthelasma.
   - Upper chest and face for spider naevi.
   - Axilla for hair loss, acanthosis nigricans.
   - Breast for gynaecomastia.
6. Inspect the abdomen, looking for the following signs:
   - Movements.
   - Any obvious mass.
   - Visible veins (check direction of flow, which is usually away from the umbilicus).
   - Visible peristalsis.
   - Hernial orifices (ask the patient to cough at this stage).
   - Expansile pulsations of aortic aneurysm.
7. Ask the patient whether the abdomen is sore at any part.
8. Palpation: kneel on the floor or sit on a chair before you begin palpation. At all times look at the patient's eyes to check whether he or she winces in pain. Begin with superficial pain and begin in the least tender area. Palpate in all the quadrants (remember that there are four quadrants).

9. Palpate:
   - For mass – determine its characteristics.
   - Liver (percuss for upper border using heavy percussion, for lower border using light percussion).
   - Kidneys (bimanual palpation, demonstrate ballottement).
   - Groin for lymph nodes.
   - Check hernial orifices.
   - Test for expansile pulsation of an aortic aneurysm.
10. Percuss, looking for shifting dullness (at this stage, when the patient is lying on his or her right side, seize the opportunity to examine for a small spleen and for pitting oedema over the sacral region). Remember that abdominal percussion should follow adequate inspection and percussion.
11. Auscultate:
    - Over an enlarged liver for bruit.
    - Over a suspected aortic aneurysm.
    - For bowel sounds.
12. Tell the examiner that you would like to perform a rectal examination and examine the external genitalia.
13. Examine the legs for oedema.

Case 111

HEPATOMEGALY

INSTRUCTION

Examine this patient's abdomen.

SALIENT FEATURES

History

- Shortness of breath, leg oedema (heart failure).
- History of alcohol ingestion, cirrhosis.
- History of malignancies (secondaries in the liver).
- History of leukaemia or lymphoma.

Examination

- Enlarged liver: comment on its size, tenderness, surface (smooth or irregular); percuss the upper border (normally in the fifth intercostal space in the right midclavicular line) and auscultate for bruit (*N Engl J Med* 1962; **266:** 554–5; *JAMA* 1968; **206:** 2518–20; *Postgrad Med* 1977; **62:** 131–4).
- Remember: how far the liver extends below the costal margin is of less importance than 'liver span', particularly in patients with emphysema or flattened diaphragms.

Note. By percussion, the mean liver size is 7 cm for women and 10.5 cm for men. A liver span 2–3 cm larger or smaller than these values is considered abnormal. The liver size depends on several factors including age, sex, body size, shape and the examination technique utilized (e.g. palpation versus percussion versus radio-graphic) (*Ann Intern Med* 1969; **70:** 1183–9).

Proceed as follows:
- Look for the following signs:
  - Spleen for ascites.
  - Signs of cirrhosis.
  - Lymph nodes.
  - Raised JVP.
  - Hepatic flap.
- At this stage you may be asked to look for nervous system signs of alcoholism (peripheral neuropathy, proximal myopathy, cerebellar syndrome, bilateral sixth cranial nerve palsy as in Wernicke's encephalopathy, recent memory loss and confabulation in Korsakoff's psychosis).

DIAGNOSIS

This patient has a nodular, hard hepatomegaly (lesion) which indicates secondaries in the liver. I would like to look for a primary, particularly in the gastrointestinal tract (aetiology).

QUESTIONS

What does a tender liver indicate?

A stretch of its capsule due to a *recent* enlargement, as in cardiac failure or acute hepatitis.

What are the common causes of a palpable liver in the UK?

- Cardiac failure (firm, smooth, tender, mild to massive enlargement).
- Cirrhosis (non-tender, firm; in later stages the liver decreases in size).
- Secondaries in the liver (enlarged with rock-hard or nodular consistency).

ADVANCED-LEVEL QUESTIONS

Mention some less common causes of hepatomegaly.

- Leukaemia and other reticuloendothelial disorders.
- Infections – glandular fever, infectious hepatitis.
- Primary biliary cirrhosis.
- Haemochromatosis.
- Sarcoid, amyloid.
- Tumours – hepatoma, hydatid cysts.

Note. The liver may be felt without being enlarged in the following circumstances: increased diaphragmatic descent, presence of emphysema with an associated depressed diaphragm, thin body habitus with a narrow thoracic cage, presence of a palpable Riedel's lobe and right-sided pleural effusion.

In which condition does a pulsatile liver occur?

Tricuspid regurgitation.

What does a hepatic arterial bruit over the liver indicate?

The hepatic arterial bruit has been described in alcoholic hepatitis, primary or metastatic carcinoma. Although reported to occur in cirrhosis, it is rare without associated alcoholic hepatitis (*Lancet* 1966; **ii:** 516–19).

What does the presence of an abdominal venous hum indicate?

It is virtually diagnostic of portal venous hypertension (usually due to cirrhosis) (*Br Heart J* 1950; **12:** 343–50). When present together with the hepatic arterial bruit in the same patient, it suggests cirrhosis with either alcoholic hepatitis or cancer.

What do you know about Cruveilhier–Baumgarten syndrome?

It is the presence of the abdominal venous hum in portal hypertension secondary to cirrhosis (*Am J Med* 1954; **17:** 143–50).

What does a hepatic friction rub indicate?

In a young woman it could be due to gonococcal perihepatitis (Fitz-Hugh–Curtis syndrome) and in others it could indicate hepatic neoplasm with inflammatory changes or infection in or adjacent to the liver. The presence of a hepatic rub with a bruit usually indicates cancer of the liver (*JAMA* 1979; **241:** 1495), whereas the presence of the hepatic rub, bruit and abdominal venous hum indicates that a patient with cirrhosis has developed a hepatoma.

Dame Sheila Sherlock, Emeritus Professor of Medicine, Royal Free Hospital, London, is a doyen of liver diseases.

Hans Popper (1903–1988), Professor of Pathology at Chicago and the founding dean of Mount Sinai School of Medicine in New York; he is regarded as the founding father of hepatology.

Howard Clarence Thomas, contemporary Professor of Medicine, St Mary's Hospital Medical School, Paddington, London; his main interest is viral hepatitis.

Case 112

CIRRHOSIS OF THE LIVER

INSTRUCTION

Examine this patient's abdomen.

SALIENT FEATURES

History

- History of fatigue, weight loss, jaundice.
- History of alcohol abuse.
- History of hepatitis B, intravenous blood products.
- History of intravenous drug abuse.
- Mental status changes (hepatic encephalopathy).
- History of drugs (methyldopa, amiodarone, methotrexate).
- History of Wilson's disease, α_1-antitrypsin deficiency.

Examination

- In the hands:
  - Clubbing, leukonychia.
  - Dupuytren's contracture (see Fig. 90), palmar erythema.
  - Spider naevi, tattoos, hepatic flap, pallor.
  - Scratch marks, generalized pigmentation.
- Eyes and face: icterus, cyanosis, parotid enlargement.
- Chest: spider naevi, loss of axillary hair, gynaecomastia.
- Abdomen:
  - Splenomegaly (seldom more than 5 cm below the costal margin).
  - Ascites.
  - Hepatomegaly (particularly in alcoholic liver disease).
- Loss of hair on the shins.
- Leg oedema.
- Tell the examiner that you would like to look for testicular atrophy.

DIAGNOSIS

This patient has spider naevi, gynaecomastia, splenomegaly, parotid enlargement (lesions) due to cirrhosis of the liver caused by alcohol abuse (aetiology). The patient has hepatic flap indicating liver cell failure (functional status).

QUESTIONS

What is cirrhosis?

Cirrhosis is defined pathologically as a diffuse liver abnormality characterized by fibrosis and abnormal regenerating nodules.

Mention a few causes of cirrhosis of the liver.

- Alcohol dependence.
- Hepatitis B virus infection (look for tattoos).
- Lupoid hepatitis.
- Primary biliary cirrhosis.
- Haemochromatosis.
- Drugs – methyldopa, amiodarone, methotrexate.
- Metabolic: Wilson's disease, α_1-antitrypsin deficiency.
- Cryptogenic.

How would you investigate this patient?

- FBC including haemoglobin and platelet count.
- Liver function tests including γ-glutamyl transpeptidase (GGT).
- Prothrombin time.
- Hepatitis B markers.
- Serum autoantibodies.
- Serum iron and ferritin.
- Serum α-fetoprotein.
- Ascitic fluid analysis.
- Ultrasonography of the liver.

Why does this patient have a low serum albumin concentration?

Albumin is synthesized in the liver. In cirrhosis there is liver cell failure, causing impaired synthesis.

What are the major sequelae of cirrhosis?

- Portal hypertension.
- Variceal haemorrhages.
- Hepatic encephalopathy.
- Ascites and spontaneous bacterial peritonitis.
- Hepatorenal syndrome.
- Coagulopathy.
- Hepatocellular carcinoma.

ADVANCED-LEVEL QUESTIONS

What are the poor prognostic factors?

- Encephalopathy.

- Low serum sodium concentration, less than 120 mmol/l (not due to diuretic therapy).
- Low serum albumin level, less than 25 g/l.
- Prolonged prothrombin time.

What factors can precipitate hepatic encephalopathy in a patient with previously well-compensated hepatic cirrhosis?

- Infection.
- Diuretics, electrolyte imbalance.
- Diarrhoea and vomiting.
- Sedatives.
- Upper gastrointestinal haemorrhage.
- Abdominal paracentesis.
- Surgery.

How would you manage variceal bleeding in cirrhosis?

- Blood transfusion to replace falling haematocrit.
- Early endoscopy to confirm the bleeding site.
- Endoscopic sclerotherapy with octreotide (*N Engl J Med* 1995; **333**: 555–60).
- Intravenous vasopressin is less effective than sclerotherapy.
- Endoscopic ligation (*N Engl J Med* 1999; **340**: 988–93).
- Balloon tamponade is effective in temporarily stopping bleeding while awaiting more definitive therapy.
- Combination of vapreotide (a somatostatin analogue) and endoscopic treatment (*N Engl J Med* 2001; **344**: 23–8).
- Transjugular intrahepatic portosystemic stent-shunt (*N Engl J Med* 1994; **330**: 165–71).
- Combination of nadolol and isosorbide mononitrate (*N Engl J Med* 1996; **334**: 1624–9).

Case 113

JAUNDICE

INSTRUCTION

Would you like to ask this patient a few questions and perform a relevant examination?

SALIENT FEATURES

Proceed as follows:

Ask the patient about the following:

- His or her age (hepatitis is more common in the young and carcinoma in the elderly).

- Sore throat and rash (infectious mononucleosis).
- Occupation (Weil's disease in sewerage and farm workers).
- Contact with jaundice (hepatitis A).
- Drug history (oral contraceptives, phenothiazines).
- Blood transfusions, injections, arthritis, urticaria (hepatitis B).
- Alcohol consumption.
- Pruritus (cholestasis due to hepatitis A, primary biliary cirrhosis).
- Colour of the urine.
- Colour of the stools (pale stools in obstructive jaundice).
- Abdominal pain (cholecystitis, gallstones, cholangitis, carcinoma of the pancreas).
- Past history (recurrent jaundice, as in Dubin–Johnson syndrome).
- Fever, rigors and abdominal pain (suggests cholangitis).

Examination

- Examine the following:
  - Hands (clubbing, palmar erythema, Dupuytren's contracture).
  - Sclera (to confirm the icterus).
  - Conjunctiva (for pallor).
  - Neck (lymph nodes).
  - Upper chest (spider naevi, loss of axillary hair and gynaecomastia).
  - Abdomen (hepatomegaly, splenomegaly, Murphy's sign, palpable gallbladder, ascites).
  - Legs (for pitting oedema).
- Tell the examiner that you would like to investigate as follows:
  - Examine the urine.
  - Perform a per rectum examination.

Remember. The most important question to answer in the evaluation of any jaundiced patient is 'Will this patient require surgery to relieve biliary obstruction?'

DIAGNOSIS

This patient is markedly icteric and has spider naevi and gynaecomastia (lesions) due to alcoholic liver disease (aetiology).

QUESTIONS

What do you understand by the term 'jaundice'?

It is the yellowish discoloration of skin, sclera and mucous membrane due to the accumulation of bile pigments. It is usually clinically manifest when the serum bilirubin concentration is at least 7–8 mg/dl.

How would you differentiate jaundice from carotenaemia?

The discoloration of carotenaemia is differentiated from jaundice by the absence of yellow colour in the sclera and mucous membranes, normal urine colour and the presence of yellow–brown pigmentation of carotenoid pigment in the palms, soles and nasolabial folds.

What is Murphy's sign and what does it indicate?

It is the tenderness elicited on palpation at the midpoint of the right subcostal margin on inspiration. It is a sign of cholecystitis.

Have you heard of Courvoisier's law?

It states that in a patient with obstructive jaundice a palpable gallbladder is unlikely to be due to chronic cholecystitis.

What is Charcot's fever?

Intermittent fever associated with jaundice and abdominal discomfort in a patient with cholangitis and biliary obstruction.

How would you investigate this patient?

- Urine for bile pigments.
- FBC.
- Serum haptoglobulin, reticulocyte count and Coombs' test (if you suspect haemolysis).
- Liver function tests (serum albumin, bilirubin, enzymes).
- Prothrombin time.
- Viral studies (hepatitis antigen and antibodies, Epstein–Barr virus antibodies).
- Ultrasonography of the abdomen (if you suspect cholestatic jaundice).
- Special investigations: mitochondrial antibodies, endoscopic retrograde cholangiopancreatography (ERCP), CT of the abdomen, liver biopsy.

ADVANCED-LEVEL QUESTIONS

What do you know about Dubin–Johnson syndrome?

It is a rare benign condition characterized by jaundice and pigmentation secondary to a failure of excretion of conjugated bilirubin. The liver is stained by melanin in the centrilobular zone. The bromsulphthalein test shows a late secondary rise at 90 minutes.

Mention a few causes of postoperative jaundice.

Causes of postoperative jaundice (usually occurring in the first 3 postoperative weeks) include:

- Resorption of haematomas, haemoperitoneum, haemolysis of transfused erythrocytes (particularly when stored blood products are used), haemolysis due to glucose-6-phosphate dehydrogenase deficiency.
- Impaired hepatocellular function due to halogenated anaesthetics, sepsis, hepatic ischaemia secondary to perioperative hypotension.
- Extrahepatic biliary obstruction due to biliary stones, unsuspected injury to biliary tree.

How does estimation of serum bilirubin concentration help in discerning the aetiology of jaundice?

Normal serum bilirubin concentration is no greater than 1.5 mg/dl and consists predominantly of the unconjugated form. When jaundice is primarily due to haemolysis or a disorder of bilirubin conjugation, the unconjugated form constitutes at least 85% of the total. With normal liver function, haemolysis alone does not produce a serum bilirubin level greater than 4 mg/dl. A rise in serum bilirubin levels of up to 2 mg/dl per day is compatible with extrahepatic cholestasis, but a greater rate indicates haemolysis, hepatitis or hepatic cell necrosis. The serum bilirubin level of patients with pure biliary obstruction seldom exceeds 30 mg/dl; a greater value indicates that there is associated hepatocellular jaundice as well.

A. Gilbert (1858–1927), Professor of Medicine at l'Hôtel Dieu in Paris.

P.S.A. Weil (1848–1916), Professor of Medicine in Tartu, Estonia and Berlin.

J.B. Murphy (1857–1916), Professor of Surgery at Northwestern University in Chicago.

J. Courvoisier (1843–1918), Professor of Surgery, Basel, Switzerland.

I.N. Dubin, Professor of Pathology, Pennsylvania, and F.B. Johnson, pathologist, Veterans Administration Hospital, Washington.

Case 114

ASCITES

INSTRUCTION

Examine this patient's abdomen.

SALIENT FEATURES

History

- History of abdominal distension, dyspnoea.
- History of pain in the abdomen (spontaneous bacterial peritonitis, malignancy).
- History of heart failure, renal failure or liver disease.
- History of TB (peritoneal tuberculosis).
- History of malignancy (mesothelioma, metastatic spread from primary tumours).

Examination

- Full flanks and umbilicus.
- Presence of shifting dullness (always percuss with your finger parallel to the level of fluid).
- If the ascites is gross, use the 'dipping' method of palpation to feel the liver and spleen.
- Look for stigmata of underlying disease (e.g. signs of cirrhosis, cardiac failure, renal failure or malignancy).

Proceed as follows:
Check for sacral oedema and swollen ankles.

DIAGNOSIS

This patient has marked ascites and leg oedema with splenomegaly (lesions) due to portal hypertension, the cause of which needs to be investigated (aetiology).

QUESTIONS

What are the causes of a distended abdomen?
Fat, fluid, faeces, flatus and fetus.

What do you understand by the term 'ascites'?
It is the pathological accumulation of fluid in the peritoneal cavity.

What are the common causes of ascitic fluid?
• Portal hypertension with cirrhosis.
• Abdominal malignancy.
• Congestive cardiac failure.

What investigations would you perform to determine the underlying cause?
Diagnostic paracentesis for proteins and malignant cells, ultrasonography of the abdomen, peritoneal biopsy or laparoscopy if the cause remains unclear.

What is the difference between an exudate and a transudate?
An exudate has a protein content of over 25 g/l.

ADVANCED-LEVEL QUESTIONS

What are the mechanisms of ascites formation in cirrhosis?
• It is caused by a combination of liver failure and portal hypertension. Liver failure decreases renal blood flow, resulting in retention of salt and water.
• Secondary hyperaldosteronism due to increased renin release and decreased metabolism of aldosterone by the liver.
• Decreased metabolism of aldosterone by the liver.
• Decreased metabolism of antidiuretic hormone.
• Hypoalbuminaemia which decreases colloid oncotic pressure.
• Lymphatic obstruction, resulting in a 'weeping' liver.
• More recently, overproduction of nitric oxide has been proposed to be important in the pathogenesis of ascites, sodium and water retention and haemodynamic abnormalities in cirrhosis (*N Engl J Med* 1998; **339:** 533–41). Inhibition of nitric oxide synthesis improves sodium and water excretion in cirrhotic rats with ascites.

What is the relationship between ascites and chronic liver disease?
• Ascites indicates decompensation of previously asymptomatic chronic liver disease.
• Ascites occurs in about half of the patients within 10 years of a diagnosis of compensated cirrhosis.
• The development of fluid retention in patients with chronic liver disease is a poor prognostic sign – only half of these patients survive beyond 2 years.

What do you know about the serum–ascites albumin gradient?
It is calculated by subtracting the ascitic fluid albumin concentration from the serum albumin concentration from samples obtained at the same time. This gradient correlates directly with portal pressure; those whose gradient exceeds 1.1 g/dl have portal hypertension and those with gradients of less than 1.1 g/dl do not. The accuracy of such determinations is 97%.

How would you manage a patient with cirrhosis and ascites?

The most important treatments are sodium restriction and diuretics (*N Engl J Med* 1994; **330**: 337–42):

- Sodium restriction to 88 mmol per day; only 15% of these patients lose weight or have a reduction in ascitic fluid with this therapy alone.
- Fluid restriction is usually not necessary unless the serum sodium concentration drops below 120 mmol/l.
- When the patient has tense ascites, 5 litres or more of ascitic fluid should be removed to relieve shortness of breath, to diminish early satiety and to prevent pressure-related leakage of fluid from the site of a previous paracentesis.
- Diuretic therapy should be initiated immediately, before which the serum sodium concentration of a random urine sample should be measured. Serial monitoring of urinary sodium concentration helps to determine the optimal dose of diuretic; doses are increased until a negative sodium balance is achieved. The most effective diuretic regimen is a combination of spironolactone and furosemide (frusemide). More than 90% of patients respond to this therapy.
- Diuretic-resistant ascites:
  - Therapeutic paracentesis with infusion of salt-free albumin (reported to decrease hospital stay).
  - Peritoneovenous shunting, e.g. LeVeen shunt, limited by the high rate of infection and disseminated intravascular coagulation.
  - Transjugular intrahepatic portosystemic stent shunt (TIPS) is a non-surgical side-to-side shunt consisting of a stented channel between a main branch of the portal vein and the hepatic vein. The stent shunt is associated with an operative mortality rate of 1% compared with 5–39% for surgical shunts (*N Engl J Med* 1995; **332**: 1192–7).
  - Extracorporeal ultrafiltration of ascitic fluid with reinfusion.
  - Liver transplantation.

In patients with cirrhosis and refractory or recurrent ascites would you prefer paracentesis or TIPS?

A recent study suggests that, in comparison with large volume paracentesis, the creation of a TIPS can improve the chance of survival without liver transplantation in these patients (*N Engl J Med* 2000; **342**: 1701–7). These investigators defined the ascites as refractory when the patients did not respond to diuretic therapy (a dose of at least 300 mg of spironolactone per day or 120 mg furosemide (frusemide) per day). Patients were excluded from the study if they had hepatic encephalopathy of grade 2 or higher, a serum bilirubin concentration of more than 86 μmol/l, portal vein thrombosis or a serum creatinine concentration of more than 3 mg/dl (265 μmol/l). TIPS is ineffective in those patients with associated intrinsic renal disease.

What are the complications of ascites?

- Respiratory embarrassment may complicate large amounts of ascites.
- Spontaneous bacterial peritonitis is seen in cirrhotics (suspect when there is an ascitic fluid leukocyte count of 500 cells per μl, or more than 250 polymorphonuclear cells per μl; empirical therapy with a non-nephrotoxic broad-spectrum antibiotic should be initiated immediately).

Mention some uncommon causes for ascitic fluid.
- Nephrotic syndrome.
- Constrictive pericarditis.
- Tuberculous peritonitis.
- Chylous ascites.
- Budd–Chiari syndrome.
- Meigs' syndrome.

What do you know about the pathogenesis of ascites in cirrhotics?
Two theories have been proposed (*N Engl J Med* 1982; **307**: 1577):

- Underfilling theory: this suggests that the primary abnormality is inappropriate sequestration of fluid within the splanchnic vascular bed due to portal hypertension. This results in a decrease in intravascular volume and the kidney responds by retaining salt and water.
- Overflow theory: this suggests that the primary abnormality is inappropriate retention of salt and water by the kidney in the absence of volume depletion.

G. Budd (1808–1882), Professor of Medicine at King's College, London.

H. Chiari (1851–1916), Professor of Pathology at the German University in Prague.

J.V. Meigs (1892–1963), Professor of Gynaecology at Harvard, Massachusetts General Hospital.

H.H. LeVeen, gastroenterologist at the Veterans Administration Hospital in New York.

Sometime during the rule of Tiberius (25–50 AD), the physician Celsus wrote about oedema. 'A chronic malady may develop in patients who collect water under their skin. The Greeks call this hydrops. There are three types: a) Sometimes the water is all drawn within and is called ascites, b) sometimes the body is rendered uneven by swellings arising here and there and all over. The Greeks call this hyposrka and c) sometimes the belly is tense. The Greeks call this tympanites (adapted from *BMJ* 1999; **318**: 1610–3).'

Case 115

HAEMOCHROMATOSIS

INSTRUCTION

Examine this patient's abdomen.
Look at this patient.

SALIENT FEATURES

History
- Family history.
- Skin tan.
- Shortness of breath (cardiac failure).
- Diabetes (pancreatic involvement).

- Joint pain (present in 50% of cases): pseudogout usually affects the second and third metacarpophalangeal joints. Any small joint may be involved.
- Melaena, haematemesis (bleeding from varices).

Examination

- The patient is a pigmented male over 30 years of age.
- Palmar erythema, spider naevi.
- Jaundice.
- Ascites, hepatomegaly (firm, regular).
- Loss of secondary sexual hair.

Proceed as follows:

Tell the examiner that you would like to investigate as follows:

- Look for testicular atrophy (due to iron deposition affecting hypothalamo-pituitary function).
- Examine the heart for dilated cardiomyopathy, cardiac failure.
- Check urine for sugar, looking for evidence of diabetes mellitus (present in 80% of cases).

Remember. Such patients develop cirrhosis and hepatocellular carcinoma.

DIAGNOSIS

This male patient has generalized hyperpigmentation, hepatomegaly and signs of liver cell disease (lesions) due to haemochromatosis which may be hereditary (aetiology).

ADVANCED-LEVEL QUESTIONS

Does this disease run in families?

Yes, and it is an autosomal recessive condition. Two mutations of the *HFE* gene (*845A (C282Y)* and *187C (H63D)*) account for 90% of the cases of European extraction. It is closely associated with human leukocyte antigen HLA-A3 and to a lesser extent with HLA-B14 antigen. The responsible alleles are on the short arm of chromosome 6 (*Nat Genet* 1996; **13:** 399–408). Asymptomatic close relatives of patients with hereditary haemochromatosis, in particular siblings, should be advised to undergo screening, i.e. measurements of serum ferritin and iron, and saturation of iron-binding capacity. Recent data have shown that hereditary haemochromatosis can occur in adults who do not have pathogenic mutations on the gene on chromosome 6 (*N Engl J Med* 1999; **341:** 725–32; *N Engl J Med* 1999; **341:** 718–24). A substantial number of homozygous relatives of these patients (more commonly men) have disease-related conditions such as cirrhosis, hepatic fibrosis, elevated aminotransferase and haemochromatotic arthropathy that have yet to be detected clinically (*N Engl J Med* 2000; **343:** 1529–35). Also, 10% or more of the patients with clinically severe hereditary haemochromatosis do not have either mutation. These facts limit the value of diagnostic DNA testing.

What is the mechanism of increased iron uptake?

Iron absorption is mediated by the duodenal metal transporter, DMT-1 (also called NRAMP-2). It has been suggested that increased NRAMP-2 mRNA expression in the duodenal mucosa of patients with hereditary haemochromatosis may promote duodenal uptake of iron and result in iron overload (*Lancet* 1999; **353**: 2120–3).

What is the benefit of early identification?

Early venesection has shown benefits, particularly in those who have not developed diabetes mellitus or cirrhosis. Early venesection prevents progression of hepatic disease and may consequently prevent the complication of hepatocellular carcinoma.

How would you confirm your diagnosis?

- Transferrin saturation is increased.
- Serum ferritin levels are raised.
- Liver biopsy to measure iron stores is a definitive test.

How would you manage such a patient?

- Avoidance of alcohol and Indian balti curries which are prepared in cast iron cookware (*BMJ* 1995; **310**: 1368).
- Avoidance of uncooked shellfish and marine fish since patients are susceptible to fatal septicaemia from the marine bacterium *Vibrio vulnificus*.
- Venesection prolongs life and often reverses tissue damage. Initially, weekly venesection for 2 years (as 50 g iron or more is removed) and then once every 3 months. Many manifestations improve (insulin requirements often diminish) except for testicular atrophy and chrondrocalcinosis.

What is the commonest cause of death in patients with hereditary haemochromatosis?

The most common cause of death is hepatocellular carcinoma, for which the risk is 200-fold greater than in the general population. Depletion of iron, and even reversal of cirrhosis, do not totally prevent the occurrence of this fatal neoplasm. Patients diagnosed in the subclinical, precirrhotic stage and treated by regular phlebotomy have a normal life expectancy (*N Engl J Med* 1985; **313**: 1256–62).

Mention a few causes of generalized pigmentation.

Common causes are sun tan and race.

Uncommon causes are as follows:

- Liver disease: haemochromatosis in males; primary biliary cirrhosis in females.
- Addison's disease.
- Uraemia.
- Chronic debilitating conditions such as malignancy.

The term 'haemochromatosis' was first used by von Recklinghausen (see p. 199) in 1889 to describe autopsy findings in men with cirrhosis associated with massive deposition of iron in the hepatocytes (von Recklinghausen FD 1889 Ueber Hämochromatose. *Tageblatt Versamml Dtsch Naturforsch Aertze Heidelberg* **62**: 324–5).

The inherited nature of haemochromatosis was first recognized by Sheldon in 1935 (Sheldon JH 1935 *Haemochromatosis*. Oxford University Press, London).

Case 116

PRIMARY BILIARY CIRRHOSIS

INSTRUCTION

Examine this patient's abdomen.

SALIENT FEATURES

History

- Pruritus (affecting half the patients) – more common in men.
- Fatigue (commonest symptom).
- Lethargy and pain in the right upper quadrant (in a quarter of the patients).
- Symptoms of hepatic decompensation (jaundice, ascites, variceal haemorrhage) in a fifth of patients.
- Steatorrhoea.

EXAMINATION

- Usually occurs in middle-aged women.
- Clubbing.
- Generalized pigmentation.
- Xanthelasma (may occur at any stage but more common in advanced disease).
- Icterus.
- Scratch marks.
- Hepatosplenomegaly (common in early stages).

Proceed as follows:
- Look for xanthomata over joints, skin folds and sites of trauma to the skin.
- Remember that there may be clinical features of other autoimmune diseases such as rheumatoid arthritis, dry mouth of Sjögren's syndrome, systemic sclerosis, CREST syndrome (see p. 506), Hashimoto's thyroiditis, dermatomyositis.
- Check for proximal muscle weakness due to osteomalacia.
- Examine for peripheral neuropathy.
- Tell the examiner that you would like to test for high serum levels of alkaline phosphatase and antimitochondrial antibodies (present in 95% of the patients, with the M2 antibody being more specific; it is almost always negative in extra-hepatic obstruction).

DIAGNOSIS

This middle-aged woman has generalized pigmentation, jaundice, xanthelasmata and pruritus with hepatosplenomegaly (lesions) due to primary biliary cirrhosis (aetiology). She is in liver cell failure as evidenced by the hepatic flap (functional status).

ADVANCED-LEVEL QUESTIONS

How does primary biliary cirrhosis present?

Classically, it presents with itching in a middle-aged woman. However, in 50% of cases there may be no liver symptoms. There are 4 phases:

1. Asymptomatic with normal liver tests

Antibodies to pyruvate dehydrogenase complex (antimitochondrial antibodies, AMA) are detectable. Approximately three quarters of these patients develop symptoms of PBC in 2 years; 83% developed abnormal liver function tests at a median period of 5 years from first detection of AMA (*Lancet* 1996; **348:** 1399–402). Most patients have liver histology compatible with or diagnostic of PBC. In one series none had died from liver disease 12 years after AMA detection (*J Hepatol* 1994; **20:** 707–13).

2. Symptomless with abnormal liver tests

Circulating AMA are present. More than half have established fibrosis at diagnosis. Up to 80% of patients develop symptoms or signs of PBC during the first 5 years of follow-up. The median time from diagnosis to death is 8–12 years.

3. Symptomatic

Lethargy and pruritus are prominent, and time to death or transplantation is 5–10 years.

4. Decompensated primary biliary cirrhosis

Signs include ascites, variceal haemorrhage and jaundice. The mean time to death or transplantation is 3–5 years.

What diseases are associated with primary biliary cirrhosis?

- Common (up to 80%): sicca syndrome (p. 339).
- Frequent (~20%): arthralgia, fibrosing alveolitis, Raynaud's syndrome, sclerodactyly, thyroid disease.
- Rare (<5%): Addison's disease, glomerulonephritis, hypertrophic pulmonary osteoarthropathy, myasthenia gravis, systemic lupus erythematosus, thrombocytopenic purpura, vitiligo.

Is primary biliary cirrhosis associated with cancer?

It is estimated that these patients have a 20-fold increased relative risk of developing hepatocellular carcinoma and increased risk of cancer overall (*Hepatology* 1997; **26:** 1138–42).

How would you investigate this patient?

Liver function tests

Normal in presymptomatic stage, characteristically cholestatic pattern (raised alkaline phosphatase, 5-nucleotidase and γ-glutamyl transpeptidase); serum aminotransferases may be slightly raised but rarely exceed 5 times the upper limit of normal. Serum bilirubin is normal initially but rises as disease progresses. Once serum bilirubin exceeds 170 μmol/l, the estimated survival is less than 18 months (*Gut* 1979; **20:** 137–40).

Hepatic synthetic function

Well preserved until late stages; a prolonged prothrombin time may indicate malabsorption of vitamin K due to cholestasis.

Serum lipids

Hypercholesterolaemia is common. Lipoprotein lp(a) is low; HDL cholesterol is increased in the early stages but falls as the disease progresses.

Immunological tests

IgM and IgG are elevated; complement activation although C3 levels are normal; several antibodies are elevated but antibodies to components of the nuclear pore complex and AMA are very closely elevated with PBC. AMA is found in 96% of patients with PBC but the E2 subtype is specific to PBC. Autoimmune cholangitis is a variant of PBC which has characteristic histological features of PBC but is negative for AMA in serum (*Gut* 1997; **30:** 440–42). The AMA are directed against the mitochondrial pyruvate dehydrogenase complex.

Histology

Non-suppurative destructive cholangitis or granulomatous cholangitis.

Is liver biopsy necessary to confirm the diagnosis?

Although liver biopsy is routinely used to confirm the diagnosis, the need for this procedure for either diagnosis or prognosis is questionable (*Lancet* 1997; **350:** 875–9). The very close association between histology and E2 AMA in PBC means that liver histology is not required unless clinical and serological features are equivocal. The presence of cirrhosis is of very little value in determining the prognosis, and clinically significant portal hypertension (ascites, variceal haemorrhage) may occur during the early histological stages.

What is the mechanism for itching in these patients?

The itching used to be ascribed to retention of bile acids with cholestasis, but recent work has emphasized the importance of naturally occurring opioid tone characterized by an increase in the concentration of endogenous opioid receptors and upregulation of opioid receptors (*Gut* 1996; **38:** 644–5). These findings have led to the use of opioid antagonists for treatment of pruritus.

What drugs have been used to control pruritus?

Colestyramine is first line, rifampicin and ursodeoxycholic acid are second line, and naloxone, nalmefene and propofol are third line agents used to treat pruritus.

What drugs have been used to treat this condition?

Ursodeoxycholic acid, corticosteroids, ciclosporin, azathioprine, tacrolimus, methotrexate, colchicines.

What is the rationale behind bile salt therapy?

Hepatocytes affected by autoimmune processes are further injured by endogenous bile acids (such as chenodeoxycholic acid and cholic acid) which accumulate due to associated cholestasis. Partial replacement of water-soluble bile acids such as ursodeoxycholic acid may reduce pruritus and damage to the liver cell.

Is there a cure for primary biliary cirrhosis?

Liver transplantation is the only known cure. Five-year survival following transplantation exceeds 80%. It is associated with a rapid resolution of lethargy and itching, and bone loss slows after the first year. Although the quality of life is not normal, it is usually excellent.

When is liver transplantation indicated?

Indications for liver transplantation are either symptoms (e.g. intractable pruritus, lethargy) or signs and symptoms of end-stage liver disease: increasing jaundice with serum bilirubin >170 μmol/l, estimated survival less than one year, intractable ascites, encephalopathy, fasting serum albumin <30 g/l, progressive muscle loss, recurrent spontaneous bacterial peritonitis, increasing osteoporosis, hepato-pulmonary syndrome, early, incidental hepatocellular carcinoma and unacceptable quality of life.

What factors predict survival after transplantation?

Serum urea and albumin, presence of ascites, Child's grade, and United Network for Organ Sharing Status (reflecting whether the patient is at home, in a general hospital bed or intensive care unit) are predictors of survival after transplantation (*Hepatology* 1997; **25**: 672–7).

What do you understand by secondary biliary cirrhosis?

It is that which occurs secondary to large duct obstruction and is usually due to extrahepatic obstruction such as bile duct stricture, gallstones or sclerosing cholangitis.

Professor Peter Brunt, contemporary gastroenterologist and liver physician, Aberdeen Royal Infirmary, is also the personal physician to the Queen and is an astute clinician. He is the President of the Association of Physicians of Great Britain, a society founded by Osler.

Roger Williams, Professor at King's College, London, and Sir Roy Calne, Professor of Surgery, Cambridge, pioneered liver transplantation in the UK.

Thomas E. Starzl, surgeon, Pittsburgh, USA, is an internationally known pioneer in liver transplantation.

Case 117

WILSON'S DISEASE

INSTRUCTION

Look at this patient's eyes.

SALIENT FEATURES

History

- History of consanguinity.
- In young adult or child – hepatitis, haemolytic anaemia, portal hypertension or neuropsychiatric abnormalities.
- In adolescents – presents as liver disease.
- In adults <40 years of age consider chronic or fulminant hepatitis.

Examination

Greenish yellow to golden-brown pigmentation at the limbus of the cornea, called the Kayser–Fleischer ring. The ring is most marked at the superior and inferior poles of the cornea and is due to the deposition of copper in Descemet's membrane in the cornea. (It is often apparent only on slit-lamp examination. It may be absent in patients with hepatic manifestations only but is present in those with neuropsychiatric disease.)

Proceed as follows:
Look for the following:

- Jaundice (look at the sclera).
- Sunflower cataracts.
- Hepatomegaly.
- Signs of liver cell failure.
- Neurological manifestations – tremor, chorea, mask-like facies with a vacuous smile.

DIAGNOSIS

This patient has a classical Kayser–Fleischer ring with jaundice and hepatomegaly (lesions) due to Wilson's disease (aetiology) and does not have a hepatic flap (functional status).

ADVANCED-LEVEL QUESTIONS

Is Kayser–Fleischer ring pathognomonic of Wilson's disease?
No, it is also seen in primary biliary cirrhosis, chronic active hepatitis with cirrhosis, cryptogenic cirrhosis and long-standing intrahepatic cirrhosis of childhood.

At what age do the neurological manifestations usually manifest?
They usually appear between 12 and 30 years of age. The most frequent first neurological symptom is difficulty in speaking or writing while in school.

What do you know about the inheritance of the disease?
Autosomal recessive inheritance; the gene *ATP7B* is located on chromosome 13, often associated with a family history of consanguinity. The disease is caused by mutations encoding a copper-transporting P-type ATPase (Wilson's disease protein, WNDP). Approximately 27 mutations have been reported; the most common, His1069Gln, is present in about a third of the patients of European extraction.

What do you know about the pathophysiology of this disease?
The precise defect is not known. The major aberration is excessive absorption of copper from the small intestine with decreased excretion of copper by the liver, resulting in an increase in tissue deposition, particularly in the brain, cornea, liver and kidney. The animal models of this condition are the Long–Evans cinnamon rat and the toxic milk mouse, which are currently undergoing evaluation to determine the precise defect in Wilson's disease.

What are the biochemical changes in Wilson's disease?
- Low serum caeruloplasmin level (caeruloplasmin is the copper-carrying protein).
- Serum copper concentration may be high, low or normal.

- Orally administered radiolabelled copper is incorporated into caeruloplasmin.
- Increased urinary excretion of copper.

How is the diagnosis of a suspected case confirmed?
By the demonstration of one of the following:

- Kayser–Fleischer rings and a serum caeruloplasmin level lower than 20 mg/l.
- Serum caeruloplasmin concentration of less than 200 mg/l and copper concentration in a liver biopsy sample greater than 250 µg/g on a dry-weight basis.

How would you treat such a patient?
Penicillamine removes and detoxifies deposits of copper. Treatment is lifelong and continuous.

What are the clinical stages of Wilson's disease?
Wilson's disease progresses through four clinical stages:

- Stage I: characterized by asymptomatic accumulation of copper in the liver which begins when the patient is born.
- Stage II: the patient is either asymptomatic or manifests with haemolytic anaemia or liver failure.
- Stage III: copper accumulates in the brain.
- Stage IV: progressive neurological disease.

> Samuel Alexander Kinnier Wilson (1877–1937) qualified in Edinburgh and worked at the National Hospital, Queen Square, London, as a neurologist (Wilson SAK 1912 Progressive lenticular degeneration. A familial nervous disease associated with cirrhosis of liver. *Brain* **34**: 295).
>
> Bernard Kayser (1869–1954) and Bruno Fleischer, both German ophthalmologists, described the same condition in 1902 and 1903 respectively.

Case 118

SPLENOMEGALY

INSTRUCTION

Examine this patient's abdomen.

SALIENT FEATURES

History

- Fatigue (due to anaemia).
- Night sweats, low-grade fever (due to hypermetabolic state caused by overproduction of WBCs in chronic myeloid leukaemia, CML).
- Abdominal fullness (due to splenomegaly).
- Bleeding, bone pain (myeloproliferative disorders due to bone marrow infiltration).

- History of leukaemia.
- History of myelofibrosis.
- History of residence in endemic areas of malaria, kala-azar.
- Family history of Gaucher's disease.
- History of fever (infectious mononucleosis, infective endocarditis).
- Blurred vision, respiratory distress, priapism (due to leukostasis in CML).
- Occasionally transverse myelitis (due to myelopoiesis in epidural space).

Examination

- Massive spleen. There may be associated anaemia.
- Start low while examining for the spleen and be gentle during palpation. Even if you are certain it is the spleen, you must go through the motions of ruling out a palpable kidney: do a bimanual palpation and check for ballottement; feel for the splenic notch; auscultate for splenic rub.

Proceed as follows:
- Look for enlarged lymph nodes and anaemia.
- Remember that the spleen must be at least two or three times its usual size before it can be felt.
- Remember that, normally, the spleen does not extend beyond the anterior axillary line and lies along the 9th, 10th and 11th ribs. The spleen percussion sign is a useful diagnostic technique (*Ann Intern Med* 1967; **67**: 1265).

DIAGNOSIS

This patient has massive splenomegaly (lesion), probably due to a myelo-proliferative disorder (aetiology).

QUESTIONS

What is your diagnosis?
Myeloproliferative disorder:
- Myelofibrosis, particularly in males.
- Chronic myeloid leukaemia, particularly in females.

How would you confirm your diagnosis?
Bone marrow examination.

ADVANCED-LEVEL QUESTIONS

In which other conditions is a massive spleen palpable?
- Malaria.
- Kala-azar.
- Gaucher's disease.

In which conditions is a moderately enlarged spleen (two to four finger-breadths or 4–8 cm) felt?
- Portal hypertension secondary to cirrhosis.
- Lymphoproliferative disorders such as Hodgkin's disease and chronic lymphatic leukaemia.

In which common conditions would the spleen be just palpable?

- Lymphoproliferative disorders.
- Portal hypertension secondary to cirrhosis.
- Infectious hepatitis.
- Glandular fever (infectious mononucleosis).
- Subacute endocarditis.
- Sarcoid, rheumatoid arthritis, collagen disease, idiopathic thrombocytopenia, congenital spherocytosis and polycythaemia rubra vera.
- Slender young women (*Ann Intern Med* 1967; **66**: 301).

What do you know about the genetics of chronic myelocytic leukaemia?

The fusion of c-*abl* (normally present on chromosome 9) with *bcr* sequences on chromosome 22 is pathognomonic of the chronic phase of chronic myelocytic leukaemia (the Philadelphia chromosome). The p53 gene appears to be the culprit in cases of myeloid blast transformation and there are structural alterations of *RB1* or N-*ras* in less than 10% of the cases with myeloid blast crisis.

What do you understand about the terms 'myeloid metaplasia' and 'extramedullary haematopoiesis'

'Myeloid metaplasia' and 'extramedullary haematopoiesis' are used interchangeably. They describe the process of ectopic haematopoietic activity that may occur in any organ system but predominantly affects the liver and spleen. It may or may not be associated with bone marrow fibrosis (myelofibrosis). The term 'myelofibrosis with myeloid metaplasia' is usually used to describe idiopathic myelofibrosis or agnogenic myeloid metaplasia (*N Engl J Med* 2000; **342**: 1255–65).

What do you understand by the term 'chronic myeloid disorders'?

Chronic myeloid disorders include:

- Chronic myeloid leukaemia.
- Myelodysplastic syndrome.
- Atypical chronic myeloid disorder.
- Chronic myeloproliferative disease: polycythaemia vera, essential thrombocythaemia, myelofibrosis with myeloid metaplasia. Essential thrombocythaemia in turn includes agnogenic myeloid metaplasia, post-polycythaemic myeloid metaplasia and post-thrombocythaemic myeloid metaplasia.

What is the treatment of Gaucher's disease?

Enzyme replacement therapy with glucocerebrosidase (alglucerase) is beneficial (*N Engl J Med* 1991; **324**: 1464–70; *N Engl J Med* 1992; **327**: 1632–6).

P.C.E. Gaucher (1854–1918), Professor of Dermatology in France.

Sir David Weatherall, FRS, contemporary Regius Professor of Medicine, Oxford, who has the unique distinction of being both a molecular biologist and an astute clinician.

The 1902 Nobel Prize was awarded to Sir Donald Ross (1857–1932; born in Almora, India), University of Liverpool, for his work on malaria, in which he showed how it enters the organism and thereby laid the foundation for successful research on this disease and methods of combating it.

Case 119

FELTY'S SYNDROME

INSTRUCTION

Examine this patient's abdomen.

SALIENT FEATURES

History

- Fever, weight loss.
- Rheumatoid arthritis.
- Leg ulcers, hyperpigmentation.

Examination

- Mild to moderate splenomegaly.
- Rheumatoid arthritis.

Proceed as follows:

Look for the following signs:

- Anaemia.
- Vasculitis.
- Diffuse pigmentation.
- Leg ulcers.

DIAGNOSIS

This patient has moderate splenomegaly with rheumatoid arthritis (lesions) due to Felty's syndrome.

ADVANCED LEVEL QUESTIONS

What is Felty's syndrome?

It is a rare complication of rheumatoid arthritis in which there is leukopenia with selective neutropenia and splenomegaly. The bone marrow is typically hyperplastic. The disease typically manifests late in the course of 'burnt-out' joint disease. The prognosis is poor because of recurrent Gram-positive infections. The 'large granular lymphocyte syndrome', a pre-malignant disorder of the T lymphocyte, may mimic Felty's syndrome in rheumatoid arthritis.

Note. Splenectomy does not prevent sepsis and may hasten the onset of malignancy.

What do you understand by the term 'hypersplenism'?

It implies removal of erythrocytes, granulocytes or platelets from the circulation by the spleen. Removal of the spleen is indicated when the underlying disorder cannot be corrected.

Criteria for hypersplenism include the following:

- Enlarged spleen.
- Destruction of one or more cell lines in the spleen.
- Normal bone marrow.

What are the indications for splenectomy?

- Hereditary spherocytosis in children.
- Autoimmune thrombocytopenia or haemolytic anaemia not controlled by steroids.
- To ameliorate hypersplenism in Gaucher's disease, thalassaemia, hairy cell leukaemia.
- Symptoms due to massive organomegaly.

What are the characteristic cells in a peripheral blood smear following splenectomy?

The presence of Howell–Jolly bodies (in all), siderocytes and spur cells (in 25% of patients).

What are the causes of asplenia?

Causes of asplenia include:

- Diminished function: sickle cell disease, thalassaemia, coeliac disease, SLE, lymphoma, leukaemia, amyloidosis.
- Surgical removal: hereditary spherocytosis, thalassaemia, lymphoma, idiopathic thrombocytopenia, traumatic rupture.

To which infections is the asplenic patient susceptible?

- *Streptococcus pneumoniae*, *Haemophilus influenzae* B, *Neisseria meningitidis* and malaria parasites pose a significant risk.
- Less common organisms include babesiasis, caused by tick-borne protozoa, and infection with *Capnocytophaga canimorus* following a dog bite.

What precautions would you advise an asplenic patient in the outpatient clinic?

Vaccination
- Pneumococcal vaccine – a single injection; booster doses at 5–10-year intervals.
- Hib vaccine – a single dose at the same time as pneumococcal immunization.
- Meningococcus groups A and C vaccine (although the majority of infections are due to group B strains for which there is no vaccine of proven efficacy).

Antibiotic prophylaxis
Phenoxymethylpenicillin or amoxicillin.

Foreign travel
Antimalarial chemoprophylaxis, other precautions (insect repellants, screens at night).

Augustus R. Felty (1895–1964) was a physician at Hartford Hospital, Hartford, Connecticut. He described this syndrome while he was working at the Johns Hopkins Hospital, Baltimore.

Case 120

POLYCYSTIC KIDNEYS

INSTRUCTION

This patient gives a history of intermittent haematuria; obtain a brief history and examine this patient's abdomen.

SALIENT FEATURES

History

- Acute loin pain and/or haematuria (owing to haemorrhage into a cyst, cyst infection or urinary stone formation).
- Loin or abdominal discomfort (due to increasing size of kidneys).
- Family history of polycystic kidney disease (as the condition is autosomal dominant with nearly 100% penetrance).
- Complications of hypertension.
- Stroke (due to ruptured berry aneurysm).
- Family history of brain aneurysm (the prevalence of intracranial aneurysms increases from 5% to 20% when there is a family history).

Examination

- Arteriovenous fistulas in the arms or subclavian dialysis catheter (remember that in the UK polycystic kidneys constitute the third most common cause for chronic renal failure after glomerulonephritis and pyelonephritis).
- Palpable kidneys (confirm by bimanual palpation and ballottement; there is a resonant note on percussion due to overlying colon; the hand can get between the swelling and the costal margin).

Proceed as follows:
- Look for the following signs:
  - Enlarged liver due to cystic disease.
  - Transplanted kidney may be palpable in either iliac fossa.
  - Third nerve palsy (berry aneurysms are associated with polycystic kidneys).
  - Look for anaemia (due to chronic renal failure) or polycythaemia (due to increased erythropoiesis).
  - Check the blood pressure (hypertension develops in 75% of cases).
- Tell the examiner that you would like to investigate as follows:
  - Look at the ECG for left ventricular hypertrophy (it appears that LVH occurs to a greater degree for a given rise in blood pressure in ADPKD compared with other renal disorders and with essential hypertension).
  - Microscopic haematuria.

Remember. Polycystic kidney disease is a misnomer as it is a systemic disorder affecting many organs.

DIAGNOSIS

This patient has polycystic kidney disease (lesion and diagnosis) and is currently on dialysis as evidenced by the arteriovenous fistula in the arm (functional status).
  Read: *N Engl J Med* 1993; **329**: 332.

QUESTIONS

How may polycystic disease present?

Haematuria, hypertension, urinary tract infection, pain in the lumbar region, uraemic symptoms, subarachnoid haemorrhage associated with berry aneurysm, and complications of associated liver cysts.

Is the kidney involvement usually unilateral or bilateral?

The disease is universally bilateral; unilateral cases reported probably represent multicystic renal dysplasia.

ADVANCED-LEVEL QUESTIONS

What do you know about the prevalence of this disease?

Autosomal dominant polycystic kidney disease (ADPKD) is one of the most common hereditary disorders, being 10 times more common than sickle cell disease, 15 times more common than cystic fibrosis and 20 times more common than Huntington's disease. It has a worldwide distribution. In the white population the disease appears to occur in about 1 in 400 to 1 in 1000 people (*Acta Med Scand* 1957; **328**: 1–255). Although the disease is rare in Africa and less common in American blacks than whites, the incidence of end-stage renal disease due to autosomal dominant polycystic kidney disease is similar in blacks and whites. ADPKD is an important cause of renal failure with 77% of patients dying or reaching end-stage renal disease by the age of 70 years (*Kidney Int* 1992; **41**: 1311–19).

In which other conditions may bilateral renal cysts be observed in an ultrasonographic study?

Multiple simple cysts, autosomal recessive polycystic kidney disease in children, tuberous sclerosis and von Hippel–Lindau syndrome.

What are the criteria for diagnosis of polycystic kidney disease using ultrasonography?

The presence of at least two renal cysts (unilateral or bilateral) in individuals at risk and younger than 30 years may be regarded as sufficient to establish a diagnosis; among those aged 30–59 years the presence of at least two cysts in each kidney; and among those aged 60 years and above at least four cysts in each kidney should be required (*Lancet* 1994; **343**: 824–7).

How would you like to manage this patient?

- FBC, urea and electrolytes, serum creatinine, urine microscopy, urine culture.
- Ultrasonography of the kidneys to confirm the diagnosis. Ultrasound may be equivocal in subjects under the age of 20 years.
- Contrast-enhanced spiral CT head scan or MRI as a screening test for intracranial aneurysms in patients aged 18–40 years and with a family history of intracranial aneurysms or subarachnoid haemorrhage (*N Engl J Med* 1992; **327**: 953–5).

In which other organs are cysts seen in this condition?

Liver (in 30% of cases), spleen, pancreas, lungs, ovaries, testes, epididymis, thyroid, uterus, broad ligament and bladder.

What are the neurological manifestations of this condition?

Subarachnoid haemorrhage from an intracranial berry aneurysm, causing death or neurological lesions in about 9% of patients. About 8% of patients with ADPKD have an asymptomatic intracranial aneurysm; the prevalence is twice as high in those with a family history of such aneurysms or of subarachnoid haemorrhage.

What is the pathology?

Cysts develop in Bowman's capsule and at other levels in the nephron, displacing kidney tissue.

What cardiovascular manifestations have been reported in these patients?

- Mitral valve prolapse in 26%.
- Other lesions commonly seen are mitral, aortic and tricuspid valve regurgitation.

What are the renal manifestations of this disease?

- The main structural change is the formation of cysts. Cysts enlarge, lose their tubular connection and become isolated from the glomerulus, requiring trans-epithelial transport of solutes and fluids for further expansion. Cyst fluids have different compositions, some having high and others low sodium concentration.
- One of the earliest and most consistent functional abnormalities is a decrease in renal concentrating ability.
- There may be altered endocrine function as reflected by increased secretion of both renin (causing increased predilection to hypertension) and erythropoietin (resulting in better maintained haematocrit in renal failure, unlike in renal failure due to other causes; rarely can result in polycythaemia).

What are the causes of abdominal pain in this disease?

Infected cyst, haemorrhage into cyst or diverticular perforation.

What are the complications of polycystic kidney disease?

Renal complications

- Hypertension (intrarenal activation of the renin–angiotensin system is said to be the main mechanism and hence ACE inhibitors are first line agents to control blood pressure).
- Pain – back pain or abdominal pain. (Cyst decompression may help to relieve pain but does not alter the rate of progression.)
- Gross or microscopic haematuria.
- Cyst infection (lipophilic antibiotics against Gram-negative bacteria such as cotrimoxazole, fluoroquinolones penetrate the cysts better and are preferred to standard antibacterial agents).
- Renal calculi (seen in 10–20% of patients with ADPKD; are frequently radiolucent and composed of uric acid).
- Urinary tract infection including pyelonephritis.
- Proteinuria.

- Renal failure (once the GFR falls below 50 ml/minute the rate of progression is more rapid than in other primary renal disorders and is about 5 ml/minute every year). About one half of the patients have normal life with adequate renal function.

Extrarenal manifestations
- Cystic: cysts in the liver, ovary, pancreas, spleen and central nervous system. Unlike renal cyst formation, liver cysts seem to be influenced by female hormones. Whilst men and women have the same frequency of liver cysts, massive liver cysts are almost exclusively found in women.
- Non-cystic:
  - Cardiac valvular abnormalities – mitral valve prolapse (seen in ~20% of patients with ADPKD), aortic valve abnormalities.
  - Intracranial saccular aneurysm or berry aneurysm. Magnetic resonance angiography is the most reliable technique of non-invasive screening among such patients.
- Gastrointestinal – colonic diverticula, hernias of the anterior abdominal wall.

What do you know about the genetic transmission of this disease?
Polycystic kidney disease is an autosomal dominant disorder. Mutations in at least three different genes can lead to autosomal dominant polycystic kidney disease (ADPKD). The *PKD1* gene is located on chromosome 16 (*Cell* 1994; **77**: 881–4). The protein product of *PKD1*, polycystin-1, is an integral membrane glycoprotein involved in cell-to-cell and/or cell-to-matrix interaction (*J Am Soc Nephrol* 1995; **6**: 1125–33). The *PKD2* gene is situated on chromosome 4 and its protein product is similar to the alpha1 subunit of voltage-activated calcium and sodium channels, suggesting a related role for polycystin-2 (*Science* 1996; **272**: 1339–42). The polycystins interact through their C-terminal cytoplasmic tails which suggests that *PKD1* and *PKD2* may function through a common signalling pathway (*Nat Genet* 1997; **16**: 179–83). At least one other gene containing mutations that lead to ADPKD is known to exist; its chromosomal location is not known.

Among the European ADPKD population, *PKD1* is the cause in about 85% of families and *PKD2* the cause in about 15%. Compared with individuals affected by *PKD2*, those with *PKD1* have more severe disease with a higher prevalence of hypertension, an increased risk of progression into renal failure and shorter life expectancy. Although *PKD2* is clinically milder than *PKD1* it has a deleterious impact on overall life expectancy and cannot be regarded as a benign disorder (*Lancet* 1999; **353**: 103–7).

What do you know about screening in this condition?
- The children and siblings of patients with established ADPKD should be offered screening.
- Affected individuals should have their blood pressure checked regularly and offered genetic counselling.
- Genetic linkage analysis can be utilized in many families. Ultrasound is usually not useful before the age of 20 years.

What are the poor prognostic factors in ADPKD?
Patients are liable to progress more rapidly if they are male, or have polycystin-1 mutations, early onset hypertension, episodes of gross haematuria (*J Am Soc*

Nephrol 1997; **8:** 1560–7), or family history of hypertension in the unaffected patient (*J Am Soc Nephrol* 1995; **6:** 1643–8), but these only account for a fraction of the variability of disease progression.

What are the causes of death in these patients?

One third of adult patients die from renal failure; another third die from the complications of hypertension (including heart disease, intracerebral haemorrhage and rupture of berry aneurysm). The remaining third die from unrelated causes.

Sir W. Bowman (1816–1892), Surgeon at the Royal London Ophthalmic Hospital.

E.L. Potter (1901–), US pathologist. She also described Potter's syndrome with renal agenesis and characteristic of epicanthic folds, receding jaw and low set ears with less cartilage than usual.

O.Z. Dalgaard's study in 1957 clarified the autosomal dominant pattern of inheritance of the disease.

Case 121

TRANSPLANTED KIDNEY

INSTRUCTION

Examine this patient's abdomen.

SALIENT FEATURES

History

- History of chronic renal failure – determine duration, aetiology (diabetes, hypertension, glomerulonephritis).
- History of haemodialysis.
- History of arteriovenous fistula.
- History of transplanted kidney.

Examination

- Laparotomy scar (comment on the scar).
- Arteriovenous fistulas in arms.
- Transplanted kidney felt in either right or left iliac fossa.

Proceed as follows:

- Tell the examiner that you would like to look for other signs of uraemia (see pp 585–8).
- Do know the differential diagnosis for masses in the right/left iliac fossa (see p. 331).

DIAGNOSIS

This patient has a transplanted kidney (lesion) probably due to diabetic nephropathy as evidenced by the sugar-free drinks by the bedside (aetiology).

QUESTIONS

Mention a few indications for renal transplantation.

End-stage renal diseases; the most common diseases that result in referral of patients for transplantation include:

- Diabetes mellitus with renal failure.
- Hypertensive renal disease.
- Glomerulonephritis.

ADVANCED-LEVEL QUESTIONS

Would you refer a patient for renal transplantation before instituting haemodialysis?

Referral for renal transplantation need not be delayed until the patient has begun dialysis. It is acceptable and, in fact, usually preferable to refer the patient to a renal transplant unit before dialysis is required. With judicious planning on the part of the general practitioner, renal physician and transplant surgical team, transplantation can be performed before dialysis is even required.

In which age group is transplantation preferred to dialysis?

Infants and children have a high morbidity rate on long-term haemodialysis or peritoneal dialysis. Thus, renal transplantation from parents or siblings improves growth and allows a more normal lifestyle.

Is there any advantage to HLA matching before transplantation?

Kidneys from living related donors who are HLA identical and also red blood cell ABO matched have a 90% survival rate at 1 year; less well matched grafts tend to have a somewhat lower survival rate. Kidney transplants from matched cadaver donors survive nearly as long, especially if the recipient does not contain antibodies to donor antigens.

There is some evidence that HLA mismatching has a greater effect on living related than it does on cadaveric donor kidney transplantation. Recent evidence has shown that HLA-matched kidneys, particularly for DR, B and A antigens, are associated with long-term survival of the patient. Complete matching of DR, B and A loci is associated with the best chance of success. HLA-DR matching appears to have the greatest impact on survival, followed by B, and lastly the A loci (*N Engl J Med* 1994; **331**: 803–5).

Should repeated blood transfusions be avoided in a patient waiting for a renal transplant?

If the anaemia is well tolerated and is due to the renal failure *per se*, blood transfusion should be avoided as it carries a risk of HLA sensitization. Pretreatment of recipients with multiple blood transfusions from the *donor* tends to increase graft survival, in contrast to the deleterious effect on bone marrow engraftment.

What other factors are known to cause sensitization to HLA antigens?
Pregnancy, previously failed transplant.

What drugs are used for post-transplant immunosuppression?
Steroids, azathioprine and ciclosporin – used independently or in combination. Newer drugs include FK 506, rapamycin, sirolimus, mycophenolate mofetil, and daclizumab.

What are the contraindications for kidney transplantation?
- A positive cross-match by cytotoxicity testing between recipient serum and donor cells is considered to be a contraindication for transplantation.
- Presence of HIV or other infectious agents on donor screening.

What are the complications of renal transplantation?
- Opportunistic infection, e.g. cytomegalovirus, *Pneumocystis*.
- Premature coronary artery disease.
- Hypertension – primarily to ciclosporin.
- Lymphomas and skin cancers.
- *De novo* glomerulonephritis in the transplanted kidney.
- Complications of steroid therapy, e.g. aseptic necrosis of bone.

What do you know about warm ischaemic time?
Shorter warm ischaemic time of the transplanted kidney is associated with longer survival of the recipient. However, a slight increase in the duration of cold ischaemia justifies HLA-matching before kidney transplantation because of higher rates of survival, a lower incidence of the episodes of rejection and lower risk of loss as a result of rejection (*N Engl J Med* 2000; **343:** 1078–84).

What is the survival rate following kidney transplant?
The 2-year kidney graft survival rate for living related donor transplantation is 85%, whereas in cadaveric donor transplantation it is about 70%.

What do you know about rejection of the transplanted kidney?
It may be acute or chronic and must be suspected when the graft is tender, the urine output is falling or the creatinine concentration is rising. It is a complex process in which both cell-mediated immunity and circulating antibodies play a role. Evaluation of suspected rejection usually requires graft biopsy.

- Acute rejection is characterized by a lymphocytic interstitial infiltrate with destruction of epithelial cells. It usually responds to treatment which includes high-dose methyl prednisolone, antilymphocytic globulin and anti-T-lymphocyte monoclonal antibody (OKT3) administration.
- Chronic rejection shows histological features of interstitial fibrosis, atrophy of tubules and proliferation of the arterial intima. There is no specific treatment and general management of chronic renal failure should be reinstituted.

Is there any advantage of renal transplantation as compared to long-term dialysis in end-stage renal disease?
The benefits of renal transplantation include better quality of life (*Am J Kid Dis* 1990; **15:** 201–8), reduced medical expenses (*Semin Nephrol* 1992; **12:** 284–9) and about a 68% reduction in the long-term risk of death (*N Engl J Med* 1999; **341:** 1725–30).

What is the role of pancreas–kidney transplantation in patients with diabetes mellitus and end-stage renal failure?

Pancreas transplantation in type I diabetes can reverse the lesions of diabetic nephropathy but reversal requires more than 5 years of normoglycaemia (*N Engl J Med* 1998; **339**: 69–75). Simultaneous pancreas–kidney transplantation prolongs survival in patients with diabetes and end-stage renal failure (*Lancet* 1999; **353**: 1915–19).

Does acute myocardial infarction influence long-term survival among patients on long-term dialysis?

Patients on dialysis who have an acute myocardial infarction have high mortality from cardiac causes and poor long-term survival (*N Engl J Med* 1998; **339**: 799–805).

In the 1920s, Alexis Carrel developed the technique of vascular anastomoses which made possible David Hume's and Joseph Murray's human allograft attempts in the early 1950s.

Joseph E. Murray (1919–), Professor of Surgery, Brigham and Women's Hospital and Harvard Medical School, was awarded the 1990 Nobel Prize for Medicine for his pioneering work on organ transplantation along with Thomas E. Donnall (1920–) of the Fred Hutchinson Cancer Research Centre, Seattle, Washington, USA (Murray JE, et al. Prolonged survival of human-kidney homografts by immunosuppressive drug therapy. *N Engl J Med* 1963; **268**: 1315–23).

In 1966, Terasaki and co-workers reported the association between HLA matching and outcome in patients receiving cadaveric organs (*Ann N Y Acad Sci* 1966; **129**: 500–20).

The observation by Schwartz and Damasheck that 6-mercaptopurine was effective in blocking primary but not secondary antibody response in rabbits paved the way for drug-induced immunosuppression in the late 1950s (*Nature* 1959; **183**: 1682–3).

Case 122

ABDOMINAL AORTIC ANEURYSM

INSTRUCTION

Examine this patient's abdomen.
This patient presented with low back pain; examine the abdomen.

SALIENT FEATURES

History

- Remember, three quarters of the patients are asymptomatic.
- Vague abdominal pain.
- History of embolization.
- Family history of rupture of abdominal aneurysm.
- History of smoking.

Examination

- Large expansile pulsation along the course of the abdominal aorta.
- Auscultate for bruit over the aneurysm and over the femoral pulses.
- 'Trash' foot – digital infarcts in patient with easily palpable pulses (suggests either a popliteal or abdominal aneurysmal source of emboli) (*BMJ* 2000; **320:** 1193–6).
- Examine all peripheral pulses.

Proceed as follows:
- Tell the examiner that you would like to check the following:
  - Urine for sugar.
  - Blood pressure.
  - Serum cholesterol.
- Remember that:
  - Popliteal artery aneurysms often coexist and, in fact, their presence should prompt the physician to look for an abdominal aortic aneurysm.
  - Ninety per cent of atherosclerotic abdominal aortic aneurysms are present below the origin of the renal arteries and can involve the aortic bifurcation.
  - The infrarenal aorta is normally 2 cm in diameter; when it exceeds 4 cm an aneurysm is said to exist.
  - True arterial aneurysms are defined as a 50% increase in the normal diameter of the vessel.
  - The aneurysmal process may affect any medium or large sized artery.
  - The vessels most commonly affected are the aorta and iliac arteries, followed by popliteal, femoral and carotid arteries.

DIAGNOSIS

This patient has a large pulsatile mass in the epigastrium (lesion) due to an aneurysm of the abdominal aorta (aetiology).

Read classic reviews on this subject: *N Engl J Med* 1993; **328:** 1167; *BMJ* 2000; **320:** 1193–6.

QUESTIONS

Which investigations would you perform to confirm your diagnosis?

- B mode ultrasonography of the abdomen – a simple, cheap and accurate screening test.
- Large aneurysms require angiography.
- Magnetic resonance imaging is useful, particularly as it does not require administration of contrast.
- Remember that plain abdominal radiography shows a calcified aneurysmal aortic wall in only half the cases.

ADVANCED-LEVEL QUESTIONS

How would you manage an abdominal aneurysm?

- Pooled data suggest that aortic aneurysms of more than 55 mm carry a high risk of rupture and hence should be referred to the vascular surgeon for surgery if there are no confounding factors that increase the risk of surgery.

- The UK small aneurysm trial studied 1090 patients with an aortic diameter of 40–50 mm and found a 30-day mortality of 5.8%, mean annual risk of rupture for small aneurysms of 1%, and no difference in survival between the treatment groups at two, four or six years (*Lancet* 1998; **352:** 1649–55). Smaller aneurysms must be followed up; they enlarge at a rate of about 0.5 cm a year. In selected cases an endovascular prosthesis is preferred.

What factors predispose to rupture of the abdominal aneurysm?

- Diameter of the aneurysm.
- History of smoking.
- Diastolic blood pressure.
- COAD.
- Family history of ruptured aneurysm.
- Rate of expansion.
- Inflammatory aneurysms.

What is the prognosis of aneurysms greater than 55 mm?

The mortality rate for a patient undergoing elective surgery is less than 5%, whereas that for a ruptured aneurysm is nearly 90%.

In 1951, C. Dubost from Paris performed the first successful aortic resection for aneurysm.

Case 123

UNILATERAL PALPABLE KIDNEY

INSTRUCTION

Examine this patient's abdomen.

SALIENT FEATURES

History

- Nephrectomy.
- Congenital absence of kidney.
- History of azotaemia, dialysis.

Examination

One kidney is palpable (bimanually ballottable; there is a transverse band of colonic resonance on percussion and you will be able to insinuate your fingers between the mass and costal margin).

Proceed as follows:

Look carefully for arteriovenous fistulas in the arms, haemodialysis catheters in the subclavian region.

DIAGNOSIS

This patient has a unilateral palpable kidney (lesion) which may be due to either polycystic kidney disease or renal neoplasm (aetiology).

QUESTIONS

What are the common causes of a palpable kidney?
• Polycystic kidney disease.
• Renal carcinoma.
• Hydronephrosis.
• Renal cyst.
• Hypertrophy of the solitary functioning kidney.

What changes can occur in a kidney when the other is removed?
Long-term renal function remains stable in most patients with a reduction in renal mass of more than 50%. However, these patients are at increased risk for proteinuria, glomerulopathy and progressive renal failure. Hence it is important to monitor patients with remnant kidneys. Problems are most frequent in those in whom the amount of renal tissue removed is greatest and who have survived the longest (*N Engl J Med* 1991; **325:** 1058).

Leon Fine, contemporary Professor and Chair of Medicine, University College Hospital, London.

Graeme Catto, contemporary Professor of Renal Medicine and Dean, Aberdeen Medical School.

H.A. Lee, retired Professor of Renal Medicine, Portsmouth, University of Southampton, who is also interested in metabolism.

Case 124

ABDOMINAL MASSES

INSTRUCTION

Examine this patient's abdomen.

SALIENT FEATURES

Patient 1

The patient has an epigastric mass. Differential diagnosis:

• Carcinoma of the stomach: look for supraclavicular lymph nodes, hepatomegaly; comment on pallor and asthenia.
• Carcinoma of the pancreas: look for jaundice.

- Aneurysm of the abdominal aorta: look for pulsatile mass; check femoral and foot pulses; auscultate over the mass and the femoral pulses (see p. 328).
- Retroperitoneal lymphadenopathy (lymphoma).

Patient 2

The patient has a mass in the right iliac fossa. Differential diagnosis:

- Crohn's disease: look for mouth ulcers; tell the examiner that you would like to look for fistulas and take a history for chronic diarrhoea (see p. 575).
- Carcinoma of the caecum: look for hard mass, lymph nodes.
- Look for lymph nodes elsewhere (see pp 569–71); feel for liver and spleen; examine the drainage area of iliac lymph nodes (such as the leg, perianal area, external genitalia; do a rectal examination).
- Transplanted kidney: comment on the laparotomy scars, stigmata of renal failure and artificial arteriovenous fistulas.
- Appendicular abscess.
- Ileocaecal abscess, particularly in Asians.
- Ovarian tumours (must be mentioned as a differential diagnosis in female patients).

Less common causes of masses in the right iliac fossa:
- Amoebiasis.
- Carcinoid (ileal).
- Actinomycosis.
- Ectopic kidney.

Patient 3

The patient has a mass in the left iliac fossa. Differential diagnosis:

- Diverticular abscess: look for a tender, mobile mass.
- Carcinoma of the colon: look for hepatomegaly; tell the examiner that you would like to do a per rectum examination.
- Faecal mass (the mass may be moulded by pressure).
- Ovarian tumour (in females).
- Iliac lymph nodes: look for other lymph nodes, liver and spleen; examine the drainage areas.
- Transplanted kidney: comment on the laparotomy scar, look for signs of renal failure, arteriovenous fistulas (see pp 603–5).

Note. The investigation of first choice in such patients is abdominal ultrasonography.

Robin Warren, Pathologist at Royal Perth Hospital in Western Australia, and Barry J. Marshall discovered that *Helicobacter pylori* causes peptic ulcer disease (*Lancet* 1983; i: 1273–5). In 1984, Marshall infected himself by drinking a pure culture of *H. pylori*. After feeling fine for 5 days he experienced nausea and vomiting. Histology confirmed acute gastritis. In 1995 he received the Albert Lasker Clinical Medical Research Award. *H. pylori* has also been implicated in the causation of gastric cancer in Japanese people.

HISTORY

Ask the patient whether he or she has any pain, stiffness or difficulty in dressing or walking.

EXAMINATION

- *Look* at posture, gait and joint deformity.
- *Feel* for temperature, tenderness, joint fluid and crepitus of movement of the joints.
- *Move*: check passive and active movements of the joints; test stability of the joints.
- *Measure* muscle wasting and shortening of the limb.

Examination of the hands

1. Ask the patient, 'Are your hands painful?'.
2. Inspect for joint deformity:
   - Swan-neck deformity (flexion at the distal interphalangeal joints and hyperextension of the proximal interphalangeal joints).
   - Boutonnière deformity (flexion of the proximal interphalangeal joints and hyperextension of the distal interphalangeal joint).
   - Z deformity of the thumb.
   - Ulnar deviation of the fingers.
3. Examine the nails:
   - Nail fold infarcts (rheumatoid arthritis).
   - Nail pitting, onycholysis, ridging, hyperkeratosis, discoloration (psoriasis).
4. Comment on the following:
   - Wasting of small muscles of the hand, in particular those of the dorsum of the hand.
   - Heberden's nodes, i.e. bony nodules at the distal interphalangeal joints (osteoarthroses).
   - Bouchard's nodes, i.e. bony nodules at the proximal interphalangeal joints (osteoarthroses).
   - Spindle-shaped deformity of the fingers.
   - Gouty tophi.
5. Examine the palms:
   - Wasting of the thenar or hypothenar eminence.
   - Thickening of the palmar fascia – Dupuytren's contracture (rheumatoid arthritis).
   - Palmar erythema (rheumatoid arthritis).
   - Tap over the flexor retinaculum to detect median nerve entrapment (Tinel's sign).
6. Get the patient to perform the following movements:
   - Unbuttoning of clothes.
   - Pincer movements.

- Hand grip.
- Abduction of the thumb.
- Writing.

7. Test sensation of the index and little fingers.
8. Examine the elbows for the following signs:
   - Rheumatoid arthritis.
   - Gouty tophi.
   - Psoriatic plaques.
9. Tell the examiner that you would like to examine the other joints.

Note. When asked to examine the hands, consider the possibility of arthropathy, myopathy, neuropathy, a peripheral nerve lesion or acromegaly.

> W. Heberden, Sr. (1710–1801), an English physician.
>
> C.J. Bouchard (1837–1915), a French physician.

Examination of the knees

1. Ask the patient if the joints are sore.
2. Expose both knees and lower thighs fully with the patient lying supine.
3. Look for:
   - Quadriceps wasting.
   - Swelling of the joint.
4. Feel:
   - Temperature.
   - Synovial thickening.
   - Do the patellar tap (ballottement): fluid from the suprapatellar bursa is forced into the joint space by squeezing the lower part of the quadriceps and then the patella is pushed posteriorly with the fingers; this test indicates fluid in the synovial cavity.
5. Movement:
   - Test passive flexion and extension – make a note of the range of movements and feel for crepitus.
   - Gently extend the knee and examine for fixed flexion deformity.
   - Test the medial and lateral ligaments by steadying the thigh with the left hand and moving the leg with the right laterally and medially when the knee joint is slightly flexed – movement of more than 10 degrees is abnormal.
   - Test the cruciate ligaments by steadying the foot with your elbow and moving the leg anteriorly and posteriorly with the other hand – laxity of more than 10 degrees is abnormal.
6. Ask the patient to lie on his or her stomach and feel the popliteal fossa when the knee is extended.

Examination of the feet

1. Look:
   - For skin rash, scars.
   - At the nails for changes of psoriasis.

- At the forefoot for hallux valgus, clawing and crowding of the toes (rheumatoid arthritis).
- At the callus over the metatarsal heads which may occur in subluxation.
- At both the arches of the foot, in particular medial and longitudinal (flat foot, pes cavus).

2. Palpate:
- Ankles for synovitis, effusion, passive movements at the subtalar joints (inversion and eversion) and talar joint (dorsiflexion and plantar flexion); remember that tenderness on movement is more important than the range of movement.
- Metatarsophalangeal joints for tenderness.
- Individual digits, for synovial thickening.
- Bottom of heel, for tenderness (plantar fasciitis), and Achilles tendon for nodules.

Case 125

RHEUMATOID HANDS

INSTRUCTION

Examine this patient's hands.

SALIENT FEATURES

History

Painful swollen joints, morning stiffness.

Examination

Ask the patient for permission to examine her hands and then ask whether the hands are sore.

Proceed as follows:
- Comment on deformities (Fig. 1) such as the following:
  - Subluxation at the metacarpophalangeal joint.
  - Swan-neck deformity.
  - Boutonnière deformity (hyperextension at the terminal interphalangeal joint and flexion at the proximal interphalangeal joint).
  - Z deformity of the thumb.
  - Dorsal subluxation of the ulna at the carpal joint.
- Comment on the following signs:
  - Nail-fold infarcts and vasculitic skin lesions.
  - Palmar erythema.
  - Wasting of the first dorsal interossei and other small muscles of the hand.

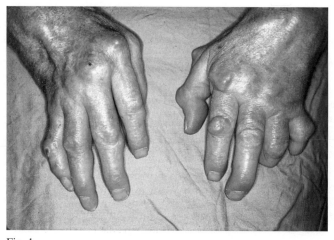

Fig. 1

- Test grip and pincer movements. Quickly test for abductor pollicis brevis and interossei, and pinprick sensation over index and little fingers. The median nerve may be involved if there is associated carpal tunnel syndrome.
- Examine the elbow for rheumatoid nodules.
- Ask the patient to perform simple tasks involving hand function, such as unbuttoning her clothes, or writing.
- Tell the examiner that you would like to examine other joints.
- Highlight the following points:
  - Whether terminal interphalangeal joints are spared or affected.
  - Whether the arthritis is active (if the joints are inflamed) or inactive.

DIAGNOSIS

This patient has swan-neck deformity of the fingers (lesions) due to rheumatoid arthritis (aetiology) with marked active arthritis of the interphalangeal joints, and is unable to button her clothes (functional status).

QUESTIONS

What is the significance of rheumatoid arthritis?
The presence of nodules indicates seropositive and more aggressive arthritis.

Where else are nodules found?
Flexor and extensor tendons of the hand, sacrum, Achilles tendon, sclera, lungs and myocardium.

What are the skin lesions in rheumatoid arthritis?
Vasculitis, nail-fold infarcts.

What are the causes of anaemia in rheumatoid arthritis?
- Anaemia of chronic disease.
- Megaloblastic anaemia due to folate deficiency or associated pernicious anaemia.
- Felty's syndrome.
- Drugs: non-steroidal anti-inflammatory drugs (NSAIDs) causing iron deficiency anaemia; bone marrow suppression caused by gold.

What factors have been implicated in anaemia of chronic disease?
- Decreased production of red blood cells:
  - Due to inadequate iron: impaired absorption and transport, failure to release iron stores.
  - Due to decreased concentration or marrow resistance to erythropoietin.
  - Ineffective erythropoiesis.
  - Abnormal development of erythroid progenitor cells.
- Increased destruction of red cells.

What is Felty's syndrome?
It is seen in some patients with severe rheumatoid arthritis and consists of spleno-megaly, anaemia, leukopenia and thrombocytopenia (hypersplenism), and leg ulcers. Splenectomy ameliorates hypersplenism. Felty's syndrome is associated with positive rheumatoid factor.

What are the pulmonary manifestations of rheumatoid arthritis?
- Pleural effusion or pleurisy (seen in 25% of men with rheumatoid arthritis).
- Rheumatoid nodules.
- Fibrosing alveolitis.
- Caplan's syndrome (rheumatoid arthritis coexists with rounded fibrotic nodules 0.5–5 cm in diameter, mainly in the periphery of lung fields in coal-worker's pneumoconiosis).

What are the eye manifestations of rheumatoid arthritis?
- Episcleritis.
- Scleritis.
- Scleromalacia, scleromalacia perforans.
- Keratoconjunctivitis sicca.
- Sjögren's syndrome (see above).

What precautions are necessary before upper gastrointestinal endoscopy or general anaesthesia?
It is prudent to take a cervical spine radiograph to rule out atlanto-axial subluxation.

Which joints are commonly affected in rheumatoid arthritis?
Wrists, proximal interphalangeal joints and metacarpophalangeal joints of the hands, metatarsophalangeal joints and knees.

What is palindromic rheumatoid arthritis?
Palindromic onset is seen in some patients with recurrent episodes of joint stiffness and pain in individual joints lasting only a few hours or days. Hydroxychloroquine may be of value in preventing recurrences.

ADVANCED-LEVEL QUESTIONS

How would you treat the arthritis?
Prescribe NSAIDs (ibuprofen is the safest at conventional doses) including aspirin. If, after 1 month of NSAIDs, the symptoms persist with no sign of remission then a second-line drug should be added. Second-line drugs include hydroxy-chloroquine, sulfasalazine and penicillamine. Low-dose methotrexate and gold salts are used to prevent disease progression. Treatment with monoclonal antibody to tumour necrosis factor (etanercept, infliximab) produces significant improvement in the severity of arthritis. Etanercept is a fusion protein of the ligand binding region of the TNF receptor that is linked to the Fc portion of the human IgG, and infliximab is a chimeric (mouse and human) monoclonal antibody against TNF. These TNF inhibitors have surprisingly few side effects. The most common reactions are at the injection site (in the case of etanercept) and hypersensitivity reactions (in the case of infliximab). TNF-α inhibitors suppress disease activity only during treatment and thus relapses are inevitable once the treatment is discontinued (*N Engl J Med* 2000; **343**: 1640–1).

If the patient is known to experience gastric distress with NSAIDs, what precautions would you take while prescribing them?
Prophylaxis for NSAID-associated gastric distress may be attempted with con-current administration of an H_2-receptor blocker (such as ranitidine), omeprazole or

misoprostol. The latter is a prostaglandin analogue which has been shown to protect the gastric mucosa.

What are the neurological manifestations of rheumatoid arthritis?

- Peripheral neuropathy – glove-and-stocking sensory loss.
- Mononeuritis multiplex.
- Entrapment neuropathy, e.g. carpal tunnel syndrome.
- Cervical disease or atlanto-axial subluxation may cause cervical myelopathy.

What are the causes of proteinuria in patients with rheumatoid arthritis?

- Drug therapy: gold salts, penicillamine.
- Amyloidosis.

What is Sjögren's syndrome?

- The association of keratoconjunctivitis sicca (lack of lacrimal secretion) and xerostomia (dry mouth due to lack of salivary gland secretion) in association with a connective tissue disorder, usually rheumatoid arthritis. This syndrome may be associated with autoimmune thyroid disease, myasthenia gravis or autoimmune liver disease.
- The Schirmer filter paper test provides a crude measure of tear production. Filter paper is hooked over the lower eyelid; in normal people at least 15 mm is wet after 5 minutes, whereas in patients with keratoconjunctivitis sicca it is less than 5 mm.
- Anti-Ro (SSA) and anti-SS-B antibodies may be seen in this syndrome.
- Treatment is symptomatic with artificial tears (hypromellose drops or 1% methyl-cellulose), artificial saliva and NSAIDs for the arthritis.

What are the criteria for rheumatoid arthritis?

American Rheumatism Association criteria:

1. Morning stiffness for at least 1 hour for a duration of 6 weeks or more.
2. Swelling of at least three joints for 6 weeks or more.
3. Swelling of wrist, metacarpophalangeal or proximal interphalangeal joints for 6 weeks or more.
4. Symmetry of swollen joint areas for 6 weeks or more.
5. Subcutaneous nodules.
6. Positive rheumatoid factor.
7. Radiographic features typical of rheumatoid arthritis, i.e. erosions and periarticular osteopenia.

When four or more of the above criteria are met, there is 93% sensitivity and 90% specificity. It is important to note that the diagnosis of rheumatoid arthritis should not be made on the basis of these criteria alone if another systemic disease associated with arthritis is definitely present.

What are the poor prognostic factors?

- Systemic features: weight loss, extra-articular manifestations.
- Insidious onset.
- Rheumatoid nodules.
- Presence of rheumatoid factor more than 1 in 512.

- Persistent activity of the disease for over 12 months.
- Early bone erosions.

What are the factors leading to ulnar deviation of the hands?
- In the normal grip the fingers move to ulnar deviation.
- Weakening of radial sides of the joint capsule and the radial insertion of the interossei ligaments.
- The volar supports of the flexor tendon sheath are weakened by inflammation, allowing the tendon to bow in the direction of the ulna during gripping.
- Ulnar displacement of the extensor tendons in early deviation makes them slip, if the dorsal metacarpophalangeal joint is taut, and thereby exacerbates the development of ulnar deviation by acting as a bowstring.
- The joint capsules of metacarpophalangeal joints are weaker on radial sides than on ulnar sides.

A.B. Garrod coined the term 'rheumatoid arthritis' in 1858.

H.S.C. Sjögren, a Swedish ophthalmologist, described this condition in 1933.

A. Caplan, a British physician, was an industrial officer in the Welsh coal mines.

In 1931, Philip S. Hench (1896–1965) of the Mayo Clinic observed that arthritic pain temporarily decreased in pregnant women. For the next 8 years he studied the phenomenon that allergic conditions such as asthma, hay fever and food sensitivity were also lessened in the presence of jaundice or pregnancy. He reasoned that a steroid hormone may be responsible, since hormone levels are high in the blood during pregnancy (Hench PS 1953 A reminiscence of certain events before, during and after the discovery of cortisone. *Minn Med* **36**: 705–10).

Edward Kendall (1886–1972), Chief of the Division of Biochemistry, suggested the name 'corsone' on a piece of paper but Hench amended this to 'cortisone', and thus the steroid hormone was 'baptized'. The 1950 Nobel Prize for Medicine was jointly awarded to Kendall, Hench and Tadeus Reichstein (1897–) of Basel University, Switzerland, for their discoveries relating to the hormones of the adrenal cortex, their structure and biological effects (*Lancet* 1999; **353**: 1370).

Sir John Vane, showed that inhibition of prostaglandin synthesis was central to both the actions and side effects of aspirin (*Proc R Coll Physicians Edinb* 2000; **30**: 191–8).

Case 126

ANKYLOSING SPONDYLITIS

INSTRUCTION

Examine this patient's back.
Examine this patient.

SALIENT FEATURES

History
- Back stiffness and back pain – worse in the morning, improves on exercise and worsens on rest.

- Symptoms in the peripheral joints (in ~40%), particularly shoulders and knees.
- Onset of symptoms is typically insidious and in the third to fourth decade.
- Extra-articular manifestations: red eye (uveitis), diarrhoea (GI involvement), history of aortic regurgitation, pulmonary apical fibrosis (worse in smokers).

Examination

- 'Question mark' posture (due to loss of lumbar lordosis, fixed kyphoscoliosis of the thoracic spine with compensatory extension of the cervical spine).
- Protuberant abdomen.

Proceed as follows:

- Ask the patient to look to either side – the whole body turns when the patient does this.
- Examine the cervical, thoracic and lumbar spines (remember that cervical spine involvement occurs later in the disease and results in pain and a grating sensation on movement of the neck).
- Measure the occiput-to-wall distance (inability to make contact when heel and back are against the wall indicates upper thoracic and cervical limitation).
- Perform Schober's test – this involves marking points 10 cm above and 5 cm below a line joining the 'dimple of Venus' on the sacral promontory. An increase in the separation of less than 5 cm during full forward flexion indicates limited spinal mobility.

Note. Finger–floor distance is a simple indicator but is less reliable because good hip movement may compensate for back limitation.

- Examine for distal arthritis (occurs in up to 30% of patients and may precede the onset of the back symptoms). Small joints of the hand and feet are rarely affected.
- Measure chest expansion with a tape (less than 5 cm suggests costovertebral involvement).
- Tell the examiner that you would like to examine the following:
  - Eyes for iritis, anterior uveitis (seen in 20% of patients).
  - Heart for aortic regurgitation (seen in 4% of patients who have had the disease for over 15 years), cardiac conduction defects.
  - Lungs for mild restrictive disease, apical fibrosis, apical cavities and secondary fungal infection.
  - Central nervous system such as tetraplegia, etc.
  - Foot for Achilles tendinitis and plantar fasciitis.

Remember:

- The four 'A's of ankylosing spondylitis: **a**pical fibrosis, **a**nterior uveitis, **a**ortic regurgitation, **A**chilles tendinitis.
- That psoriasis and Reiter's syndrome can also cause sacroiliitis.

DIAGNOSIS

This patient has fixed kyphoscoliosis of the thoracic spine with loss of lumbar lordosis (lesion) due to ankylosing spondylitis (aetiology) on Schober's test; spinal movements are severely diminished (functional status).

Read classic review: *BMJ* 1995; **310**: 1321–4.

QUESTIONS

What investigations would you like to perform in this patient?

Anteroposterior view of sacroiliac joints and lateral radiographs of lumbar spine: the earliest changes are erosions and sclerosis of the sacroiliac joints. Later in the disease syndesmophytes may be found in the lumbosacral spine. In severe disease, involvement progresses up the spine, leading to a 'bamboo spine'. The New York criteria (1966) for the diagnosis of ankylosing spondylitis require a combination of clinical and radiographic features, but the diagnosis should be suspected on the basis of inactivity, spinal stiffness, and pain, with or without additional features.

In which other seronegative arthritic disorders is low back pain a feature?

Sacroiliitis is often seen in Reiter's syndrome, psoriatic arthritis, juvenile chronic arthritis and intestinal arthropathy.

How would you manage a patient with ankylosing spondylitis?

- Encourage exercise, particularly physical therapy, to preserve back extension.
- NSAIDs, in particular indometacin (indomethacin). Phenylbutazone is reserved for resistant cases.
- Surgical therapy, consisting of vertebral wedge osteotomy, is occasionally indicated.

ADVANCED-LEVEL QUESTIONS

What genetic counselling would you give this patient?

In HLA-B27 positive patients, the siblings have a 30% chance of developing this disease. Hence children of such patients who develop symptoms such as joint pains or sore eyes should be referred to a rheumatologist.

What is the natural history of the disease?

About 40% go on to develop severe spinal restriction; about 20% have significant disability; early peripheral joint disease, particularly of the hip, indicates a poor prognosis.

What is the risk in those with a 'bamboo' cervical spine when driving?

Increased susceptibility to whiplash injury and restricted lateral vision.

What therapy may the patient have received in the past if the blood film shows a leukaemic picture?

In the past, patients were treated with irradiation of the spine. However, such patients tend to develop leukaemia several years after therapy.

The term 'ankylosing spondylitis' derives from the Greek words, *ankylos* (bent or crooked) and *spondylos* (vertebra). Past names have included Marie–Strümpell disease and von Bechterew's disease.

The first clinical report of ankylosing spondylitis (1831) concerned a man from the Isle of Man. Vladimir von Bechterew of St Petersburg, Russia, described a series of cases between 1857 and 1927. Adolf Strümpell (1853–1926) of Erlangen, and Pierre Marie (1853–1940) of Paris, independently described this condition in 1897 and 1898 respectively.

H.C. Reiter (1881–1969), a German physician.

Achilles is a figure from Greek mythology who was a hero of the Trojan War. His mother dipped him into the river Styx, holding him by his heel, to make him invulnerable to attack. He slew Hector in this war, but was himself slain, wounded in his vulnerable heel by Paris.

Case 127

PSORIATIC ARTHRITIS

INSTRUCTION

Examine this patient's hands.

SALIENT FEATURES

History
- Cutaneous psoriasis with itching in a fifth of the patients.
- Joint pain, joint stiffness worse in the morning.

Examination
Distal interphalangeal joint involvement.

Proceed as follows:
- Tell the examiner that you would like to:
  - Examine the nails, looking for pitting, onycholysis, discoloration, thickening (nails are involved in 80% of patients with psoriatic arthritis).
  - Look for psoriatic plaques in the extensor aspects of elbows, scalp, sub-mammary region, umbilicus and natal cleft; describe these as reddish plaques with well-defined edges and silvery white scales.
- Comment on the fingers, which are sausage shaped due to tenosynovitis.

DIAGNOSIS

This patient has nail pitting, psoriatic plaques and distal interphalangeal arthropathy (lesion) due to psoriasis (aetiology) and has good hand function (functional status).

ADVANCED-LEVEL QUESTIONS

What are the patterns of joint involvement seen in psoriasis?
The patterns include (*Acta Derm Venereol* 1961; **41**: 396–403):

- Asymmetrical terminal joint involvement.
- Symmetrical joint involvement as seen in rheumatoid arthritis.
- Sacroiliitis: this differs from ankylosing spondylitis, most notably in that the syndesmophytes tend to arise from the lateral and anterior surfaces of the vertebral bodies and not at the margins of the bodies.
- Arthritis mutilans – complicated by the 'telescoping' of digits.

What are the radiological features of psoriatic arthritis?
- 'Fluffy' periostitis.
- Destruction of small joints.
- 'Pencil and cup' appearance, osteolysis and ankylosis in arthritis mutilans.
- Non-marginal syndesmophytes in spondylitis (*Q J Med* 1977; **46**: 411).

What is the prognosis?

Deforming and erosive arthritis is present in 40% of cases, and 11% of patients are disabled by their arthritis (*Lancet* 1988; **ii:** 375).

Case 128

PAINFUL KNEE JOINT

INSTRUCTION

Examine this patient's leg.
Examine this patient's joints.
Examine this patient's knee joint.

SALIENT FEATURES

History

- Painful knee joint.
- Take a history of trauma and fever.
- History of rheumatoid arthritis, gout or haemophilia.

Examination

- Pain on movement of the joint (take care not to hurt the patient).
- Swelling of the joint (you must demonstrate fluid in the joint).
- Check both active and passive movements.
- Look for disuse atrophy of the muscles around the joint.

Proceed as follows:

Tell the examiner that you would like to investigate as follows:

- Examine other joints.
- Obtain radiographs of the knee (anteroposterior and lateral views).
- Analyse the joint fluid for cells, sugar, protein and culture.

DIAGNOSIS

This patient has a painful knee joint with restricted movement (lesion and functional status) following trauma while playing rugby (aetiology).

QUESTIONS

What are the common causes of a painful knee joint?

- Rheumatoid arthritis.
- Osteoarthrosis.

- Trauma.
- Septic arthritis (will require emergency removal of the pus to prevent joint damage).
- Viral infection.
- Gout.
- Pseudogout.
- Haemophilia.

ADVANCED-LEVEL QUESTIONS

What is palindromic rheumatoid arthritis?
Palindromic onset of rheumatoid arthritis refers to acute recurrent arthritis, usually affecting one joint, with symptom-free intervals of days to months between attacks. This term was introduced by P.S. Hench (see p. 340) and E.F. Rosenberg.

A patient with a painful knee joint and a unilateral facial nerve palsy is seen by you in the outpatient department. Six weeks before this she developed an annular rash after a camping trip in Europe. What is your diagnosis and what confirmatory test would you carry out?
The diagnosis is Lyme disease and the confirmatory test is an antibody titre against *Borrelia burgdorferi*. The disease was first recognized in Lyme, Connecticut, USA.

Case 129

OSTEOARTHROSIS

INSTRUCTION

Look at this patient's hands.
Examine this patient's joints.

SALIENT FEATURES

History
- Age.
- Pain in the joints.
- Stiffness after a period of inactivity.
- Impairment of gait due to joint pain.

Examination
- Heberden's nodes (bony swellings) at the terminal interphalangeal joints.
- Squaring of the hands due to subluxation of the first metacarpophalangeal joint.

Proceed as follows:

Tell the examiner that you would like to examine the hips and knees as these joints are usually involved (feel the knee for crepitus: it may be red, warm and tender, and have an effusion).

DIAGNOSIS

This elderly patient has Heberden's nodes and squaring of the hands with involvement of the interphalangeal joints of the hands (lesions) due to osteoarthrosis (aetiology) and is unable to button his clothes (functional status).

Read review: *BMJ* 1995; **310:** 457–60; *N Engl J Med* 1989; **320:** 1322; *Am J Med* 1987; **83** (suppl 5A): 5.

QUESTIONS

Which other joints are frequently involved?
Spine, in particular cervical and lumbar spines.

Mention the types and a few causes of osteoarthrosis.
• Primary.
• Secondary:
  – Trauma – affects athletes, pneumatic drill workers, anyone doing work involving heavy lifting.
  – Inflammatory arthropathies – rheumatoid arthritis, septic arthritis, gout.
  – Neuropathic joints – in diabetes mellitus, syringomyelia, tabes dorsalis.
  – Endocrine – acromegaly, hyperparathyroidism.
  – Metabolic – chondrocalcinosis, haemochromatosis. .

What are Heberden's nodes?
Bony swellings seen at the terminal interphalangeal joints in osteoarthrosis.

What are Bouchard's nodes?
Bony swellings at the proximal interphalangeal joints in osteoarthrosis.

ADVANCED-LEVEL QUESTIONS

What are the typical radiological features?
• Subchondral bone sclerosis and cysts.
• Osteophytes.

What will the synovial aspirate show?
Fewer than 100 white blood cells per millilitre.

What do you understand by the term 'nodal osteoarthrosis'?
Nodal osteoarthrosis is a primary generalized osteoarthrosis with characteristic features. It occurs predominantly in middle-aged women and is autosomal dominant. It characteristically affects the terminal interphalangeal joints with the development of Heberden's nodes. The arthritis may be acute and, although there may be marked deformity, there is little disability. It can also affect the carpometacarpal joints of the thumbs, spinal apophyseal joints, knees and hips.

How would you manage a patient with osteoarthrosis?

- Change in lifestyle: maintain optimal weight, encourage exercise, use appropriate footwear.
- Drugs: simple analgesics, rubifacients, NSAIDs for acute flare-ups, intra-articular corticosteroid injections for acute flare-ups or patients unfit for surgery.
- Surgery: arthroscopic removal of loose body, arthroscopic washout or radio-isotope synovectomy for persistent synovitis, joint replacement for hip and knee.

William Heberden (1710–1801) was a London physician who described the nodes as 'little hard knobs' and this was first published posthumously in 1802.

J.K. Spender (1886), of Bath, introduced the term 'osteoarthritis'. Archibald E. Garrod, from London, established the modern usage and clinical differentiation from rheumatoid arthritis in 1907.

In 1884, C.J. Bouchard (1837–1915) described nodes adjacent to the proximal interphalangeal joints identical to those at the distal interphalangeal joints.

Case 130

GOUT

INSTRUCTION

Examine this patient's hands or examine the feet.

SALIENT FEATURES

History

- Usually acute pain at the base of great toe, worse at night and associated with redness.
- Occasionally multiple joints involved.
- Systemic symptoms, e.g. low-grade fever.

Examination

Chronic tophaceous deposit (Fig. 2) with asymmetrical joint involvement.

Proceed as follows:
- Tell the examiner that you would like to proceed as follows:
- Examine the helices of the ears, olecranon bursae and Achilles tendons for tophi.
- Examine the feet or hands.

Note. Uric acid crystals are negatively birefringent, needle shaped and may be deposited in bursae and bone marrow. They are demonstrable in synovial fluid within leukocytes and free in the fluid during attacks of gouty arthritis. They react with nitric acid and ammonium hydroxide to give a purple colour (murexide test).

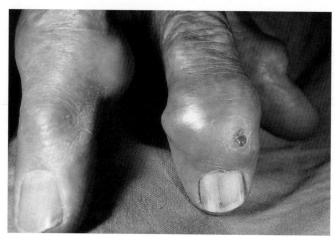

Fig. 2

DIAGNOSIS

This patient has a painful great toe with swelling of the joint (lesion) due to gout (aetiology) and is unable to walk because of the pain (functional status).

QUESTIONS

What is the basic pathophysiology of gout?

Gout is a metabolic disorder of purine metabolism. It is characterized by hyperuricaemia due to either overproduction (75%) or underexcretion (25%) of uric acid.

What are the different clinical manifestations of gout?

- Asymptomatic hyperuricaemia.
- Acute arthritis.
- Chronic arthritis.
- Chronic tophaceous gout.

How would you treat an acute attack of gout?

Prescribe an NSAID such as indometacin (indomethacin). Refractory gout may require steroids.

What factors may precipitate acute gouty arthritis?

Drugs (diuretics, aspirin), copious consumption of alcohol, dehydration, surgery, fasting, food high in purines (sweetbreads, liver, kidney and sardines).

ADVANCED-LEVEL QUESTIONS

Under what circumstances would you treat hyperuricaemia?

Frequent attacks of acute arthritis, renal damage and consistently raised serum uric acid levels. Before attempting to lower serum uric acid levels it is prudent to use colchicine to prevent acute attacks.

What is the drug of choice for controlling hyperuricaemia?
Allopurinol (a xanthine oxidase inhibitor).

What drugs would you use if the patient was allergic to allopurinol?
Uricosuric drugs such as probenecid, sulfinpyrazone.

What is pseudogout?
Pseudogout is an acute arthritis resulting from the release of calcium pyrophosphate
dihydrate crystals (deposited in the bone and cartilage) into the synovial fluid.

> Gout was recognized as early as the 4th century BC. Two concepts have prevailed: that
> it occurs mainly in sexually active mature men and that gastronomic and sexual
> excesses may precipitate acute attacks. Antonj van Leewenhoeck (1632–1723) described
> the microscopic appearance of urate crystals from gouty tophus. In 1847, Alfred Garrod,
> in London, identified uric acid in the serum of a gouty man.
>
> James Wyngaarden, contemporary Professor of Medicine, Duke University, USA, whose
> chief interest is metabolic and genetic diseases.

Case 131

CHARCOT'S JOINT

INSTRUCTION

Examine this patient's joints.
Examine the locomotor system in this patient.

SALIENT FEATURES

History
- History of diabetes (*Medicine* 1972; **51**: 191–210).
- Gait deformity.
- Loss of pain threshold.
- Atrophy of muscles of the joint.

Examination
- Enlargement of the affected joint (compare with the other side).
- Instability of the joint, in particular hypermobility of the joint.
- May be warm, swollen and tender in the early stages.
- Enlargement and crepitus may be present in the later stages.

Proceed as follows:
- Check sensation in the affected limb.
- Tell the examiner that you would like to investigate as follows:
  - Do a thorough neurological examination, looking for loss of proprioception,
    and/or pain sensation, and vibratory sensation with a 128 Hz tuning fork.

–Examine the urine for sugar (looking for evidence of diabetes mellitus).
–Ask for lancinating pains, check posterior column signs and look for Argyll Robertson pupil (tabes dorsalis).
–Check for dissociated sensory loss (syringomyelia).
–Test muscle strength.

DIAGNOSIS

This patient has Charcot's joint (lesion) due to diabetes mellitus (aetiology) and has marked deformity of the joint with restricted movement (functional status).

QUESTIONS

What do you understand by the term 'Charcot's joint'?

It is a chronic progressive degenerative arthropathy resulting from a disturbance in the sensory innervation of the affected joint. It is a neuropathic arthropathy which represents a complication of various disorders affecting the nervous system. It results in gross deformity, osteoarthrosis and new bone formation from repeated trauma.

Mention a few conditions responsible for the development of Charcot's joints.

- Diabetic neuropathy – affecting tarsal joints, tarsometatarsal, metatarsophalangeal joints.
- Tabes dorsalis – affecting knee, hip, ankle, lumbar and lower dorsal vertebrae.
- Syringomyelia – affecting shoulder, elbow, cervical vertebra.
- Myelomeningocele – affecting ankle, tarsus.
- Miscellaneous: hereditary sensory neuropathies, peripheral nerve injury, congenital insensitivity to pain, leprosy.

Jean Martin Charcot (1825–1893) was a French neurologist. He was a Professor of Pathology in 1872 and Professor of Nervous Diseases in 1882. The other conditions that bear his name include the following: Charcot's fever (intermittent fever due to cholangitis), Charcot's triad (intention tremor, nystagmus and scanning speech in multiple sclerosis), Charcot–Leyden crystals (seen in the sputum of asthmatics), Charcot–Marie–Tooth disease (peroneal muscular atrophy), Charcot–Wilbrand syndrome (visual agnosia).

Case 132

STILL'S DISEASE

INSTRUCTION

Examine this patient's joints.
Look at this patient.

SALIENT FEATURES

History

- Maculopapular rash.
- History of fever in the initial stages of the disease.
- Joint pains, swelling, determine onset and course.

Examination

- Micrognathia.
- Joints usually involved are upper cervical apophyseal joints, carpometacarpal joints and terminal interphalangeal joints.
- Splenomegaly and lymph node enlargement.

DIAGNOSIS

This patient has micrognathia, arthropathy of terminal interphalangeal joints and a past history of maculopapular rash (lesion) due to Still's disease (aetiology).
    Read *BMJ* 1995; **310:** 728–31.

ADVANCED-LEVEL QUESTIONS

What do you know about juvenile chronic arthritis?

The diagnosis is made when a child aged less than 16 years has arthritis for at least 6 weeks with no other apparent cause. After 6 months of disease three major patterns are seen:

- Still's disease (10–20% of cases) is defined as arthritis associated with daily temperature spikes to 39.4°C (103°F) for at least 2 weeks with or without maculopapular rash.
- Polyarticular juvenile chronic arthritis (15–25%) in which five or more joints are affected. Early fusion of the mandible and cervical spine result in a receding chin and early fusion of the cervical spine.
- Pauciarticular juvenile chronic arthritis (60–75%) which affects four or less joints; iritis is common in girls, whereas sacroiliitis is common in boys.

What are the complications of juvenile chronic arthritis?

- Pain, lethargy, anorexia and irritability.
- Joint contractures.
- Anaemia.
- Chronic anterior uveitis.
- Growth disturbance.
- Amyloidosis.
- Joint failure.

How would you treat a patient with juvenile chronic arthritis?

- Education about the disease, counselling and social support.
- Physical and occupational therapy: monitoring and recording range of movement of joints, exercises to increase range of movement and muscle bulk, hydrotherapy, splinting.

- NSAIDs: naproxen, ibuprofen, piroxicam, indometacin (indomethacin), diclofenac.
- Intra-articular steroids: triamcinolone, methylprednisolone acetate.

What is the risk of treating young children with salicylates?

Reye's syndrome has been reported in children treated with aspirin for fever accompanying viral infections such as influenza. Children with juvenile chronic arthritis who are treated continuously for long periods have not been shown to have an increased incidence of this syndrome (*Pediatrics* 1980; **66:** 859).

What are the poor prognostic factors?

- Chronic and polyarticular arthritis, particularly in patients with a systemic or pauciarticular onset.
- Polyarticular onset and a positive test for immunoglobulin rheumatoid factor.

Which drugs have been used in the treatment of resistant juvenile rheumatoid arthritis?

- Penicillamine.
- Hydroxychloroquine.
- Methotrexate (long-term therapy should be avoided as it is known to cause hepatic fibrosis) (*N Engl J Med* 1992; **326:** 1077).

Sir George Fredrick Still (1868–1941), a London physician, described 12 children (in 1897) who had a polyarthritis which he stated should be distinguished from rheumatoid arthritis, and a further six children with a disease indistinguishable from adult rheumatoid arthritis. The distinctive findings in the first group included splenomegaly, lymphadenopathy, frequent occurrence of pericarditis and a predilection for cervical spine involvement. He also noted that fever and growth retardation were prominent features (Still GF 1897 On a form of chronic joint disease in childhood. *Med Chir Trans* **80:** 47). The rash, however, was first described by Eric G.L. Bywaters.

R.D.K. Reye (1912–1977), an Australian histopathologist.

EXAMINATION OF THE THYROID

INSTRUCTION

Examine the thyroid.
Test this patient's thyroid status.
Look at this patient's neck.

SALIENT FEATURES

1. *Introduce yourself* to the patient and, while shaking hands, note whether the palms are warm and sweaty.

2. *Inspection of the neck:*
   - Look for the JVP.
   - Scars of surgery (often missed by candidates).
   - Enlarged cervical lymph nodes.
   - Goitre.

3. *Palpation* (always begin by palpating from behind):
   - Seat the patient comfortably.
   - Comment first on exophthalmos.
   - While palpating the gland, ensure that there is a glass of water to swallow.
   - Palpate the thyroid and note the following:
     - Size – specify the World Health Organization grade (see below).
     - Mobility.
     - Texture – simple or nodular (solitary or multiple)?
     - Tenderness.
   - Pemberton's sign (on raising the arms above the head, patients with retro-sternal goitres may develop signs of compression, i.e. suffusion of the face, syncope or giddiness).
   - Palpate cervical lymph nodes.
   - Feel the carotid arteries.
   - Palpate for tracheal deviation.
   - Percuss for retrosternal extension.
   - *Auscultate over the gland for bruit*, carotid bruits.
   - Test sternomastoid function (this muscle may be infiltrated in thyroid malignancy).

4. *Thyroid function* should then be assessed:
   - Eye signs:
     - Lid lag.
     - Exophthalmos.
     - Lid retraction (sclera visible above the cornea).
     - Extraocular movements.
   - Hands:
     - Pulse for tachycardia or atrial fibrillation.
     - Tremor.

– Acropachy or clubbing.
– Palmar erythema (thyrotoxicosis).
– Supinator jerks (inverted in hypothyroidism).
– Proximal weakness in the upper arm.
- Skin: look for pretibial myxoedema.
- Elicit the ankle jerks.

If you are permitted to ask questions, enquire about shortness of breath, dysphagia, iodine-containing medications and possible exposure to radiation.

QUESTIONS

How would you grade the size of the goitre?
WHO grading of goitre (*Lancet* 2000; **355:** 106–10):

Grade 0:   No palpable or visible goitre.
Grade 1:   Palpable goitre (larger than terminal phalanges of examiner's thumbs).
          1A   Goitre detectable only on palpation.
          1B   Goitre palpable and visible with neck extended.
Grade 2:   Goitre visible with neck in normal position.
Grade 3:   Large goitre visible from a distance.

What is the significance of the thyroid bruit?
The thyroid bruit is almost pathognomonic of Graves' disease and occurs only rarely in patients with colloid goitres or other thyroid disorders.

In 1915, Kendall isolated a crystalline product named thyroxine (Kendall EC 1915 The isolation in crystalline form of the compound containing iodine which occurs in the thyroid. *JAMA* **64:** 2042).

In 1927, Harrington and Barger synthesized thyroxine (Harrington CR, Barger G 1927 Chemistry of thyroxine. *Biochem J* **21:** 169).

In 1952, Gross and Pitt-Rivers identified tri-iodothyronine (Gross J, Pitt-Rivers R 1952 The identification of 3,5,3' L-triiodothyronine in human plasma. *Lancet* i: 439).

In 1946, H.S. Pemberton described the sign of the 'submerged' goitre (Pemberton HS 1946 Sign of submerged goitre. *Lancet* **251:** 509).

Case 133

GRAVES' DISEASE

INSTRUCTION

Look at this patient.
Determine this patient's thyroid status.

SALIENT FEATURES

Patient is fidgety and restless.

Proceed as follows:

History

- Easy irritability, nervousness, insomnia.
- Fatigue.
- Weight loss with increased appetite.
- Frequent defaecation.
- Oligomenorrhoea.
- Dislike for hot weather, heat intolerance, excessive sweating.
- Palpitations, dyspnoea.
- Family history of thyroid disease.
- Proximal muscle weakness, muscle atrophy, periodic paralysis (particularly in patients of Oriental extraction).

Examination

Hands:
- While shaking hands with the patient note the warm sweaty palms.
- Look for tremor, thyroid acropachy, onycholysis (Plummer's nails), vitiligo and palmar erythema.
- Check pulse (for tachycardia or the irregularly irregular pulse of atrial fibrillation).

Eyes:
- Comment on proptosis (after looking at the eyes from behind and above).
- Check for lid lag.
- Check for scars of previous tarsorrhaphy.

Neck:
- Mention previous thyroidectomy scar if present.
- Examine the neck for goitre and auscultate over the gland.

Chest:
- Gynaecomastia can occur in men due to increased oestrogen production.
- Examine the cardiovascular system: sinus tachycardia, widened pulse pressure, loud first heart sound, third heart sound, systolic murmur, atrial fibrillation.

Lower limbs:
- Examine the shins for pretibial myxoedema (bilateral pinkish brown dermal plaques).
- Test for proximal myopathy with hyper-reflexia.

Tell the examiner:
That you would like to check for thyroid-stimulating antibodies, TsAb, which give near 100% detection rate in Graves' patients.

DIAGNOSIS

This patient has tremor, proptosis and lid lag (lesions) due to autoimmune Graves' disease (aetiology), and is in fast atrial fibrillation and hyperthyroid (functional status).

QUESTIONS

How would you confirm the diagnosis in this patient?
Serum thyroxine (T_4), serum thyroid-stimulating hormone (TSH) levels and thyroid autoantibodies.

What are the causes of hyperthyroidism?
- Primary: Graves' disease, toxic nodule, multinodular goitre, Hashimoto's thyroiditis, iodine-induced, excess thyroid hormone replacement, postpartum thyroiditis.
- Secondary: pituitary or excess TSH hypersecretion, hydatidiform mole, struma ovarii, factitious.

What are the components of Graves' disease?
Hyperthyroidism with goitre, eye changes and pretibial myxoedema – they run independent courses.

ADVANCED-LEVEL QUESTIONS

What happens to radioactive iodine uptake in Graves' disease?
Radioactive iodine uptake increases in Graves' disease.

Which is the best laboratory test to diagnose hyperthyroidism?
Serum TSH measurement is the single most reliable test to diagnose all common forms of hyperthyroidism, particularly in an outpatient setting (*Arch Intern Med* 2000; **160:** 1573–5). Typically, serum concentrations are less than 0.1 mIU/l in Graves' disease, toxic adenoma, nodular goitre, subacute and lymphocytic (silent, postpartum) thyroiditis, iodine-induced hyperthyroidism and exogenous thyroid hormone excess. To diagnose hyperthyroidism accurately, TSH assay sensitivity, the lowest reliably measured TSH concentration, must be 0.02 mIU/l or less. Some less sensitive TSH assays cannot reliably distinguish hyperthyroidism from euthyroidism. Free T_4 and T_3 concentrations should be measured when less sensitive TSH assays are utilized. In rare types of TSH-mediated hyperthyroidism (pituitary adenomas and selective pituitary resistance to thyroid hormone) serum TSH alone will not suffice and again free T_4 and T_3 concentrations should be measured.

What are the causes of isolated TSH suppression?

- Mild (subclinical) hyperthyroidism.
- Recovery from overt hyperthyroidism.
- Non-thyroidal illness (which can cause a low serum free T_4).
- Pregnancy during the first trimester.
- Medications such as dopamine and glucocorticoids.

Mention a few causes of hyperthyroidism with reduced iodine uptake.

- Thyroiditis.
- Malignancy of thyroid.
- Struma ovarii.

What drugs are used in the treatment of thyrotoxicosis?

- Carbimazole.
- Methimazole.
- Propylthiouracil.

What are the disadvantages of antithyroid drugs?

- High rates of relapse once treatment is discontinued.
- Occasionally complicated by troublesome hypersensitivity reaction and very rarely by life-threatening agranulocytosis and hepatitis.

What are the advantages and disadvantages of radioactive iodine, compared with partial thyroidectomy for thyrotoxicosis?

Both radioactive iodine therapy and surgical thyroidectomy are extremely effective and usually result in permanent cure. Patients will require lifelong thyroxine replacement. Thyroid surgery is expensive, inconvenient and occasionally complicated by injury to surrounding structures in the neck in less skilled hands, and by the risks of anaesthesia. In Graves' disease the indications for surgery include: a large goitre, the patient's preference, drug non-compliance and disease relapse when radioiodine is not available.

Radioactive iodine, although safe, may not be acceptable to patients who are sensitive to the calamities of Chernobyl and Hiroshima.

What are the contraindications to radioiodine therapy?

- Breastfeeding and pregnancy.
- Situations in which it is clear that the safety of other persons cannot be guaranteed.
- Patients who are incontinent who are unwilling to have a urinary catheter.
- Allergy to iodine.

What are the indications for radioiodine therapy in hyperthyroidism?

- Hyperthyroidism due to Graves' disease with moderate goitre (40–50 g), with no significant eye signs and first presentation.
- Toxic multinodular goitre in older persons complicated by heart failure or atrial fibrillation.
- Toxic adenoma, usually with mild hyperthyroidism.
- Ophthalmopathy with thyroid dysfunction with stable eye disease.
- Ablation therapy in those with severe manifestations such as heart failure, atrial fibrillation or psychosis.

What advice would you give to patients who are administered radioiodine?

- Depending on the dose, they should avoid journeys on public transport, stay off work, avoid places of entertainment or close contact with other people for up to 12 days and avoid non-essential close personal contact with children and pregnant women for up to 27 days.
- Patients should be warned that in the first fortnight after administration of therapy they may experience palpitations or other exacerbations of symptoms, particularly when not euthyroid before treatment.
- The importance of regular follow-up should be emphasized, as should the need to report the recurrence of thyrotoxic symptoms or the development of hypothyroidism.
- Patients should be informed that atrial fibrillation often reverts to normal rhythm and that digitalis may then be discontinued.
- Patients should be reminded to avoid pregnancy for 4 months after radioiodine therapy.

Is there an increased frequency of cancer in patients with Graves' disease?

There is little evidence to suggest an increased frequency of thyroid cancer in patients with Graves' disease.

Does thyrotoxicosis affect the bone?

Yes, chronic thyrotoxicosis is associated with osteoporosis.

If a patient with thyrotoxicosis develops muscle weakness following oral carbohydrate or intravenous dextrose, which condition comes to mind?

Hypokalaemic periodic paralysis, which occurs particularly in Asian men. These attacks may last for 7–72 hours.

What is the effect of iodine on thyroid status?

It may cause transient hypothyroidism (Wolff–Chaikoff effect) or hyperthyroidism (Jod–Basedow phenomenon).

What is the prevalence of hyperthyroidism?

The prevalence is 0.2% in the adult population; the prevalence of mild (subclinical) hyperthyroidism, where serum TSH is less than 0.1 mIU/l and free T_4 and T_3 are normal, is 0.1–6% of the adult population.

What do you know about amiodarone-induced hyperthyroidism?

Amiodarone, which contains 37% iodine, can induce hyperthyroidism; this disorder is more common in iodine-deficient areas (*Ann Intern Med* 1984; **101:** 28–34) and in patients with nodular goitres and thyroid autoantibodies. There are two mechanisms by which amiodarone may cause hyperthyroidism: thyroid destruction due to an iodine-associated increase in circulating interleukin-6 (*J Clin Endocrinol Metab* 1994; **78:** 423–7) or an increase in thyroid hormone synthesis. Amiodarone-induced hyperthyroidism sometimes responds to thionamide antithyroid drugs but may also be very resistant to treatment. A combination of potassium perchlorate and carbimazole should be tried; steroids may be effective, particularly if interleukin-6 concentrations are high, which suggests a destructive thyroiditis. In resistant cases, total thyroidectomy should be considered (*Lancet* 1997; **349**: 339–43).

Robert James Graves (1796–1853) was a Dublin physician who described this condition. In 1835 he described three patients and wrote of one patient, 'It was now observed that the eyes assumed a singular appearance for the eyeballs were apparently enlarged, so that when she slept or tried to shut her eyes her lids were incapable of closing, when the eyes were open, the white sclerotic could be seen, to a breadth of several lines all around the cornea' (Graves R 1835 *London Med Surg J* **7**(Part II): 516). Graves' disease is also termed Basedow's or Parry's disease.

Case 134

EXOPHTHALMOS

INSTRUCTION

Examine this patient's face.
Perform a general examination of this patient.

SALIENT FEATURES

History

- Obtain a history of thyrotoxicosis (see p. 355).
- History of smoking (ophthalmopathy is more common in cigarette smokers, *Lancet* 1991; **338**: 25–7).

Examination

- Prominent eyeballs.
- Look at the patient's eyes from behind and above for proptosis.
- Comment on lid retraction (the sclera above the upper limbus of the cornea will be seen); this is Dalrymple's sign.
- Comment on the sclera visible between the lower eyelid and the lower limbus of the cornea (i.e. comment on the exophthalmos). Most patients have bilateral exophthalmos with unilateral prominence.
- Check for lid lag (ask the patient to follow your finger and then move it along the arc of a circle from a point above her head to a point below the nose – the movement of the lid lags behind that of the globe); this is von Graefe's sign. Voluntary staring can result in a false lid lag, and the patient must be suitably relaxed before eliciting this sign.
- Check for extraocular movements and comment on the cornea.
- Look for the following:
  - Signs of thyrotoxicosis (fast pulse rate, tremor and sweating).
  - Goitre (listen for a bruit).
  - Post-thyroidectomy scar.

DIAGNOSIS

This patient has marked exophthalmos with ophthalmoplegia (lesions) with signs of thyrotoxicosis (functional status) due to Graves' disease (aetiology).

ADVANCED-LEVEL QUESTIONS

What eye signs of thyroid disease do you know?

Werner's mnemonic, **NO SPECS** (*J Clin Endocrinol Metab* 1977; **44:** 203–4):

No signs or symptoms.
Only signs of upper lid retraction and stare, with or without lid lag and exophthalmos.
Soft tissue involvement.
Proptosis.
Extraocular muscle involvement.
Corneal involvement.
Sight loss due to optic nerve involvement.

How would you investigate this patient?

- History and clinical examination for signs of thyrotoxicosis and thyroid enlargement and bruit.
- Serum T_4, triiodothyronine (T_3), TSH.
- Thyroid antibodies.

Mention the factors implicated in the phenomenon of lid lag.

- Sympathetic overstimulation, causing overaction of Müller's muscle.
- Myopathy of the inferior rectus causing overaction of superior rectus and levator muscles.
- Restrictive myopathy of the levator muscle.

What is euthyroid Graves' disease?

The patient will be clinically and biochemically euthyroid but will have manifestations of Graves' ophthalmopathy. A thyrotrophin-releasing hormone (TRH) stimulation test will show a flat response curve.

What would you recommend if a patient with unilateral exophthalmos is clinically and biochemically euthyroid?

- Ophthalmological referral.
- Ultrasonography of the orbit.
- CT scan of the orbit.

How is proptosis quantified?

It is assessed using a Hertel's exophthalmometer. The upper limit of normal is subject to ethnic variation: usually, more than 20 mm is considered as proptosis.

How would you manage a patient with Graves' ophthalmopathy?

The single most important aspect is a close liaison between the physician and the ophthalmologist.

Severe Graves' disease and visual loss should be treated immediately with high doses of corticosteroids, orbital irradiation and plasma exchange as an adjunct and, if there is no improvement within 72–96 hours, orbital nerve decompression by surgical removal of the floor and medial wall of the orbit is necessary.

Moderate ophthalmopathy improves substantially in 2–3 years in most patients. In the interim the patient is treated symptomatically:

- Pain and grittiness is treated with methylcellulose eye drops by day and a lubricating eye ointment at night.
- Exposure keratitis may be relieved by lateral tarsorrhaphy, surgery of the lower eyelid.
- Diplopia may be relieved by prisms or surgery of the extraocular muscles.
- Static or worsening ophthalmopathy is an indication for steroids, orbital decompression or orbital irradiation.
- Patients should be advised to stop smoking.

Mild ophthalmopathy should be rectified by cosmetic eyelid surgery. It is important to remember that patients can be distressed by their appearance. During the early acute phase patients will have considerable symptomatic relief from the following measures:

- Elevating the head at night.
- Diuretics to reduce oedema.
- Tinted glasses for protection from the sun, wind and foreign bodies.

What is the role of radioiodine in thyroid eye disease?

- Firstly, since radioiodine treatment carries a substantial risk of exacerbating preexisting thyroid eye disease, it should be avoided as far as possible in patients with active or severe ophthalmopathy, in whom medical therapy with a thionamide drug such as carbimazole is preferable. Radioiodine may be used in patients with mild eye disease but adjuvant oral corticosteriods should be prescribed (*N Engl J Med* 1998; **338**: 73–8).
- Secondly, patients without clinical evidence of thyroid disease have a small risk of developing ophthalmopathy and a very low risk of developing severe eye disease. It is prudent to warn all patients of this complication, but the risks do not justify denying most patients the benefits of definitive treatment with radioiodine when indicated. In addition, the risks do not justify the routine use of corticosteroids in patients without ophthalmopathy (*BMJ* 1999; **319**: 68–9).
- Thirdly, smoking, a raised serum triiodothyronine concentration, and uncorrected hypothyroidism are also factors which can exacerbate thyroid eye disease. Therefore, to reduce the risk of thyroid eye disease, patients should be encouraged to stop smoking, be rendered euthyroid with a thionamide before radioiodine, and be monitored closely to detect and treat early hypothyroidism or persistent hyperthyroidism.

Mention the less important eponyms related to thyroid eye disease.

These include:

- Infrequent blinking – Stellwag's sign.
- Tremor of closed eyelids – Rosenbach's sign.
- Difficulty in everting upper eyelid – Gifford's sign.
- Absence of wrinkling of forehead on sudden upward gaze – Joffroy's sign.
- Impaired convergence of the eyes – Möbius' sign.
- Weakness of at least one of the extraocular muscles – Ballet's sign.
- Paralysis of extraocular muscles – Jendrassik's sign.

- Poor fixation on lateral gaze – Suker's sign.
- Dilatation of pupil with weak adrenaline solution – Loewi's sign.
- Jerky pupillary contraction to consensual light – Cowen's sign.
- Increased pigmentation of the margins of eyelids – Jellinek's sign.
- Upper lid resistance on downward traction – Grove's sign.
- Abnormal fullness of the eyelid – Enroth's sign.
- Unequal pupillary dilatation – Knie's sign.
- When the eyeball is turned downwards, there is arrest of the descent of the lid, spasm and continued descent – Boston's sign.
- When the clinician places his or her hand on a level with the patient's eyes and then lifts it higher, the patient's upper lids spring up more quickly than the eyeball – Kocher's sign.

J. Dalrymple (1804–1852), an English ophthalmologist.

Exophthalmos associated with goitre and non-organic heart disease was first described by English physician Caleb Hillard Parry (1775–1822) in a paper published posthumously in 1825. He graduated in medicine from Edinburgh and practised in Bath. He described hyperthyroidism before Graves' disease.

In 1977, Solomon et al presented the evidence that three independent autoimmune diseases tended to occur concomitantly in the same euthyroid Graves' ophthalmopathy: idiopathic hyperthyroidism, Hashimoto's thyroiditis and Graves' ophthalmopathy.

Anthony Toft, an endocrinologist at Edinburgh Royal Infirmary, is past President of the Royal College of Physicians of Edinburgh.

Case 135

HYPOTHYROIDISM

INSTRUCTION

Obtain a history and perform relevant general examination.

SALIENT FEATURES

History

- Dryness of skin.
- Hair dryness or loss.
- Cold intolerance.
- Change in the voice (hoarse, husky).
- Lethargy, undue tiredness.
- Constipation.
- Moderate weight gain in spite of loss of appetite.
- Menstrual irregularity, especially menorrhagia.
- Infertility.
- Depression.

- Dementia.
- Muscle cramps.
- Oedema.
- Radioiodine therapy for previous Graves' disease (the patient may have associated eye signs of Graves' disease).
- Medications and other compounds such as lithium carbonate and iodine-containing compounds (e.g. amiodarone, radiocontrast agents, expectorants containing potassium iodide, and kelp).
- Family history of thyroid dysfunction, pernicious anaemia, diabetes mellitus, primary adrenal insufficiency.
- Obtain history of hypercholesterolaemia, angina pectoris and hypertension (remember, hypertension occurs in 10% of these patients and disappears with thyroxine replacement).

Examination

- Coarse, dry skin (look for yellowish tint of carotenaemia – 'peaches and cream' complexion).
- 'Dirty elbows and knees' sign (Ber A 1954 The sign of 'dirty' knees and elbows. *Acta Endocrinol* (Copenh) **16**: 305).
- Puffy lower eyelids.
- Loss of outer third of eyebrows, xanthelasma.

Proceed as follows:
- Examine the neck for goitre and the scar of previous thyroidectomy. The typical Hashimoto gland is firm and lobulated.
- Slow pulse.
- Check the ankle jerks, looking for delayed relaxation.
- Look for:
  - Proximal muscle weakness.
  - Cerebellar signs.
  - Carpal tunnel syndrome.

DIAGNOSIS

This patient has delayed ankle jerks, puffy lower eyelids, slow pulse and hoarse, husky voice (lesions) indicating that he has hypothyroidism (functional status); the cause needs to be determined (aetiology).

QUESTIONS

How is delayed relaxation best elicited in the ankle?
Get the patient to kneel on a chair with his hands holding the back of the chair and then elicit the jerks on either side.

What are the causes of goitre?
- Idiopathic (majority).
- Hashimoto's thyroiditis.
- Graves' disease.

- Iodine deficiency (simple goitre).
- Puberty, pregnancy, subacute thyroiditis, goitrogens (lithium, phenylbutazone).

What is the thyroid status in Hashimoto's disease?
Hypothyroidism (usually).

What is the single best clinical indicator for hypothyroidism?
Delayed ankle jerks.

What is the best laboratory indicator for hypothyroidism?
Elevated serum TSH levels. When there is a suspicion of pituitary or hypothalamic disease, the serum free T_4 concentration should be measured in addition to serum TSH levels. Serum triiodothyronine concentrations are a poor indicator of hypothyroid state and should not be used.

What are the laboratory changes in hypothyroidism?
- Hypercholesterolaemia.
- Hyponatraemia.
- Anaemia.
- Elevations of creatinine phosphokinase and lactate dehydrogenase.
- Hyperprolactinaemia.

What are the causes of isolated TSH elevation?
- Mild (subclinical) hypothyroidism.
- Recovery from hypothyroxinaemia of non-thyroidal illnesses.
- Medications such as amiodarone or lithium (*Arch Intern Med* 2000; **160:** 1573–5).

What are the causes of isolated TSH suppression?
- Mild (subclinical) hyperthyroidism.
- Recovery from overt hyperthyroidism.
- Non-thyroidal illness which cause low serum free thyroxine concentration.
- Pregnancy during first trimester.
- Medications such as dopamine and glucocorticoids.

How would you investigate a simple goitre?
Estimation of serum T_3, T_4, TSH and thyroid antibodies.

What is the cause for delayed relaxation in hypothyroidism?
The exact cause is not known. It is probably due to decreased muscle metabolism.

How would you manage this patient with hypothyroidism?
Oral thyroxine replacement therapy for life. The therapeutic dose varies between 100 and 200 µg per day taken as a single dose. Dose adjustments are made once in 3 weeks. The dose is adjusted depending on the clinical response and suppression of raised serum TSH levels. Lack of response to thyroxine suggests:

- Non-thyroid related disease.
- Poor compliance.
- Underlying psychiatric abnormalities.
- Presence of pernicious anaemia.
- Associated autoimmune disease such as Addison's disease.

What is the hazard in treating the elderly?

Rapid T_4 replacement may precipitate angina and myocardial infarction. The starting dose in the elderly is 50 µg per day.

What are the cardiovascular manifestations of hypothyroidism?

- Bradycardia.
- Mild hypertension.
- Pericarditis and pericardial effusion.
- High low-density lipoprotein, low high-density lipoprotein levels, hypercholesterolaemia.
- Diminished cardiac output and cardiac failure.
- Coronary artery disease.
- ECG changes: low-voltage T and P waves, prolongation of QT interval.

What are the neurological manifestations of hypothyroidism?

- Delayed deep tendon reflexes (Woltman's sign).
- Carpal tunnel syndrome, peripheral neuropathy.
- Myxoedema madness.
- Myxoedema coma.
- Pseudodementia.
- Deafness to high tones (Trotter's syndrome) (Trotter WR 1960 The association of deafness with thyroid dysfunction. *Br Med Bull* **16**: 92).
- In Pendred's syndrome, babies are born with a goitre, deafness and mental retardation.
- Cerebellar syndrome (*Lancet* 1960; **ii:** 225).
- Hoffmann's syndrome, i.e. muscle aches with myotonia in myxoedema. In infants, muscle involvement may result in Kocher–Debré–Sémélaigne syndrome or 'infant Hercules'.

What do you understand by subclinical hypothyroidism?

This is a condition in which serum thyroxine levels are low normal, and serum TSH is moderately raised (grade 1: 5–10, grade 2: 10.1–20, grade 3: >20). All these patients should be treated.

What other conditions are associated with Hashimoto's thyroiditis?

- Addison's disease.
- Diabetes mellitus.
- Graves' disease.
- Hypoparathyroidism.
- Premature ovarian failure.
- Pernicious anaemia.
- Rheumatoid arthritis.
- Sjögren's syndrome.
- Ulcerative colitis.
- SLE.
- Haemolytic anaemia.

What do you understand by the term 'sick euthyroid syndrome'?

In severe acute non-thyroidal illness or following surgery, changes in pituitary–thyroid function result in altered thyroid indices but, despite this, patients remain euthyroid. On recovery from the illness, the indices of thyroid function return to normal (*N Engl J Med* 1995; **333**: 1562–3). The changes in thyroidal indices include:

- Decrease in extrathyroidal conversion of thyroxine T_4 to triiodothyronine (T_3), the active form of the thyroid hormone.
- A decrease in thyrotrophin secretion, which causes decreased thyroidal secretion and, in time, decreases in serum T_4 concentrations and further decreases in serum T_3 concentrations – the latter due to both decreased secretion of T_3 by the thyroid and diminished availability of T_4 for peripheral conversion to T_3.
- Decreased production or diminished affinity for thyroidal hormones of one or more major serum thyroid hormone-binding proteins – thyroxine-binding globulin, transthyretin and albumin. These decreases can result in decreased serum total thyroxine levels but not in free T_4 or T_3. Serum concentrations of reverse T_3 (which is inactive) are increased because its deiodination is impaired.

What is the prevalence of hypothyroidism?

The prevalence is 2% of the adult population, whereas that of mild (subclinical) hypothyroidism is 5–17% (subclinical hypothyroidism is when serum TSH is elevated with a normal free T_4 concentration).

The complete clinical description of myxoedema was first given by Gull in 1873, but it was Ord in 1878 who coined the word myxoedema when, at autopsy, he found extensive deposits of mucin in the skin of the feet (Ord WM. On myxoedema, a term proposed to be applied to an essential condition in the 'cretinoid' affection occasionally observed in middle-aged women. *Med Chir Trans* 1878; **61**: 57).

W.W. Gull (1816–1890), FRS, graduated from Guy's Hospital in London and was created a Baronet when he treated the then Prince of Wales, who had typhoid. He was a good teacher and said that 'Savages explain, science investigates' (Gull WW. On a cretinoid state supervening in adult life in women. *Trans Clin Soc London* 1873; **7**: 180–5).

Emil Theodor Kocher (1841–1917), Swiss Professor of Surgery in Berne, was awarded the Nobel Prize in 1909 for his work on the physiology, pathology and surgery of the thyroid gland. He was the first to excise the thyroid gland for goitre and described myxoedema following thyroidectomy – 'cachexia strumipriva'. His name is associated with: (1) Kocher forceps; (2) Kocher's transverse cervical incision for thyroidectomy; (3) Kocher's operation for the wrist; (4) Kocher's oblique right subcostal incision for gallbladder surgery; (5) Kocher manoeuvre for reduction of a dislocated shoulder; and (6) Kocher syndrome describing splenomegaly and lymphadenopathy with thyrotoxicosis.

R. Debré and G. Sémélaigne were both French physicians (Debré R, Sémélaigne G. Syndrome of diffuse muscular hypertrophy in infants causing athletic appearance. Its connection with congenital myxoedema. *Am J Dis Child* 1935; **50**: 1351).

H. Hashimoto (1881–1934), a Japanese surgeon.

Johann Hoffmann (1857–1919), a German neurologist.

In 1948, H.E.W. Roberton, a general practitioner in New Zealand, was the first to recognize post-partum thyroid disease – he successfully treated lassitude and other symptoms of hypothyroidism related to the post-partum period with thyroid extract.

Case 136

MULTINODULAR GOITRE

INSTRUCTION

Examine this patient's neck.

SALIENT FEATURES

History

- Stridor (trachea must be narrowed to 20–30% for this symptom).
- Hoarseness of voice (due to pressure on recurrent laryngeal nerve; suggests thyroid malignancy).
- Acute painful enlargement (suggests bleeding into thyroid nodule).
- Suffusion of face when the patient raises the arms above the head (suggests substernal goitre).
- Dysphagia.
- Deafness (if due to eighth cranial nerve involvement suggests Pendred's syndrome; rare).
- Symptoms of thyroid hyper- or hypofunction.

Examination

- Middle-aged or elderly patient.
- Multinodular goitre.
- Atrial fibrillation.
- Signs of thyrotoxicosis (see p. 355).

DIAGNOSIS

This patient has a multinodular goitre (lesion) and is hyperthyroid with atrial fibrillation (functional status).

QUESTIONS

What is the natural history of thyrotoxicosis in nodular goitre?

It is permanent and there are no spontaneous remissions; therefore, antithyroid drugs to decrease thyroid hormone secretion are not an appropriate long-term therapy.

How would you investigate a nodular goitre?

- Serum thyrotrophin and free thyroxine should be measured to identify those with subclinical or overt hyperthyroidism.
- *Ultrasonography* of the thyroid gland indicates whether the goitre is *cystic* or *solid*.
- If nodule is solid, perform a radioisotope scan to indicate whether it is hot or cold.
- If cold nodule, fine-needle aspiration.

- Patients with features of tracheal compression (inspiratory stridor and dyspnoea) should undergo CT or MRI of the neck and upper thorax, and pulmonary function tests, especially flow-volume loop studies. When CT is used, iodinated contrast agents should not be given because of the risk of inducing hyperthyroidism.

How would you treat such a patient?
- Beta-blockers to control thyrotoxicosis.
- Warfarin in atrial fibrillation to prevent embolic complications.
- Radioiodine for hyperthyroidism.
- Surgery if the patient refuses radioiodine, for large multinodular goitres or malignancy.

What are the indications for treatment of patients with non-toxic multinodular goitre?
- Compression of the trachea or oesophagus and venous outflow obstruction.
- Growth of the goitre, especially where there is intrathoracic extension.
- Neck discomfort or cosmetic issues.

What treatment options are available for non-toxic multinodular goitre?

Surgery

Standard therapy, especially when rapid decompression of vital structures is required. It allows pathological examination of the thyroid. Disadvantages include postoperative tracheal obstruction, recurrent laryngeal nerve injury, hypo-parathyroidism, hypothyroidism and goitre recurrence.

Thyroxine

Alternative to surgery in young patients with small goitres. Its disadvantage is that it causes only a small decrease in thyroid volume; long-term efficacy is not known; decrease in bone mineral density in postmenopausal women; possible cardiac side effects.

Radioiodine

An alternative to surgery in elderly patients and in those with cardiopulmonary disease. It results in a substantial decrease in thyroid volume and improvement of compressive symptoms in most patients. Disadvantages include: it only causes a gradual decrease in thyroid volume; radiation thyroiditis (usually mild); radiation-induced thyroid dysfunction (hyperthyroidism in 5%, hypothyroidism in 20–30%); possible risk of radiation-induced cancer (*N Engl J Med* 1998; **338:** 1438–47).

What treatment options are available for toxic multinodular goitre?
Treatment is always indicated when overt hyperthyroidism is present. In cases of subclinical hyperthyroidism, treatment is advisable in elderly patients and in younger ones who are at risk for cardiac disease or osteoporosis. The treatment options available are:

Antithyroid drugs

Valuable as pretreatment for surgery; valuable before and after radioiodine treatment in elderly patients and those with concurrent health problems; long-term treatment is recommended only when other therapies cannot be used. The disadvantages are that the treatment is lifelong and there are adverse effects such as agranulocytosis.

Surgery

Should be considered for large goitres when rapid relief is needed. The other advantage is that it provides tissue for a pathological diagnosis. Disadvantages include surgical mortality and morbidity; hypothyroidism, persistence or recurrence of hyperthyroidism.

Radioiodine

An appealing option in the majority of the patients because it is highly effective for reversal of hyperthyroidism. The disadvantages include a gradual diminution of the hyperthyroid state, more than one dose may be necessary, hypothyroidism (<20%); theoretical risk of radiation-induced cancer (*N Engl J Med* 1998; **338:** 1438–47).

ADVANCED-LEVEL QUESTIONS

How do you differentiate between Graves' disease and toxic nodular goitre?

Graves' disease	Toxic nodular goitre
Younger age group	Older individuals
Diffuse goitre	Nodular enlargement of the gland
Eye signs common	Eye signs rare
Atrial fibrillation uncommon	Atrial fibrillation common
	(about 40% of the patients)
Other autoimmune diseases common	Other autoimmune diseases uncommon

What factors influence the decision to proceed to radiotherapy?

Patient's age, sex, diagnosis, severity of hyperthyroidism, presence of other medical conditions, access to radioiodine (I-131), and patient and doctor preference.

Case 137

ADDISON'S DISEASE

INSTRUCTION

Look at this patient, who presented with weakness, loss of appetite and weight loss.

SALIENT FEATURES

History

- Dizziness, syncope.
- Skin pigmentation (ask if the patient has been sitting in the sun).

- Ask questions regarding fatigue, weakness, apathy, anorexia, nausea, vomiting, weight loss and abdominal pain.
- Depression.

Examination

The striking abnormality is hyperpigmentation.

Proceed as follows:
- Examine for hyperpigmentation:
  - The hand: compare the creases with your own.
  - The mouth and lips for pigmentation.
  - Areas not usually covered by clothing: nipples, areas irritated by belts, straps, collars or rings.
- Look for vitiligo.
- Tell the examiner that you would like to investigate as follows:
  - Examine the blood pressure, in particular for postural hypotension.
  - Look for sparse axillary and pubic hair.
  - Examine the abdomen for adrenal scar (if the scar is pigmented, think of Nelson's syndrome and examine field defects).
- If you suspect Addison's disease, tell the examiner that you would like to do a short ACTH (1–24) test (Synacthen test).

DIAGNOSIS

This patient has postural hypotension, marked hyperpigmentation and sparse axillary hair (lesion) due to autoimmune Addison's disease (aetiology). The patient has marked hypoadrenalism (functional status).

QUESTIONS

What is the size of the heart in Addison's deficiency?
The heart is small.

Mention some causes of hyperpigmentation.
- Suntan.
- Race.
- Uraemia.
- Haemochromatosis.
- Primary biliary cirrhosis.
- Ectopic ACTH.
- Porphyria cutanea tarda.
- Nelson's syndrome.
- Malabsorption syndromes.

Mention some causes of Addison's disease.
- Idiopathic (80%).
- Tuberculosis.
- Metastasis.
- HIV infection.

Which conditions may be associated with Addison's disease?
Graves' disease, Hashimoto's thyroiditis, primary ovarian failure, pernicious anaemia, polyglandular syndromes.

ADVANCED-LEVEL QUESTIONS

What are the components of Schmidt's syndrome?
Addison's disease and hypoparathyroidism.

What do you know about polyglandular syndromes?
They are autoimmune in nature and are of two types:

- Type I: chronic mucocutaneous candidiasis, hypoparathyroidism and Addison's disease.
- Type II: Addison's disease, insulin-dependent diabetes and thyroid disease (hyperthyroidism or hypothyroidism). This syndrome is also known as autoimmune polyendocrinopathy–candidiasis–ectodermal dysplasia.

What are the features of Allgrove's syndrome?
Adrenal insensitivity to ACTH (resulting in cortisol deficiency), achalasia, alacrima and neurological disease.

How would you investigate this patient?
- FBC (for lymphocytosis, eosinophilia).
- Electrolytes (for hyponatraemia, hyperkalaemia, hyperchloraemic acidosis, hypercalcaemia).
- Blood glucose, looking for hypoglycaemia.
- Short ACTH (1–24) (Synacthen) test; if positive, follow up with a prolonged ACTH stimulation test.
- ACTH and cortisol levels.
- Adrenal autoantibodies.
- CXR for tuberculosis.
- Plain radiograph of the abdomen for adrenal calcification.
- CT scan of the adrenals.

How would you manage this patient if the underlying aetiology is autoimmune?
- Replacement steroids: prednisolone 5 mg *mane* and 2.5 mg *nocte*; adjust dose depending on serum levels and clinical well-being.
- Fludrocortisone 0.025–0.15 mg daily; adjust dose depending on postural hypotension.
- Give steroid card and Medic Alert bracelet.
- Stress the importance of regular therapy, and increase the dose in the event of stress such as dental extraction or urinary tract infection. It is also important to tell the patient that this therapy is lifelong and that an ampoule of hydrocortisone should be kept at home.
- Follow up every 6 months.

Note. In addisonian crisis, intravenous fluids and hydrocortisone should be administered (after drawing a blood sample for cortisol determination).

Thomas Addison (1793–1860) qualified from Edinburgh and worked at Guy's Hospital, London. He wrote *The Constitutional and Local Effects of the Disease of the Suprarenal Capsules*. Armand Trosseau in Paris labelled the disease 'maladie d'Addison'. Addison also first described morphoea. The original description of the disease was reported in the following paper: Addison T 1855 Disease of the suprarenal capsules. *London Med Gaz* **43**: 517.

John F. Kennedy, past president of the USA, reportedly had Addison's disease and was on replacement corticosteroid therapy.

Case 138

ACROMEGALY

INSTRUCTION

Examine this patient's face.
This patient complains of excessive sweating; examine him.
Examine this patient's hands.

SALIENT FEATURES

History

- Ask the patient about old photographs of him/herself for comparison.
- Ask whether the patient has outgrown wedding ring and shoes.
- Hyperhidrosis.
- Headaches, visual field defects (depends on the size of the tumour).
- Paraesthesia and symptoms of carpal tunnel syndrome (p. 212).
- Hypertension.
- Acral and facial changes.
- Oligomenorrhoea/amenorrhoea, galactorrhoea in females.
- Impotence in males.
- Shortness of breath (cardiac failure).
- Arthritis (hands, feet, hips and knees).

Examination

Hands

- On shaking hands there is excessive sweating – moist, doughy, enveloping handshake.
- Large hands with broad palms, spatulate fingers; there is an increase in the 'volume' of the hands.

Proceed as follows:

Look for evidence of carpal tunnel syndrome (tap over the flexor retinaculum for Tinel's sign).

Face
- Prominent supraorbital ridges.
- Large nose and lips.
- Protrusion of the lower jaw (prognathism); ask the patient to clench his teeth and note the malocclusion and splaying of the teeth (i.e. interdental separation).

Proceed as follows:
Ask the patient to show his tongue and look for macroglossia and for impressions of the teeth on the edges of the tongue (see p. 616).

Test
- For bitemporal hemianopia (see pp 133–4) and optic atrophy.
- Neck for goitre.
- Axillae for skin tags (molluscum fibrosum), acanthosis nigricans (black velvety papillomas).
- Chest for cardiomegaly, gynaecomastia and galactorrhoea.
- Abdomen for hepatosplenomegaly.
- Joints for arthropathy, i.e. osteoarthrosis, chondrocalcinosis.
- Spine for kyphosis.
- Blood pressure for hypertension (present in 15% of cases).
- Tell the examiner that you would like to examine the urine for sugar (impaired glucose tolerance).

DIAGNOSIS

This patient has a protruding lower jaw, splaying of teeth and large spade-like hands (lesions) which are features of acromegaly due to a pituitary tumour (aetiology).

QUESTIONS

Would you like to ask the patient a few questions?
Ask about any increase in size of shoes, gloves and hat, and whether the wedding ring is tight to wear.

ADVANCED-LEVEL QUESTIONS

Mention some causes of macroglossia.
- Acromegaly.
- Amyloidosis.
- Hypothyroidism.
- Down's syndrome.

How can this condition present?
One third of patients notice a change in their features, one third are noticed to have a change in their features by their GP, and the remaining third have symptoms such as excessive sweating and visual difficulties.

What are the complications of acromegaly?
- Cardiomegaly and heart failure.
- Hypertension.
- Impaired glucose tolerance.

- Hypopituitarism.
- Carpal tunnel syndrome.
- Arthritis of the hip, knee and spine.
- Spinal stenosis resulting in cord compression.
- Visual field defects.

What are the indicators of disease activity?

- Symptoms such as headache, increase in size of ring, shoe or dentures.
- Excessive sweating.
- Skin tags.
- Glycosuria.
- Hypertension.
- Increased loss of visual fields.

How would you investigate this patient?

Biochemical tests

- Non-suppressibility of growth hormone levels to less than 2 ng/ml after oral administration of 100 g glucose.
- Plasma insulin-like growth factor levels (allow assessment of the efficacy of initial therapy and in the post-therapeutic period).
- Also serum T_4, prolactin, testosterone; evaluate pituitary function – static and dynamic tests.
- Calcium levels (to exclude multiple endocrine neoplasia (MEN) type 1 syndrome).

Radiography

- Pituitary fossa (enlarged sella).
- Sinuses.
- Chest (cardiomegaly).
- Hand (terminal phalangeal 'tufting').
- Foot (terminal phalangeal 'tufting', lateral view shows increased thickness of the heel pad).
- CT scan (MRI scan is more reliable).

Remember that, unlike in Cushing's disease and prolactinomas, the majority of the patients with acromegaly have macroadenomas.

Other investigations

- Formal perimetry.
- Obtain old photos.
- New photos of face, torso, hands on the chest.
- ECG.
- Triple stimulation test if hypopituitarism is suspected.

What therapeutic options are available?

- Neurosurgical intervention – typically trans-sphenoidal – is the primary therapeutic choice for almost all patients. Diaphoresis and carpal tunnel syndrome often improve within 1 day of surgery. Although growth hormone levels fall immediately, insulin-like growth factor levels fall gradually.
- Radiation therapy is a primary treatment option for a few patients who have acromegaly but are not surgical candidates.
- Octreotide and bromocriptine are valuable as adjunctive therapy.

Remember. The aim of treatment should be symptomatic control and a growth hormone concentration of less than 5 mU/l.

Mention four common causes of death in such patients.

- Cardiac failure.
- Tumour expansion (mass effect and haemorrhages).
- Effects of hypertension.
- Degenerative vascular disease.

Mention other conditions in which there is excess growth hormone secretion.

- Multiple endocrine neoplasia type 1 (parathyroid hyperplasia, pituitary tumours and gut tumours).
- McCune–Albright syndrome (polyostotic fibrous dysplasia, sexual precocity and café-au-lait spots).
- Carney complex, of autosomal dominant aetiology, which consists of multi-centric tumours in many organs (including cardiac myxomas, myxomas in breast, testes, pigmented skin lesions and pigmented nodular hyperplasia).

In 1886, Pierre Marie (1853–1940) used the term 'acromegaly' in describing two patients and reviewed eight previously published papers describing patients with presumed acromegaly (Marie P 1886 Sur deux cas d'acromegalie. Hypertrophie singulière non-congénitale des extrémités supérieures, inférieures et céphaliques. *Rev Med* **6**: 297–333). He also described Charcot–Marie–Tooth disease. In 1887, Minkowski deduced that acromegaly is related to pituitary tumour (Minkowski O 1887 Uber einen Fall von Akromegalie. *Berl Klin Wochenschr* **24**: 371–4).

In 1891, the New Syndenham Society published a translation of Marie's original paper and a review by Souza-Leite of 48 patients (Marie P, Souza-Leite JD 1891 *Essays on Acromegaly*. London: New Sydenham Society).

Fuller Albright, Professor of Endocrinology at Massachussetts General Hospital and Harvard Medical School, whose chief interest was calcium metabolism.

Case 139

HYPOPITUITARISM (SIMMONDS' DISEASE)

INSTRUCTION

Look at this patient.

SALIENT FEATURES

History

- In a male, the frequency of shaving, impotence.
- In a female, postpartum haemorrhage, amenorrhoea.
- History of radiation (e.g. proton-beam radiation) – causes hypopituitarism primarily because of its effects on hypothalamic function, whereas high-dose radiation can directly affect the pituitary.

Examination

- Patient is pale; the skin is soft.
- Paucity of axillary and pubic hair.
- Atrophy of breast (in females).
- Examine the blood pressure for postural hypotension.
- Check visual fields: bitemporal hemianopia may be present.
- Examine the fundus for optic atrophy.

Proceed as follows:

Tell the examiner that you would like to examine the external genitalia for hypogonadism (small testes).

DIAGNOSIS

This patient has pale soft skin and absence of axillary hair with atrophied breasts (lesion) due to hypopituitarism (functional status) secondary to postpartum necrosis (aetiology).

QUESTIONS

Mention a few causes of hypopituitarism.

- Iatrogenic – from surgical removal of the pituitary or irradiation.
- Chromophobe adenoma (particularly in males).
- Postpartum pituitary necrosis in females – known as Sheehan's syndrome.

Rare causes

- Craniopharyngioma.
- Metastatic tumours, granulomas (TB, sarcoid, haemochromatosis, histiocytosis X).

How would you assess such a patient?

- FBC for normochromic normocytic anaemia.
- Urea and electrolytes for hyponatraemia due to dilution. Hyperkalaemia does not usually occur because aldosterone production is not affected.
- Measurement of pituitary hormone levels (ACTH, TSH, luteinizing hormone (LH), growth hormone, prolactin).
- Measurement of target organ secretion (T_4, T_3, serum cortisol, testosterone, oestrogen and progesterone levels).
- Pituitary stimulation tests:
  - Thyrotrophin-releasing hormone (TRH) stimulation tests.
  - Tetracosactide (Synacthen) tests.
  - Insulin hypoglycaemia test.
  - Luteinizing hormone releasing hormone (LHRH) tests.
- Skull radiography.
- MRI provides the best image of parasellar lesions. The posterior pituitary usually has a high-intensity signal on sagittal MRI that is absent in central diabetes insipidus.
- Assessment of visual fields (formal perimetry).

In what order do the hormone secretions generally fail?

In general, growth hormone, follicle-stimulating hormone (FSH) and LH secretions become deficient early, followed by TSH and ACTH. Last of all, antidiuretic hormone (ADH) secretions diminish and fail.

How would you treat such patients?

The mainstay of therapy is lifetime replacement of end-organ hormone deficiencies (thyroid, adrenal and gonads).

Does hypopituitarism affect life expectancy?

Even when hormonal replacement therapy (adrenal, gonadal and thyroid) is carried out in an adequate manner, there is a two-fold risk of death in patients with hypopituitarism (*J Clin Endocrinol Metab* 1996; **81:** 1169–72). It has been suggested that this is due to untreated growth hormone deficiency.

ADVANCED-LEVEL QUESTIONS

What is the Houssay phenomenon?

Houssay showed that diabetes of pancreatectomized dogs improved after hypophysectomy. A diminishing requirement of insulin by diabetics may be a sign of hypopituitarism with diminished secretion of growth hormone and ACTH (and thus corticosteroids). Similarly, diabetes due to acromegaly may improve with pituitary surgery or octreotide therapy.

> Morris Simmonds of Hamburg described this condition in 1914.
>
> Bernardo Alberto Houssay (1889–1971), an Argentinian physiologist in Buenos Aires, was awarded the Nobel Prize for his discovery of the part played by the hormone of the anterior pituitary lobe in the metabolism of sugar. The other half of the Nobel Prize was awarded to Carl and Gerty Cori of St Louis, Missouri, USA, who were awarded the prize for their discovery of the course of the catalytic conversion of glycogen.

Case 140

GYNAECOMASTIA

INSTRUCTION

Look at this patient's chest.

SALIENT FEATURES

History

- Take a drug history – oestrogens, digoxin, spironolactone, cimetidine, diazepam, alkylating agents; methyldopa, clomifene.
- Ask the patient if it is painful.

Examination

Unilateral or bilateral enlargement of the breasts in a male patient.

Proceed as follows:
- Palpate to confirm the presence of glandular tissue.
- Tell the examiner that you would like to look for stigmata of cirrhosis of the liver.

DIAGNOSIS

This patient has gynaecomastia (lesion) due to spironolactone therapy (aetiology), which is cosmetically distressing to the patient (functional status).
Read: *N Engl J Med* 1993; **328**: 490.

QUESTIONS

Mention the physiological causes of gynaecomastia.
- Newborn.
- Adolescence.
- Ageing.

Mention a few pathological causes.
- Chronic liver disease.
- Thyrotoxicosis.
- Klinefelter's syndrome.
- Viral orchitis.
- Renal failure.
- Neoplasms (bronchogenic carcinoma, testicular carcinoma, hepatoma).
- Bulbospinal muscular atrophy or Kennedy's syndrome (a defect in the androgen receptor gene alters function of motor neurons; 50% of patients have gynaecomastia).
- Drugs associated with gynaecomastia include:
  - Antibiotics: isoniazid, ketoconazole, metronidazole, miconazole.
  - Cardiovascular drugs: atenolol, captopril, digoxin, enalapril, methyldopa, nifedipine, spironolactone, verapamil.
  - Antiulcer drugs: cimetidine, ranitidine, omeprazole.
  - Psychoactive drugs: diazepam, tricyclic antidepressants.

ADVANCED-LEVEL QUESTIONS

How would you investigate such a patient?
- CXR for metastatic or bronchogenic carcinoma.
- Plasma human chorionic gonadotrophin (β-hCG) – detectable levels implicate a testicular tumour or lung or liver neoplasm.
- Plasma testosterone and luteinizing hormone in the diagnosis of hypogonadism.
- Serum oestradiol (usually normal).
- Other: serum prolactin, serum thyroxine and TSH, and chromosomal analysis for Klinefelter's syndrome.

What are the causes of a feminizing state?

- Absolute increase in oestrogen formation by tumours.
- Increased availability of oestrogen precursors, e.g. as a result of cirrhosis.
- Increased extraglandular oestrogen synthesis.
- Relative increase in ratio of oestrogen to androgen, e.g. as a result of testicular failure.
- Drugs.

Ancient Egyptian sculptures and paintings suggest that the pharaoh Tutankhamen (1357–1339 BC) had gynaecomastia.

Case 141

CARPOPEDAL SPASM (POST-THYROIDECTOMY HYPOPARATHYROIDISM)

INSTRUCTION

Look at this patient's hands.

SALIENT FEATURES

History

- History of thyroid surgery.
- Paraesthesias of fingers, toes and circumoral region.
- Muscle cramping, carpopedal spasm, laryngeal stridor, convulsions.

Examination

Spasm of the hands – the fingers are extended, except at the metacarpophalangeal joints, and the thumb is strongly adducted.

Proceed as follows:
- Look at the feet for spasm and then investigate as follows:
  - Tap over the facial nerve (in front of the tragus of the ear). There is contraction of the lips and facial muscles (Chvostek's sign or Chvostek–Weiss sign).
  - Inflate the cuff just above the systolic pressure for 3 minutes; this will cause the hand to go into spasm – Trousseau's sign.
  - Look into the mouth for candidiasis (may be seen in primary hypoparathyroidism) and defective teeth.
  - Fingernails may be thin and brittle.
  - Check for thyroidectomy scar.
  - Look for cataracts.
- Tell the examiner that you would like to perform the following tests:
  - Skull radiograph (looking for basal ganglia calcification).
  - Measurement of serum calcium and magnesium levels.

–ECG for prolonged QT intervals and T-wave abnormalities.
–Slit-lamp examination for early posterior lenticular cataract formation.

DIAGNOSIS

This patient has carpopedal spasm (lesion) due to hypoparathyroidism as a complication of thyroidectomy (aetiology).

ADVANCED-LEVEL QUESTIONS

Mention any drugs that you would use cautiously in hypoparathyroidism.

Furosemide (frusemide), as it may enhance hypocalcaemia, and phenothiazine drugs, because they may precipitate extrapyramidal symptoms.

How would you manage an acute attack of hypoparathyroid tetany?

- Maintain airway.
- Slow intravenous calcium gluconate and oral calcium.
- Vitamin D preparations.
- Magnesium (if associated hypomagnesaemia).

What are the causes of hypoparathyroidism (Arch Intern Med 1979; 139: 1166)?

- Damage during thyroid or neck surgery (*Lancet* 1960; **ii:** 1432).
- Idiopathic.
- Destruction of the parathyroid gland due to the following:
  –Radioactive iodine therapy.
  –External neck irradiation.
  –Haemochromatosis and Wilson's deficiency.
  –Metastatic disease from the breast, lung, lymphoproliferative disorder.
- Dysembryogenesis (DiGeorge syndrome).
- Polyglandular autoimmune syndrome (PGA type 1) which is also known as autoimmune polyendocrinopathy–candidiasis–ectodermal dystrophy (APECD) (see p. 371).

What are the biochemical features of hypoparathyroidism?

Typically, low serum calcium, high serum phosphate and normal alkaline phosphatase levels and reduced urine calcium excretion.

What do you know about pseudohypoparathyroidism?

It is a condition characterized by end-organ resistance to parathyroid hormone. The biochemistry is similar to that of idiopathic hypoparathyroidism except that patients with pseudohypoparathyroidism do not respond to injected parathyroid hormone. These patients are moon faced, short statured and mentally retarded and may have short fourth or fifth metacarpals. Patients without hypocalcaemia but who have these phenotypic abnormalities are said to have 'pseudopseudohypoparathyroidism'.

What are the main physiological effects of parathyroid hormone?

It results in a net increase of ionized calcium in the plasma as a result of:

- Increased bone osteoclastic activity resulting in increased delivery of calcium and phosphorus to the extracellular compartment.

- Enhanced renal tubular absorption of calcium.
- Inhibits the absorption of phosphate and bicarbonate by the renal tubule.
- Stimulates the synthesis of 1,25-dihydrocholecalciferol (vitamin D) by the kidney.

Franz Chvostek (1835–1884) was Professor of Medicine in Vienna, Austria.

Nathan Weiss (1851–1883), an Austrian physician.

Armand Trousseau (1801–1867), a Parisian physician, was the first to refer to adrenal insufficiency as Addison's disease.

Case 142

CARCINOID SYNDROME

INSTRUCTION

Look at this patient who was told by her GP that she has a 'nervous bowel'.

SALIENT FEATURES

History
- Confirm a history of chronic intermittent diarrhoea.
- Flushing attacks, which may be associated with increased lacrimation and periorbital oedema. Flushing may be provoked by eating, exertion, excitement or ethanol.
- Wheeze (due to bronchoconstriction during flushing attacks).

Examination
- Flushed face ('fire-engine' face).
- Telangiectasia.

Proceed as follows:
- Listen to the chest for wheeze (bronchial carcinoid).
- Listen to the heart (right-sided murmurs in intestinal, gastric, hepatic and ovarian carcinoid, left-sided murmurs in bronchial carcinoid).
- Look for hepatomegaly (nodular and firm due to metastases, may be pulsatile due to tricuspid regurgitation).

DIAGNOSIS

This patient has facial flushing and tricuspid regurgitation (lesion) due to carcinoid syndrome (aetiology) and is in cardiac failure (functional status).

Classic reference: *Am J Med* 1956; **20**: 520–32.

ADVANCED-LEVEL QUESTIONS

What are the cardiac lesions seen in metastatic carcinoid from the liver?

- Right-sided valvular lesions, including tricuspid stenosis or regurgitation, and pulmonary stenosis or regurgitation. (**Note:** bronchial carcinoids metastasize to the left side of the heart.)
- Endocardial fibrosis.

How is the diagnosis confirmed?

Raised urinary levels of 5-HIAA (hydroxyindoleacetic acid).

How are these tumours treated?

- Emergency treatment includes prednisolone.
- Severe diarrhoea: hydration, diphenoxylate with atropine, cyproheptadine or methysergide.
- Octreotide (a somatostatin analogue) is associated with a significant reduction in 5-HIAA concentration.
- Surgery is useful for localized carcinoid.
- Chemotherapy in advanced disease (fluorouracil, streptozocin, dacarbazine).
- Interferon-α may be useful in those who do not respond to surgery and octreotide treatment (*Digestion* 1994; **55** (suppl 3): 64–9).

Case 143

OBESITY

INSTRUCTION

Look at this patient.

SALIENT FEATURES

History

- Family history of obesity (parental obesity more than doubles the risk of adult obesity among both obese and non-obese children under 10 years of age, *N Engl J Med* 1997; **337:** 869–73).
- History of sleep apnoea, snoring and insomnia.
- History of hypertension, diabetes, hyperlipidaemia, cardiovascular disease.
- Gastro-oesophageal reflux.
- History of gallstones (cholesterol gallstones more prevalent in obesity).
- History of endometrial cancer in women (two to three times more common in obese than in lean women).
- History of breast cancer (risk increases with body mass index in postmenopausal women).

- Cancer of gallbladder and biliary system (obese women have a higher incidence).
- Cancer of colon, rectum and prostate, and renal cell cancer (*N Engl J Med* 2000; **343:** 1305–11) (higher in obese men).

Examination

Patient has excessive adipose tissue.

Proceed as follows:
- Measure the height and body weight (to determine body mass index).
- Check blood pressure (the prevalence of hypertension is approximately three times higher in the obese than the non-obese).
- Examine the joints to exclude osteoarthrosis.
- Examine skin for intertrigo in redundant folds of skin (fungal and yeast infections of skin are also common).
- Tell the examiner that you would like to:
  - Assess urine sugar (the prevalence of diabetes is three times higher in overweight than in non-overweight persons).
  - Check serum lipids (these patients often have an adverse pattern of plasma lipoproteins that generally improves with weight loss).
  - Assess pulmonary function (sleep apnoea).
  - Exclude secondary causes (hypothyroidism, Cushing's syndrome, polycystic ovary syndrome).

DIAGNOSIS

This patient has gross obesity (lesion) of genetic origin, complicated by hypertension and osteoarthrosis.

ADVANCED-LEVEL QUESTIONS

Is obesity of genetic origin?

Although many obese individuals are blamed for being obese – by their friends, physicians, family and by themselves – increasingly it has been shown that genetic influences have a substantial influence on body mass index. The *ob* gene is an adipocyte-specific gene that encodes leptin, a protein that regulates body weight. Animals with mutations in the *ob* gene are obese and lose weight when given leptin (*Nature* 1994; **372:** 425–32). In humans, serum leptin concentrations correlate with the percentage of body fat, suggesting that most obese people are insensitive to endogenous leptin (leptin resistance).

What is the body mass index?

It is a measure to determine the presence of excessive adipose tissue and is calculated by dividing the body weight in kilograms by the height in metres squared. The normal spread of the body mass index is from 20 to 25 kg/m^2.

What is morbid obesity?

It is relative weight greater than 200% and is associated with a ten-fold increase in mortality rate.

Mention some adverse health consequences of obesity.

Obese people have a greater risk for diabetes mellitus, stroke, coronary artery disease, premature mortality, thromboembolism, gallstones, reflux oesophagitis, sleep apnoea, polycythaemia, and cancer of the colon, rectum, prostate, uterus, breast and ovary. The risk of death from all causes is increased and the risk associated with a high body mass index is greater for whites than blacks (*N Engl J Med* 1999; **341:** 1097–105). Also, higher maternal weight before pregnancy increases the risk of late fetal death although it protects against delivery of a small-for-gestational age infant (*N Engl J Med* 1998; **338:** 147–52).

What patterns of obesity correlate with premature coronary artery disease?

Central obesity (abdomen and flank) and when there is excessive visceral fat within the abdominal cavity rather than subcutaneous fat around the abdomen.

How would you manage such patients?

- Multidisciplinary approach to weight loss: hypocaloric diets, exercise, social support.
- Drugs: orlistat (orlistat partially inhibits the absorption of dietary fat by binding to pancreatic lipase in the gastrointestinal tract) (*Lancet* 1998; **352:** 167–73).
- Surgery: vertical banded gastroplasty, gastric bypass operations.

What are the mechanisms of obesity?

- Insensitivity to leptin, presumably in the hypothalamus.
- Neuropeptide Y-induced hyperphagia.
- Deficiency of production or action of anorexigenic hypothalamic neuropeptides.
- Increased secretion of insulin and glucocorticoid.
- Mutation in the gene for PPAR-Υ accelerates differentiation of adipocytes and may cause obesity (*N Engl J Med* 1998; **339:** 953–9). PPAR-Υ is peroxisome proliferator-activated receptor-Υ and is a nuclear receptor through which the thiazolidinedione class of antidiabetic drugs acts.

Mention some syndromes in which obesity is a prominent feature.

Cushing's syndrome (see pp 385–7), Laurence–Moon–Biedl syndrome (see pp 536, 537), pickwickian syndrome (see pp 290–1), Alstrom's syndrome, Prader–Willi syndrome.

What is the link between obesity and diabetes?

Fat cells release free fatty acids and tumour necrosis factor-alpha which cause insulin resistance, and leptin causes insulin sensitivity. A new protein called resistin that is secreted by fat cells causes insulin resistance. A group of antidiabetic drugs, the thiazolidinediones, reduces insulin resistance by suppressing the expression of resistin by the fat cells (*Nature* 2001; **409:** 307–12).

Case 144

CUSHING'S SYNDROME

INSTRUCTION

Examine this patient.
Look at this patient's face.

SALIENT FEATURES

History

- History of steroid therapy.
- Central weight gain.
- Hirsutism (see pp 428–31).
- Easy bruising.
- Acne.
- Weakness of muscle.
- Menstrual disturbance.
- Loss of libido.
- Depression, sleep disturbances.
- Back pain due to spinal osteoporosis.

Examination

Moon-like facies (Fig. 3), acne, hirsutism and plethora (due to telangiectasia).

Proceed as follows:

- Examine the following:
  - The mouth for superimposed thrush.
  - The interscapular area for 'buffalo hump'.
  - Increased fat pads and bulge above supraclavicular fossae (more specific for Cushing's syndrome).
  - The abdomen for thinning of skin and purple striae (also seen over the shoulders and thighs) – said to be present on almost all patients (Fig. 4).

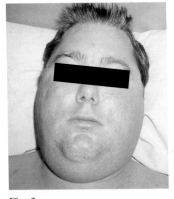

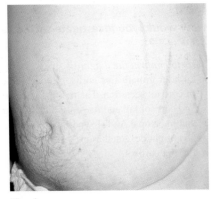

Fig. 3   Fig. 4

- The limbs for bruising, wasting of the limbs, weakness of the muscles of the shoulders and hips – get the patient to squat (proximal myopathy).
- Ask the patient whether she has back pain and then examine the spine, looking for evidence of osteoporosis and collapse of vertebra, kyphoscoliosis.
- Measure the blood pressure.
- Tell the examiner you would like to:
  - Test the urine for glucose.
  - Check visual fields (for pituitary tumour).
  - Examine the fundus for optic atrophy, papilloedema, signs of hypertensive or diabetic retinopathy.

Note. Hirsutism is not common in Cushing's syndrome caused by exogenous steroids because they suppress adrenal androgen secretion.

Also comment on signs of asthma, rheumatoid arthritis, SLE, fibrosing alveolitis (as these are conditions that are treated with long-term steroids).

DIAGNOSIS

This patient has moon-like facies, acne and supraclavicular pads of fat (lesions), which are features of Cushing's syndrome caused by long-term steroid therapy (aetiology) for asthma. The patient is now steroid dependent and is disabled by proximal myopathy and kyphoscoliosis due to osteoporosis (functional status).

QUESTIONS

Mention some causes of Cushing's syndrome.
- Steroids, including adrenocorticotrophic hormone (ACTH).
- Pituitary adenoma (Cushing's disease).
- Adrenal adenoma.
- Adrenal carcinoma.
- Ectopic ACTH (usually by small cell carcinoma of the lung).

What is the difference between Cushing's disease and Cushing's syndrome?
Cushing's disease is increased production by the adrenals secondary to excess pituitary ACTH, whereas Cushing's syndrome is caused by excess steroid from any cause.

How would you investigate such a patient (J Clin Endocrinol Metab *1999; 84: 440–8*)?

Tests to confirm the diagnosis
- 24-hour urinary free cortisol: this is the most direct and reliable practical index of cortisol secretion. The reason is that plasma concentrations of corticotrophins and cortisol fall and rise episodically, in normal subjects, in Cushing's syndrome and in ectopic ACTH syndrome.
- Overnight dexamethasone test.
- Plasma cortisol.

Tests to determine the site of hormone production

- Low- and high-dose dexamethasone test: low-dose dexamethasone fails to suppress urinary steroid secretion in Cushing's disease whereas high-dose dexamethasone (2 mg q6h for 2 days) suppresses at least 50% of urinary steroid secretion.
- CXR for carcinoma of the bronchus.
- Plain radiograph of the abdomen for adrenal calcification.
- Ultrasonography of the abdomen for adrenal tumours.
- If Cushing's disease is suspected:
  - Plasma ACTH, radiography of pituitary, MRI gadolinium enhancement, and bilateral measurement of corticotrophin in the inferior petrosal sinus.
  - Corticotrophin-releasing hormone (CRH) test (helpful in distinguishing pituitary-led Cushing's disease from ectopic corticotrophin secretion).
- Inferior petrosal sinus sampling is used to distinguish primary and ectopic sources of ACTH when the source of the ACTH is not obvious based on clinical circumstances, biochemical evaluation and imaging studies.

How would you manage Cushing's syndrome?

- Cushing's disease: trans-sphenoidal microadenomectomy, pituitary irradiation, total bilateral adrenalectomy.
- Adrenal tumour: surgical resection, mitotane therapy, resection of recurrent tumour.
- Ectopic ACTH: surgical resection of tumour.
- Taper corticosteroid therapy.

ADVANCED-LEVEL QUESTIONS

What is pseudo-Cushing's syndrome?

In chronic alcoholics and patients with depression there may be increased urinary excretion of steroids, absent diurnal variation of plasma steroids and a positive overnight dexamethasone test. All these investigations return to normal on discontinuation of alcohol or improvement of emotional status.

What do you know about Nelson's syndrome?

It is a syndrome that occurs after bilateral adrenalectomy and is characterized by a rapidly growing pituitary adenoma, very high ACTH levels and hyperpigmentation. As the incidence may be as high as 50%, patients with Cushing's disease who have undergone adrenalectomy should be followed by regular plasma ACTH levels and imaging for pituitary tumours.

Harvey Williams Cushing (1869–1939) was Professor of Surgery at Harvard. He was awarded the Pulitzer Prize for his biography of Osler (Cushing H 1932 The basophil adenomas of the pituitary body and their clinical manifestation. *Bull Johns Hopkins Hosp* **1**: 137).

Christopher Edwards, contemporary Principal, Imperial College, London; his chief interest is metabolism of steroids.

INSTRUCTION

Would you like to perform a general examination of this patient?
Look at this patient.

SALIENT FEATURES

History

- Ask whether or not the rash itches.
- Ask where the rash started and ask the patient to describe its evolution.
- Take a drug history (e.g. ampicillin, cephalosporins).
- History of fever (viral exanthems).
- Mucosal involvement.

Examination

Reddish, blotchy maculopapular rash over the trunk (check the chest, back and axillae) and limbs.

Proceed as follows:
- Palpate the surface of the rash to confirm your inspectory findings.
- Check the mucous membranes of the mouth.
- Tell the examiner that you would like to examine for lymph nodes (glandular fever) – some examiners may expect you to examine the lymph nodes as part of the general examination. If lymph nodes are palpable, then examine all groups (cervical, supraclavicular, axillary and inguinal).

Note. Avoid waffling descriptions such as 'skin rash'.

DIAGNOSIS

This patient has a maculopapular rash (lesion) due to ampicillin ingestion (aetiology), which usually resolves on discontinuing the drug (functional status).

QUESTIONS

What is your differential diagnosis?

- Drug-induced rash.
- Glandular fever (rash seen in only 3% of patients with infectious mononucleosis but approaches 100% when these patients were administered ampicillin).
- Viral exanthems (measles, rubella).

What is your differential diagnosis when the rash is associated with lymphadenopathy?

- Glandular fever.
- Lymphoproliferative disorders such as Hodgkin's disease.
- HIV infection.

Case 146

PURPURA

INSTRUCTION

Examine this patient's skin.

SALIENT FEATURES

History

- Take a drug history – steroids, anticoagulants, carbimazole, phenylbutazone, chloramphenicol, gold salts.
- Age (senile purpura) see Figure 5.
- History of chronic liver disease.
- History of mouth ulcers (severe neutropenia).

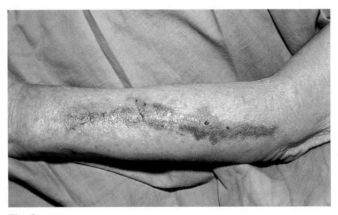

Fig. 5

Examination

Small circumscribed areas of bleeding into the skin – purpura or larger lesions – bruises or ecchymoses.

Proceed as follows:
- Look for an underlying cause:
  - Comment on the patient's age – consider senile purpura.
  - Comment on the distribution – Henoch-Schönlein purpura is seen over the buttocks and lower limbs (see pp 399–401).
- Look for the following signs:
  - Rheumatoid arthritis, in which the purpura is drug induced (steroids, gold).
  - Anaemia (leukaemia, marrow aplasia or infiltration).
  - Chronic liver disease.
  - Ulcers in the mouth (severe neutropenia).
  - Bleeding gums, corkscrew hair and perifollicular haemorrhages of scurvy (particularly in the elderly).
  - Stigmata of Ehlers–Danlos syndrome.
  - Bleeding from multiple venepuncture sites (disseminated intravascular coagulation).
- Tell the examiner that you would like to examine for spleen, liver and lymph nodes.

DIAGNOSIS

This patient has purpura (lesion) which is due to ingestion of steroids (aetiology) and is cosmetically unacceptable to the patient (functional status).

QUESTIONS

What are the common causes of purpura?
- Senile purpura, due to senile changes in the vessel walls.
- Purpura induced by steroids or anticoagulants.
- Thrombocytopenia due to leukaemia and marrow aplasia.

What are causes of bruising?
- Thrombocytopenia: idiopathic thrombocytopenic purpura, marrow replacement by leukaemia or secondary infiltration.
- Vascular defects: senile purpura, steroid-induced purpura, Henoch–Schönlein purpura, scurvy, von Willebrand's disease, uraemia.
- Coagulation defects: haemophilia, anticoagulants, Christmas disease.
- Drugs: thiazides, sulphonamides, phenylbutazone, sulphonylureas, sulindac, barbiturates.

ADVANCED-LEVEL QUESTION

What do you know about Moschcowitz's syndrome?
Moschcowitz's syndrome, or thrombotic thrombocytopenic purpura, is an acute disorder characterized by thrombocytopenic purpura, microangiopathic haemolytic anaemia, transient and fluctuating neurological features, fever and renal impairment.

E. Moschcowitz (1879–1964), New York physician.

In 1951, William Harrington, then a trainee in haematology at the Barnes Hospital in St Louis, Missouri, had severe thrombocytopenia immediately after voluntarily receiving plasma from a patient with the disease, establishing beyond doubt that a plasma factor causes the destruction of platelets in chronic idiopathic thrombocytopenic purpura.

Case 147

PSORIASIS

INSTRUCTION

Look at this patient.
Do a general examination.

SALIENT FEATURES

History

- Symptoms (itching, pain, flexural intertrigo, limitation of manual dexterity), cosmetic problems or both.
- Joint pains (see p. 343 for psoriatic arthropathy; psoriatic arthritis may be found in 10–15% of patients).
- Family history (30% of patients have a family history).
- Aggravating factors (emotional stress, overuse of alcohol, streptococcal infections, drugs such as beta-blockers or lithium).

Examination

Well-demarcated salmon pink plaques with silvery white scales (Fig. 6) over extensor surfaces, scalp, navel and natal cleft. Patients often tend to have a pink or red line in the intergluteal fold.

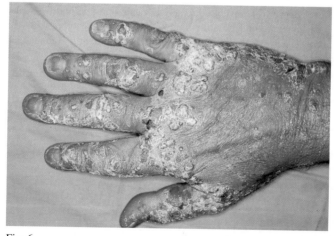

Fig. 6

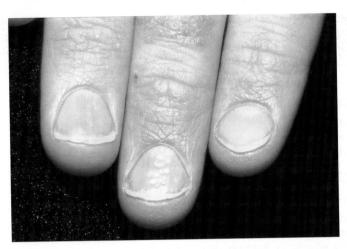

Fig. 7

Proceed as follows:
Look at the nails for pitting (Fig. 7) and onycholysis (separation of the nail plate from the bed; see Fig. 56, p. 489).

DIAGNOSIS

This patient has silvery white scales and nail pitting (lesion) due to psoriasis (aetiology), with considerable itching (functional status).

QUESTIONS

How common is this condition?
It affects 1–2% of the population of the UK.

What are the typical features of psoriatic plaques?
Distinguishing features include:

- Silvery colour of the scaling.
- The moist red surface on removal of the scales (Bulkeley's membrane).
- Capillary bleeding when individual silvery scales are plucked from the plaque (Auspitz's sign).
- New skin lesions at the site of trauma (Koebner's phenomenon).

ADVANCED-LEVEL QUESTIONS

How is the severity of involvement usually estimated?
- The patient's own perception of the disability.
- Objective assessment of disability.

It is usually estimated by using the Psoriasis Area and Severity Index which takes into consideration the area of involvement, thickness, redness and scaling. The maximal score on this index is 72, with mild, moderate and severe having scores of <10, 10–50 and >50 respectively.

What are the types of psoriasis?

Depending on the natural history:
- Type 1: young patients with a strong family history have a more aggressive disorder.
- Type 2: older patients with no family history have a more indolent course.

Depending on the nature of the skin lesion:
- Chronic plaque psoriasis.
- Inverse psoriasis: plaques evolve in the intertriginous areas and thus lack the typical silver scale appearance because of moisture and maceration.
- Guttate psoriasis: numerous small papular lesions with silvery scaling evolve suddenly over the body surface.
- Pustular psoriasis – localized or generalized: superficial pustules may stud the plaques.
- Erythrodermic psoriasis: generalized erythema and scaling; can be life-threatening.

What do you know about the genetics of psoriasis?
Polygenic inheritance is likely, although it has been located to the distal end of the long arm of chromosome 17 in several kindreds.

What do you know about the pathology of plaque psoriasis?
- Hyperproliferation of the epidermis.
- Inflammation of the epidermis and dermis.

What do you understand by the term 'Koebner's phenomenon'?
Injury or irritation of psoriatic skin tends to provoke lesions of psoriasis in the site in some patients – this is known as Koebner's phenomenon.

Mention a few exacerbating factors.
- Drugs: beta-blockers, ACE inhibitors, lithium, indometacin, antimalarials, alcohol.
- Psychological factors.
- Infection: β-haemolytic streptococci, HIV virus (pre-existing psoriasis may become more refractory to therapy and plaque psoriasis may change to the guttate form in patients with HIV positivity).
- Injury to the skin: mechanical injury, sunburn.

How would you manage a patient with psoriasis (N Engl J Med 1995; 332: 581)?
- Educate the patient to understand that there is no cure and that only suppression of the disease is possible.
- Indications for treatment include symptoms (itching, pain, flexural intertrigo, limitation of manual dexterity), cosmetic problems or both.
- Initial treatment is topical when less than 20% of the body is involved.
  – Topical therapy in some form is usually the mainstay of treatment and includes:
  – Emollients (soft yellow paraffin or aqueous cream).

- Keratolytic agents (salicylic acid).
- Coal tar is usually used in combination with ultraviolet B phototherapy (PUVA B) – Goeckerman treatment.
- Dithranol (often used according to the Ingram regimen – a daily coal tar bath, ultraviolet B phototherapy and 24-hour application of a dithranol paste containing salicylic acid).
- Topical steroids.
- Calcipotriol (vitamin D_3) is known to act locally to increase extracellular calcium concentrations, which leads to increased keratinocyte differentiation and decreased proliferation and scaling. It is an excellent alternative to steroids.
- Systemic therapy:
  - Phototherapy (ultraviolet B radiation) – narrowband ultraviolet B has replaced broadband ultraviolet B as it induces longer remissions and fewer burns (*BMJ* 2000; **320**: 850–3).
  - Photochemotherapy (methotrexate with ultraviolet A therapy).
  - Methotrexate.
  - Etretinate (vitamin A derivative), retinoids.
  - Systemic steroids.
  - Ciclosporin, tacrolimus or mycophenolate mofetil.
- Novel approach: anti-CD4 monoclonal antibody.

What are the indications for systemic treatment?
- Failure of topical therapy.
- Repeated hospital admissions for topical treatment.
- Extensive plaque psoriasis in the elderly.
- Generalized pustular or erythrodermic psoriasis.
- Severe psoriatic arthropathy.

What underlying condition would you suspect when psoriasiform lesions are seen on the nose, ears, fingers and toes?
Such lesions are paraneoplastic eruptions associated with squamous cell carcinoma of the oropharynx, tracheobronchial tree and oesophagus – this is known as Bazex syndrome.

B. Russell, in 1950, proposed that psoriasis be known by the eponym Willan–Plumbe syndrome (Russell B 1950 Lepra, psoriasis, or the Willan–Plumbe syndrome. *Br J Dermatol Syphilis* **62**: 359–61). The first clear descriptions were by Willan (1808) and Plumbe (1824).

Case 148

BULLOUS ERUPTION

INSTRUCTION

Look at this patient.

SALIENT FEATURES

History

- Onset and blisters.
- History of mucosal involvement (mouth ulcers).
- Drug history.

Examination

- Bullous eruption.
- Crusts or superficial erosions (these suggest a preceding fluid-filled lesion).

Proceed as follows:
- Comment on the distribution: knees, thighs, forearms and umbilicus in the elderly (pemphigoid).
- Look in the mouth for ulceration; if the blisters break easily, leaving denuded skin, it is more likely to be pemphigus.
- Tell the examiner that a biopsy of the skin is essential to confirm the diagnosis.

DIAGNOSIS

This patient has a bullous eruption (lesion) due to sulphonamides (aetiology) which is widespread with involvement of mucous membrane (functional status).

QUESTIONS

What do you understand by the term 'bulla'?
It is a circumscribed elevation of the skin, larger than 0.5 cm, containing fluid.

How would you confirm the diagnosis?
Biopsy of a fresh blister (less than 12 hours old) with a portion of perilesional skin for histology and immunofluorescence studies.

ADVANCED-LEVEL QUESTIONS

Mention a few blistering conditions.
- Common: friction, insect bites, drugs, burns, impetigo, contact dermatitis.
- Uncommon:
  - Autoimmune bullous diseases (pemphigoid, pemphigus vulgaris, dermatitis herpetiformis, immunoglobulin A mediated diseases, bullous erythema multiforme, epidermolysis bullosa acquisita).

– Porphyria cutanea tarda.
– Paraneoplastic pemphigus.

How would you manage a patient with pemphigus vulgaris?

Barrier nursing, antibiotics, intravenous fluids, large doses of systemic steroids, usually with immunosuppressive drugs – azathioprine, cyclophosphamide or methotrexate – which act as steroid-sparing agents. Other drugs used include dapsone, nicotinamide, gold and ciclosporin.

What are the forms of pemphigus?

There are two main forms; both occur commonly in middle age. These include:

- Pemphigus vulgaris and its variant pemphigus vegetans. The vulgaris form begins in the mouth in over 50% of cases.
- Pemphigus foliaceus and its variant pemphigus erythematosus. These are more superficially blistering conditions. The foliaceus form may be drug induced, e.g. penicillamine toxicity, or associated with autoimmune disease.

What are the characteristics of pemphigus vulgaris?

Pemphigus vulgaris is characterized by bullae in the epidermis. It is often preceded by bullae in the mucous membrane. Superficial separation of the skin after pressure, trauma or on rubbing the thumb laterally on the surface of uninvolved skin may cause easy separation of the epidermis (Nikolsky's sign). Biopsy shows disruption of epidermal intercellular connections called acanthocytolysis. Immunofluorescence shows intercellular deposition of immunoglobulin G in the epidermis.

What are the characteristics of bullous pemphigoid?

It is a relatively benign condition. Characteristically, tense blisters are present in the flexural areas and trunk, typically in the elderly (Fig. 8). The bullae are subepidermal and eosinophil rich; immunoelectronmicroscopy shows deposits of immunoglobulin G and complement 3 (C3) in the lamina lucida of the basement membrane. The disease has a chronic course marked by exacerbation and remission. Therapy involves systemic glucocorticoids and/or immunosuppressives.

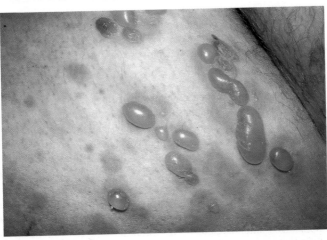

Fig. 8

What do you know about herpes gestationis?

It is a self-limiting disease with the initial appearance of bullae in the periumbilical region, trunk and extremities, usually in the fifth or sixth month of pregnancy. Pruritus is typically severe. It may recur in subsequent pregnancies. Menses and oestrogen are known to precipitate flare-ups. The blisters are eosinophil rich and subepidermal, with C3 in the basement membrane and serum complement-fixing immunoglobulin antibody. Corticosteroids, usually systemic, are the treatment of choice.

What do you know about the pathogenesis of pemphigus?

In pemphigus vulgaris autoantibodies bind to the surface of the keratinocytes whereas in pemphigus foliaceus the antibodies have specificity for keratinocytes in the subcorneal region. The antibodies in pemphigus foliaceus are directed against desmoglein 1 (*J Clin Invest* 2000; **105:** 207–13) whereas in pemphigus vulgaris they are directed against desmoglein 3 (*J Clin Invest* 1997; **99:** 31–40). The desmogleins are desmosomal glycoproteins in the cadherin family of cell adhesion molecules. There is strong evidence that the endemic form of pemphigus foliaceus is initiated by an environmental vector whose antigens mimic those of desmoglein (*N Engl J Med* 2000; **343:** 23–30; *N Engl J Med* 2000; **343:** 31–5).

How would you manage generalized forms of autoimmune bullous disease?

- The treatment of patients with autoimmune blistering diseases is grounded in clinical experience rather than randomized controlled trials.
- Systemic steroid therapy is usually chosen first to treat patients with generalized forms of any autoimmune bullous disease except those mediated by immunoglobulin A. Topical steroids have little, if any, value in the treatment of such patients, although they are sometimes effective in patients with localized disease.
- Other immunosuppressive drugs: Many patients with moderate to severe pemphigus, bullous pemphigoid, cicatricial pemphigoid or epidermolysis bullosa acquisita require a second immunosuppressive drug (such as azathioprine or cyclophosphamide), either for its corticosteroid-sparing effect or to achieve complete remission. The specific choice is a matter of personal experience, concern over the relative toxic effects, and possible contraindications. Some patients have been treated successfully with prednisone and ciclosporin, but the latter alone is not beneficial. Low-dose methotrexate plus prednisone may benefit patients with pemphigus or bullous pemphigoid.
- Dapsone and related drugs: Dapsone is the drug of choice for patients with dermatitis herpetiformis or linear immunoglobulin A dermatosis who are not allergic to sulphonamides. It inhibits the chemotaxis of neutrophils, reducing their accumulation in the upper dermis and thus diminishing tissue inflammation. The response is rapid, with most lesions resolving within 48–72 hours. Alternatives to dapsone include sulfapyridine, sulfoxone sodium and sulfamethoxypyridazine. Dapsone is effective as monotherapy in only a minority of patients with bullous pemphigoid.
- Chrysotherapy: systemic gold is rarely used as an alternative or adjunct to prednisone therapy in patients with pemphigus because it is efficacious in only a subgroup of patients and carries the potential risk of side-effects on prolonged administration.

- Plasmapheresis is used in patients with severe pemphigus unresponsive to conventional therapy and high titres of pemphigus autoantibodies. Plasmapheresis may also be beneficial in patients with bullous pemphigoid even in the absence of detectable autoantibodies, although its mechanism of action in such patients is not known.
- Gluten-free diets in dermatitis herpetiformis.
- Other therapies: extracorporeal absorption of antibodies for pemphigus, combination tetracycline and nicotinamide in bullous pemphigoid, colchicine in immunoglobulin A dermatosis.

P.V. Nikolsky (b. 1858), Professor of Dermatology, first in Warsaw and later in Rostov.

Pemphigus – from the Greek *pemphix*, meaning blister or bubble.

Case 149

HENOCH–SCHÖNLEIN PURPURA

INSTRUCTION

Look at this patient's legs.

SALIENT FEATURES

History

Ask the patient about the following:

- Upper respiratory tract infection.
- Joint pains (knees and ankles are commonly involved).
- Abdominal pain.
- The rash – its onset and evolution.
- Recent drug ingestion.

Examination

Purpuric rash over the legs (Fig. 9) and buttocks.

Proceed as follows:
- Tell the examiner that you would like to examine the rest of the body – including arms, body, scalp and behind the ears – for distribution of rash.
- Examine the mouth to confirm or rule out involvement of mucous membranes.
- Tell the examiner that you would like to examine the urine for haematuria.

DIAGNOSIS

This patient has purpuric rash over the legs and buttocks with renal involvement (lesions) due to Henoch–Schönlein purpura (aetiology). I would like to know his

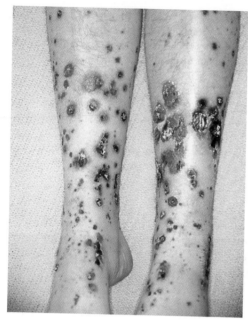

Fig. 9

24-hour urine output and levels of urea and electrolytes to determine renal function (functional status).

ADVANCED-LEVEL QUESTIONS

What do you know about Henoch–Schönlein purpura?

Henoch–Schönlein or anaphylactoid purpura is a distinct, self-limiting vasculitis which occurs in children and young adults. It is a disorder characterized by non-thrombocytopenic purpura, arthralgia, abdominal pain and glomerular nephritis. It is due to circulating immune complexes containing immunoglobulin (Ig) A. It usually lasts between 1 and 6 weeks and subsides without sequelae if renal involvement is mild. The presence of IgG indicates a worse prognosis. Adults are more likely to develop renal involvement (*Lancet* 1992; **339:** 280).

What investigations would you like to perform?

• Examine the urine for haematuria and proteinuria.
• Antinuclear factor.
• Venereal Disease Research Laboratory test.
• Skin biopsy to detect arteriolar and capillary vasculitis.

What is the differential diagnosis?

• Drug-induced purpura.
• SLE.
• Gonococcal arthralgia.
• Keratoderma blenorrhagicum.
• Secondary syphilis.

How would you classify vasculitis clinically?
- Purpuric disorders: Henoch–Schönlein purpura, leukocytic vasculitis.
- Microscopic polyarteritis: polyarteritis nodosa.
- Aortic type: Takayasu disease, polyarteritis nodosa (in the latter, the subclavian artery is spared).
- Pulmonary type: Wegener's granulomatosis, Churg–Strauss syndrome.

How would you treat this patient?
Patients with IgA nephropathy and increased urinary protein excretion (1.0–3.5 g daily) and plasma creatinine concentrations of 133 μmol/l (1.5 mg/dl) or less may benefit from a 6-month course of steroid treatment (*Lancet* 1999; **353:** 883–7). Steroids, plasma exchange, immunoglobulins and cytotoxic agents have all been used in complicated cases and there are no data from controlled trials (*Lancet* 2000; **356:** 562).

This disorder was first reported in the English literature by Willan in 1808.

Eduard Heinrich Henoch (1820–1910) qualified in Berlin, where he ran the neurology department; he studied under Schönlein and eventually became a paediatrician. In 1874 he reported the coexistence of purpura and gastrointestinal haemorrhage.

Johannes Lucas Schönlein (1793–1864) was initially Professor of Medicine in Würzburg but, because of his liberal views, he was dismissed; he eventually became Professor of Medicine, first in Zurich and then in Berlin. In 1837 he reported the coexistence of purpura and arthritis.

Anthony Fauci, contemporary Director of the National Institute of Allergy and Infectious Diseases and Director of AIDS Research, NIH, Bethesda, whose chief interests include immunological disorders including AIDS.

Case 150

ICHTHYOSIS

INSTRUCTION

Look at this patient.
Examine this patient's skin.
Perform a general examination on this patient.

SALIENT FEATURES

History
- Take a family history of the disorder.
- Ask whether or not it is of recent onset (underlying malignancy).

Examination
Rough, dry skin with fish-like scales (Fig. 10).

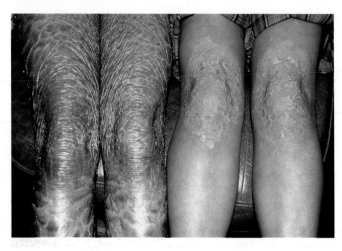

Fig. 10

Proceed as follows:
Examine the palms for dry skin and hyperkeratotic creases.

Note. Although ichthyosis is said not to be increased in frequency in HIV/AIDS, it may be more severe when associated with this condition.

DIAGNOSIS

This patient has rough, dry skin with fish-like scales (lesion) due to ichthyosis (aetiology), which causes severe itching and may be cosmetically unacceptable (functional status).

ADVANCED-LEVEL QUESTIONS

What do you know about ichthyosis?

Ichthyosis can be classified as follows:

1. *Inherited* ichthyosis is present from birth or childhood and may be apparent only in winter.
   - Ichthyosis vulgaris: present from childhood; autosomal dominant; spares flexural areas; associated with atopy.
   - X-linked ichthyosis: present from birth; over the trunk; associated with corneal opacities.
   - Lamellar ichthyosis: autosomal recessive; present from birth; seen over the body, palms and soles; associated with ectropion.
   - Epidermolytic hyperkeratosis: autosomal dominant; present since birth; predominant flexural involvement.
2. *Metabolic* ichthyosis:
   - Refsum's disease – a metabolic disorder of lipid metabolism.
3. *Malignancy* – as a cutaneous marker:
   - Hodgkin's disease.
   - Multiple myeloma.
   - Breast cancer.

How would you manage such patients?

Regular use of emollients and moisturizing creams. Creams containing urea are useful.

S. Refsum, a Norwegian physician.

Case 151

HEREDITARY HAEMORRHAGIC TELANGIECTASIA (RENDU–OSLER–WEBER DISEASE)

INSTRUCTION

Examine the patient's face and obtain a relevant history.
Perform a general examination.
Look at this patient's face.

SALIENT FEATURES

History

- Does it run in the family (autosomal dominant)?
- Is there a history of gastrointestinal bleeding?
- Is there a history of epistaxis?
- Is there a history of repeated blood transfusions?
- Is there a history of dyspnoea, fatigue, cyanosis or polycythaemia? (pulmonary arteriovenous malformations).
- Is there a history of headaches, subarachnoid haemorrhage? (cerebral arteriovenous malformations).

Examination

- Punctiform lesions and dilated small vessels present on the face, in particular around the mouth (Fig. 11).
- The patient may be pale (due to iron deficiency anaemia).

Proceed as follows:

- Look into the patient's mouth and inspect the tongue and palate for telangiectasia.
- Examine the nail beds, arms, trunk for telangiectasia.
- Examine the chest for bruits (pulmonary arteriovenous malformations with a predilection for lower lobes).
- Look for signs of cardiac failure caused by left-to-right shunting and hepatic bruits (both due to hepatic arteriovenous malformations) (*N Engl J Med* 2000; **343**: 938–52).

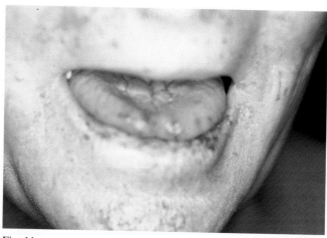

Fig. 11

DIAGNOSIS

This patient has multiple telangiectases around the mouth and on the tongue and lips (lesion), probably hereditary in nature (aetiology). The patient is severely anaemic, probably as a result of upper gastrointestinal bleeding, and is currently receiving a blood transfusion (functional status).

QUESTIONS

What do you understand by the term 'telangiectasia'?

Telangiectasia is a cluster of dilated capillaries and venules. In this disorder telangiectases consist of focal dilatations of postcapillary venules.

Mention a few conditions in which telangiectases are seen.

Of the face:
- Those who work outdoors in a temperate or cold climate (e.g. farmers).
- In mitral stenosis.
- Myxoedema.
- Transitory phenomenon during pregnancy.

Of other sites:
- Secondary to irradiation.
- Scleroderma (CREST syndrome).
- Dermatomyositis.
- SLE.
- Acne rosacea.
- Lupus pernio.
- Polycythaemia.
- Necrobiosis lipoidica diabeticorum.

ADVANCED-LEVEL QUESTIONS

What do you know about the genetics of hereditary telangiectasia?

Mutations in two genes, endoglin-β (at chromosome 9q3; *Nat Genet* 1994; **6:** 205–9) and activin receptor-like kinase 1 ALK-1 (*Nat Genet* 1996; **13:** 189–95), are known to cause HHT. Each encodes a protein expressed on vascular endothelial cells and involved in signalling by members of the transforming growth factor (TGF)-β superfamily. It is interesting that heterozygote endoglin-knockout mice develop a phenotype (*J Clin Invest* 1999; **104:** 1343–51) similar to that of humans who are heterozygous for a null mutation in the endoglin-β gene: the hereditary haemorrhagic telangiectasia. These heterozygous mice develop nose bleeds and cutaneous telangiectasia, and curiously the ears are more commonly affected than in human beings.

What do you know about the pathology of the condition?

In the skin

- The small telangiectases are focal dilatations of postcapillary venules with prominent stress fibres in the pericytes along the luminal border.
- In fully developed telangiectasia, there is marked dilatation of the venules, which are also convoluted. They extend along the entire dermis, with excessive layers of smooth muscle devoid of elastic fibres. These often are directly connected to dilated arterioles.
- Mononuclear cells, predominantly lymphocytes, accumulate in the perivascular space.

In the lungs, liver and brain

Arteriovenous malformations lack capillaries and consist of direct connections between arteries and veins.

What are the clinical criteria for diagnosing hereditary haemorrhagic telangiectasia (HHT)?

Shovlin criteria

- Recurrent epistaxis.
- Telangiectasia at a site other than in the nasal mucosa.
- Evidence of autosomal dominant inheritance.
- Visceral involvement.

The diagnosis of HHT is definite if three criteria are present. A diagnosis of HHT cannot be established in patients with only two criteria, but should be recorded as possible or suspected to maintain a high index of clinical suspicion. If fewer than two criteria are present, HHT is unlikely, although children of affected individuals should be considered at risk in view of age-related penetration in this disorder (*Am J Med Genet* 2000; **91:** 66–7).

What are the complications of hereditary telangiectasia?

- Epistaxis (usually begins by the age of 10 years and age 21 in most; it becomes more severe in later decades in about two thirds of affected patients; *N Engl J Med* 1995; **333:** 918–24).
- Gastrointestinal haemorrhage (usually does not manifest until the fifth or sixth decade). Arteriovenous malformations, angiodysplasias and telangiectases are present in the stomach, duodenum, small bowel, colon and liver.

- Iron deficiency anaemia.
- Haemoptysis, cyanosis, clubbing, cerebral abscess and embolic stroke due to pulmonary arteriovenous malformations.
- Headache and subarachnoid haemorrhage.
- High-output cardiac failure is almost always associated with shunts from the hepatic artery to the hepatic veins (*N Engl J Med* 2000; **343:** 931–6).

How would you manage such patients?

- Anaemia: ferrous sulphate, multiple blood transfusions.
- Epistaxis: oestrogen, cauterization, septal dermatoplasty, laser ablation and trans-catheter embolotherapy of arteries leading to the nasal mucosa.
- Cutaneous telangiectasia: cosmetic therapy with topical agents, laser ablation.
- Pulmonary arteriovenous malformations: embolotherapy, surgical resection or ligation of arterial supply.
- Gastrointestinal telangiectasia: blood transfusions, photocoagulation, oestrogen–progestogen therapy.
- Brain and spinal cord arteriovenous malformations: embolotherapy, neurosurgery, stereotactic surgery.
- Active bleeding: epsilon aminocaproic acid (*N Engl J Med* 1994; **330:** 1789; *N Engl J Med* 1994; **330:** 1822).

This condition was described by H.J.L.M. Rendu, a French physician, in 1896, by Sir William Osler in 1901, and by F. Parkes Weber, a London physician, in 1936.

Case 152

HERPES LABIALIS

INSTRUCTION

Look at this patient's mouth.

SALIENT FEATURES

History

- Pain, itching, burning lasting several hours.
- Vesicles.
- Sore mouth.
- Fever.
- Gum swelling.
- Mouth ulcers.

Examination

Small vesicles with an erythematous base on the lips and around the mouth.

Proceed as follows:
Look for vesicles in the mouth (gingiva, tongue, soft and hard palate) and pharynx.
Tender anterior cervical lymph nodes.

DIAGNOSIS

This patient has small vesicles around the mouth (lesion) due to herpes labialis
(aetiology), which is causing severe itching (functional status).

QUESTIONS

What usually causes a 'cold sore'?
Herpes simplex virus (HSV) type I: in children it causes asymptomatic gingivosto-
matitis; in adults there may be severe stomatitis with mouth ulcers, local lymph
node enlargement and systemic features.

What do you know about HSV-II?
HSV-II causes genital infection, called vulvovaginitis. Women with genital herpes
ought to have cervical screening as a link with carcinoma of the cervix is suspected.
There has recently been a dramatic increase in the prevalence of HSV-II infection
(*N Engl J Med* 1997; **337:** 1105–11).

ADVANCED-LEVEL QUESTIONS

What are the complications of herpes infection?
- Erythema multiforme.
- Disseminated infection in the immunocompromised individual.
- Herpes keratitis, scarring and visual impairment.
- Herpes simplex encephalitis (propensity for the temporal lobe).
- Herpetic whitlow (infection of the finger; Fig. 12).

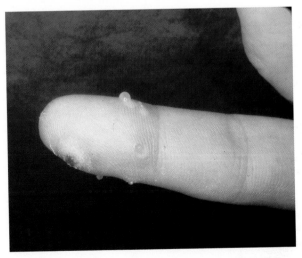

Fig. 12

- Herpes gladiatorum (infection of the skin, described among wrestlers).
- Visceral infections, especially in viraemia in HIV (oesophagitis, pneumonitis, hepatitis).
- Neonatal HSV infection (neonates less than 6 weeks of age); usually visceral and/or central nervous system infection.
- Herpes simplex meningitis.

How would you confirm your clinical diagnosis?

- Scrapings of the base of the lesions stained with either Wright, Giemsa (Tzanck preparation) or Papanicolaou's stain will demonstrate characteristic giant cells or intranuclear inclusions of herpes infection (does not differentiate from zoster infection).
- Isolation of virus in tissue culture.
- Demonstration of HSV antigens in scrapings from lesions.

How would you treat herpes labialis?

Aciclovir cream applied locally.

What drugs are available for herpes simplex infections?

- Mucocutaneous herpes: topical aciclovir, foscarnet.
- Eye infections: idoxuridine, trifluorothymidine, topical vidarabine. Prophylactic use of aciclovir can prevent recurrent ocular HSV disease (*N Engl J Med* 1998; **339**: 300–6).
- Encephalitis: intravenous aciclovir.
- Neonatal infections: high-dose intravenous vidarabine and aciclovir.

In a patient suspected of herpes encephalitis, which test allows early detection?

HSV DNA polymerase chain reaction (PCR) in the cerebrospinal fluid.

Case 153

HERPES ZOSTER SYNDROME (SHINGLES)

INSTRUCTION

Look at this patient.

SALIENT FEATURES

History

- Pain, particularly in the ophthalmic branch of the trigeminal nerve (Fig. 13) and in the lower thoracic dermatomes (postherpetic neuralgia occurs in about 50% of patients with zoster over the age of 60 years).
- Past history of chickenpox.

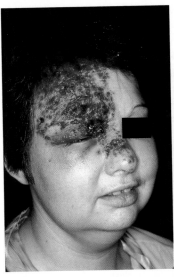
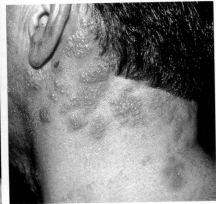

Fig. 13   Fig. 14

- Presence of an underlying immunocompromised state (e.g. recurrent zoster indicates a poorer prognosis in patients with established AIDS). Zoster occurs at least seven times more frequently in homosexual men with HIV infection than in HIV-negative controls.

Examination

- Vesicular rash along a dermatome (usually affects thoracic and lumbar dermatomes).
- Enlargement of a draining lymph node.

Proceed as follows:
Remember that the virus affects both the posterior horn of the spinal cord and the skin supplied by sensory fibres that pass through the diseased root ganglion (Fig. 14).

DIAGNOSIS

This patient has a vesicular rash along the 6th thoracic dermatome (lesion) due to herpes zoster (aetiology), and has severe local pain (functional status).

ADVANCED-LEVEL QUESTIONS

In which layer of the skin are the vesicles formed?
They are formed in the prickle-cell layer of the epidermis as a result of the 'balloon degeneration' of cells and serous exudation from the corium.

How does this condition present?
Pain in the distribution of the dermatome; malaise; fever, followed a few days later by a rash in the same distribution as the pain. The rash starts as macules, then forms vesicles and then pustules.

Which nerve is affected when the lesions are present on the tip of the nose?

The ophthalmic division of the trigeminal nerve.

How would you confirm the diagnosis?

The diagnosis is usually clinical. It is confirmed by rising viral titres and isolation of the virus from the blister. The Tzanck smear demonstrates a multinucleated giant cell and viral inclusions when material scraped from the floor of a vesicle is stained with Wright's stain. The Tzanck test can be positive in infections with herpes simplex, herpes zoster and varicella.

How would you manage such a patient?

- Topical idoxuridine 5% solution if caught in the first 36 hours of the eruption.
- Pain relief, including amitriptyline in severe cases.
- Intravenous aciclovir in the immunocompromised individual (*N Engl J Med* 1994; **330**: 896).
- Interferon appears to be effective in limiting zoster in patients with cancer.

Is varicella-zoster immune globulin (VZIG) useful in preventing zoster eruptions?

There are no known means of effectively preventing zoster eruptions; however, results on the effectiveness of the recently developed live attenuated varicella vaccine are awaited. Although there is considerable controversy, with arguments for and against universal vaccination, the American Academcy of Pediatrics has recently adopted a position in support of universal vaccination of healthy nonimmune children and adults.

What are the complications of herpes zoster?

- Corneal ulcerations.
- Gangrene of the affected area.
- Phrenic nerve palsy.
- Meningoencephalitis.
- Ramsay Hunt syndrome.
- Postherpetic neuralgia – intrathecal methyl prednisolone is an effective treatment for postherpetic neuralgia (*N Engl J Med* 2000; **343**: 1514–19).
- Disseminated zoster including pneumonia.

What are the features of herpes zoster in patients with HIV infection?

It is usually unidermatomal and uneventful. However, it may be multidermatomal, disseminated recurrent, or chronically persistent as a hyperkeratotic nodular lesion.

How does the varicella zoster virus affect the central nervous system in patients with AIDS?

In acquired immune deficiency syndrome the virus may cause the following:

- Multifocal encephalitis.
- Ventriculitis.
- Acute haemorrhagic meningomyeloradiculitis.
- Focal necrotizing myelitis.
- Vasculitis of the leptomeningeal arteries.

J. Ramsay Hunt (1874–1937), a US neurologist.

Case 154

LICHEN PLANUS

INSTRUCTION

Look at this patient's skin.

SALIENT FEATURES

History

- Itching.
- Drug ingestion (thiazides, phenothiazines, gold, organic mercurials, chloroquine, mepacrine, methyldopa, quinine, chlorpropamide, tolbutamide, proton pump inhibitors).
- Occupational history (whether the patient is in contact with colour film developer).
- Hepatitis C (erosive lichen planus is more common).

Examination

Papular, purplish, flat-topped eruption with fine white streaks (Wickham's striae) over the anterior wrists and forearms, sacral region, ankles, legs and penis.

Proceed as follows:
- Look into the mouth (buccal mucosa, tongue, gum or lips) for a lace-like pattern of white lines and papules. (Remember that oral lichen planus must be differentiated from leukoplakia.)
- Examine the scalp for cicatricial alopecia.
- Examine the nails for longitudinal ridging, pterygium formation from the cuticle, 20-nail dystrophy with roughened nail surface and brittle free nail edge, total nail loss.
- Comment on eruptions that are present along linear scratch marks (Koebner's phenomenon).
- Comment on the residual hyperpigmented macules that lichen planus leaves in its wake.

Note. The three cardinal features of lichen planus are the typical skin lesions, histopathological features of T-cell infiltration of the dermis in a band pattern, and IgG and C3 immunofluorescence at the basement membrane of the dermis.

DIAGNOSIS

This patient has violaceous, flat-topped eruptions (lesion) due to lichen planus (aetiology) with several scratch marks indicating moderately severe pruritus (functional status).

ADVANCED-LEVEL QUESTIONS

Mention a few conditions that present as white lesions in the mouth.
- Leukoplakia.
- Candidiasis.
- Aphthous stomatitis.
- Squamous papilloma.
- Verruca vulgaris.
- Secondary syphilis.

Mention a few conditions in which ulcers can be found in the mouth.
- Erosive lichen planus.
- Pemphigus vulgaris.
- Recurrent aphthous ulcers.
- Behçet's disease.
- Stevens–Johnson syndrome.
- Recurrent herpes simplex.

What is the prognosis in lichen planus?

Lichen planus is a benign condition which lasts for months to years. It may be recurrent. Oral lesions may be persistent.

How would you manage these lesions?

- Local measures: local steroid creams or intralesional steroids.
- General measures: PUVA, isotretinoin, dapsone.
- Ultraviolet light to control pruritus
- Mucous membrane lesions: corticosteroids or 'swish and spit' ciclosporin.

L.F. Wickham (1860–1913), a French dermatologist.

H. Koebner (1838–1904), a German dermatologist.

Case 155

VITILIGO

INSTRUCTION

Look at this patient.

SALIENT FEATURES

History

- Ask whether or not the disorder runs in the family (familial in 36% of cases).
- Other autoimmune disorders (hypothyroidism, hyperthyroidism, thyroiditis, Addison's disease, diabetes mellitus, pernicious anaemia).

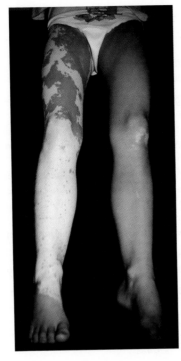

Fig. 15

Examination

- Hypopigmented patches (Fig. 15) which are distributed symmetrically; sometimes the border may be hyperpigmented. The distribution often includes wrists, axillae, perioral, periorbital and anogenital skin.
- White hairs in the vitiliginous area.
- Some spontaneous repigmentation in sun-exposed regions (in a third of cases).

Proceed as follows:

Look at the scalp for alopecia and white hair.

Note. Scratching when the disease is active may induce lesions along the scratch marks; this is termed isomorphic response or Koebner's phenomenon.

DIAGNOSIS

This patient has vitiligo (lesion) which is of autoimmune origin (aetiology) and can be cosmetically distressing to the patient (functional status).

ADVANCED-LEVEL QUESTIONS

Mention some associated conditions.

Organ-specific autoimmune conditions:

- Thyroid disease – Graves' disease, myxoedema, Hashimoto's disease.
- Pernicious anaemia.

- Diabetes mellitus.
- Alopecia areata.
- Addison's disease.

Which fungal condition can be mistaken for vitiligo?
Pityriasis versicolor (caused by the fungus *Malassezia furfur*).

How would you manage such patients?
- Cosmetics are useful for concealing disfiguring patches.
- When less than 20% of the skin is involved, topical methoxsalen with long-wavelength ultraviolet A (UVA) is used, followed by thorough washing and application of an SPF 15 sunscreen.
- When more than 20% of the skin is affected, oral methoxsalen with UVA.
- When vitiligo is extensive, good cosmetic results may be obtained by 'de-pigmenting' normal skin with a bleaching agent like hydroquinone.
- New lesions of vitiligo may benefit from topical steroids.
- Newer therapies include epidermal autografts and cultured epidermis combined with PUVA.

Note. On the whole, treatment of vitiligo remains unsatisfactory.

Mention a few conditions in which hypopigmentation is common.
- Hypopituitarism.
- Albinism.
- Phenylketonuria.
- Leprosy.
- Burns.
- Radiodermatitis.
- Piebaldism (an autosomal dominant condition manifested by a white forelock).
- Ash leaf spots (tuberous sclerosis).
- Leukoderma (a disorder that occurs as a complicaton of lichen planus, lichen simplex chronicus, atopic dermatitis and discoid lupus erythematosus).

What is the histology of vitiligo?
Characteristically, there is partial or complete loss of pigment-producing melanocytes in the epidermis. In contrast, some forms of albinism have melanocytes but no melanin pigment is produced because of lack of, or a defect in, the tyrosinase enzyme.

Why are melanocytes progressively lost in this condition?
The various theories of pathogenesis include:

- Autoimmune destruction due to circulating antibodies against the melanocytes and impaired cell-mediated immunity.
- Self-destruction by toxic intermediates of melanin production.
- Neurohumoral factors.

Case 156

RAYNAUD'S PHENOMENON

INSTRUCTION

Examine this patient's hands.

SALIENT FEATURES

History

Ask the patient about the following:

- Whether the condition is precipitated by cold, emotion and relieved by heat.
- The different phases of Raynaud's phenomenon (in idiopathic Raynaud's disease the cold dead-white hands (ischaemia) become blue (stasis) and finally red (reactive hyperaemia) and painful.
- Sensory changes secondary to vasospasm (numbness, stiffness, aching pain).
- Occupation (polishing tools, vibrating tools).
- Dysphagia (CREST syndrome).
- Butterfly rash, arthralgia, xerostomia (SLE, collagen vascular disorder).
- Use of electrically heated gloves.

Examination

- Hands may be painful – ask the patient.
- The hands and fingers are cyanosed and cold, or may be warm and red or blue (Fig. 16). The thumbs are rarely affected.

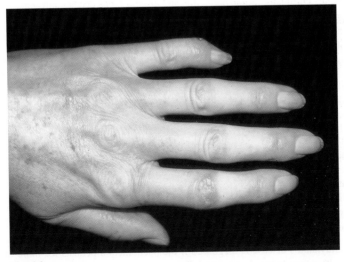

Fig. 16

Proceed as follows:

- Examine the hands carefully for signs of scleroderma (tightening of skin, telangiectasia; Fig. 16).
- Examine the face for tightening of skin around the mouth (scleroderma), butterfly rash (SLE).
- Tell the examiner that you would like to examine upper limb pulses and blood pressure in both upper limbs (useful in the detection of cervical rib).

DIAGNOSIS

This patient has cold, blue hands (lesion) due to Raynaud's phenomenon (aetiology) and is unable to continue her occupation, which requires using a vibratory hand drill (functional status).

Read: *BMJ* 1991; **303:** 913; *BMJ* 1995; **310:** 795–8.

ADVANCED-LEVEL QUESTIONS

What are the causes of Raynaud's phenomenon?

Immunological and connective tissue disorders
- Scleroderma.
- SLE.
- Dermatomyositis.
- Rheumatoid arthritis.
- Mixed connective tissue disorders.

Obliterative arterial disease
- Atherosclerosis.
- Thoracic outlet syndrome, cervical rib.

Occupational
- Vibration, causing white fingers.
- Cold injury, e.g. from handling frozen commodities.
- Vinyl chloride.

Drugs
- Beta-blockers.
- Bromocriptine.
- Sulfasalazine.
- Ergot alkaloids.
- Combination of bleomycin and vincristine (as for testicular cancer).

Miscellaneous
- Cold agglutinins.
- Cryoglobulins.
- Idiopathic.

Note. Raynaud's disease is diagnosed if the phenomenon persists for more than 3 years without evidence of associated disease.

What investigations would you perform to look for autoimmune rheumatic disease in a patient with Raynaud's phenomenon?

- FBC, ESR.
- Total immunoglobulin and electrophoresis strip.
- Urine analysis.
- Nail-fold capillaroscopy.
- Chest radiography.
- Renal and liver function tests.
- Test for antinuclear antibody.
- *H. pylori* (one paper suggested that eradication of *H. pylori* ameliorates Raynaud's phenomenon; *Dig Dis Sci* 1998; **43:** 1641).
- Hand radiography.

What drugs have been used to treat Raynaud's syndrome?

Nifedipine, nitrates, stanazolol, inositol nicotinate, naftidrofuryl oxalate, prostaglandin 12, moxisylyte (thymoxamine), guanethidine, prazosin.

What is the role of surgery in treating Raynaud's disease?

Dorsal sympathectomy may be indicated in patients resistant to medical therapy with severe, frequent attacks, and if trophic changes have occurred, interfering with work.

Do you know of any other vasospastic conditions?

- White finger syndrome.
- Livedo reticularis.
- Erythromelalgia.
- Chilblains.

Maurice Raynaud (1834–1881) described the sign in 1862. He was a physician at Hôpital Lariboisière, Paris. (Raynaud M (1888) On local and symmetrical gangrene of the extremities. In: Barlow T (translator) *Selected Monographs*, vol. 121. London: New Sydenham Society.)

Case 157

SYSTEMIC LUPUS ERYTHEMATOSUS

INSTRUCTION

Examine this patient's face (usually young women).

SALIENT FEATURES

History

- Fatiguability and tiredness (suggests anaemia).
- Joint symptoms, particularly small joints (90% of patients).
- Gangrene of the digits (vasculitis).

- Skin rash (butterfly rash on face) in sun-exposed areas, livedo reticularis, alopecia, Raynaud's phenomenon.
- Mouth ulcers.
- Hypertension, oedema (suggesting renal involvement).
- Fever, enlargement of lymph nodes.
- Bleeding from gums, excessive menstrual bleeding, purpura (due to thrombocytopenia).
- Neuropsychiatric symptoms, seizures.
- History of remissions and exacerbations.
- Drug history (hydralazine, procainamide, minocycline).

Examination

Butterfly rash – follicular plugging, scales, telangiectasia and scarring affecting the bridge of the nose and cheeks (the patient may be cushingoid due to steroids).

Proceed as follows:
- Examine the following:
  - Conjunctiva for anaemia (often Coombs' test positive).
  - Mouth ulcers (seen in one third of cases).
  - Scalp for alopecia.
  - Sun-exposed areas and elbows for vasculitic rash, subcutaneous nodules.
  - Nails for splinter haemorrhages, nail-fold capillaries and periungual infarcts.
  - Hands for palmar erythema, Raynaud's phenomenon, arthritis.
  - Knees for vasculitic rash.
  - Feet for secondary oedema (secondary to nephrotic syndrome).
- Tell the examiner that you would like to examine the urine for proteinuria.

Note. SLE principally affects skin, joints, kidney and serosal membranes.

DIAGNOSIS

This patient has a butterfly rash of the face with telangiectasia (lesion) due to systemic lupus erythematosus (aetiology) and has renal failure, probably due to lupus nephritis, as evidenced by the haemodialysis catheter (functional status).
Read: *BMJ* 1995; **310**: 1257–61; *N Engl J Med* 1994; **330**: 187.

ADVANCED-LEVEL QUESTIONS

What is the histology of the skin rash in SLE?
- Liquefactive degeneration of the basal layer of the epidermis together with oedema at the dermoepidermal junction. Immunofluorescence microscopy shows deposition of immunoglobulin and complement along the dermoepidermal junction.
- Oedema of the dermis accompanied by infiltrates of perivascular mononuclear cells.
- Vasculitis with fibrinoid necrosis of the vessels.

What are the skin manifestations of SLE?
Butterfly rash, periungual erythema, nail-fold telangiectasia, alopecia, livedo reticularis, hyperpigmentation, urticaria, purpura, scarring eruption of discoid lupus.

What are the criteria for diagnosis of SLE?

Any four of the following 11 criteria are required to make a diagnosis (*Arthritis Rheum* 1982; **25**: 1271):

- Malar rash.
- Discoid rash.
- Photosensitivity.
- Oral ulcers.
- Arthritis – nonerosive arthritis.
- Serositis – pleuritis, pericarditis.
- Renal involvement – proteinuria, cellular casts (nephritis is more common in patients with anti-native DNA).
- Neurological involvement – seizures, psychosis.
- Haematological involvement – haemolytic anaemias, leukopenia, thrombocytopenia.
- Antinuclear antibody – seen in over 95% of patients.
- Immunological disorder – positive LE cell, anti-DNA antibody, false-positive syphilitic serology.

Note. American Rheumatic Association (ARA) criteria are intended to provide a degree of diagnostic certainty, primarily for research purposes. It is often possible to be reasonably confident about a diagnosis of SLE on less strict clinical grounds. A diagnosis of SLE is usually made when patients have three or four typical manifestations, such as a characteristic skin rash, thrombocytopenia, serositis or nephritis and antinuclear antibodies (*Medicine* 1993; **72**: 113). Polyarthritis and dermatitis are the most common manifestations. It should be noted that antibodies to double-stranded DNA and the so-called 'Smith antigen' (Sm) are virtually diagnostic of SLE.

What do you know about SLE in older patients?

The initial presentation of idiopathic SLE usually occurs between the first and fourth decades of life. However, about 10% of cases may first occur in patients over 60 years of age. Patients with SLE after the age of 50 years less often present with malar rash, arthritis and nephritis.

The diagnosis of SLE in older patients must be one of exclusion. The frequency of low titres on antinuclear antibody tests increases with advancing age, and a positive test may be associated with malignant disease or chronic infection.

What do you know about drug-induced lupus erythematosus?

- Procainamide is responsible for the majority of the cases. Other causes include hydralazine, isoniazid.
- Drugs causing a lupus-like syndrome do not seem to aggravate primary SLE.
- Although multiple organs are affected, nephritis and central nervous system features are not ordinarily present.
- Antihistone antibodies are characteristic of drug-induced lupus, but are not specific for this syndrome; anti-native DNA is almost never detected.
- Clinical manifestations and many laboratory features return to normal after the offending drug is withdrawn.

How useful is the detection of antinuclear antibodies in the diagnosis of SLE?

The detection of antinuclear antibodies (ANAs) is a sensitive screening test for SLE. Since ANAs occur in 95% of the patients, it is hard to be certain of the diagnosis in their absence. The degree of positivity is diagnostically important. Serum dilutions below which normal serum may be positive for these antibodies vary in different laboratories. Titres that are less than two times higher than the normal limit in any laboratory ought to be viewed sceptically. The positive predictive value of the test increases with higher titres.

How would you manage a patient with SLE?

- Avoidance of sunlight provocation. In Britain, patients should avoid being outside from 11am to 3pm from March to September and should wear protective clothing, including hats; patients should holiday in temperate latitudes or during the winter. In addition, sun block creams such as titanium dioxide (rather than barrier cream) are essential.
- Avoidance of drug provocation – penicillin, sulphonamides.
- Encourage the patient to join the Lupus Society.
- Educate the patient to understand that no therapy is curative and that medical treatment is largely empirical, selected on the basis of specific manifestations (see table below).

Disease manifestations	Treatment
Serological abnormalities and minor cytopenia unaccompanied by symptoms	No treatment
Rash and mild systemic symptoms	Antimalarial drugs
Mild or moderate arthritis, fever, pleuropericarditis	NSAIDs or low-dose prednisolone
Malaise, weight loss and lymphadenopathy	Low-dose steroids
High fever, active inflammatory glomerulonephritis, severe thrombocytopenia, severe haemolytic anaemia and most neurological disturbances	High-dose prednisolone (>60 mg per day for 4–6 weeks)
Rapidly progressive renal disease	Intravenous administration of bolus doses of 1000 mg methylprednisolone
Lupus nephritis with high histological activity score	Oral or intravenous cyclophosphamide or mycophenolate mofetil with high-dose steroids (N Engl J Med 2000; 343: 1156–62)
Thromboembolism with antiphospholipid	Long-term anticoagulation antibody
Severe disease	Experimental treatments*

*Experimental treatments include apheresis, intravenous gammaglobulin, ciclosporin, immunoadsorption, photochemotherapy, nodal irradiation, various monoclonal antibodies and autologous haemopoietic stem-cell infusion (Lancet 2000; 356: 701–7).

What are the patterns of lupus nephritis?

The World Health Organization's morphological classification of lupus nephritis describes five patterns:

- Normal by light, electron and immunofluoroscence microscopy (rare).
- Mesangial lupus glomerulonephritis.
- Focal proliferative glomerulonephritis.
- Diffuse proliferative glomerulonephritis.
- Membranous glomerulonephritis.

Note. None of these patterns is specific for lupus.

What are the common causes of death in SLE?

The most common causes of death are renal failure and intercurrent infections, followed by diffuse central nervous system disease.

R.R.A. Coombs (b. 1921), Professor of Immunology at Cambridge, is reported to have said 'red blood cells were primarily designed by God as tools for the immunologist and only secondarily as carriers of haemoglobin'.

Ferdinand von Hebra (1816–1880) from Vienna described an eruption that occurs 'mainly on the face, on the cheeks and nose in a distribution not dissimilar to a butterfly' in 1845.

Pierre Louis Alphée Cazenave (1795–1877) from Paris first used the term 'lupus érythémateux' in 1851.

Sir William Osler (1849–1919) first described the systemic manifestations of systemic lupus erythematosus under the name exudative erythema between 1895 and 1904.

Case 158

PHLEBITIS MIGRANS

INSTRUCTION

Look at this patient's leg: he has had similar such lesions at different sites at intervals.

SALIENT FEATURES

History

- Time course, pain and tenderness of skin lesions.
- Ask the patient about local trauma (including intravenous infusions).
- Gastrointestinal malignancies (pancreatic or gastric cancer).
- History of oral contraceptives.

Examination

Inflamed superficial leg veins.

Proceed as follows:

Tell the examiner that you would like to investigate for the underlying malignancy, usually carcinoma of the pancreas or stomach (Trousseau's sign) (*N Engl J Med* 1994; **327**: 1163–4; *N Engl J Med* 1992; **327**: 1128–33).

DIAGNOSIS

This patient has migratory phlebitis (lesion) and I would like to investigate for an underlying pancreatic or gastric malignancy (aetiology).

ADVANCED-LEVEL QUESTIONS

In which other condition is superficial phlebitis a prominent sign?
Thromboangiitis obliterans.

Is superficial thrombophlebitis associated with deep vein thrombosis?
It may be associated with occult deep vein thrombosis in about 20% of cases, although pulmonary emboli are rare.

Is phlebitis more frequently associated with plastic venous catheters or with steel intravenous needles?
It is more likely to be associated with plastic catheters, but this may be because a catheter remains in the vein for a longer period.

How is superficial phlebitis treated?
- Local heat, elevation of the leg, and NSAIDs.
- When phlebitis is very extensive or in proximity to the saphenofemoral junction, ligation and division of the saphenous vein at the saphenofemoral junction (as pulmonary embolism may result if the phlebitis of the saphenous vein extends into the deep vein).
- Septic thrombophlebitis, which is usually due to *Staphylococcus aureus*, requires excision of the involved vein up to its junction with an uninvolved vein in order to control infection.

What other dermatoses complicate pancreatic disease?
- Panniculitis.
- 'Bronze' pigmentation of haemochromatosis.
- 'Necrolytic migratory erythema' of glucagonoma syndrome.
- Cutaneous haemorrhage of acute pancreatitis – 'bruising' of the left flank (Grey Turner's sign) or umbilicus (Cullen's sign).

What is relationship between venous thromboembolism and cancer?
Cancer risk is increased in patients with venous thromboembolism. A recent study reported a dichotomous pattern of risk with time (*Lancet* 1998; **351**: 1077–80). These investigators found that in the first year after admission for venous thromboembolism there was a four-fold increase over rates in the general population, particularly for cancers of the brain, liver, pancreas, ovary, and Hodgkin's disease and polycythaemia vera. This study also reported that thromboembolism was a marker of long-term risk of cancer: there was a 30% increased overall incidence of malignancy over a 10-year period. Another study reported that cancer diagnosed at the

same time as or within one year of an episode of venous thromboembolism is associated with advanced stage and poor prognosis (*N Engl J Med* 2000; **343:** 1846–50). Yet another study reported that the risk of newly diagnosed cancer after a first episode of venous thromboembolism is elevated during at least the following two years. Subsequently, the risk seems to be lower among patients treated with oral anticoagulants for six months than those treated for six weeks (*N Engl J Med* 2000; **342:** 1953–8).

Armand Trousseau (1801–1867), physician at the Hôtel-Dieu in Paris, noted the sign as his death warrant, confirming his suspicion of an underlying malignancy in 1865. (Trousseau A 1872 Phlegmasia albia dolens. In: *Lectures on clinical medicine, delivered at the Hôtel-Dieu, Paris*, pp. 281–295. London: New Wydenham Society).

G. Grey Turner (1877–1951), Professor of Surgery, Hammersmith Hospital, London.

T.S. Cullen (1868–1953), Canadian born, Professor of Gynaecology, Johns Hopkins Hospital, Baltimore, USA.

Case 159

ERYTHEMA MULTIFORME

INSTRUCTION

Perform a general examination.

SALIENT FEATURES

History

- History of preceding sore throat or cold.
- Drug history (barbiturates, sulphonamides, phenytoin, penicillins).
- Blister-like skin rash with intense itching.
- Mouth ulcers (mucosal involvement suggests Stevens–Johnson syndrome).

Examination

- Target-shaped lesions (Fig. 17), usually over the limbs. A classical target lesion consists of three concentric zones of colour change – typically there is a central, dark, purple area or blister surrounded by a pale, oedematous round zone which in turn is surrounded by a peripheral rim of erythema.
- Pleomorphic eruption with macules, papules and bullae.

Proceed as follows:
- Look at the mucous membranes of the mouth and eyes (Stevens–Johnson syndrome).
- Tell the examiner that you would like to examine the external genitalia for ulcers.

Note. Erythema multiforme is a cell-mediated hypersensitivity reaction to many different immunological insults, including drugs and infectious agents such as

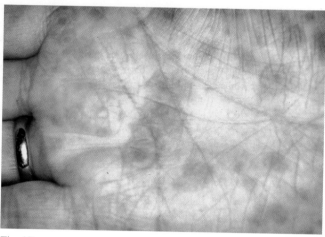

Fig. 17

viruses (most notably herpes simplex). In its so-called 'minor' form, it is manifested by heterogeneous cutaneous eruption, at times bullous.

DIAGNOSIS

This patient has target-shaped lesions (lesion) due to sulphonamides (aetiology) which usually resolve on discontinuing the drug (functional status).

QUESTIONS

What is the underlying aetiology?
- Infections (herpes simplex, mycoplasma, streptococci).
- Drug hypersensitivity (sulphonamides, penicillin, barbiturates, salicylates, antimalarials).
- Collagen vascular disorder (SLE, dermatomyositis, periarteritis nodosa).
- Malignancy (carcinomas and lymphomas).
- Multiple myeloma.
- Idiopathic – in 50% of cases no cause may be found.

ADVANCED-LEVEL QUESTIONS

How would you investigate this patient?
- Viral titres, in particular for herpes simplex type 1.
- Complement fixation test for mycoplasma.
- Antistreptolysin O (ASO) titres.

If the above are negative:

- Serum(s) antibodies.
- Protein electrophoresis, urine for Bence-Jones protein.

What is the histology of erythema multiforme?

- Early lesions: superficial perivascular lymphocytic infiltrate with oedema of the dermis, accompanied by degeneration and necrosis of keratinocytes and margination of lymphocytes at the dermoepidermal junction.
- Late lesions: upward migration of lymphocytes into the epidermis; discrete and confluent portions of the epidermis necrose resulting in blister formation and subsequently erosions (due to sloughing of the epidermis).
- Target lesions: characterized by central necrosis surrounded by perivenular inflammation.

What do you understand by the term 'Stevens–Johnson syndrome'?

Stevens–Johnson syndrome, also referred to as erythema multiforme major, is characterized by fever and mucous membrane involvement (usually oral cavity, eye and genital) in addition to the eruptions of erythema multiforme.

How would you manage a patient with erythema multiforme and Stevens–Johnson syndrome?

- Symptomatic treatment with antipyretics, intravenous fluids and antibiotics.
- Systemic corticosteroids, although the role of steroids is controversial.
- Other immunosuppressive drugs used in recurrent erythema multiforme and Stevens–Johnson syndrome include levamisole, azathioprine, dapsone, thalidomide, high-dose intravenous immunoglobulin and ciclosporin.
- Aciclovir is recommended by some authors as a therapeutic trial in any patient with severe recurrent erythema multiforme, even if no preceding herpes simplex infection has been documented.
- Other therapeutic options:
  - Localized care including use of antibiotic creams, ointments, sterile dressings, special beds containing beads, amnion dressings on denuded skin.
  - Ophthalmological care includes use of artificial tears and topical vitamin A.
  - Extensive denudation of the skin is best treated in a burns unit.

Erythema multiforme is a self-limiting condition, but Stevens–Johnson syndrome may be fatal.

F.C. Johnson (1894–1934) and A.M. Stevens (1884–1945), both American paediatricians, described this condition in 1922 in a paper entitled *A new eruptive fever with tonsillitis and ophthalmia* (*Am J Dis Child* 1922; **24**: 526–33).

H. Bence-Jones (1814–1873), English physician, St George's Hospital, London.

Case 160

ERYTHEMA AB IGNE

INSTRUCTION

Examine this patient's legs.
Examine this patient's abdomen.

SALIENT FEATURES

History

Ask the patient whether she exposed the affected area to heat.

Examination

Reticular erythematous or pigmented rash, usually on the forelegs (or abdomen), known as 'Granny's tartan' (Fig. 18).

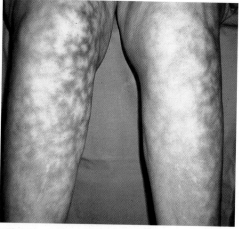

Fig. 18

Proceed as follows:
- Look for features of hypothyroidism (pulse, ankle jerks).
- Tell the examiner that you would like to proceed as follows:
  - Measure T_4 and thyroid-stimulating hormone (TSH) levels.
  - Investigate for chronic pancreatitis and intra-abdominal malignancy.

Note. If the rash is present over the anterior abdominal wall or lumbar region, it is very likely that there is an intra-abdominal malignancy or chronic pancreatitis (*Lancet* 1997; **350:** 1379–85; *J R Soc Med* 1984; **77:** 299–31).

DIAGNOSIS

This patient has a reticular pigmented rash (lesion) on the abdomen due to local heat from a hot-water bottle (aetiology); I would like to exclude an underlying intra-abdominal malignancy.

ADVANCED-LEVEL QUESTIONS

What do you know about erythema ab igne?

It is dusky discolouration of the skin which is associated with repeated exposure to heat. Typically the heat is not painful (<45°) and does not burn the skin but produces a net-like reticulated pigmentation. It is usually found on the front of the lower legs of the elderly who sit in front of open fireplaces or on the abdomen or back of patients with chronic conditions who seek relief of pain by the long-term application of hot-water bottles or heating pads (*Lancet* 1998; **351:** 677).

How may erythema ab igne be complicated?

Epitheliomas may develop in keratoses, which form in later stages of this condition.

What other reticulated rashes do you know of?

- Livedo reticularis (Fig. 19), seen in the following conditions:
  - Polyarteritis nodosa.
  - SLE.
  - Occult malignant neoplasm.
  - Atherosclerotic microemboli to the skin.
  - Physiological in young women (it is most apparent on the thighs of young females playing outdoor sports on a cold day).
- Cutis marmorata, seen in children.

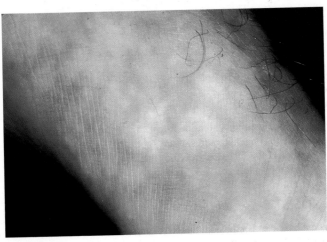

Fig. 19

Mention some skin abnormalities related to heat or cold.
- Erythema ab igne.
- Livedo reticularis (due to cold in young women).
- Raynaud's phenomenon.
- Chilblains.

Case 161

HIRSUTISM

INSTRUCTION

Examine this patient.

SALIENT FEATURES

History

- Age of onset.
- Rate of progression of hirsutism.
- History of thinning of scalp hair, or deepening of voice.
- History of obesity.
- Drug history (corticosteroids, androgens, phenytoin, minoxidil, diazoxide, ciclosporin).
- Take a menstrual history – oligomenorrhoea, infertility, acne, seborrhoea, voice change suggest polycystic ovaries.
- Family history (familial).

Examination

Excessive hair growth, particularly over the face (Fig. 20) and upper and lower limbs.

Proceed as follows:
Tell the examiner that you would like to:

- Check the blood pressure and urine for sugar.
- Comment on cushingoid features, if any.
- Look for signs of virilization (receding hairline, muscular development, breast atrophy, clitoromegaly).

DIAGNOSIS

This patient has hirsutism (lesion) due to polycystic ovarian disease (aetiology) that is cosmetically unacceptable (functional status).

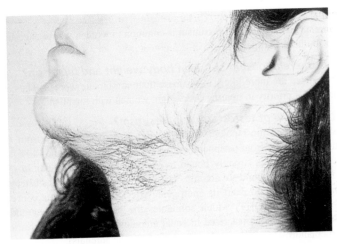

Fig. 20

Read reviews: *N Engl J Med* 1994; **331**: 1015; *BMJ* 1990; **301**: 619; *N Engl J Med* 1995; **333**: 853–61.

QUESTIONS

What do you understand by the term 'hirsutism'?
Hirsutism is the male pattern of hair growth in women and consists of excessive *terminal* hair (androgen-sensitive hair). It is abnormal, particularly on the chin, sternum, upper abdomen and upper back in women. Terminal hair may normally occur on the arms, legs, upper lip, linea alba and periareolar area in women. The degree of hirsutism can be assessed by the Ferriman–Gallwey Score, a simple, semiquantitative method of recording distribution and severity of excess body hair (*J Clin Endocrinol Metab* 1961; **21**: 1440–7).

Why do you want to take a menstrual history?
If menstruation is normal, it indicates that there is no increase in testosterone production. However, if menstruation is abnormal, the commonest cause is polycystic ovary disease (POCD or Stein–Leventhal syndrome), which is the underlying cause in 92% of women with hirsutism (the popular belief that most cases of hirsutism are idiopathic is incorrect).

ADVANCED-LEVEL QUESTIONS

What other causes of hirsutism can you tell us?
- Cushing's syndrome.
- Adrenal or ovarian tumours.
- Acromegaly.
- Drugs:
  – Those that increase *vellus* growth: phenytoin, minoxidil, diazoxide, ciclosporin.
  – Those that increase *terminal* hair growth: androgens.

- Familial.
- Ethnic: a 'male-pattern' of hirsutism is common in women whose ancestors hail from southern Europe.

What is the relationship between body weight and hirsutism?

Hirsute women are more likely to be obese than non-hirsute women. Thus, weight loss must be a priority in treating overweight women with hirsutism.

What is the role of testosterone in hirsutism?

Testosterone is the most potent androgen and is derived directly from ovarian secretion (60%) and from peripheral conversion of androstenedione (40%). About 65% of testosterone is strongly bound to sex hormone-binding globulin (SHBG) and 33% is weakly bound to albumin. The remaining 2% is free testosterone and can enter target cells to exert its androgenic effect. In the skin it is converted to dihydrotestosterone (DHT) which stimulates the hair follicle. Other androgens include androstenedione (secreted in equal amounts by adrenals and ovaries) and dehydroepiandrosterone (derived exclusively from the adrenals).

What is the pathophysiology of POCD?

It is due to an abnormality of pulsatile secretion of gonadotrophin-releasing hormone (GnRH) causing increased luteinizing hormone (LH) and follicle-stimulating hormone (FSH) secretion. This results in hyperplasia of the ovarian thecal cell leading to multiple follicular cysts and excessive androgen synthesis and anovulation. (Remember that POCD is the association of hyperandrogenism with chronic anovulation in women without specific underlying diseases of adrenals or pituitary glands.)

How would you investigate a patient with suspected POCD?

- Ovarian ultrasonography is the most accurate investigation; typically it shows thickened capsules, multiple 3–5 mm cysts and a hyperechogenic stroma.
- Biochemistry:
  - Total testosterone levels may be normal, but free androgens are raised.
  - Sex hormone-binding globulin (SHBG) level is low.
  - LH:FSH ratio is raised, usually greater than 2:1, but FSH level is low or normal.
  - Mild hyperprolactinaemia is common and rarely exceeds 1500 mU/l.

Is glucose metabolism affected in POCD?

POCD is associated with hyperinsulinaemia and insulin resistance, and consequently patients may have impaired glucose tolerance. The site of insulin resistance in these patients is skeletal muscle and fatty tissue but not hepatic resistance (the latter being a feature of non-insulin-dependent diabetes mellitus). It is believed that full expression of polycystic ovary disease requires the interaction of insulin abnormality with an underlying disorder of androgen biosynthesis, and that an abnormality of insulin alone is unlikely to cause hyperandrogenism.

How would you treat hirsutism?

- Treatment is directed towards the underlying cause of hyperandrogenism.
- Mild hyperandrogenism which is idiopathic or mild POCD: oral contraceptives.
- Severe hirsutism: antiandrogens (spironolactone, cyproterone acetate, flutamide), finasteride (5α-reductase inhibitor) prevent the cutaneous conversion of testosterone to active dihydrotestosterone, GnRH analogues (leuprolide, nafarelin).

- Local treatment: shaving, epilation, laser-assisted epilation (phototricholysis), waxing, electrolysis or bleaching.

I.F. Stein (1887–), a US gynaecologist and M.L. Leventhal (1901–1971), a US obstetrician (Stein IF, Leventhal ML 1935 Amenorrhea associated with bilateral polycystic ovaries. *Am J Obstet Gynecol* **29**: 181–91).

Case 162

ACANTHOSIS NIGRICANS

INSTRUCTION

Perform a general examination.

SALIENT FEATURES

History

- Age (>40 years of age, more likely to be associated with malignancy; more likely to be associated with endocrinopathies in younger individuals).
- Diabetes.
- Carcinoma of the stomach or other neoplasms (in 80% of cases the cancer is abdominal and in 60% of cases the cancer is in the stomach) – symptoms of weight loss, asthenia and decreased appetite.
- Diabetes mellitus (insulin resistant diabetes).
- Endocrinopathies: acromegaly, Cushing's disease, polycystic ovaries, hypothyroidism, hyperthyroidism.

Examination

Black, velvety overgrowth seen in the axillae (Fig. 21), neck, umbilicus, nipples, groin or facial skin.

Proceed as follows:

- Look for the following signs:
  - Tripe palms (roughness of the palmar and plantar skin).
  - Filiform growths around the face and mouth and over the tongue (when mouth and tongue are involved it is highly suggestive of an underlying neoplasm).
- Tell the examiner that you would like to investigate for underlying malignancy, in particular adenocarcinoma of the stomach and for endocrine disorders (diabetes, Cushing's syndrome, acromegaly).
- Comment if the patient is obese or non-obese (when pigmented verrucous areas develop in the body folds of non-obese individuals about 80–90% have an underlying gastric cancer).

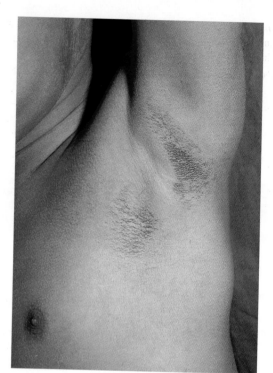

Fig. 21

DIAGNOSIS

This patient has a velvety black overgrowth in the axillae (lesion) and I would like to exclude an underlying adenocarcinoma, particularly of the stomach (aetiology).

Read: *Int J Dermatol* 1976; **15:** 592; *N Engl J Med* 1987; **317:** 1582.

ADVANCED-LEVEL QUESTIONS

What is the histology of acanthosis nigricans?

- Undulating epidermis with numerous sharp peaks and valleys.
- Variable amount of hyperplasia, hyperkeratosis and slight pigmentation of the basal cell layer (but no melanocytic hyperplasia).

With which conditions is acanthosis nigricans associated?

Benign conditions

- Diabetes associated with marked insulin resistance.
- Cushing's syndrome.
- Acromegaly.
- Stein–Leventhal syndrome.

Malignant conditions (due to abnormal production of epidermal growth factors)
- Adenocarcinomas (usually stomach, gastrointestinal tract, and uterus; less commonly lung, ovary, breast and prostate).
- Lymphomas (rarely).

What is the relationship between the course of the skin lesion and the underlying malignancy?

The acanthosis nigricans may precede the neoplasm by more than 5 years. In about two thirds of cases the course parallels that of the tumour, including remission with cure.

Mention some cutaneous manifestations of visceral malignancy.

- Dermatomyositis (in individuals older than 40 years the prevalence of internal malignancy, particularly lung and breast cancer, is increased).
- Migratory thrombophlebitis.
- Ichthyosis (when acquired suggests gastrointestinal leiomyosarcoma, lymphoma, multiple myeloma).
- Paget's disease of the nipple.
- Tylosis or palmar hyperkeratosis (suggests oesophageal cancer).
- Leser–Trélat sign, which is the sudden appearance of multiple seborrhoeic keratoses and suggests underlying cancer in the elderly.
- Necrotic migratory erythema suggests alpha-cell tumours of the pancreas secreting glucagons.
- Bazex's syndrome or acrokeratosis paraneoplastica suggests malignancy of the upper respiratory tract, particularly squamous cell carcinomas of the mouth, pharynx, larynx, oesophagus and bronchus.
- Lymphomatoid papulosis is cutaneous lymphoid infiltration associated with T-cell lymphomas or Hodgkin's disease.

Acanthosis is hyperplasia of the stratum spinosum of the epidermis.

Case 163

LIPOATROPHY

INSTRUCTION

Look at this patient.
Look here (the examiner pointing at the patient's thighs).

SALIENT FEATURES

History

- Whether the patient is taking insulin for diabetes.
- Past history of renal disease (mesangiocapillary glomerulonephritis).
- History of HIV and whether patient is receiving antiretroviral agents.

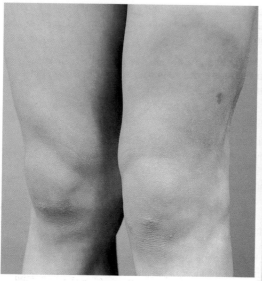

Fig. 22

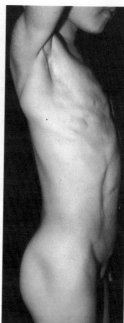

Fig. 23

Examination

Atrophy of the subcutaneous fat leading to disfiguring excavations and depressed areas (Figs 22 and 23).

DIAGNOSIS

This patient has atrophy of subcutaneous fat or lipoatrophy (lesion) due to local injection of subcutaneous insulin (aetiology).

ADVANCED-LEVEL QUESTIONS

With which conditions is lipoatrophy associated?
- Mesangiocapillary glomerulonephritis.
- Localized scleroderma.
- Morphoea.
- Chronic relapsing panniculitis.
- HIV.

What advice would you give this patient on insulin?
The insulin should be changed to a more purified form. The purified form should be injected directly into the atrophic area, which often results in the restoration of the local contours.

What is the mechanism of lipoatrophy atrophy?
This complication results from an immune reaction.

Can lipohypertrophy occur with insulin injections?

Yes, as a consequence of the pharmacological effects of insulin being repeatedly deposited in the same location. Rotation of injection sites can prevent this complication. It can occur with purified insulins and responds best to liposuction.

What is the relationship between lipoatrophy and HIV?

Patients infected with HIV-1 receiving antiretroviral therapy have been reported to have abnormal fat distribution including (a) lipoatrophy or loss of subcutaneous fat, and (b) central or visceral fat accumulation. Typically these patients have wasting of face and limbs along with adipose tissue accumulations in the abdomen and back of the neck, the latter giving a 'buffalo hump' appearance. It was initially considered to be caused only by HIV-1 protease inhibitors but subsequently has been found in patients who have never received these agents and, moreover, there is no reversion of the lipodystrophy following withdrawal of protease inhibitors. More recently, lipoatrophy has been associated with nucleoside reverse transcriptase inhibitors (NRTIs) and is said to be due to interference with lipid metabolism and the mitochondrial toxicity of these agents (*Lancet* 2001; **357**: 592–8).

The 1923 Nobel Prize in Medicine was awarded for the discovery of insulin to a Canadian surgeon, Sir Fredrick G. Banting (1891–1941) and Scottish physiologist, John J.R. Macleod (1876–1935) working in Toronto. Banting shared his monetary prize with Charles Best whereas Macleod shared his prize with J.J. Collip (the latter purified insulin to the point that it could be used in humans). Macleod corrected Banting's deficiencies on carbohydrate metabolism and provided him with laboratory support including the services of a graduate student in physiology, viz. Charles Best. Macleod was from Aberdeen.

Case 164

LUPUS PERNIO

INSTRUCTION

Look at this patient's face.

SALIENT FEATURES

History

- Shortness of breath, cough, chest discomfort.
- Fatigue, weight loss, malaise, anorexia.

Examination

Reddish blue or violaceous plaques on the nose (Fig. 24), cheeks, ears and fingers, with telangiectasia over and around the plaques (Fig. 25).

Proceed as follows:

Tell the examiner that you would like to do radiography for hilar adenopathy.

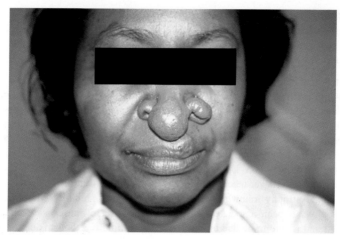

Fig. 24

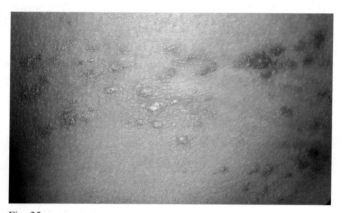

Fig. 25

DIAGNOSIS

This patient has violaceous plaques on his face (lesion) due to sarcoidosis (aetiology) which are cosmetically disfiguring (functional status). (James DG & Jones Williams W 1984 *Sarcoidosis and other Graulomatous Disorders*. Philadelphia: WB Saunders.)

ADVANCED-LEVEL QUESTIONS

What is the differential diagnosis of such a lesion?

- Rhinophyma (see Fig. 36, p. 455).
- Lupus vulgaris.
- Leprosy.

What are the cutaneous manifestations of sarcoid?
- Erythema nodosum (see Fig. 48, p. 480).
- Micropapular sarcoid (Fig. 25).
- Scar infiltration.
- Sarcoid plaques of limbs, shoulders, buttocks and thighs.

How may sarcoid present?
- Acute sarcoidosis usually presents in the third decade, characterized by erythema nodosum, parotid enlargement and hilar lymphadenopathy.
- Chronic sarcoidosis usually presents in the fifth decade with an insidious onset characterized by fatigue, dyspnoea, arthralgia and lupus pernio. Bone cysts are another feature.

How would you investigate such a patient?
- FBC and ESR (leukopenia, eosinophilia and raised ESR).
- CXR. There are three stages of sarcoidosis depending on the radiographic findings: Stage I, bilateral hilar adenopathy alone; Stage II, both hilar adenopathy and lung parenchymal involvement; Stage III, parenchymal involvement alone.
- Slit-lamp examination of the eyes.
- Kviem's test (the antigen is cultured in human spleen and thus, increasingly, it is recommended that this test should not be performed because of the risk of transmitting viral infections).
- Mantoux test (skin anergy is present in 70%).
- Serum angiotensin-converting enzyme levels (raised in 40–80% with active disease, although this finding is neither sensitive nor specific enough to have diagnostic significance).
- Lung function tests (usually restrictive changes with decreased lung volumes and diffusing capacity; occasionally airflow obstruction).
- Serum calcium levels (hypercalcaemia in 10% of patients).
- Gallium-67 scan.
- Bronchoalveolar lavage (usually characterized by an increase in lymphocytes and a high CD4:CD8 ratio).
- Histological confirmation: transbronchial lung biopsy; biopsy of lymph node, skin, liver, gums and minor salivary glands (presence of non-caseating granulomas with typical manifestations is generally required for diagnosis of sarcoidosis; fibrotic response develops over time).

What is the prognosis and treatment of sarcoidosis?
- Acute sarcoidosis usually regresses spontaneously within 2 years and does not recur; it may not require treatment.
- Chronic sarcoidosis may require systemic cortiocosteroids in order to prevent serious disability and even death from respiratory failure.

What is the treatment of cutaneous sarcoid?
Monthly intralesional triamcinolone injections, topical and systemic steroids, hydroxychloroquine, allopurinol, thalidomide, and tranilast (*N Engl J Med* 1997; **336**: 1224–34).

What are the specific indications for systemic steroids in sarcoidosis?
- Progressive deterioration in lung function, particularly transfer factor and vital capacity. Serial evaluation should be performed every 2 months initially, gradually

increasing the intervals between follow-up to about 4–5 months; patients should be followed for at least 2 years after steroids are stopped.
- CNS involvement.
- Hypercalcaemia.
- Severe ocular disease.
- Hepatitis.
- Cutaneous lesions.
- Constitutional symptoms.
- Symptomatic pulmonary lesions.

What are the ocular manifestations of sarcoidosis?
- Anterior uveitis, seen in about 5% of all cases:
  - Acute.
  - Chronic – mutton fat keratic precipitates, iris nodules.
- Retinal vasculitis, neovascularization (*Br J Ophthalmol* 1981; **65**: 348–58).
- Vitreous opacities.
- Choroidal granulomata.
- Optic nerve granuloma.

What is Löfgren's syndrome?
Erythema nodosum, hilar adenopathy and polyarthralgias in a patient with sarcoidosis.

What is the source of the raised angiotensin-converting enzyme level in sarcoidosis?
It is derived from the cell membranes of epithelioid cells in the sarcoid granuloma and its synthesis is controlled by epithelioid cells.

What is Blau's syndrome?
It is a multisystem granulomatous disorder of the skin, eyes and joints that resembles childhood sarcoidosis. It was described by Edward Blau, a Wisconsin paediatrician (*Lancet* 1999; **354**: 1035).

Is there any relationship between viral infections and sarcoid?
Variant human herpes virus-8 DNA sequences have been found in sarcoid tissue. Also, 16s ribosomal RNA genes of mycobacteria are more frequently found in sarcoid tissue but this does not indicate infection by a particular mycobacteria species (*Lancet* 1997; **350**: 655–61).

M.A. Kviem (b. 1892), a Norwegian pathologist.

C.P.M. Boeck (1845–1917), Professor of Medicine and dermatologist in Oslo, Norway, first described the disease as 'multiple benign sarcoid'.

S. Löfgren, a Swedish physician.

D. Geraint James, contemporary Professor of Medicine, Royal Free Hospital, London; his chief interest is sarcoidosis. His wife, Dame Sheila Sherlock, is a renowned hepatologist.

C. Mantoux (1877–1947), a French physician from Cannes, who showed that his intradermal test was more sensitive than the older Pirquet subcutaneous tests using tuberculin.

James DG & Jones Williams W (1984) *Sarcoidosis and other Granulomatous Disorders*. Philadelphia: WB Saunders.

Case 165

XANTHELASMA

INSTRUCTION

Examine this patient's eyes.

SALIENT FEATURES

History

- Jaundice, generalized pigmentation, itching (primary biliary cirrhosis).
- Family history of hyperlipidaemia.
- History of diabetes, hypertension.
- Symptoms of hypothyroidism (see pp 362–3).
- History of oral contraceptives.

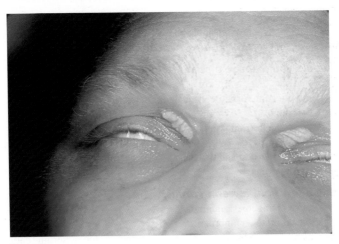

Fig. 26

Examination

Xanthelasmata (flat yellow nodules or plaques) seen on eyelids and around both eyes, particularly on the inner canthus (Fig. 26).

Proceed as follows:

- Look for the following signs:
  - Corneal arcus.
  - Jaundice, generalized pigmentation, scratch marks (primary biliary cirrhosis).
  - Tendon xanthomata.
  - Palmar xanthomata.

- Tell the examiner that you would like to check the following:
  - Urine sugar.
  - Blood pressure.
  - Pulse and ankle jerks (hypothyroidism).

Remember. Blood lipids can often be normal.

DIAGNOSIS

This patient has xanthelasmata on the eyelids (lesions) and I would like to test serum lipids to exclude an underlying lipid disorder (aetiology).

ADVANCED-LEVEL QUESTIONS

In which conditions are xanthelasmata seen?
Those in which there is an increase in serum cholesterol:

- Type IIb hyperlipidaemia – increased cholesterol and triglycerides.
- Type IIa hyperlipidaemia – increased cholesterol only.
- Type III hyperlipidaemia – equal increase in cholesterol and triglycerides.

Mention a few secondary causes of hyperlipidaemia.
Diabetes mellitus, hypothyroidism, nephrotic syndrome, cholestatic jaundice, excess alcohol intake, oral contraceptives.

How would you manage a patient with hyperlipidaemia?
- Lifestyle advice.
- Dietary modification (usually adequate for those whose cholesterol level is in the range 6.5–8 mmol/l).
- Avoidance of alcohol, smoking, oestrogens and thiazides.
- Exercise.
- Control of hypertension and diabetes.
- Lipid-lowering drugs.

Mention a few lipid-lowering drugs.
- Ion exchange resin: colestyramine.
- Fibrates: bezafibrate, gemfibrozil.
- Sitostanol-ester margarine (a plant sterol that reduces serum cholesterol concentration by inhibiting cholesterol absorption).
- Hydroxymethylglutaryl (HMG) coenzyme A (CoA) reductase inhibitors: simvastatin, pravastatin, lovastatin. These drugs block the endogenous synthesis of cholesterol and reduce levels of low-density lipoprotein cholesterol.
- Nicotinic acid derivatives: nicotinic acid, probucol.

Are HMG CoA reductase inhibitors useful in patients with hypercholesterolaemia and coronary heart disease?
Yes, the Scandinavian Simvastatin Survival Study (the 4S trial) demonstrated a survival benefit from lowering cholesterol with simvastatin in patients with coronary disease (*Lancet* 1994; **344**: 1383–9). In the LIPID study (Long-Term Intervention with Pravastatin in Ischemic Heart Disease), a major secondary prevention trial, pravastatin administered to 9000 patients with unstable angina or acute myocardial

infarction significantly reduced total mortality by 23%, coronary heart disease mortality by 24%, the need for coronary revascularization, the number of admissions to hospitals (*Lancet* 2000; **355**: 1871–5) and the risk of stroke by 20% (*N Engl J Med* 2000; **343**: 317–26). The Lescol in Severe Atherosclerosis (LISA) study evaluated fluvastatin in patients with coronary artery disease and hypercholesterolaemia and found that it reduced cardiac events by 71%.

What is the role of HMG CoA reductase inhibitors in patients with hypercholesterolaemia and no signs of coronary heart disease?

A recent study from Scotland showed that treatment with pravastatin significantly reduced the incidence of myocardial infarction (30% reduction) and death from cardiovascular causes (33% reduction) without adversely affecting the risk of death from non-cardiovascular causes in men with moderate hypercholesterolaemia and without a history of myocardial infarction (*N Engl J Med* 1995; **333**: 1301–7).

What is the role of HMG CoA reductase inhibitors in patients with coronary artery disease and 'average' cholesterol levels?

The CARE study (Cholesterol and Recurrent Events Trials Investigators) found that pravastatin lowered rates of coronary events (including fatal events and non-fatal myocardial infarction) in the majority of the patients with coronary disease who have average cholesterol levels (*N Engl J Med* 1996; **335**: 1001–9).

What is the effect of statins on elevated triglyceride concentrations?

Serum triglyceride concentrations are reduced by all statins, with atovastatin and simvastatin having the greatest effect. The higher the baseline concentration of triglycerides, the greater is the reduction induced by statin therapy.

Mention some adverse effects of statins.

- Common: gastrointestinal upset, myalgias and hepatitis.
- Rare: rash, myopathy, peripheral neuropathy, insomnia, bad dreams, difficulty in sleeping or concentrating.

What is the effect of meals on statin absorption?

Lovastatin is better absorbed when taken with food whereas pravastatin is best taken on an empty stomach or at bed time. Food has less of an effect on the absorption of other statins.

Why are all statins best given in the evening?

Because the rate of endogenous cholesterol synthesis is higher at night.

A patient with hypercholesterolaemia on treatment with statins requires further lowering of LDL cholesterol. If the patient's serum HDL is low, what is the preferred second drug you would choose to add to the patient's antilipid regimen?

Nicotinic acid is the preferred second drug. Nicotinic acid usually increases serum HDL concentrations by 30%, fibrates by 10–15%, statins by 5–10% and bile acid resins by 1–2% (*N Engl J Med* 1999; **341**: 498–511).

James Scott, FRS contemporary Professor and Chairman of the Department of Medicine at Hammersmith Hospital, London, is a physician, biochemist and molecular biologist. He has made a considerable contribution to lipid and cardiovascular research.

Case 166

NECROBIOSIS LIPOIDICA DIABETICORUM

INSTRUCTION

Look at this patient's legs.
Examine this patient's back.

SALIENT FEATURES

History

History of diabetes (according to a recent study from Ireland only a minority of the patients have diabetes; *Br J Dermatol* 1999; **40:** 283–6).

Examination

- Usually seen in females (two to four times more frequently than in men).
- Sharply demarcated oval plaques seen on the shin (Fig. 27), arms or back.
- The plaques have a shiny surface with yellow waxy atrophic centres and brownish red margins with surrounding telangiectasia.

Proceed as follows:
Tell the examiner that you would like to check the urine for sugar.

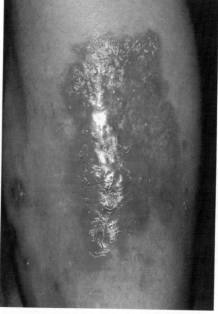

Fig. 27

DIAGNOSIS

This patient has plaques with yellow waxy centres on the shins (lesions) due to diabetes mellitus (aetiology) which are cosmetically disfiguring (functional status).

N Engl J Med 1993; **329:** 320; a classical photograph of the lesion; candidates are encouraged to refer to this photograph.

ADVANCED-LEVEL QUESTIONS

What is the histology of these lesions?
Collagen degeneration surrounded by epithelioid and giant cells.

What may complicate the condition?
Ulceration of the plaque.

What treatment is available for such lesions?
- Good diabetic control.
- Whirlpool therapy, occlusive dressings, aspirin, pentoxifylline.
- Local steroids.
- Excision and skin grafting.
- Hyperbaric oxygen (*Diabetes Metab* 1998; **24:** 156–9).

What other skin lesions are usually seen on the shins?
- Erythema nodosum (see p. 480).
- Pretibial myxoedema (see p. 514).
- Diabetic dermopathy.
- Erythema ab igne (see pp 426–7).
- Livedo reticularis.

What are the other skin lesions seen in diabetes?
- Granuloma annulare.
- Chronic pyogenic infections and carbuncles (indicating poor control).
- Eruptive xanthomata (from hypertriglyceridaemia associated with poor glycaemic control; see pp 448–9).
- Xanthelasmata (see p. 439).
- Lipoatrophy and lipohypertrophy (see pp 433–5).
- Leg ulcers and gangrene.
- Acanthosis nigricans (see pp 431–3).
- 'Pebbles' on the dorsal aspect of the fingers (*Postgrad Med* 2000; **107:** 207–10).
- Peripheral anhidrosis (due to autonomic neuropathy).
- Vulval candidiasis.

Case 167

RADIOTHERAPY MARKS

INSTRUCTION

Look at this patient's chest.

PATIENT 1

Salient features

History
- History of breast cancer.
- Ask about chemotherapy and schedule of radiotherapy.

Examination
- Telangiectasia over the chest wall.
- There may be a unilateral mastectomy.

Diagnosis

This patient has telangiectasia and a unilateral mastectomy (lesion), indicating that she has had radiotherapy (aetiology) for breast cancer in the past.

PATIENT 2

- India ink marks over the chest (Fig. 28).
- Localized erythema in the same region.

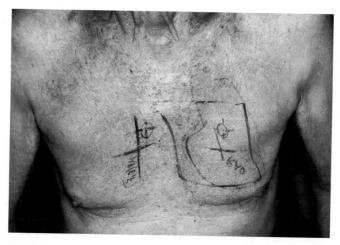

Fig. 28

Diagnosis

This patient has India ink marks over the chest with localized erythema (lesion) indicating that she is currently undergoing radiotherapy treatment (aetiology).

ADVANCED-LEVEL QUESTIONS

Which other normal tissues, apart from the skin, are affected by radiation therapy?

Tissues that exhibit early or late damage from radiation therapy include mucosa, spinal cord, bone marrow and lymphoid system. To minimize these effects, radiation is normally delivered in a fractionated manner to allow recovery of normal host tissues (but not of tumour).

What modalities may be used to minimize the side-effects of radiation?

- Fractionation of dose.
- Rendering the tumour more sensitive to radiotherapy by prior chemotherapy and thereby reducing the dose.
- Regional hyperthermia (40–42°C), particularly in superficial tumours and relatively bulky non-vascular tumours.
- Radiolabelled antibodies which deliver high levels of radiation locally to the tumour bed.

How is radiotherapy usually delivered?

It is usually delivered either as brachytherapy (where the radiation source is close to the tumour) or as teletherapy (where supervoltage radiotherapy is usually delivered with a linear accelerator).

In which conditions is radiotherapy beneficial?

Malignant conditions

- Radiotherapy as the sole agent with a curative intent: in Hodgkin's disease, some neoplasms of brain and spinal cord, oral cavity, pharynx, oesophagus, laryngeal tumours permitting cure without loss of voice, tumours of cervix and vaginal cavity.
- Radiation with surgery: in cancers of lung, breast, urinary bladder, seminomas, ovary, uterus, sarcomas of soft tissue and testicular seminomas.
- Radiation as adjuvant to chemotherapy: lymphomas, lung cancers and childhood cancers.
- Radiation as palliative therapy for pain and/or dysfunction: superior vena caval obstruction, dysphagia of terminal illness, upper airway obstruction, spinal cord compression, pericardial tamponade secondary to malignant pericardial tumours.

Non-malignant conditions

- Exophthalmos.
- Rheumatoid arthritis (total lymphoid irradiation is an experimental therapeutic procedure).
- Ankylosing spondylitis, where local external irradiation of an involved peripheral joint or injected radiation synovectomy can be valuable in ameliorating pain and allowing mobility. Spinal irradiation is no longer used because of the risk of haematological malignancy.

- Intracoronary radiation can significantly reduce restenosis rates after angioplasty (*Circulation* 2000; **101:** 360–5).

What are the side-effects of radiotherapy?

- Acute toxicity: systemic symptoms including malaise, fatigue, anorexia, nausea and vomiting; diarrhoea and local skin and mucosal changes. Bone marrow suppression may occur following irradiation to the pelvis and long bones.
- Long-term toxicity: cutaneous hyperpigmentation, impaired function of irradiated viscera, bone necrosis, myelopathy and secondary malignancies.

> The use of irradiation began shortly after the discovery of X-rays by Roentgen in 1895 (*Lancet* 1997; **349** (suppl II): 1–3).
>
> Allen Lichter is radiation oncologist and Dean of the University of Michigan School of Medicine (Lichter AS, Lawrence TS 1995 Recent advances in radiation oncology. *N Engl J Med* **332:** 371–7). He was recently nominated by the Institute of Medicine, National Academy of Sciences, USA, for his contributions which include three-dimensional treatment planning and conformal radiotherapy of cancers.

Case 168

TENDON XANTHOMATA

INSTRUCTION

Look at this patient's hands.

SALIENT FEATURES

History

- Family history of hyperlipidaemia.
- History of premature coronary artery disease.

Examination

Tendon xanthomata seen on the extensor tendons and becoming more prominent when the patient clenches his fist (Fig. 29).

Proceed as follows:

- Look at other tendons, particularly the patellar and Achilles tendon.
- Look at the eyes for xanthelasmata (see Fig. 26, p. 439) and corneal arcus.
- Tell the examiner that you would like to:
  - Check fasting lipids, in particular for an increase in cholesterol level
  - Screen family members for hypercholesterolaemia (*BMJ* 2000; **321:** 1497–500; *Lancet* 2001; **357:** 165–8).

DIAGNOSIS

This patient has tendon xanthomata (lesion) due to hypercholesterolaemia (aetiology).

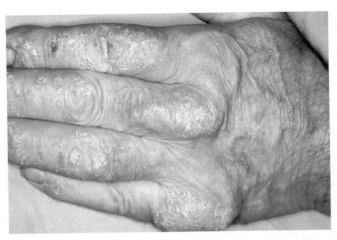

Fig. 29

QUESTIONS

In which condition are these seen?
Familial hypercholesterolaemia, an autosomal dominant trait with an excess of low-density lipoprotein (LDL) or β-lipoprotein in the blood. It occurs in 1 in 200–500 of the population.

ADVANCED-LEVEL QUESTIONS

What is the basic defect?
Goldstein and Brown, in 1975, showed that this condition was due to a defect or deficiency in LDL cell receptors.

At what age do these patients manifest the condition?
Homozygotes usually have xanthomata at birth or as children. They have a predisposition to ischaemic heart disease, which usually results in death before the age of 30 years. About 50% of heterozygotes also present by the same age.

What are xanthomata?
Xanthomata are tumour-like collections of foamy histiocytes within the dermis. There are five types of xanthoma:

- Eruptive xanthoma (seen in types I, IIb, III, IV, V).
- Tuberous xanthoma (types IIa, III, rarely IIb, IV).
- Tendon xanthoma (types IIa, III, rarely IIIb).
- Palmar xanthoma (types III, IIa, associated with primary biliary cirrhosis).
- Xanthelasma (types IIa, III; also without lipid abnormalities).

Is there any treatment for familial hypercholesterolaemia?
One view is that in these patients statin treatment should be started when boys are in their late teens and women from their late twenties. If the family history is particularly adverse, however, then there is an increasing tendency for paediatricians to commence treatment (*Lancet* 2001; **357:** 574).

Michael S. Brown (b. 1941) and Joseph L. Goldstein (b. 1940), both of the University of Texas Health Science Centre in Dallas, were awarded the 1983 Nobel Prize for their discoveries concerning the regulation of cholesterol metabolism.

Case 169

ERUPTIVE XANTHOMATA

INSTRUCTION

Examine this patient's skin.
This uncontrolled diabetic has developed a profuse eruption; what are these lesions?

SALIENT FEATURES

History

- Duration and treatment of diabetes.
- History of hyperlipidaemia.
- Rash – duration, onset and evolution and associated symptoms such as itching.

Examination

Multiple, itchy, red–yellow vesicles or nodules which are seen over extensor surfaces, i.e. buttocks, back, knees and elbows (Fig. 30).

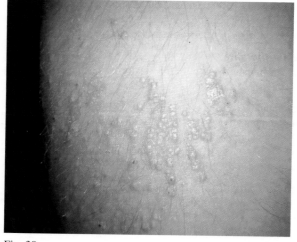

Fig. 30

Proceed as follows:
Tell the examiner that you would like to:

- Examine the fundus for lipaemia retinalis.
- Check the urine for sugar.
- Do a lipid profile (remember that eruptive xanthomata signify hyper-triglyceridaemia).

DIAGNOSIS

This patient has eruptive xanthomata (lesion) due to hypertriglyceridaemia (aetiology).

ADVANCED-LEVEL QUESTIONS

In which conditions are eruptive xanthomata seen?
- Type IV hyperlipidaemia.
  - Familial hypertriglyceridaemia.
  - Lipoprotein lipase deficiency.
  - Apolipoprotein CII deficiency.
- Type I hyperlipidaemia – chylomicronaemia.
- Type V hyperlipidaemia – increased levels of triglycerides and chylomicrons.

Mention some other causes of hypertriglyceridaemia.
- Primary hypertriglyceridaemia (usually greater than 500 mg/dl): familial hyper-triglyceridaemia, familial combined hyperlipidaemia.
- Secondary hypertriglyceridaemia: diet, obesity, excess alcohol intake, diabetes mellitus, hypothyroidism, uraemia, dysproteinaemias, drugs (beta-blockers, oral contraceptives and oestrogens, retinoids).

What is the relationship between hypertriglyceridaemia and coronary artery disease?
The relationship of hypertriglyceridaemia with coronary artery disease is less clear than that with hypercholesterolaemia, but is said to increase risk when levels are greater than 500 mg/dl, when other risk factors are present or in familial combined hyperlipidaemia.

Of what are patients particularly at risk when serum levels of triglycerides are markedly raised (>1000 mg/dl)?
They are more susceptible to acute pancreatitis and hyperchylomicronaemia.

How would you manage a patient with raised levels of serum triglycerides?
- Diet: restrict dietary fat, decrease intake of alcohol and simple sugars.
- Weight loss if the patient is overweight.
- Exercise.
- Discontinuation of drugs, e.g. beta-blockers.
- Control secondary causes.
- Niacin or gemfibrozil may be used for elevated triglycerides (>200 mg/dl) regardless of LDL or HDL cholesterol.

Case 170

PALMAR XANTHOMATA

INSTRUCTION

Examine this patient's hands.

SALIENT FEATURES

History

Family history of hyperlipidaemia and coronary artery disease.

Examination

Yellowish-orange discolorations over the palmar and digital creases.

Proceed as follows:
- Look for the following signs:
  - Xanthelasmata around the eyes.
  - Tuboeruptive xanthomata around the elbows and knees.
  - Signs of primary biliary cirrhosis (p. 310)
- Tell the examiner that this patient probably has a type III hyperlipidaemia.

Note. A more generalized form may be associated with monoclonal gammopathy of myeloma or lymphoma.

ADVANCED-LEVEL QUESTIONS

How would you classify hyperlipidaemia?

Fredrickson classification, depending on laboratory findings:

- Type I: raised levels of chylomicrons and triglycerides, normal cholesterol concentration (pancreatitis, eruptive xanthomata and lipaemia retinalis).
- Type IIa: raised LDL and cholesterol levels, normal concentration of triglycerides (premature coronary artery disease, tendon xanthomata and arcus corneae).
- Type IIb: raised levels of LDL, very low density lipoprotein (VLDL), cholesterol and triglycerides (premature coronary artery disease).
- Type III: raised β-VLDL (cholesterol-rich) remnants, cholesterol and triglycerides (premature coronary artery disease, peripheral vascular disease, palmar and tuberous xanthomata).
- Type IV: raised VLDL and triglycerides, normal cholesterol (premature coronary artery disease – in some forms, risk of developing chylomicronaemia syndrome).
- Type V: raised chylomicrons, VLDL, cholesterol and triglycerides (pancreatitis, eruptive xanthoma, lipaemia retinalis).

What are the causes of hypercholesterolaemia?

- Primary hypercholesterolaemia: familial hypercholesterolaemia, familial combined hyperlipidaemia, polygenic hypercholesterolaemia.

- Secondary hypercholesterolaemia: biliary cirrhosis, hypothyroidism, nephrotic syndrome, diet, drugs (thiazides, beta-blockers, oestrogens).

What is the histology of xanthomas?

Xanthomas are collections of foamy histiocytes within the dermis. These cells have abundant and finely vacuolated cytoplasm giving them a foamy appearance. Cholesterol (both free and esterified), triglycerides and phospholipids are present within the cell. Often the cells are surrounded by inflammatory cells and fibrosis about the central zone of lipid-laden cells.

Case 171

PSEUDOXANTHOMA ELASTICUM

PATIENT 1

Instruction

Look at this patient's fundus.

Salient features

History

- Family history (either autosomal recessive, which is most common, or autosomal dominant; the gene for both forms has been mapped to chromosome 16, *Hum Mol Genet* 1997; **6**: 1823).

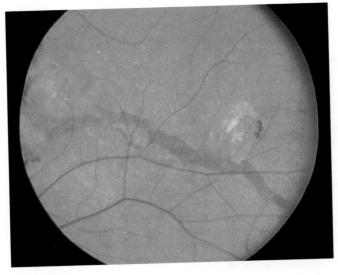

Fig. 31

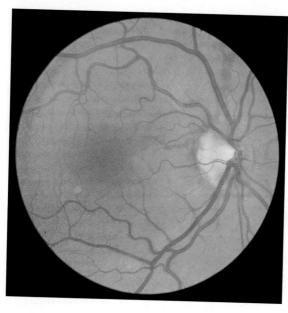

Fig. 32

- Upper gastrointestinal haemorrhage, myocardial infarction, stroke and intermittent claudication, visual loss.
- Hypertension (due to involvement of renal vasculature).

Examination

Fundus shows angioid streaks, i.e. linear grey or dark red streaks with irregular edges which lie beneath the retinal vessels (Figs 31 and 32; roughly 50% of patients with angioid streaks have pseudoxanthoma elasticum, whereas 85% of those with pseudoxanthoma have angioid streaks).

Proceed as follows:

- Look at the neck (Fig. 33), antecubital fossae, axillae (Fig. 34), groin and periumbilical region for loose 'chicken skin' appearance of skin.

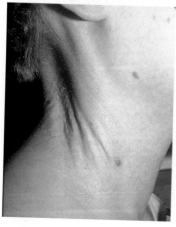

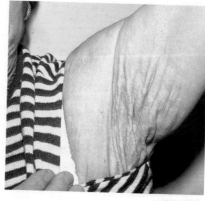

Fig. 33

Fig. 34

- Examine peripheral pulses (absent pulses due to peripheral arterial involvement but acral ischaemia is uncommon due to development of collaterals).

PATIENT 2

Instruction

Look at this patient.

Salient features

Small yellow papules arranged in a linear or reticular pattern in plaques on the neck, axillae, cubital fossae, periumbilical region and groin.

Proceed as follows:
Tell the examiner that you would like to examine the fundus.

Diagnosis

This patient has angioid streaks on fundoscopy and 'chicken-skin' appearance in the neck and axillae (lesions) due to pseudoxanthoma elasticum (aetiology).

Read: *N Engl J Med* 1993; **333**: 1240; *N Engl J Med* 1997; **337**: 828 (candidates are encouraged to refer to this picture for characteristic features of this disease).

ADVANCED-LEVEL QUESTIONS

In which other conditions are angioid streaks seen?

- Regularly seen in: Paget's disease, sickle cell disease.
- Occasionally seen in: Ehlers–Danlos syndrome, hyperphosphataemia, lead poisoning, trauma, pituitary disorders and intracranial disorders.

What are angioid streaks caused by?

They are caused by abnormal elastic tissue in the Bruch's membrane of the retina.

Which fundal finding is virtually pathognomonic of pseudoxanthoma elasticum?

'Leopard skin spotting' changes which consist of yellowish mottling of the posterior pole temporal to the macula. These may antedate angioid streaks.

What is the triad of pseudoxanthoma elasticum, angioid streaks and vascular abnormalities known as?

Groenblad–Strandberg syndrome.

What are the cardiovascular manifestations of this condition?

- Mitral valve prolapse.
- Restrictive cardiomyopathy.
- Renovascular hypertension.
- Premature coronary artery disease resembling accelerated atherosclerosis due to calcification of the internal elastic laminae of arteries. Arterial grafts should not be used for coronary artery bypass surgery in these patients because of possible calcification of the internal elastic laminae of the internal mammary artery.
- Peripheral vascular disease.

What are the gastrointestinal manifestations of this disease?

Gastrointestinal haemorrhage, particularly during the first decade. Bleeding complications can be prevented by avoiding aspirin in patients with pseudoxanthoma elasticum.

What are the causes of visual loss in pseudoxanthoma elasticum?

Macular involvement by a streak; disciform scarring secondary to choroidal haemorrhage or traumatic macular haemorrhage.

What are the cutaneous histological features of pseudoxanthoma elasticum?

The histological diagnosis is made by doing 4 mm punch biopsy of scars or flexural skin of the neck or axillae in patients who have angioid streaks on fundoscopy but no visible skin lesions. The Verhoeff–van Gieson stain (for elastic tissue) reveals characteristic fragmentation and clumping of elastic tissue in middle and deep dermis. The von Kossa stain (for calcium) shows staining of calcified elastic tissue in the middle and deep dermis. Calcified elastic tissue is the hallmark of pseudoxanthoma elasticum. An arteriolar sclerosis develops in the media of muscular arteries and arterioles and as a result the lumen may become progressively and concentrically narrowed.

K.W.L. Bruch (1819–1884), Professor of Anatomy at Giessen, Germany.

E.E. Groenblad, Swedish ophthalmologist and J. Strandberg, Swedish dermatologist.

T.L. Terry (1899–1946), Head of Ophthalmology at Harvard University, described angioid streaks in Paget's disease.

Case 172

ROSACEA

INSTRUCTION

Look at this patient.

SALIENT FEATURES

History

• Intermittent facial flushing.
• Blushing of the face by caffeine, alcohol or spicy foods.
• History of unilateral headaches (an increased incidence of migrainous headaches accompanying rosacea has been reported).

Examination

Red patch with telangiectasia, acneiform papules, and pustules overlying the flush areas of the face, i.e. cheeks, chin and nose (Fig. 35). (The papules and pustules distinguish it from the rash of SLE.)

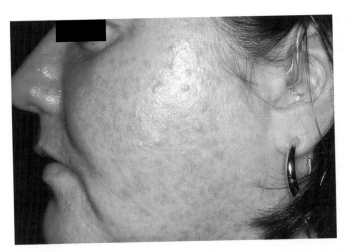

Fig. 35

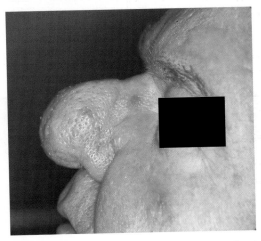

Fig. 36

Proceed as follows:

- Comment on the following:
  - Rhinophyma (Fig. 36; irregular thickening of the skin of the nose with enlarged follicular orifices).
  - Blepharitis, conjunctivitis.
- Tell the examiner that you would like to obtain an ophthalmological evaluation for chalazion and progressive keratitis which can lead to scarring and blindness.

DIAGNOSIS

This patient has a red patch on the face with papules and pustules (lesion) due to rosacea (aetiology) which is cosmetically disfiguring (functional status).

ADVANCED-LEVEL QUESTIONS

How would you distinguish rosacea from acne?

Rosacea is distinguished from acne by age (middle-aged and older people), the presence of a vascular component (i.e. rosy hue, erythema and telangiectasia) and the absence of comedones.

How would you manage such a patient?

- Avoid factors that provoke facial flushing.
- Tetracycline or metronidazole.
- Hydrocortisone cream.
- Retinoids – in resistant disease.
- Yellow light laser for telangiectasia.
- Surgical removal for rhinophyma.

What are the causes of red face in an adult?

Malar rash of SLE, heliotrope rash of dermatomyositis, seborrhoeic dermatitis and perioral dermatitis.

> It has been suggested that the painter Rembrandt had rosacea, which he depicted in his self-portrait (*Lancet* 1997; **350**: 1835–7).

Case 173

DERMATITIS HERPETIFORMIS

INSTRUCTION

Look at the skin of this patient, who in the past had chronic diarrhoea.

SALIENT FEATURES

History

- History of diarrhoea.
- History of gluten intolerance (although these patients rarely have gross malabsorption).
- Ask the patient whether the rash itches.

Examination

Dry, itchy vesicles and urticarial plaques occurring bilaterally and symmetrically over the extensor surfaces, elbows, knees, posterior neck, back and buttocks.

Proceed as follows:

Look for similar lesions on the scalp, face, neck, shoulders, buttocks, knees and calves.

DIAGNOSIS

This patient has itchy vesicles on the elbows (lesion) due to dermatitis herpetiformis (functional status).

ADVANCED-LEVEL QUESTIONS

From which other itchy skin disorder should dermatitis herpetiformis be differentiated?
Scabies.

What are the extracutaneous manifestations of dermatitis herpetiformis?
- Gluten-sensitive enteropathy (frequent, asymptomatic).
- Thyroid dysfunction (especially hypothyroidism).
- Lymphoma (especially gastrointestinal).

How would you investigate such a patient?
- Skin biopsy: fibrin and neutrophils accumulate selectively at the *tips of dermal papillae*, forming small microabscesses. Subepidermal vesicle with neutrophilic infiltrate. Immunofluorescence demonstrates granular dermal papillary immunoglobulin (Ig) A deposits.
- Circulating anti-endomysium antibodies are present in all cases.
- Jejunal biopsy: patchy abnormality showing subtotal villous atrophy with increased lymphocyte infiltration in the epithelium.
- Therapeutic test: dapsone dramatically reduces itching in 72 hours, often providing confirmation before the biopsy result is available.
- HLA-B8 and HLA-DRw3 are positive in more than 80% of patients.

How would you treat such a patient?
- Gluten restriction (*Br J Dermatol* 1994; **131:** 541).
- Dapsone or sulfapyridine – neither drug should be given to a patient with glucose-6-phosphate deficiency. Treatment is lifelong; there is usually a rapid relapse if the drug is stopped.

In which foods is gluten found?
Wheat, barley and rye (rice and maize are permitted in these patients).

Is it advisable for these patients to add oats to their gluten-free diets?
Moderate amounts of oats can be ingested without harmful effects in coeliac disease (*N Engl J Med* 1995; **333:** 1033–7; *BMJ* 1996; **313:** 1300–1) and in dermatitis herpetiformis (*N Engl J Med* 1997; **337:** 1884–7; *Gut* 1998; **43:** 490–3). Oats do not contain gliadin but have avenin. However, avenin comprises only 5–15% of the total seed protein content. Thus, even if avenin in oats were as toxic as gliadin in wheat (a fact that is not universally conceded), the ingestion of large quantities of oats would be required to bring about an equivalent effect, in terms of the amount of protein ingested.

What do you know about gluten?
Gluten is the protein component that persists following the removal of water and starch from defatted flour. Gliadin is a class of protein found in the gluten fraction

of flour. There are four gliadin fractions (α, β, γ and ω). α-Gliadin is injurious to the small intestinal mucosa, although there is some disagreement about the toxicity of other peptides. Patients with dermatitis herpetiformis develop IgA and IgG antibodies to gliadin and reticulin (the latter a component of the anchoring fibrils that tether the epidermal basement membrane to the upper dermis).

What are the benefits of a gluten-free diet?

It gradually improves skin lesions, improves any associated manifestations of malabsorptive enteropathy and may reduce the late risk of intestinal lymphoma. It also normalizes histological abnormalities. (**Note.** An elemental diet lacking protein has been reported to benefit patients with dermatitis herpetiformis even in the presence of a gluten challenge.)

Dermatitis herpetiformis was first described in 1884 by L.A. Duhring (1845–1913), Professor of Diseases of the Skin at the University of Pennsylvania. He studied dermatology in Paris, London and Vienna, and wrote the first American textbook of dermatology. Others believe that dermatitis herpetiformis was first described by F. von Hebra, who also wrote a textbook of dermatology.

Samuel J. Gee (1839–1911) of St Bartholomew's Hospital, London, provided the first thorough description of coeliac sprue in 1888 (Gee S 1888 On the coeliac affection. *St Barth Hosp Rep* **24**: 17–20). Dutch paediatrician, W.K. Dicke, astutely observed that wheat and rye were harmful in children with this disease (Dicke WK 1950 *Coeliac disease: investigation of the harmful effects of certain types of cereal on patients with coeliac disease*. Doctoral thesis, University of Utrecht, The Netherlands). Parveen Kumar, contemporary Physician, St Bartholomew's Hospital, London, has made major contributions to gastroenterology and, together with Michael Clark, also a physician at St Bartholomew's Hospital, has made a major contribution to medical education. The book entitled *Clinical Medicine*, which they edited, is the most popular medical textbook in the UK (*N Engl J Med* 1995; **333**: 1075–6).

Case 174

HAIRY LEUKOPLAKIA

INSTRUCTION

Look at this patient's tongue.

SALIENT FEATURES

History

- Usually asymptomatic.
- Patients may complain of pain or voice changes.
- Tell the examiner that you would like to know whether the patient is immunocompromised (due to HIV or immunosuppressive treatment, particularly in kidney transplant recipients).

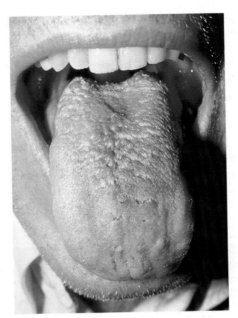

Fig. 37

Examination

Shaggy, hairy, white lesions on the lateral margins of the tongue (remember that hairy leukoplakia does not affect the vaginal or anal mucosa) (Fig. 37).

Note. Oral hairy leukoplakia may be difficult to distinguish from oral candidiasis but, in contrast to oral candidiasis, it does not rub off, does not respond to antifungal therapy and may change its appearance daily.

DIAGNOSIS

This patient has whitish hairy lesions on the lateral edges of the tongue (lesions) which is oral hairy leukoplakia caused by the Epstein–Barr virus (aetiology).

QUESTIONS

What is the cause of this lesion?

Hairy leukoplakia is caused by the Epstein–Barr virus (*N Engl J Med* 1985; **313:** 1564–71).

ADVANCED-LEVEL QUESTIONS

What is the significance of this lesion?

In HIV-seropositive subjects, usually it is a harbinger of rapid progression to AIDS. It is rarely seen in non-HIV-immunosuppressed patients.

What are the histological features of this condition?

- Hyperkeratosis.
- Hyperplasia and ballooning of prickle cells (acanthosis).
- Depletion of Langerhans' cells.

How would you treat this condition?

Treatment is seldom indicated, but ganciclovir or aciclovir may be helpful if the patient has discomfort. Podophyllin and retinoin have also been used (*Lancet* 1996; **348:** 729–33).

P. Langerhans (1847–1888), German pathologist and dermatologist.

Oral 'hairy' leukoplakia was initially reported in the Lancet in 1984 (*Lancet* 1984; ii: 831–4).

Case 175

KAPOSI'S SARCOMA

INSTRUCTION

Look at this skin lesion.

SALIENT FEATURES

History

- Determine whether the patient is immunocompromised (due to HIV or therapy following organ transplantation).
- If lesions are present in the mouth, ask the patient whether there is any difficulty in eating (the gingival margin may make oral hygiene difficult because of secondary infection and pain).

Examination

Plum-coloured violet plaques, either solitary or in crops, on the limbs, mouth, tip of the nose and palate (Figs 38 and 39).

Proceed as follows:

Tell the examiner that you would like to check HIV antibody titres (Kaposi's sarcoma has an estimated prevalence of 10–20% in HIV-positive patients and was one of the first diseases to define AIDS in 1981).

Read recent review: *N Engl J Med* 2000; **342:** 1027.

DIAGNOSIS

This patient has Kaposi's sarcoma (lesion) which has been shown to be caused by human herpes virus 8 (aetiology) in patients with AIDS.

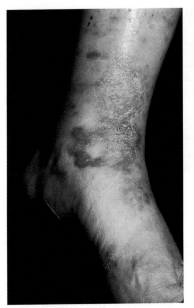

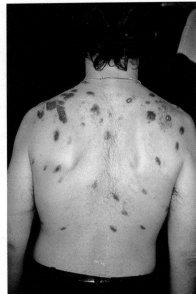

Fig. 38   Fig. 39

ADVANCED-LEVEL QUESTIONS

What are the varieties of Kaposi's sarcoma?

- Classic Kaposi's sarcoma (Fig. 40): initially described in Jews; indolent; found on the legs of elderly men; confined to the skin and may be present for decades; not fatal.
- African variety (Fig. 41): violaceous skin plaques; black under Negroid skin; an aggressive invasive tumour which is ultimately fatal. It occurs in children and

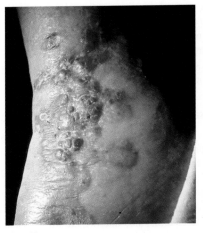

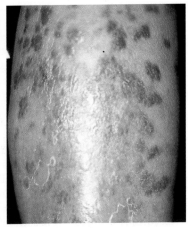

Fig. 40   Fig. 41

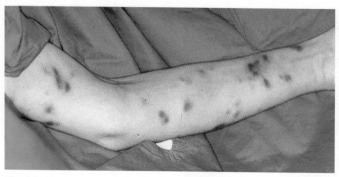

Fig. 42

younger men. In the former it is often associated with generalized lymph-adenopathy.

- AIDS-associated Kaposi's sarcoma (Fig. 42): found in approximately one third of patients with AIDS and more common in homosexuals. The cutaneous lesions respond to α-interferon and cytotoxic chemotherapy. About one third develop a second malignancy such as lymphoma, myeloma or leukaemia. Patients eventually die from secondary infection seen in AIDS rather than as a direct consequence of Kaposi's sarcoma.

- Transplantation-associated Kaposi's sarcoma, particularly in patients on high-dose immunosuppressive therapy; the lesions often regress when therapy is stopped. Transmission of human herpes virus 8 infection occurs from renal transplant donors to recipients and is a risk factor for Kaposi's sarcoma (*N Engl J Med* 1998; **339:** 1358–63).

What is the aetiology of Kaposi's sarcoma?

The aetiology is not known but epidemiological data support a viral infection (*N Engl J Med* 1995; **332:** 1181–5; *N Engl J Med* 1998; **332:** 1186–91). Recent reports indicate a herpes-like virus (human herpes virus 8, HHV08). This new agent has been detected in all forms of Kaposi's sarcoma. Between 70% and 100% of patients with Kaposi's sarcoma have antibodies to human herpes virus 8 (compared with 1–5% of the general population). Seroconversion may occur several months before the appearance of Kaposi's sarcoma.

What is the histology of Kaposi's sarcoma?

Histologically, all varieties are similar.

- The early or 'patch' stage: similar to granulation tissue and characterized by jagged, thin-walled, dilated vascular spaces in the epidermis with interstitial inflammatory cells and extravasated red cells (with haemosiderin deposition).

- Later or 'nodular' lesions: features are more characteristic at this stage and comprise spindle-shaped stromal cells with irregular slit-like spaces filled with red blood cells and lined by recognizable endothelium, intertwined with normal vascular channels.

Is there any difference in the prognosis of AIDS depending on whether the patient has oral or cutaneous Kaposi's sarcoma?

It has been reported that there is a greater mortality risk with oral as compared with cutaneous Kaposi's sarcoma, independent of the CD4 count (*Lancet* 2000; **356:** 2160).

How would you manage Kaposi's sarcoma in patients with HIV infection?

* Baseline treatment includes an antiretroviral agent such as zidovudine, which has no direct effect on Kaposi's sarcoma but diminishes the degree of immuno-suppression. Retinoic acid is a promising alternative.
* Localized mucocutaneous lesions respond well to radiotherapy, cryotherapy, surgical excision, intralesional vinblastine or sclerosing solutions, bleomycin or interferon-α.
* Interferon-α as systemic treatment is effective in 40–50% of patients with indolent Kaposi's sarcoma and a CD4 count above 0.4×10^9 cells per litre who have few systemic symptoms and no opportunistic infections.
* Radiation therapy.
* Combination therapy of surgery, chemotherapy and radiation, or with chemo-therapy alone.
* Relatively marrow-sparing chemotherapy (bleomycin, vincristine or low-dose doxorubicin) is used when other treatment fails in patients with aggressive Kaposi's sarcoma (*Lancet* 1997; **350:** 1363). Complete or partial remission may be obtained in over three quarters of those with Kaposi's sarcoma; shorter survival is associated with low CD4 cell count.

Mortiz Kaposi (1837–1902), a Hungarian dermatologist, in 1872 described five men with 'idiopathic multiple pigmented sarcoma'. He also described the rash in SLE as 'butterfly rash' in 1875 (Kaposi M 1872 Idiopathisches multiples Pigmentsarkom der Haut. *Arch Dermatol Syph* **4**: 265–73).

Case 176

PEUTZ–JEGHERS SYNDROME

INSTRUCTION

Look at this patient's face.

SALIENT FEATURES

History

* Pain in the abdomen due to intestinal intussusception.
* Gastrointestinal haemorrhage in the upper gastrointestinal tract, or rectal bleeding.
* Family involvement (autosomal dominant).

Examination

Pigmented freckles around the lips.

Proceed as follows:

Look in the mouth for similar pigmentation and anaemia.

DIAGNOSIS

This patient has pigmented freckles around the lips (lesions) due to Peutz–Jeghers syndrome (aetiology).

ADVANCED-LEVEL QUESTIONS

What are the types of colonic polyps?

- Tubular adenomas: over 60% are in the rectosigmoid colon and may cause bleeding or obstruction. The risk of malignancy correlates with size. The tubular adenoma is removed endoscopically. Follow-up surveillance is by colonoscopy every 2 years.

- Villous adenomas are usually found in the left colon and have a high risk of malignancy. Polyps larger than 2 cm have a 50% risk of malignancy. They may present with hypokalaemia due to potassium loss in the stools. They are removed by colonoscopic resection.

- Hyperplastic polyps are benign and rarely undergo malignant change. They are usually detected as an incidental finding at colonoscopy.

What is the histology of polyps in Peutz–Jeghers syndrome?

The polyps, which are large and pedunculated, histologically show an arborizing network of connective tissue and well-developed smooth muscle which extends into the polyp and surrounds normal abundant glands lined by normal intestinal epithelium rich in goblet cells. Polyps are distributed in the small bowel (100%), stomach (25%) and colon (30%).

What do you know about the genetics of Peutz-Jeghers syndrome?

The gene has been identified and found to encode the serine threonine kinase LKB1 or STK11. Dutch investigators recently studied the original kindred described by Peutz and reported that in this family clinical features included gastrointestinal polyposis, mucocutaneous pigmentation, nasal polyps and rectal polyps. They found that in this family longevity was reduced by intestinal obstruction and malignant transformation. They found an inactivating germline mutation in the LKB1 gene (*Lancet* 1999; **353:** 1211–15).

What polyposis syndromes do you know?

Familial adenomatous polyposis (FAP) and variants

- FAP: an autosomal dominant condition in which the defect is localized to the APC gene on chromosome 5q21 (*N Engl J Med* 1993; **329:** 1982). There are several thousand polyps in the colon. The polyps appear between the age of 10 and 35 years. The potential malignant change is 100% by the age of 40 years, hence all relatives ought to be screened annually from the age of 12 years and all patients should have prophylactic colectomy by the age of 30. Recently, a protein assay has been developed that can diagnose the genetic defect in 87% of such families, and 150 mg sulindac twice daily has been shown to reduce the number and size of the adenomatous polyps in the rectum (*N Engl J Med* 1993; **328:** 1313). Another promising drug is celecoxib, a cyclo-oxygenase-2 inhibitor (*N Engl J Med* 2000; **342:** 1946–52), which leads to a significant reduction in the number of colorectal polyps. Calcium supplementation has been shown to reduce the risk of recurrent colorectal adenomas (*N Engl J Med* 1999; **340:** 101–7).

- Gardner's syndrome: a variant of FAP in which affected members develop extra-intestinal soft tissue tumours (osteomas, lipomas, dermoid tumours) and pigmentation of fundi.
- Turcot's syndrome: central nervous system gliomas may also develop. Disruption of any of the three genes – *APC, hMLH1* or *hPMS2* – can lead to Turcot's syndrome (*N Engl J Med* 1995; **332:** 839–47).

Other polyposis syndromes

- Familial juvenile polyposis: autosomal dominant condition occurring in children and teenagers. It may cause gastrointestinal bleeds, abdominal pain, diarrhoea and intussusception. There is an increased incidence of malignant change in the interspersed adenomatous polyps.
- Peutz–Jeghers syndrome: characterized by mucocutaneous melanosis with gastro-intestinal hamartomas. The inheritance is autosomal dominant. The intestinal polyps may give rise to haematemeis, melaena or rectal bleeding, anaemia or intussusception, depending on their location. These polyps are usually found in the ileum and jejunum and they rarely undergo malignant change; however, these patients tend to have an increased incidence of other malignancy, both of gastro-intestinal tract (stomach and duodenum) and other viscera (lung, breasts, pancreas and gonads).
- Cronkhite–Canada syndrome: sporadic, colonic, small bowel or gastric polyps associated with ectodermal changes such as hyperpigmentation, nail atrophy and alopecia.
- Cowden's disease: autosomal dominant; multiple gastrointestinal hamartomas with warty papules on the mucosa, and skin malformations.

What do you know about the genetics of colorectal cancer?

Three separate research groups reported the location of the gene on chromosome 2 in familial colonic cancer, which, it is claimed, may predispose to up to 15% of colorectal cancer. Screening in colorectal cancer should include colonoscopy, and in women pelvic ultrasonography. Those who develop colorectal cancer should be treated by subtotal colectomy.

This condition was originally described by J.L. Peutz of Holland in 1921 and rediscovered by H.J. Jeghers et al of the USA in 1949 (*N Engl J Med* 1949; **241:** 993–1005, 1031–6).

E.J. Gardner (b. 1909), US geneticist and Professor of Zoology at Utah University.

J. Turcot, Canadian surgeon, J-P. Després and F. St Pierre first described Turcot's syndrome in 1959. In 1949, H.W. Crail described a similar syndrome (*US Naval Medical Bull* 1949; **49:** 123–8).

L.W. Cronkhite, physician, Massachusetts General Hospital.

Wilma J. Canada, US radiologist.

Morrison PJ, Nevin NC 1993 Peutz–Jeghers syndrome. *N Engl J Med* 329: 774. (A classical picture of a patient with Peutz–Jeghers syndrome.)

Case 177

PYODERMA GANGRENOSUM

INSTRUCTION

Look at this patient's skin.

SALIENT FEATURES

History

- Diarrhoea (inflammatory bowel disease).
- Joint pains (rheumatoid arthritis).
- Leukaemia, multiple myeloma.

Examination

Necrotic ulcer with purplish overhanging edges, usually seen on the lower limbs or trunk (Fig. 43).

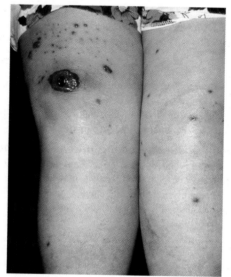

Fig. 43

DIAGNOSIS

These are necrotic ulcers (lesions), which are a feature of pyoderma gangrenosum (aetiology); I would like to investigate for underlying inflammatory bowel disease.
Read recent review: *Lancet* 1998; **351:** 581–5.

QUESTIONS

What are the variants of this condition?

Variants have been described according to the location of the lesion or the associated process, the skin lesion being similar to classical pyoderma gangrenosum:

- Peristomal pyoderma gangrenosum at the site of ileostomy or colostomy in ulcerative colitis or Crohn's disease.
- Vulvar pyoderma gangrenosum.
- Penile or scrotal pyoderma gangrenosum in adolescents and adults.
- Associated with pre-leukaemic state (the ulcer is shallow with a bullous blue-grey border).
- Pyostomatitis vegetans is an oral variant with chronic pustular and eventually vegetative lesions in the mucous membrane of the mouth.

What is the histology in this condition?

Non-specific features including massive neutrophilic infiltration, haemorrhage and necrosis of the epidermis.

How would you evaluate these patients?

- Detailed history and physical examination.
- Skin biopsy (with cultures for bacteria, fungus and virus).
- Gastrointestinal studies.
- Serology for ANCA, ANA, antiphospholipid antibody and serum protein electrophoresis.
- Complete blood count, peripheral smear and bone marrow examination.

In which conditions can pyoderma gangrenosum be seen?

- Ulcerative colitis.
- Crohn's disease.
- Chronic active hepatitis.
- Rheumatoid arthritis, seronegative arthritis associated with gastrointestinal symptoms.
- Acute and chronic myeloid leukaemia, myelocytic leukaemia, hairy cell leukaemia.
- Polycythaemia rubra vera.
- Multiple myeloma.
- IgA monoclonal gammopathy.

ADVANCED-LEVEL QUESTIONS

How would you manage these lesions?

- High-dose steroids.
- Intralesional steroids.
- Topical therapy including dressings, limb elevation, rest.
- Systemic therapy with dapsone.
- Some regress with treatment of the underlying cause.

Pyoderma gangrenosum was first described in 1930 by Brunsting, Goeckerman and O'Leary in five cases (*Arch Dermatol Syph* 1930; **22**: 655–80).

Case 178

STURGE–WEBER SYNDROME (ENCEPHALOTRIGEMINAL ANGIOMATOSIS)

INSTRUCTION

Look at this patient's face.

SALIENT FEATURES

History

- Obtain history of seizures (focal or generalized).
- Hemiparesis, hemisensory disturbance.
- Ipsilateral glaucoma.
- Mental subnormality.

Examination

- A port-wine stain is present on the face in the distribution of the first and second division of the trigeminal nerve (Fig. 44).
- Hypertrophy of the involved area of the face.

Proceed as follows:
- Look for haemangiomas of episclera and iris.

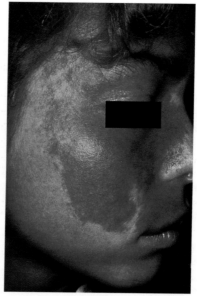

Fig. 44

- Tell the examiner that you would like to:
  - Examine the fundus for unilateral choroidal haemangiomas.
  - Do a skull radiograph for intracranial 'tramline' calcification, particularly in the parieto-occipital lobe (due to mineral deposition in the cortex beneath the intracranial angioma).
  - Check the blood pressure (may be associated with phaeochromocytoma).

DIAGNOSIS

This patient has a port-wine stain on the face in the distribution of the first two divisions of the trigeminal nerve (lesion) which is probably due to Sturge–Weber syndrome (aetiology); these lesions may be cosmetically unacceptable (functional status).

ADVANCED-LEVEL QUESTIONS

What is the inheritance in such patients?
This is the only syndrome of the phakomatoses that does not have a hereditary tendency. It occurs sporadically and there is no sexual predilection.

What are the neurological manifestations in such patients?
Jacksonian epilepsy, contralateral hemianopia, hemisensory disturbance, hemiparesis and hemianopia, low IQ.

What other ocular manifestations do you know?
Choroidal angioma, glaucoma (in 30% of cases), buphthalmos (large eye), optic atrophy.

What is the histology of port-wine stains?
They are composed of networks of ectatic vessels in the outer dermis, under a normal dermis.

How would you treat such a patient?
- Treatment is aimed at the pharmacological control of seizures.
- The patient should be referred to the ophthalmologist for management of increased intraocular pressure or choroidal angioma.
- Photothermolysis: If port-wine stains are treated in early childhood the psychological burden on the family and child may be alleviated. The 350 μs pulsed-dye laser that provides individual 585 nm pulses is the treatment of choice for most port-wine stains, particularly in children. Wavelengths of 577–590 nm are optimal as they are minimally attenuated by epidermis and dermis, and strongly absorbed by blood. Pulse durations of 0.5–5 ms produce only transmural injury to the vessel wall, by heat conduction from hot red cells, and hence prevent non-specific dermal injury. A recent study reported that there was no efficacy in treating port-wine stains with flashlamp-pumped dye laser in early childhood as compared to a later age (*N Engl J Med* 1998; **338**: 1028–33).

Otto Kalischer, a German pathologist, described post-mortem findings in a case as early as 1901.

William A. Sturge (1850–1919), a London physician, described this condition in 1879. He was attached to the Royal Free Hospital, London, and founded the Society of Prehistoric Archaeology in East Anglia.

Frederick Parkes Weber (1863–1962), a London physician, was the first to describe the radiological appearances in this condition. Two other syndromes to which Weber's name is attached are Weber–Christian disease (relapsing, febrile, nodular, non-suppurative panniculitis) and Osler–Rendu–Weber syndrome (hereditary haemorrhagic telangiectasia).

Case 179

ACNE VULGARIS

INSTRUCTION

Look at this patient.

SALIENT FEATURES

History

- Steroid ingestion.
- Isoniazid ingestion.
- Occupational exposure to oils (oil-induced acne).

Examination

- Comedones, or blackheads, usually on the chin, face, shoulders (Fig. 45) and upper chest (due to plugging of hair follicles by keratin) – these are hallmarks of acne.
- Generally found over the face, neck, chest, upper back and upper arms (areas having the most and the largest sebaceous glands).
- Whiteheads (i.e. distended sebaceous glands without a pore).
- Cysts (larger, deeper masses of retained sebum).

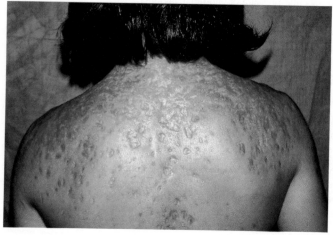

Fig. 45

- Greasy skin.
- There may be associated scarring.

Remember. Acne vulgaris is a multifactorial disease affecting the pilosebaceous follicle and characterized by open and closed comedones, papules, pustules, nodules and scars.

DIAGNOSIS

This patient has blackheads on the face with greasy skin (lesions) which is acne vulgaris caused by *Propionibacterium acnes* (aetiology) and may be cosmetically unacceptable to the patient (functional status).

Read review articles: *Lancet* 1998; **351:** 1871–6; *N Engl J Med* 1997; **336:** 1156.

ADVANCED-LEVEL QUESTIONS

What do you know about the pathogenesis of acne?

Follicular keratinization, seborrhoea and colonization of the pilosebaceous unit with *P. acnes* are central to the development of these lesions. Genetic and hormonal factors also play a role, possibly by optimizing the follicular environment for the growth of *P. acnes* or by influencing the inflammatory response and thus the nature of these lesions.

How is the severity of acne graded?

- Mild disease: open and closed comedones and some papules and pustules.
- Moderate: more frequent papules and pustules with mild scarring.
- Severe disease: all of the above plus nodular abscesses; leads to more extensive scarring, which may be keloidal in some instances.

How would you manage acne?

The aims of treatment are to prevent scarring, limit the disease duration and reduce the impact of the psychological stress that may affect over half of sufferers.

- Wash affected parts with soap not more than twice a day.
- Avoid steaming: saunas, Turkish baths.
- Dietary restriction has no role in therapy (*N Engl J Med* 1997; **336:** 1156).
- Reduce *P. acnes* proliferation:
  - Topical therapy: sulphur, benzoyl peroxide, retinoic acid, azelaic acid, erythromycin, tetracycline.
  - Systemic therapy: tetracycline, erythromycin, doxycycline, minocycline, co-trimoxazole, clindamycin, isotretinoin.
- Reduce sebum overproduction with systemic agents: oestrogens, anti-androgens, spironolactone, isotretinoin.
- Reduce inflammation:
  - Systemic agents: corticosteroids, isotretinoin.
  - Topical agents: metronidazole, intralesional steroids.
- Reduce abnormal desquamation of follicular epithelium:
  - Systemic agents: isotretinoin, antibiotics by indirect effect.
  - Topical agents: tretinoin (most effective), salicylic acid, adapalene, tazarotene, isotretinoin, antibiotics.

- Physical or surgical methods: comedo extraction, dermabrasion, chemical peeling, laser resurfacing, and punch grafts.

Have you heard of acne fulminans?

It is a rare but severe variant, seen exclusively in adolescent boys. It is due to an immune complex reaction to *P. acnes*. The lesions eventually become necrotic and form haemorrhagic crusts, causing disfigurement and scarring. There may be associated systemic features such as fever, malaise, arthralgia, arthritis and vasculitis. Osteolytic bone lesions can arise. Inpatient treatment with systemic steroids is necessary.

What do you know about acne conglobata?

It is seen in tall Caucasian males with cystic skin lesions and multiple abscess formation. It rarely regresses.

Case 180

ALOPECIA AREATA

INSTRUCTION

Examine this patient's scalp.

SALIENT FEATURES

History

- Young adult (75% of patients are below the age of 40 years).
- History of atopy.
- Ask whether there is a family history (25% give a family history).
- Ask the patient whether there are any local symptoms and if the hair loss is cosmetically unacceptable.

Examination

- Well-defined patch of hair loss (Fig. 46).
- Regrowing hair in the patch appears as a fine, depigmented downy growth.

Proceed as follows:

- Look for patches of hair loss over the eyebrows and beard area.
- Examine the nails for fine pitting, transverse lines, dystrophy, fragmentation (anonychorrhexis) and ridging and 20-nail dystrophy (roughened nail surface and brittle free nail edge; Fig. 47).
- Tell the examiner that you would like to:
  - Look for atopy.
  - Look for other autoimmune conditions including vitiligo (see below).

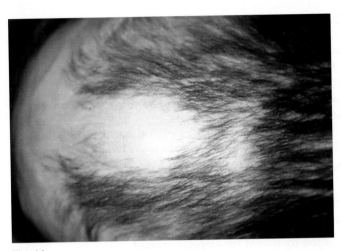

Fig. 46

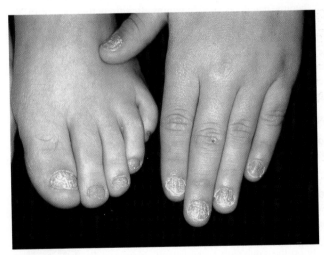

Fig. 47

DIAGNOSIS

This patient has alopecia areata (lesion) which is suspected to be of autoimmune aetiology and may be cosmetically unacceptable to the patient (functional status).

ADVANCED-LEVEL QUESTIONS

What are the signs of disease activity?

At the advancing edge, broken hairs that look like exclamation marks indicate active disease. These are very short hairs that taper and become depigmented as the scalp is approached. Plucking reveals such hair to be in the telogen phase.

Mention some associated disorders.

- Autoimmune conditions (vitiligo, thyrotoxicosis, Addison's disease, pernicious anaemia).
- Down's syndrome.
- Hypogammaglobulinaemia.

What is the difference between alopecia totalis and alopecia universalis?

Both of these conditions can occur in alopecia areata. Alopecia totalis is the loss of all scalp hair and alopecia universalis is the loss of hair from all body sites.

Is alopecia areata associated with scarring?

No.

Mention the causes of hair loss associated with scarring.

Discoid lupus erythematosus, lichen planus.

What is the treatment for alopecia areata?

- Steroids (both topical and systemic; *N Engl J Med* 1999; **341**: 964).
- PUVA therapy, but alopecia often returns after discontinuation of PUVA (*Lancet* 1997; **349**: 222).
- Dithranol is left on the scalp for 20–60 minutes.
- Topical minoxidil.
- Topical immunotherapy: dinitrochlorobenzene, squaric acid dibutylester and diphencyprone (DPCP) have been used for contact sensitization.
- Antibodies to tumour necrosis factor-α.

Cessation of treatment may be associated with recurrent hair loss.

Mention some causes of drug-induced alopecia.

Anticoagulants, retinoids, vitamin A, antithyroid drugs, oral contraceptives, anti-cancer drugs (invariably reversible).

What do you understand by the term 'trichotillomania'?

It is the self-inflicted pulling out of one's own hair and can be differentiated from alopecia areata as the hair loss is irregular and there are always growing hairs, since these cannot be pulled out until they are long enough. The patches are unilateral and are usually on the same side as the patient's dominant hand. The patient may be unaware of this habit.

What do you know about the growth of the hair follicle?

Each follicle undergoes cyclical growth controlled by a constitutional 'time clock'. It has three phases of growth (anagen), a short involutional phase (catagen) and resting (telogen) phase. The anagen phase is 3–5 years, catagen is 2–3 weeks and the telogen phase is 2–4 months. Hair found on the pillow and hairbrush is telogen hair and can be recognized by the fact that the club is depigmented as well as expanded, whereas an anagen hair obtained by traction is fully melanized.

How much hair is usually lost by a normal person?

About 70–100 hairs per day. The human scalp contains about 100 000 follicles; 5–10% are in telogen at any time, i.e. 5000–10 000. As telogen lasts for about 100 days, the number of telogen hairs pushed out each day is 70–100.

What is telogen effluvium?

It is a transitory (about 2–4 months) increase in the number of hairs in the resting (telogen) phase of the hair growth cycle. The number of hairs lost exceeds 150 per day. It is associated with high fever, stress, crash dieting, malnutrition, surgery, termination of pregnancy or oral contraceptives. The prognosis is good.

What do you know about male pattern baldness?

On the scalps of men who have a predisposition for this pattern of baldness, androgens cause a switch from terminal to vellus or vellus-like follicles and a reduction in the duration of anagen. In these individuals the concentration of the androgen receptor and 5α-reductase (converts testosterone to 5-dihydrotestosterone) activities in frontal hair follicles is greater than in occipital follicles, whereas higher activities of aromatase (involved in conversion of testosterone to oestradiol) are found in occipital follicles. This is one explanation for frontal baldness in men. Finasteride, a 5α-reductase inhibitor which does not affect the androgen receptor, results in some regrowth of hair in about 70% of men after two years of continuous use. If treatment is successful the drug is continued indefinitely because the balding process continues when it is stopped.

Case 181

ATOPIC DERMATITIS (ECZEMA)

INSTRUCTION

Look at this patient's skin.

SALIENT FEATURES

History

- Pruritus.
- Tell the examiner that you would like to know whether there is a personal or family history of atopy (asthma, allergic rhinitis, atopic dermatitis) or food allergy.

Examination

- Scratch marks.
- Hyperpigmented or hypopigmented lichenified lesions in flexures (including face, neck, upper trunk, wrists, hand, in the antecubital and popliteal folds).

DIAGNOSIS

This patient has atopic dermatitis (lesion) which is due to atopy as supported by a history of asthma (aetiology) and causes the patient severe itching (functional status).

Read review: *Lancet* 1998; **351**: 1715–21.

QUESTIONS

What are the stages of atopic dermatitis?

There are three age-related stages which are separated by remission:

1. Infantile stage (up to 2 years of age): Red, scaly, itchy crusted rash on both cheeks and extensors of the extremities. The napkin area is generally spared. Eczema of the scalp may also be seen.
2. Childhood stage (2–12 years) shows papulation (rather than exudation) in the flexural areas including neck, cubital fossa, popliteal fossa, volar aspect of wrists and ankles. The plaques show both excoriation and lichenification. In black children there may be hypopigmentation.
3. Adults (from puberty onwards): The face is commonly involved and there is lichenification of flexures including wrists, hands, fingers, ankles, toes and feet.

What are the criteria for diagnosis?

Hanifin and Rajka's major criteria require three or more of the following:

- Pruritus.
- Typical morphology and distribution: flexural lichenification in adults, facial or extensor involvement in children.
- Chronic or chronically relapsing dermatitis.
- Family or personal history of atopy (asthma, allergic rhinitis, atopic dermatitis).

Many of the minor criteria are under dispute and include ichthyosis, nipple eczema, food intolerance, keratoconus, subcapsular anterior cataracts, cheilitis, pityriasis alba and anterior neck folds. Fissuring below the auricles of the ear and diffuse scaling of the scalp may be seen in severe disease.

How would you treat such patients?

- Foods that cause itching (typically dairy products, peanuts, eggs and wheat) should be avoided.
- Patient should be instructed about skin care, including avoiding frequent baths and scratchy fabrics.
- Adequate cutaneous hydration.
- Treatment of infected skin.
- Antihistamines to control itching.
- Corticosteroid lotion, cream or ointment.
- Phototherapy with PUVA in those unresponsive to topical treatment.
- Severe recalcitrant disease: ciclosporin, azathioprine, tacrolimus, Grenz-rays.
- Investigational treatment: phosphodiesterase inhibitors, interleukin-II and thymopentin.

What is known about the genetic aspects of atopy?

A number of atopy susceptibility genes have recently been identified including interleukin-4. Several HLA class II molecules regulate the overproduction of IgE whereas others, such as the beta subunit of the IgE receptor gene (FcER1) on chromosome 11, mediate IgE effector functions. Alleles of the interleukin-4 receptor (α) are strongly associated with atopy (*N Engl J Med* 1997; **337**: 1766; *Am J Hum Genet* 2000; **66**: 517–26).

Case 182

VENOUS ULCER

INSTRUCTION

Look at this patient's leg.

SALIENT FEATURES

History

- Varicose veins – duration.
- Past history of venous thromboembolism.
- Duration of ulceration and whether this is the first episode or recurrent.
- Pain (lack of pain suggests neuropathic aetiology).
- Rheumatoid arthritis (remember, up to half the patients with rheumatoid arthritis have venous leg ulcers rather than those due to rheumatoid arthritis).

Examination

- Ulcer located on the medial aspect of leg (around the ankles) with pigmentation.
- Surrounding dermatitis and excoriation due to pruritus (stasis dermatitis).
- White atrophy with scars in the overlying skin.
- The ulcer may be secondarily infected (cellulitis or thrombophlebitis).
- Look for varicose veins.
- The range of hip, knee and ankle movement should be determined.
- Sensation should be tested with a monofilament to exclude peripheral neuropathy (see pp 349–50 for neuropathic arthritis or Charcot's joints).

DIAGNOSIS

This patient has a venous ulcer (lesion) due to varicose veins (aetiology) which has caused severe pigmentation and dermatitis around the ankles (functional status).

Read review: *BMJ* 2000; **320**: 1589–91.

ADVANCED-LEVEL QUESTIONS

What causes the surrounding pigmentation?

It occurs as a result of the extravasation of red blood cells and haemosiderin deposition.

What causes the white atrophy (atrophie blanche)?

It is due to the hyalinization of skin vessels, resulting in scars in the overlying skin.

How is the diagnosis confirmed?

- When the diagnosis is in doubt, a punch biopsy from the border (not the base) of the lesion is helpful.
- Colour duplex scanning to define underlying venous abnormality: 60% of patients have normal deep veins with isolated superficial venous incompetence.

How would you manage such an ulcer?

- Reduction of venous hypertension: elevation of the limbs, wearing support bandages, weight reduction in the obese. The mainstay of community management of venous ulcers is graduated compression bandaging (in these patients the ankle brachial pressure index must be at least 0.8). The healing rate depends on the initial size of the ulcer, but 65–70% of venous ulcers heal within 6 months.
- Infection: antibiotics for cellulitis.
- Dermatitis: zinc and salicylic acid paste.
- Skin on the lower leg must be kept moist: emollient such as simple aqueous cream or 50:50 liquid paraffin.
- Steroid cream for surrounding eczema.
- Ulcers: cleaning with potassium permanganate, debridement, skin grafting.
- Treatment of varicose veins.
- Long saphenous or short saphenous incompetence in the presence of normal deep veins may benefit from surgery to correct venous abnormality in the leg and allow ulcer healing. Patients with refluxing deep veins would benefit from compression bandaging.

Is recurrence common?

The 5-year recurrence rate of healed venous ulcers is about 40%; it is about 69% in non-compliant patients as compared to 19% of patients wearing class 2 compression hosiery.

Case 183

ARTERIAL LEG ULCER

INSTRUCTION

Look at this patient's leg.

SALIENT FEATURES

History

- Intermittent claudication.
- History of underlying cardiovascular or cerebrovascular disease.
- Pain in the distal foot when the patient is supine ('rest pain' syndrome).
- Impotence.
- Absence of bleeding from the ulcer.
- History of precipitating trauma or underlying deformity.
- History of diabetes, chronic renal failure.

Examination

- Tender, punched-out ulcers on leg (usually away from the ankle region).

- The ulcer is usually on the plantar surface over the heads of first and fifth metatarsals (uncommon on the dorsum of the foot because the pressure is less sustained and perfusion is better).
- Cold atrophic skin.
- Loss of hair.
- Thickened nails.
- Peripheral pulses are not palpable or are diminished (in diabetics and in chronic renal failure the arteries may be calcified, making the results of pulse examination less reliable).
- Pallor on elevation.
- Redness of foot on lowering the leg (dependent rubor).
- Sluggish filling of toe capillaries.

DIAGNOSIS

This patient has an arterial ulcer (lesion) due to vascular insufficiency as evidenced by the absence of popliteal pulses (aetiology).

Read reviews: *N Engl J Med* 2000; **347**: 787–93; *BMJ* 2000; **320**: 1589–91.

QUESTIONS

How would you investigate such a patient?
- X-rays may show calcification of the arteries of the leg.
- Doppler ultrasonography to define the severity of arterial involvement.
- Measurement of segmental limb pressures.
- Pulse-volume wave form and transcutaneous oxygen are particularly useful in evaluating perfusion of the diabetic foot because they are not affected by vessel calcification.
- Aortography shows narrowing and stenosis of the leg arteries.

How would you manage arterial ulcers?
- General: stop smoking; control of diabetes, obesity and hypertension.
- Limbs: should be kept warm (but avoid local heat).
- Feet: chiropodist and foot care, appropriate footwear.
- Regular exercise to promote development of anastomotic collateral vessels.
- Low-dose aspirin.
- Surgery: balloon dilatation for local iliac or femoral stenoses, aortoiliac bypass, amputation when complicated by gangrene.
- Flow-limiting arterial lesions should be evaluated and reconstructed or bypassed: prosthetic vascular grafts or autologous vein grafts may be used.

Mention other causes of leg ulcers.
- Venous ulcers (see pp 477–8).
- Neuropathic: diabetes mellitus, leprosy.
- Vasculitis: rheumatoid arthritis, SLE, pyoderma gangrenosum.
- Haematological disorders: sickle cell anaemia, spherocytosis.
- Neoplastic: basal cell carcinoma, Kaposi's sarcoma (see pp 460–3).
- Trauma or artefact.
- Infection: postcellulitis, fungal.

Case 184

ERYTHEMA NODOSUM

INSTRUCTION

Look at this patient's shins.

SALIENT FEATURES

History

- Elicit a history of:
  - Fever (may precede the skin lesions by 1–7 days).
  - Painful nodules.
  - Arthralgias.
  - Sore throat (β-haemolytic streptococcal infection).
  - Drugs (sulphonamides, oral contraceptives).
  - Gastrointestinal symptoms (*Yersinia enterocolitica* infection).
  - Infections (tuberculosis, leprosy, coccidioidomycosis, histoplasmosis).
  - Sarcoidosis.
- The lesions appear in crops, therefore there may be lesions in different stages of evolution.

Examination

Poorly defined, exquisitely tender, erythematous nodules which are better felt than seen (Fig. 48).

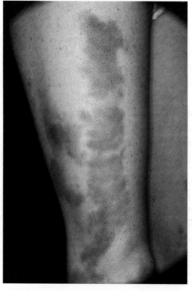

Fig. 48

DIAGNOSIS

This patient has tender erythema nodosum (lesions) on the shins due to the use of oral contraceptives (aetiology).

QUESTIONS

How can a definitive diagnosis be obtained?
By a deep wedge biopsy of the tissue.

ADVANCED-LEVEL QUESTIONS

What is the histology?
Erythema nodosum is a panniculitis, which is an inflammatory reaction in the subcutaneous fat.

- In early lesions, there is widening of the connective tissue septa owing to oedema, fibrin exudation and infiltration by neutrophils.
- Later, there is infiltration by lymphocytes, histiocytes, multinucleated giant cells and occasionally eosinophils associated with septal fibrosis.

Note. Vasculitis is absent.

Mention some examples of panniculitis.
Erythema induratum (associated vasculitis), Weber–Christian disease (relapsing febrile nodular panniculitis), factitial panniculitis.

How would you treat these patients?
- Local: hot or cold compresses.
- Systemic: NSAIDs, saturated solution of potassium iodide, corticosteroid therapy, salicylates.

F.P. Weber (1863–1962), a British physician who graduated from St Bartholomew's Hospital, London, and was a keen collector of coins and vases. He was an alpinist, like his father Sir H.D. Weber (1823–1918), who described Weber syndrome.

Henry A. Christian (1876–1951), Professor of Medicine and the first Physician-in-Chief of the Peter Bent Brigham Hospital. He also described histiocytosis X (Hand–Schüller–Christian disease).

Case 185

FUNGAL NAIL DISEASE

INSTRUCTION

Look at this patient's toenails.

SALIENT FEATURES

History

- Embarrassment from a cosmetic perspective.
- Mechanical problems including the fact that nails get snagged in clothing, etc.
- History of diabetes.

Examination

- Nails are white, green or occasionally black when the infection is superficial or proximal.
- When the infection is distal there may be onycholysis (pp 489–90).

Proceed as follows:
- Look at the fingernails.
- Tell the examiner that you would like to look for underlying immunodeficiency states and circulatory disorders (Raynaud's syndrome).

DIAGNOSIS

This patient has fungal nail disease (lesion) which is usually due to *Trichophyton* or *Candida* (aetiology), and is cosmetically unacceptable to the patient (functional status).

Read: Denning DW, Evans EGV, Kibbler CC et al (1995) Fungal nail disease: a guide to good practice. Report of a Working Group of the British Society for Medical Mycology.

ADVANCED-LEVEL QUESTIONS

What do you understand by the term 'onychomycosis'?
It refers to a fungal infection of nails.

What are the different causative organisms?
These include:

- Dermatophytes (ringworm, tinea unguium): *Trichophyton rubrum, T. interdigitale.* (Toenails are more commonly affected than fingernails.) *T. rubrum* infection is associated with distal or lateral involvement of the nail plate which spreads proximally, eventually affecting the whole nail, and this may be associated with proximal subungual nail dystrophy associated with separation of the nail from the bed. *T. interdigitale* infection, characteristically seen in patients with AIDS, produces superficial white onychomycosis with crumbly white areas on the nail surface.

- Yeasts: *Candida albicans, C. parapsilosis*. (Fingernails are more commonly affected than toenails.)
- Non-dermatophytes (moulds): *Fusarium, Scopulariopsis brevicaulis*. (Toenails are more commonly affected than fingernails.)

Does the clinical picture vary according to the nature of the infecting organism?

Yes, as follows:

- Dermatophytes: distal or lateral nail involvement spreading proximally, proximal subungual dystrophy, superficial white dystrophy, white or yellow thickened nails, crumbling of nail plate, adjacent web or skin involvement may be present.
- *Candida*: chronic paronychia, shiny red bolstered nail-fold, almost exclusively affects fingernail folds, loss of cuticle, pus exuding from under nail-fold, usually proximal nail involvement, distal nail dystrophy (associated with circulatory disorders), total dystrophic onychomycosis, nails white, green or occasionally black.
- Non-dermatophyte: superficial white onychomycosis, solitary nail involvement, colour of the nail may be influenced by the nature of infecting mould (e.g. *Fusarium* – the nails are white, *S. brevicaulis* – the nails may be white, yellow, brown or green).

What are the patterns of fungal nail involvement?

Distal lateral subungual onychomycosis, superficial white onychomycosis, proximal white subungual onychomycosis, total dystrophic onychomycosis (i.e. all the previous three sites are affected).

Is laboratory diagnosis essential before starting treatment?

Yes, for the following reasons:

- Antifungal treatment is prolonged and the causative organism may be non-fungal.
- To identify contacts of the patient.
- To exclude mixed infection.
- To optimize treatment as certain fungi are less responsive to treatment.

Mention some non-fungal nail infections.

Bacterial nail infection, e.g. *Pseudomonas aeruginosa* (green or blackish discoloration of the nails), *Staphylococcus aureus* (causes acute paronychia or whitlow).

How are specimens obtained for mycological diagnosis?

Scrapings are taken with a blunt scalpel as proximally as possible in the nail:

- In distal and lateral onychomycosis: specimens are taken from the proximal part of the diseased portion of the nail and subungual material.
- In superficial white onychomycosis: the scrapings are taken from the diseased nail surface.
- In proximal white mycosis: the scrapings are taken from the nail surface.

In the laboratory, 20–30% potassium hydroxide is added to part of the specimen to macerate nail keratin before direct microscopy and the rest of the specimen is inoculated on different media.

What is the recommended treatment for onychomycosis?

Dermatophyte infections (BMJ *1995; 311: 1277–81*)
* Localized distal nail disease: tioconazole with undecylenic acid paint, amorolfine paint weekly and 40% urea paste for dissolution.
* Proximal or extensive nail disease: terbinafine, itraconazole, griseofulvin and amorolfine nail paint. Recent data suggest that terbinafine is the treatment of choice for onychomycosis (*BMJ* 1999; **318:** 1031–5; *Lancet* 1998; **351:** 541).

Candidal infections
* Chronic paronychia (localized): imidazole creams or paints, nystatin ointment, terbinafine cream. Recent analysis found insufficient evidence on the effects of topical antifungal agents in people with frequently infected toenails (*BMJ* 2001; **322:** 288–9).
* Distal candidal nail infection: tioconazole with undecylenic acid paint, amorolfine nail paint.
* Severe candidal nail infection or severe chronic paronychia: itraconazole.

Non-dermatophyte (mould) onychomycosis
* Localized nail disease: tioconazole with undecylenic acid paint, amorolfine paint weekly, 40% urea paste for dissolution or even avulsion of the nail.
* Persistent nail disease: itraconazole.

Mention some fungal infections that do not respond to oral treatment.

Scopulariopsis, Scytalidium, Fusarium and *Acremonium*.

Case 186

LICHEN SIMPLEX CHRONICUS (NEURODERMATITIS)

INSTRUCTION

Look at this patient's skin.

SALIENT FEATURES

History

Itching (self-perpetuating scratch–itch cycle).

Examination

* Several scratch marks (due to pruritus).
* Well-circumscribed plaque with lichenified or dry, thickened, leathery skin (Fig. 49).

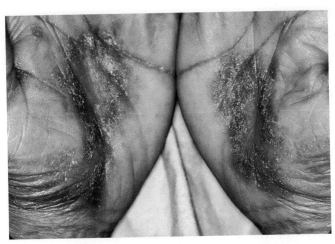

Fig. 49

Proceed as follows:
Look for similar plaques in common areas including the posterior nuchal region, wrists, perineum, dorsum of the feet or ankles.

DIAGNOSIS

This patient has lichen simplex chronicus (lesion) which is due to chronic itching and scratching (aetiology), and is cosmetically disturbing to the patient.

ADVANCED-LEVEL QUESTIONS

How would you treat such a patient?
- Break the scratch–itch–scratch cycle by administering antipruritic agents.
- High-potency topical steroids (under occlusion or intralesional injection).
- The area should be protected.
- Patient should be made aware of when he or she is scratching.

What is the prognosis?
The disease tends to remit during treatment; however, it may recur or develop at another site.

Case 187

NAIL CHANGES

INSTRUCTION

Look at these nails.

SALIENT FEATURES

Disorders of the nail bed
- Terry's nail (Fig. 50): brownish-red distal transverse band; occurs normally in the elderly; also seen in cirrhosis and congestive cardiac failure.

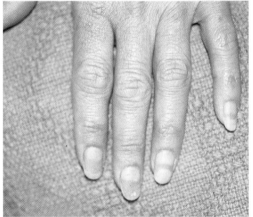

Fig. 50

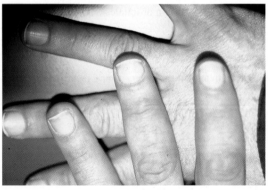

Fig. 51

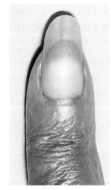

Fig. 52

- Lindsay's half-and-half nail (Figs 51 and 52): distal brown band occupying about 25–50% of the nail bed, and seen in chronic renal failure.

- Muehrcke's nail: pale transverse bands resulting from oedema of the nail bed; seen in hypoalbuminaemia.
- Onycholysis (Fig. 56, see p. 489).

Disorders of the lunula
Blue lunula: in Wilson's disease (see pp 313–5) the normally white lunula becomes blue. The lunula has the largest area in the fingers closest to the thumb; in the elderly it becomes smaller or is absent.

Disorders of the nail plate
- Clubbing (see pp 561–2).
- Leukonychia (Fig. 53): whitish discoloration which may be diffuse (liver disease, congenital, fungal), punctate or linear (Mees' lines – Fig. 54 – seen in arsenical poisoning).

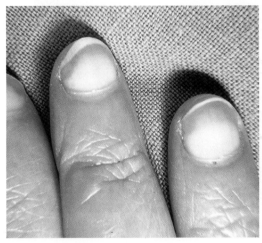

Fig. 53

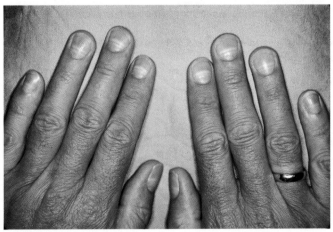

Fig. 54

- Koilonychia (spoon-shaped nails) seen in iron deficiency anaemia, thyrotoxicosis.
- Onychogryphosis: hypertrophy and thickening of the nail.
- Onychomycosis: dystrophy, destruction of the nail due to fungal or yeast infections.
- Pitting: seen in psoriasis (Fig. 7, see p. 393), alopecia areata.
- Pterygium formation: growth of the cuticle onto the nail plate.
- Longitudinal brown streaks: junctional naevi seen in black patients.
- Beau's lines (Fig. 55): transverse depression due to severe systemic illness. Allows estimation of the date of the illness. Remember, the normal nail grows at the rate of 0.1 mm per day and it takes approximately 3–4 months for the nail plate to grow out completely.

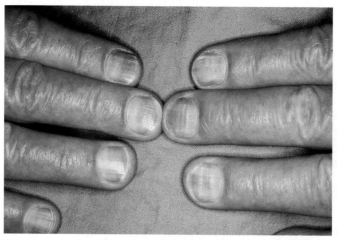

Fig. 55

Disorders of the nail-fold
- Nail-fold telangiectasia: seen in dermatomyositis, scleroderma, collagen vascular disease.
- Paronychia: may be acute or chronic, and includes the swelling and inflammation of the proximal or lateral nail-folds.

Disorders of the hyponychium
- Koenen's subungual angiofibromas (Fig. 72, see p. 513) seen in tuberous sclerosis.
- Warts.

Note. The hyponychium is the most distal region of the nail bed and marks the transition to normal skin.

Case 188

ONYCHOLYSIS

INSTRUCTION

Examine this patient's hands.

SALIENT FEATURES

History

- Take a history for excessive exposure to detergents, alkalis and keratolytic agents, and demeclocycline-induced photolysis.
- History of psoriasis (see pp 392–5).
- History of thyrotoxicosis (see pp 355–9).
- History of diabetes (fungal infection).

Examination

Distal separation of the nail plate from the nail bed. (Fig. 56)

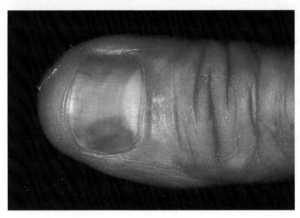

Fig. 56

Proceed as follows:
- Look for nail pitting and silvery white plaques (psoriasis).
- Glance at the neck for goitre and tell the examiner that you would like to exclude thyrotoxicosis, hypothyroidism and diabetes mellitus.
- Tell the examiner that you would like to exclude a fungal infection (see pp 482–4).

DIAGNOSIS

This patient has onycholysis (lesion), probably due to thyrotoxicosis as evidenced by tachycardia, exophthalmos and goitre (aetiology).

    Read this review for more information: *J Am Acad Dermatol* 1985; **12:** 552–60.

QUESTIONS

What nail changes are associated with psoriasis?

Yellow, friable nails with pitting and onycholysis (lifting of nail from the bed), distal subungual hyperkeratosis.

How would you manage these nail lesions?

- Manicure and careful debridement.
- Reduction of exposure to irritants (detergents, bleaches, alkalis).
- Intradermal steroids in the area of nail matrix (these are very painful injections).
- Non-surgical removal of dystrophic nails using urea ointments.

What are Plummer's nails?

This term refers to the onycholysis that occurs in hyperthyroidism, typically in the fourth finger.

S. Plummer (1874–1936), physician at the Mayo Clinic, Rochester, Minnesota, also described Plummer–Vinson syndrome (iron deficiency anaemia and dysphagia).

Case 189

MALIGNANT MELANOMA

INSTRUCTION

Look at this skin lesion.

SALIENT FEATURES

History

- Ask the patient whether the mole has changed in colour.
- Ask the patient whether the mole itches and whether it has changed in morphology.
- Does your skin have freckles or tendency to freckling?
- How many moles does your skin have? – More than 20?
- How many times in your life have you had bad sunburn (with peeling of your skin)?
- Remember MacKie's four independent risk factors for melanoma: freckles, moles (Fig. 57), atypical naevi and a history of severe sunburn (*Lancet* 1989; **ii:** 487–90).

Examination

Irregular and asymmetrical naevus, with a fuzzy border where the pigment appears to be leaking into the surrounding skin (Fig. 58). (The American Cancer Society mnemonic to suspect malignancy in a mole is ABCD: Asymmetry, Border irregular, Colour variegation and Diameter greater than 6 mm.)

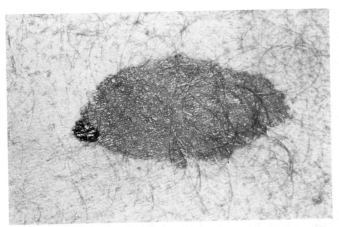

Fig. 57

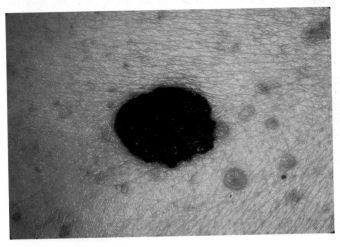

Fig. 58

Proceed as follows:
- Comment if the mole stands out from the patient's other moles.
- Comment if bleeding and ulceration are present (these are ominous signs).
- Examine regional lymph nodes and the liver (for metastatic spread).

DIAGNOSIS

This patient has a malignant melanoma (lesion) as evidenced by its irregular border and, without delay, biopsy and histological examination must be performed to exclude or confirm the diagnosis.

QUESTIONS

What are the different types of malignant melanoma?
Depending on the clinical picture and histological findings these include:

- Superficially spreading malignant melanoma (commonest type).

- Nodular malignant melanoma.
- Acral lentiginous melanomas (arising on the palms, soles and nail beds).
- Malignant melanoma on mucous membranes.
- Lentigo maligna melanoma (arising in lentigines in older individuals).
- Amelanotic (non-pigmented) melanoma.
- Miscellaneous: melanoma arising from blue naevi, congenital and giant naevocytic naevi.

ADVANCED-LEVEL QUESTIONS

What are the patterns of growth of malignant melanoma?
These include:

- Radial growth, where the growth is horizontal within the epidermis and superficial dermal layers, e.g. lentigo maligna, acral/mucosal lentiginous, superficial spreading types. During this stage of growth the tumour does not have the capacity to metastasize.
- Vertical growth occurs with time, and the melanoma grows downward into the deeper dermal layers as an expansile mass lacking cellular maturation; this correlates with the emergence of a clone of cells with metastatic potential. The nature and extent of this vertical growth phase determines the biological behaviour of malignant melanoma.

What are the predisposing factors?
These include sunlight, the presence of a pre-existing naevus (e.g. dysplastic naevus), hereditary factors.

What is the treatment of such lesions?
- Excision: following histological examination the area is usually re-excised with margins dictated by the thickness of the tumour.
- Elective lymph node dissection is controversial; in general, it is indicated only in melanomas of intermediate thickness with one draining chain of lymph nodes.
- Intralesional injection of avirulent herpes simplex virus (but capable of replication) may be of therapeutic benefit in malignant melanoma; this is currently an experimental therapy (*Lancet* 2001; **357:** 525).
- Interferon-α and vaccine therapy may reduce recurrences.

What are the prognostic factors in these patients?
- Tumour thickness: the deeper the melanoma, the more likely is metastasis. Thin melanomas (<0.76 mm) approach 100% cure rate whereas, when the depth is greater than 1.6 mm, only 20–30% survive for 5 years.
- Level of invasion.
- Sex of the patient.
- Anatomical location: melanomas in the 'TANS' areas (thorax, upper arms, neck and scalp) show a higher relative risk.

What are the melanoma-associated genes?
Candidate genes include: (a) growth regulator p16 on chromosome 9, (b) the CMM1 gene on chromosome 1p36, and (c) cyclin-dependent kinase gene CDK4 on chromosome 12q14.

Rona Mackie is contemporary professor of dermatology in Glasgow.

N Engl J Med 1994; **331**: 163. (Classical pictures of the different types of melanoma including superficial spreading melanoma lentigo maligna, nodular melanoma, subungual melanoma and amelanotic melanoma.)

Case 190

SEBORRHOEIC DERMATITIS

INSTRUCTION

Comment on this patient's skin.

SALIENT FEATURES

History

- History of itching.
- History of Parkinson's disease, strokes and HIV.

Examination

- Greasy scales overlying erythematous plaques or patches affecting the face (eyebrows, eyelids, glabella, nasolabial folds or ears; Fig. 59), submammary folds, gluteal clefts. Occasionally it is generalized.
- Severe dandruff on the scalp.

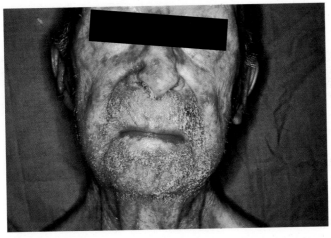

Fig. 59

Proceed as follows:

Tell the examiner that you would like to look for the underlying disorder (Parkinson's disease, HIV and strokes).

Remember that the name is misleading and the condition is unrelated to seborrhoea (excess sebum production).

DIAGNOSIS

This patient has seborrhoeic dermatitis (lesion) with Parkinson's disease, and finds the lesion cosmetically unacceptable (functional status).

ADVANCED-LEVEL QUESTIONS

What is the aetiology of this disorder?

It is based on a genetic predisposition mediated by several factors including nutritional status, infection and hormones. Its response to antifungal agents has suggested that it represents an inflammatory reaction to *Pityrosporum ovale* yeasts present in the scalp of humans.

How would you treat these skin lesions?

- Topical glucocorticoids (avoid fluorinated preparations on the face).
- Shampoos containing coal tar and salicylic acid.
- Selenium sulphide shampoos for the scalp.
- Eyelid margins respond to gentle cleaning of lid margins with undiluted Johnson and Johnson baby shampoo using a cotton swab.
- Oral ketoconazole is invaluable in the persistent seborrhoeic dermatitis of AIDS, but should rarely be used otherwise.

What is the prognosis of this condition?

There is a tendency to lifelong recurrences.

Case 191

MOLLUSCUM CONTAGIOSUM

INSTRUCTION

Look at these skin lesions.

SALIENT FEATURES

History

Ask the patient whether there are similar lesions elsewhere (particularly genitals).

Examination

- Multiple rounded, dome-shaped, waxy papules that are 2–5 mm in diameter and have central umbilication with a caseous plug.
- The common sites are face, hands, lower abdomen and genitals.

Proceed as follows:
Tell the examiner that you would like to investigate for an underlying HIV infection.

DIAGNOSIS

This patient has molluscum contagiosum (lesion) which is of viral aetiology, and you would like to rule out an underlying HIV infection as the lesions are extensive and widely distributed on the face, neck and other parts of the body.

QUESTIONS

How do these lesions spread from one part of the body to another?
Probably by autoinoculation.

How is the infection spread from one patient to another?
By direct contact.

What is the histology of these lesions?
Microscopically, they show cup-like verrucous epidermal hyperplasia. Large inclusion bodies called 'molluscum bodies' are present in the cells of the stratum corneum and granulosum. These bodies are also seen in the curd-like material that can be expressed from the central umbilication. Numerous virions are present within the molluscum bodies.

What is the aetiology of these lesions?
Molluscum contagiosum is caused by a pox virus which is characteristically brick shaped and has a central dumbbell-shaped DNA core.

How are these lesions treated?
- Curettage or applications of liquid nitrogen to freeze the lesions.
- Physical expression by squeezing.
- Phenol ablation (causes more scarring than squeezing; *BMJ* 1999; **319**: 1540).
- Light electrosurgery with a needle.
- Imiquimod cream (50%) applied three times per week eradicates about 50% of anogenital warts (*Arch Dermatol* 1998; **134**: 25–30). Imiquimod is an immune enhancing agent with antiviral and antitumour effects.
- Anecdotal reports suggest that topical cidofovir may be useful in severe molluscum contagiosum, particularly in immunodeficient individuals (*Lancet* 1999; **353**: 2042).

Note. In children these lesions tend to resolve spontaneously.

Classic picture: *N Engl J Med* 1998; **338**: 13.

Case 192

URTICARIA

INSTRUCTION

Look at the skin of this patient, who has recurrent lesions.

SALIENT FEATURES

History

- Determine physical causes that can precipitate this response (cold urticaria, dermatographism – Fig. 60, pressure, sunlight – Fig. 60, exercise, hot shower).

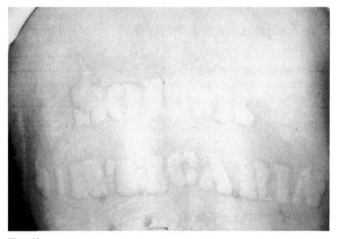

Fig. 60

- Drug history (aspirin, NSAIDs, morphine, codeine, penicillin, sulphonamides).
- Whether any foods precipitate the rash (strawberries, seafood, nuts, chocolate).
- Blood products causing these lesions.
- Wasp or bee stings.
- Viral infections and febrile illnesses.
- Ascertain whether the patient has recurrent angio-oedema.
- Obtain a history of atopy.

Examination

- Wheals that are smooth, oedematous, pink or red, and surrounded by a bright red flare. Clearing of the central area may leave an annular pattern.
- Associated scratch marks, indicating that the wheals are itchy.

Proceed as follows:
Tell the examiner that you would like to exclude infections (hepatitis, chronic sinusitis) and connective tissue disorders.

Read reviews: *BMJ* 1998; **316:** 1147; *N Engl J Med* 1995; **332:** 1767.

DIAGNOSIS

This patient has wheals (lesion) due to chronic urticaria and dermatographism (aetiology), complicated by severe itching (functional status). Tell the examiner that you would like to exclude urticarial vasculitis before making a firm diagnosis.

Notes
Systemic lupus erythematosus and Sjögren's sydrome may present with urticarial lesions, which are usually urticarial vasculitis.

Chronic urticaria is the occurrence of daily or almost daily widespread itchy wheals for at least six weeks (*N Engl J Med* 1995; **332:** 1767–72). This includes urticarial vasculitis and physical urticaria.

ADVANCED-LEVEL QUESTIONS

What do you understand by the term 'dermatographism'?
It is the presence of itchy, linear wheals with a surrounding bright red flare at sites of scratching or rubbing.

How would you investigate a patient with chronic urticaria?
- FBC and white count; if eosinophilia is present, examination of the stool for ova and parasites.
- Physical urticaria must be assessed by appropriate challenge testing.
- Serum complement C4 levels when there is a history of repeated cutaneous or mucosal angio-oedema.
- Thyroid function tests because of diagnostic overlap between chronic urticaria and thyroid disease.

How would you manage patients with chronic urticaria?
- Identify avoidable causes such as food additives. Challenge testing for food additives should be avoided in patients with a history of severe angio-oedema, asthma or episodes of anaphylaxis.
- Antihistamines: H_1 antihistamines (terfenadine, doxepin) with a low potential for sedation are first-line treatment; 2% ephedrine spray is useful for oropharyngeal oedema.
- Corticosteroids.
- A tepid shower temporarily alleviates itching.
- All patients should be advised to avoid aspirin and other NSAIDs, angiotensin-converting enzyme (ACE) inhibitors, macrolide antibiotics and imidazole antifungal agents.

Case 193

MYCOSIS FUNGOIDES (CUTANEOUS T-CELL LYMPHOMA

INSTRUCTION

Look at this patient's skin.

SALIENT FEATURES

History

- Age (usually fifth and seventh decade).
- Pruritus.

Examination

Itchy, brownish-red plaques on the hips, buttocks and interscapular region (Fig. 61).

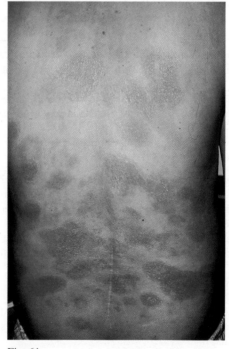

Fig. 61

Proceed as follows:

Tell the examiner that it may also involve the lymph nodes and viscera.

DIAGNOSIS

This patient has itchy brownish-red plaques with lymph node involvement (lesions), indicating mycosis fungoides (aetiology).

Read review article: *Lancet* 1996; **347:** 871–6.

ADVANCED-LEVEL QUESTIONS

How would you confirm the diagnosis?

Skin biopsy to detect Pautrier's microabscesses, atypical cells in the nests in the epidermis, atypical mononuclear cell infiltrates, large hyperchromic cells with irregular nuclei – the 'mycosis cells'. The hallmark of mycosis fungoides is the identification of the Sézary–Lautner cells. These are T helper cells (CD4 antigen positive) that characteristically form band-like aggregates within the superficial dermis and invade the dermis as single cells and small clusters (Pautrier's microabscesses).

What is the prognosis?

Very slow progression of skin lesions with eventual tumour formation and systemic dissemination of lymphoma. In most patients this process takes several weeks.

What is the differential diagnosis?

Psoriasis.

How would you treat this patient?

Treatment is palliative with steroids, chemotherapeutic agents and electron-beam therapy.

What are the stages of cutaneous T-cell lymphoma?

- Stage I: eczematoid or psoriasiform erythematous lesions.
- Stage II: infiltrated plaques.
- Stage III: nodules (Fig. 62), ulcers, tumours.

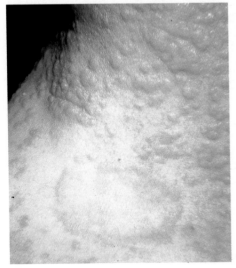

Fig. 62

- Stage IV: lymph node involvement with or without systemic dissemination.

The prognosis is good for early mycosis fungoides (*Arch Dermatol* 1996; **132:** 1309–13).

What is the treatment of mycosis fungoides?

- Various superficial treatments: topical steroids and chemotherapeutic agents (chlormethine and carmustine), PUVA and electron-beam radiotherapy improve skin disease, but none has been shown to alter the natural history of the disease.
- Novel approaches being explored include: aciclovir, interferons, retinoids, pentostatin and monoclonal antibodies directed to T-cell antigens, extracorporeal photopheresis and interferon-α (*Lancet* 1997; **350:** 32–3).

Have you heard of Sézary's syndrome?

It is a rare leukaemic, erythrodermic variant of mycosis fungoides characterized by lymphadenopathy and large mononuclear cells (Sézary cells) in the skin and blood. It is often resistant to traditional treatment and has a poor prognosis. Extracorporeal photopheresis (which consists of oral administration of methoxsalen, exposure of a lymphocyte-enriched blood fraction to ultraviolet A light and reinfusion of the cells into the patient) has recently shown promise.

Jean Louis M. Alibert, a French dermatologist, first described this condition in 1806. A. Sézary (1880–1956), a French dermatologist.

Case 194

URTICARIA PIGMENTOSA

INSTRUCTION

Look at this patient's skin.

SALIENT FEATURES

History

- Urticaria with pruritus on trauma, rubbing or heat – Darier's sign.
- Headache.
- Diarrhoea.
- Itching.

Examination

- Itchy reddish-brown macules and papules (Fig. 63).
- Telangiectasia.

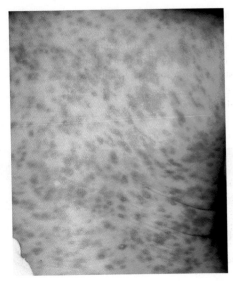

Fig. 63

Proceed as follows:
Look for hepatosplenomegaly.

DIAGNOSIS

This patient has itchy reddish-brown macules with telangiectasia and Darier's sign (lesions) indicating urticaria pigmentosa (aetiology).

ADVANCED-LEVEL QUESTIONS

What do you know about urticaria pigmentosa?
It is the cutaneous manifestation of systemic mastocytosis.

What is the histology of urticaria pigmentosa?
It varies from an increase in the number of spindle-shaped and stellate mast cells about the superficial dermal vessels to large numbers of tightly packed round-to-oval mast cells in the upper and mid dermis. Variable fibrosis, oedema and a small number of eosinophils may also be present.

What do you know about systemic mastocytosis?
It is a condition characterized by mast cell hyperplasia which, in most cases, is neither clonal nor neoplastic. It can occur at any age and is slightly more common in men. Four forms have been recognized:

- Indolent form: does not alter life expectancy and constitutes the majority of cases.
- Associated with frank leukaemia or dysmyelopoiesis: the prognosis is determined by the underlying haematological disorder.
- Aggressive form: the prognosis is determined by the extent of organ involvement.
- Mast cell leukaemia: rare, invariably fatal.

How would you manage such patients?

- H₁ blocker – for flushing and itch (e.g. clomethiazole).
- H₂ blocker – for gastric and duodenal manifestations (e.g. ranitidine, cimetidine).
- Oral sodium cromoglicate for diarrhoea and abdominal pain.
- NSAIDs for flushing not responsive to antihistamines.

F.J. Darier (1856–1938), a French dermatologist.

Case 195

DERMATOMYOSITIS

INSTRUCTION

Examine this patient.

SALIENT FEATURES

History

- The adult form usually occurs after the age of 40 years.
- Weakness of proximal muscles evolving over weeks or months: difficulty in getting up from a low chair or squatting position, climbing stairs, lifting and running.
- Inability to raise head.
- Dysphagia (due to weakness of the muscles of the pharynx).
- Dysphonia.
- Muscle pain and tenderness.
- Raynaud's phenomenon.
- Ask the patient whether the red rash is made worse by exposure to sunlight.

Skin

- Heliotrope rash or purplish-blue rash around the eyes, back of the hands, dilated capillary loops at the base of fingernails, erythema of knuckles accompanied by a raised violaceous scaly eruption (Gottron's sign; Figs 64 and 65). The erythema spares the phalanges (unlike that of systemic lupus erythematosus in which the phalanges are involved and the knuckles are spared).
- The erythematous rash may be present on the neck and upper chest (often in the shape of a V), shoulders (shawl sign), elbows, knees and malleoli.
- The cuticles may be irregular, thickened and distorted, and the lateral and palmar areas of the fingers become rough and cracked with irregular 'dirty' horizontal lines, resembling those in a mechanic's hands.

Muscles

- Proximal muscle weakness and tenderness of muscles (muscle wasting absent or minimal).
- Weakness of neck flexors in two thirds of cases.
- Intact or absent deep tendon reflexes.

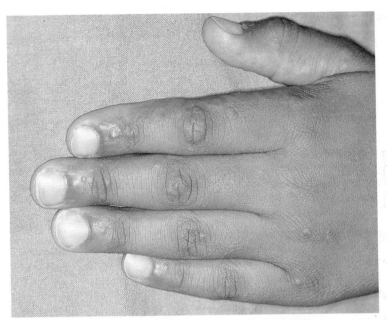

Fig. 64

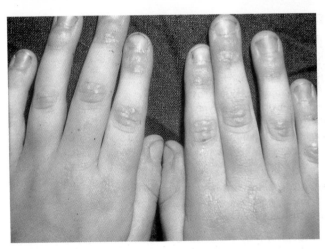

Fig. 65

Proceed as follows:
If the patient is more than 40 years old, tell the examiner that you would like to look for an underlying neoplasm.

DIAGNOSIS

This patient has Gottron's papules and proximal muscle weakness (lesion) due to dermatomyositis (aetiology).

Read review: *N Engl J Med* 1993; **325:** 1487.

QUESTIONS

What investigations would you like to perform?

- Estimation of serum creatine phosphokinase (CPK) levels (mirrors disease activity).
- EMG shows myopathic changes (spontaneous fibrillation, salvos of repetitive potentials, and short duration of polyphasic potentials of low amplitude).
- Muscle biopsy (will show necrosis and phagocytosis of muscle fibres, and interstitial and perivascular infiltration of inflammatory cells).

In which other conditions is there proximal muscle weakness with high serum creatine kinase levels?

It may be caused by drugs such as lovastatin, chloroquine and colchicine, especially in patients on chronic haemodialysis. (Remember that steroids cause proximal muscle weakness with normal serum creatine kinase levels.)

How would you treat such patients?

- Most patients respond to steroids; prednisolone is the first-line drug for the empirical treatment of polymyositis and dermatomyositis.
- Resistant cases may benefit from methotrexate, azathioprine and high-dose intravenous immunoglobulin.
- Those with an underlying neoplasm may remit after treatment of the tumour.

ADVANCED-LEVEL QUESTIONS

How would you classify polymyositis–dermatomyositis?

The classification of Bohan et al (*Medicine* 1977; **56**: 255) is as follows:

- Group I: primary idiopathic polymyositis.
- Group II: primary idiopathic dermatomyositis.
- Group III: dermatomyositis (or polymyositis) associated with neoplasia (*Mayo Clin Proc* 1986; **61**: 645).
- Group IV: childhood dermatomyositis (or polymyositis) associated with vasculitis.
- Group V: polymyositis (or dermatomyositis) with associated collagen vascular disease.

Mention a few disorders associated with myositis.

Sarcoid myositis, focal nodular myositis, infectious polymyositis (Lyme disease, toxoplasma), inclusion body myositis, eosinophilic myositis.

What do you understand by the term 'overlap syndrome'?

Overlap syndrome indicates that characteristics of two different disorders are common to both. Dermatomyositis overlaps with systemic sclerosis and mixed connective tissue disease. Specific signs of systemic sclerosis and mixed connective tissue disease, such as sclerotic thickening of the dermis, contractures, oesophageal hypomotility, microangiopathy and calcium deposits, are present in dermatomyositis. Patients with the overlap syndrome of dermatomyositis and systemic sclerosis may have a specific antinuclear autoantibody, anti-PM/Scl, directed against a nucleolar protein complex.

Heinrich Adolf Gottron (1890–1974), a German dermatologist.

Case 196

SCLERODERMA

INSTRUCTION

Look at these hands.

SALIENT FEATURES

History

- Tight skin over face and joints.
- Raynaud's phenomenon (see pp 415–7) (*BMJ* 1995; **310:** 795–8).
- Puffy hands and feet.
- Fatigue.
- Shortness of breath (lung involvement, cardiac fibrosis), dry cough.
- Gastrointestinal symptoms: dysphagia, diarrhoea, bloating and indigestion.
- Dry eyes.
- History of renal failure.

Examination

- Thickening and tightening of the skin over fingers, sclerodactyly (finger pulp atrophy; Fig. 66), beaking of nails (pseudoclubbing), atrophic nails, telangiectasia (nail-fold capillaries).

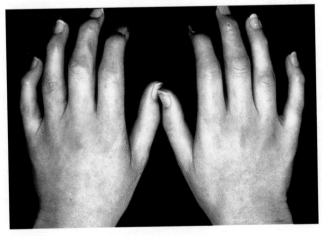

Fig. 66

- Raynaud's phenomenon.
- Subcutaneous calcification (fingers, elbows and extensor aspect of the forearms).
- Vitiligo or pigmentation.

Proceed as follows:
* Assess hand function: pincer movements, hand grip, unbuttoning of clothes, abduction of thumb and writing.
* Examine the following:
  - The joints for arthralgia or arthritis.
  - The face for microstomia, difficulty in opening the mouth, beak-like or pinched appearance of the nose, blotchy telangiectasia.
  - The abdomen for liver (primary biliary cirrhosis).

DIAGNOSIS

This patient has sclerodactyly, tightening of the skin over hands and face (lesion) due to scleroderma (aetiology). He has difficulty in buttoning his clothes and has marked dysphagia due to oesophageal involvement (functional status).

QUESTIONS

What other organ systems are involved?
* Skin: Raynaud's phenomenon; localized morphoea, local or generalized oedema, hyperpigmentation, telangiectasia, subcutaneous calcification, ulceration, particularly at the fingertips. Ten-year survival rate is 71% with skin tightness limited to fingers but 21% with diffuse truncal skin involvement. Ilioprost, a prostacyclin analogue, helps heal digital ulceration. Penicillamine improves the skin and prolongs survival in patients with early, rapidly progressive, systemic sclerosis.
* Musculoskeletal system: arthritis, myositis, myopathy, bone ischaemia with resorption of the phalanges.
* Gastrointestinal tract: dysphagia, reflux oesophagitis, large or small bowel obstruction.
* Lung: fibrosis, atelectasis, pulmonary hypertension; pneumonia.
* Kidney: glomerulonephritis, malignant hypertension (poorest prognosis with renal involvement). Angiotensin-converting enzyme (ACE) inhibitors dramatically improve renal crisis.
* Heart: myocardial fibrosis.

Remember. The prognosis is worse in those with renal disease and in males. Patients with skin and/or gut involvement without other organ disease have the best prognosis.

What are the variants of scleroderma?
CREST syndrome (see below), eosinophilic fasciitis, Thibierge–Weissenbach syndrome.

What is 'CREST' syndrome?
Calcinosis, Raynaud's phenomenon, oesophageal dysmotility, sclerodactyly and telangiectasia. It has a more favourable prognosis than systemic sclerosis, and is associated with the anticentromere antibody.

ADVANCED-LEVEL QUESTIONS

What are the criteria for diagnosis of scleroderma?
* Major criterion is proximal scleroderma (affecting metacarpophalangeals and metatarsophalangeals) (*Arthritis Rheum* 1980; **23**: 581–90).

- Minor criteria are as follows:
  - Sclerodactyly.
  - Digital tip pitting or loss of substance of distal finger pads.
  - Bibasal pulmonary fibrosis.

At least the sole major criterion or two or more minor criteria are required. These proposed criteria had a 97% sensitivity for definite systemic sclerosis and 98% specificity.

What are the subsets of scleroderma?
- Limited cutaneous scleroderma: where the skin is affected only at the extremities.
- Diffuse cutaneous scleroderma: skin of trunk and extremities affected.
- Scleroderma sine scleroderma: skin not affected, patients present with pulmonary fibrosis, scleroderma renal crisis, cardiac failure or malabsorption and pseudo-obstruction. The presence of anticentromere, scleroderma-70 and antinuclear antibodies can be helpful.

What are the causes of anaemia in such a patient?
- Iron deficiency from chronic oesophagitis.
- Folate and vitamin B_{12} deficiency from malabsorption.
- Anaemia of chronic disease.
- Microangiopathic haemolytic anaemia.

What are the phases of skin changes in scleroderma?
- An early oedematous phase (with pitting oedema of hands and possibly forearms, legs and face).
- The dermal phase.
- An atrophic phase, followed by contracture.
- Other skin changes occur, e.g. depigmentation.

What do you know about the pathogenesis of these skin changes?
The endothelial damage resulting from a circulatory protein factor has been implicated as an early component of the 'inflammatory' phase of scleroderma. Endothelial damage may result in the capillary and arteriolar abnormalities demonstrated, as well as local access of circulating proteins acting on fibroblast-enhancing collagen secretion.

How would you manage a patient with scleroderma?
- Educational and psychological support.
- Treat vascular abnormalities such as Raynaud's phenomenon.
- Symptomatic treatment, e.g. omeprazole for oesophagitis.
- Early phase of diffuse form: immunosuppressive drugs (cyclophosphamide, methotrexate, antithymocyte globulin).
- Later stages: antifibrotic drugs (penicillamine, interferon).

What is the role of prednisone in the treatment of scleroderma?
Prednisone has little or no role in the treatment of scleroderma.

What are the common fatal events in this disease?
In most cases, death results from cardiac, renal or respiratory failure.

The first reports of scleroderma were by W.D. Chowne of London in 1842, and James Startin, also from London, in 1846. The term 'sclerodermie' was suggested by E. Gintrac (1791–1877) of Bordeaux; Italian physician G.B. Fantonetti introduced the term 'skleroderma' in 1836.

Maurice Raynaud commented on the presence of Raynaud's phenomenon in scleroderma in 1863.

Heinrich Auspitz (1835–1886) reported, in 1863, on death due to renal failure in scleroderma; this was proved to be a more than chance association by H. Moore and H. Sheehan of Liverpool in 1952.

David A. Isenberg is Professor of Rheumatology, University College London.

Carol Black is Professor of Rheumatology, Royal Free Hospital.

Case 197

EHLERS–DANLOS SYNDROME

INSTRUCTION

Do a general examination.
Examine this patient's joints.

SALIENT FEATURES

History

- Family history (*JAMA* 1997; **278**: 1284–5).
- Hypermobile joints (Fig. 67).

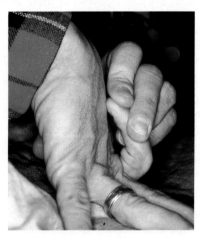

Fig. 67

- Fragile skin with impaired wound healing.
- Bleeding diathesis.

Examination

Skin

The skin over the neck, axillae and groin is smooth and elastic (Fig. 68). It can be stretched and, when released, returns immediately to its normal position. Late in the disease it becomes lax, wrinkled and hangs in folds.

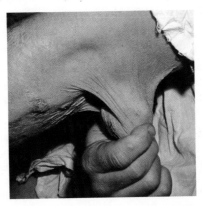

Fig. 68

Proceed as follows:

Look at bony prominences for bruising, haematomas and gaping wounds. Wounds heal to form tissue-paper or papyraceous or 'cigarette-paper' scars. Haematomas heal to form pseudotumours or nodules.

Joints

- Kyphoscoliosis.
- Hypermobility of joints (Fig. 67).

Proceed as follows:

Tell the examiner that you would like to examine the following:

- The hernial orifices.
- The heart for mitral valve prolapse and aortic regurgitation.
- The eyes for myopia, retinal detachment.

Note. The three basic clinical criteria are: (1) fragile skin; (2) bleeding diathesis; (3) hypermobile joints.

DIAGNOSIS

This patient has hypermobile joints (lesion) due to Ehlers–Danlos syndrome (aetiology).
Read the following articles: *N Engl J Med* 2000; **342:** 730; *N Engl J Med* 2000; **342:** 673–80.

ADVANCED-LEVEL QUESTIONS

What are the gastrointestinal manifestations of this syndrome?

- Marked tendency to herniate.
- Achalasia of the cardia.

- Eventration of the diaphragm.
- Megacolon.

What are the cardiovascular manifestations?
- Mitral valve prolapse.
- Aortic dissection.

What precautions would you take in managing skin wounds?
As the skin wounds tend to be gaping, they should be approximated with care; removable sutures are usually left in place for twice the usual time.

What do you know about Ehlers–Danlos syndrome?
It comprises a group of heterogeneous disorders that result from defects in collagen synthesis and vary genetically and clinically from one another (*Science* 1973; **182:** 298). The molecular defects of the following are known:

- Type VI (kyphoscoliotic type): the most common and autosomal recessive form of inheritance. There is a defect in the enzyme protein, viz. lysyl hydroxylase, which is necessary for hydroxylation of lysyl residues during collagen synthesis. Only collagen types 1 and 3 are affected, and collagen types 2, 4 and 6 are normal. The predominant clinical features are ocular fragility with rupture of the cornea and retinal detachment. Some of these patients respond to ascorbic acid.
- Type IV ('vascular type'): due to a defect in the structural gene for collagen type 3 and thus inherited as an autosomal dominant trait. As type 3 collagen is present largely in blood vessels and intestines, the typical features of this syndrome include easy bruising, thin skin with visible veins, characteristic facial features, rupture of the large arteries, uterus, colon, reducing life expectancy considerably. This is the most severe form of Ehlers–Danlos syndrome (*N Engl J Med* 2000; **342:** 673–80).
- Type VII: a defect in the conversion of procollagen to collagen, due to the mutation that affects one of the two type 1 collagen genes. Although in the single mutant allele only 50% of type 1 collagen chains are affected, heterozygotes manifest the syndrome because these abnormal chains interfere with the formation of normal collagen helices.
- Type IX: due to a defect in copper metabolism with high levels of copper in the cells but low levels of serum copper and caeruloplasmin. Because the gene influencing copper metabolism is on the X chromosome, it is inherited as an X-linked recessive trait. This disease illustrates how copper metabolism can affect connective tissue.

Note. Patients with type I, II and IV disease are often investigated for bleeding diathesis before the correct diagnosis is made. Because of joint instability and laxity, many patients with types I, II, III, VI and VII disease are investigated for developmental delay before it is recognized that they have this syndrome.

In which other condition is there a defect in collagen metabolism?
Osteogenesis imperfecta.

Note. At least some 14 types of collagen have been discerned: types 1, 2 and 3 are the interstitial or fibrillar collagen whereas types 4, 5 and 6 are amorphous and are present in the interstitial tissue and basement membranes.

What are the criteria for diagnosis of joint hypermobility?

Beighton's nine-point scoring for joint hypermobility assigns two points for each of the following four paired manoeuvres (*Ann Rheum Dis* 1973; **32:** 413–18):

- Hyperextension of the fifth metacarpophalangeal joint to 90 degrees.
- Apposition of the thumb to the volar aspect of the forearm.
- Hyperextension of the elbow beyond 10 degrees.
- Hyperextension of the knee to beyond 10 degrees.

One point is assigned for the ability to place the palms of the hands on the floor with the knees extended.

Is hypermobility advantageous to musicians?

Lax fingers and wrists are good for flautists and string players, but lax knees and spines are bad for tympanists and others who stand while they play (*N Engl J Med* 1993; **329:** 1079).

Edvard Ehlers (1863–1937), a Danish dermatologist, and H.A. Danlos, a French dermatologist, described this condition independently in 1901 and 1908 respectively. Tschernogobow in Moscow first described this syndrome in 1892 (*N Engl J Med* 2000; **342:** 730).

It is widely believed that the outstanding virtuosity of the violinist Niccolò Paganini (1782–1840) was due to remarkable flexibility of the joints of his left hand – he could span three octaves with little effort (*Arthritis Rheum* 1982; **25:** 1385–6).

Robert James Gorlin (b. 1923) described Gorlin's sign, which is the ability to touch the tip of the nose with the tongue in Ehlers–Danlos syndrome.

Case 198

TUBEROUS SCLEROSIS (BOURNEVILLE'S OR PRINGLE'S DISEASE)

INSTRUCTION

Look at this patient who has a history of seizures and mental retardation.

SALIENT FEATURES

History

- Family history (autosomal dominant inheritance with variable penetrance).
- Seizures.
- Psychomotor retardation in childhood.
- Reddened nodules (adenoma sebaceum) on the face since childhood.

Examination

- Angiofibromas (adenoma sebaceum) distributed in a butterfly pattern over the cheeks (Figs 69 and 70), chin and forehead.

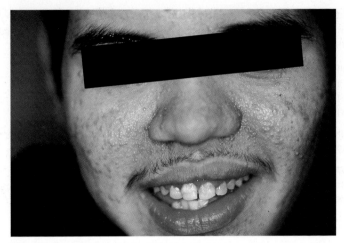

Fig. 69

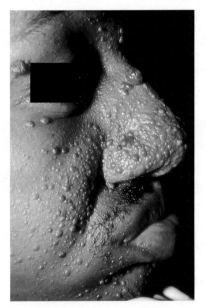

Fig. 70

- Shagreen patches (leathery thickenings in localized patches over the lumbosacral region).
- Ash-leaf patches (hypopigmented areas; Fig. 71).
- Subungual fibromas (Fig. 72).
- Examine the fundus (retinal glial hamartomas).

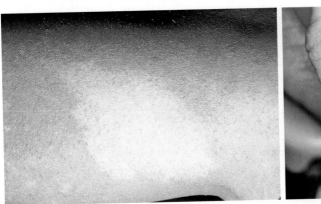
Fig. 71

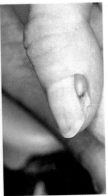
Fig. 72

DIAGNOSIS

This patient has adenoma sebaceum (lesions) due to tuberous sclerosis. I would like to know his IQ and elicit a history of seizures to determine his functional status.

ADVANCED-LEVEL QUESTIONS

What other lesions may be present?

- Hamartomas within the CNS occurring as cortical tubers and subependymal hamartomas.
- Renal angiomyolipomas.
- Cardiac rhabdomyomas and pulmonary myomas.
- Cysts in the liver, kidney and pancreas.

What is the prevalence of tuberous sclerosis?

It is estimated to be at 8 per 10 000 in Wessex (*Lancet* 1998; **351:** 1490).

How would you manage such patients?

Symptomatically, with anticonvulsant therapy for seizures and genetic counselling. When severe epilepsy and mental retardation is present the prognosis for life beyond the third decade is poor. Death usually results from seizures, associated neoplasms or intercurrent illness.

Do you know on which chromosome the gene is localized?

Linkage studies have localized the gene to chromosome 9 (TSC1) (*Science* 1997; **277:** 805–8) and chromosome 16 (TSC2) (*Cell* 1993; **75:** 1305–15). The nature of the gene on chromosome 9 is not clear whereas the gene on chromosome 16 encodes the protein tuberin. The function of this protein is unclear.

D.M. Bourneville (1840–1909), a French neurologist.

J.J. Pringle (1855–1922), an English dermatologist who was also the editor of the *British Journal of Dermatology*.

The Eker rat is an animal model of tuberous sclerosis.

Case 199

PRETIBIAL MYXOEDEMA

INSTRUCTION

Look at this patient's legs.

SALIENT FEATURES

History

As in patients with thyrotoxicosis (see p. 355).

Examination

Red thickened swelling above the lateral malleoli – peau d'orange appearance – which progresses to thickened non-pitting oedema of the feet (Fig. 73).

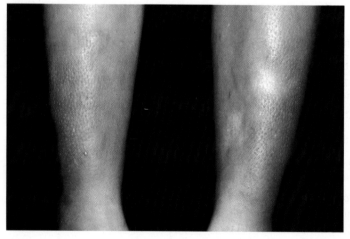

Fig. 73

Proceed as follows:

- Examine the following:
  - The hands for acropachy, palmar erythema and warm, sweaty palms.
  - The neck for goitre and thyroidectomy scar.
  - The eyes for exophthalmos.
  - The pulse for tachycardia and atrial fibrillation.
- Tell the examiner that you would like to know whether or not the patient has had any treatment, in particular radioactive iodine.

Remember. Pretibial myxoedema dermopathy is a late manifestation of Graves' disease and its onset is usually followed by the diagnosis of hyperthyroidism and ophthalmopathy.

DIAGNOSIS

This patient has pretibial myxoedema (lesion) with ophthalmopathy and signs of thyrotoxicosis (functional status) which is due to Graves' disease.

QUESTIONS

What investigations would you perform?
Serum T_4, T_3 and TSH.

How are these lesions treated?
- Intralesional steroids or fluorinated corticosteroids applied under polythene occlusion.
- Plasmapheresis.
- Cytotoxic therapy.
- Octreotide.

Note. Surgical excision should be avoided because surgical scars may aggravate the dermopathy and precipitate recurrence.

ADVANCED-LEVEL QUESTIONS

What are the types of pretibial myxoedema?
Three major classes of thyroid dermopathy have been identified (*Medicine* 1994; **73:** 1–7):

- Non-pitting oedema accompanied by hyperkeratosis, pigmentation and pinkish, brownish red or yellowish discoloration of the skin. Plaque formation and nodularity are characteristically absent in this group.
- Plaque form consisting of raised, discrete or confluent plaques.
- Nodular form, characterized by nodule formation.

Less common types:

- Elephantiasic form.
- Polypoid form.

Note. Almost all patients tend to have ophthalmopathy, which is usually severe.

What is the histology of pretibial myxoedema?
- Characteristic features include fraying and oedematous appearance on routine staining with haematoxylin and eosin, and increase of alcian blue–periodic acid–Schiff-positive mucinous material, with resultant connective tissue fibre separation.
- Review of pathology reports does not show any distinguishing microscopic characteristics for various clinical forms of this dermopathy.

What are the recommendations for screening thyroid dysfunction?
It is recommended that adults be screened for thyroid dysfunction by measurement of serum TSH concentration, beginning at the age of 35 years and every 5 years thereafter. The indication for screening is particularly compelling in women, but it may also be justified in men as a relatively cost-effective measure in the context of periodic health examination. Individuals with clinical manifestations potentially

attributable to thyroid dysfunction and those with risk factors for its development may require more frequent serum TSH testing (*Arch Intern Med* 2000; **160:** 1573–5).

How can hyperthyroidism present in the elderly?

Thyrotoxicosis can present in the elderly with atrial fibrillation, and such patients may lack other common signs of thyrotoxicosis; this is known as apathetic hyperthyroidism. Low serum TSH concentrations also constitute a risk factor for atrial fibrillation in the elderly (*N Engl J Med* 1994; **331:** 1249–52).

EXAMINATION OF THE FUNDUS

1. Tell the patient, 'Look straight ahead with your right or left (R/L) eye while I look into your L/R eye'. (The candidate need not remove his or her spectacles while the fundus is being examined.) The candidate should use his or her own R/L eye to examine the patient's R/L eye.

2. Look at the eye from a distance of at least 50 cm and check for the red reflex. (The presence of a red reflex indicates that the media in front of the retina is transparent and that the retina is firmly in apposition with the underlying choroid. Red reflex may be absent when there is a lens opacity, vitreous haemorrhage or retinal detachment.)

3. Look systematically at the following:
   - The optic discs (comment on the colour, contour, cup and lamina cribrosa).
   - The macula (one or two disc diameters away from and a little below the temporal margin of the optic disc). It appears darker than the surrounding retina, and in young individuals has a central yellow point called the fovea centralis.
   - The nasal and temporal halves of the fundus.
   - The retinal vessels (remember that the retinal artery has four main branches and the normal ratio of the artery to the vein is 2:3). The candidate should assess the transparency of the vessels (the arteries usually have a shiny central reflex stripe), the presence of pressure effects such as arteriovenous nicking, the presence of focal narrowing of arteries as well as tortuosity of the venules.

Note
- Lesions in the fundus are measured using the disc diameter as the reference size.
- Elevation of any lesion is measured by noting the difference between lens powers that focus clearly on the top of the lesion and an adjacent normal area of the fundus. Elevation of 3 dioptre lens changes is approximately equal to 1 mm in actual elevation.

Case 200

DIABETIC RETINOPATHY

INSTRUCTION

Examine the fundus in these patients.

SALIENT FEATURES

You will be expected to comment on whether there is background or proliferative retinopathy. You may have a clue about the underlying diabetes, either from a diabetic chart or from the presence of diabetic fruit juices at the bedside.

History

- Gradual or acute loss of vision.
- History of floaters.
- History of diabetes, hypertension.
- Ask about renal disease (renal–retinal syndrome of diabetes).

Examination

Patient 1 has background retinopathy (Fig. 74), caused by microvascular leakage into the retina.

- Microaneurysms, usually seen in the posterior pole temporal to the fovea.
- Dot and blot haemorrhages.
- Hard exudates.
- Cottonwool spots.

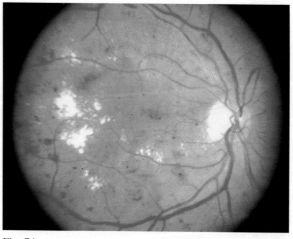

Fig. 74

DIAGNOSIS

This patient has dot and blot haemorrhages and cottonwool spots (lesions), probably due to diabetic retinopathy (aetiology), and has good visual acuity (functional status).

QUESTIONS

What symptoms will this patient have?
The patient will be asymptomatic as the macula is spared.

How would you manage such a patient?
- Treat diabetes and associated hypertension.
- Annual fundal examination.

The Early Treatment of Diabetic Retinopathy Study (ETDRS) has established that early peripheral (panretinal) argon laser photocoagulation is not indicated for mild to moderate non-proliferative retinopathy. Early treatment in the form of argon laser photocoagulation applied directly to leaking microaneurysms, as well as grid photo-coagulation applied to diffuse areas of leakage and thickening, is highly beneficial.

SALIENT FEATURES

Patient 2 has diabetic maculopathy, caused by oedema and/or hard exudates.

- Signs of background retinopathy with hard exudates or oedema of the macula.

QUESTIONS

What symptoms may this patient have?
There will be a gradual impairment of central vision, such as difficulty in reading small print or seeing road signs.

ADVANCED-LEVEL QUESTIONS

What are the signs of macular oedema?
Macular oedema includes any of the following signs:

- Retinal thickening at or within 500 μm of the centre of the macula.
- Retinal thickening of one disc area or larger, in any part of the retina which is within the one-disc diameter from the centre of the macula.
- Hard exudates at or within 500 μm of the centre of the macula.

How will you manage this patient?
Non-urgent referral to an ophthalmologist for photocoagulation which will stabilize (seldom improve) visual acuity in 50% of patients. The ability to alter the course of visual loss in diabetic macular oedema favourably is a major advance but patients must be cautioned that the most likely result of treatment is stabilization, not improvement, of visual acuity.

What is the principal mechanism of visual loss in non-proliferative retinopathy?
The principal mechanism of visual loss in non-proliferative retinopathy is macular oedema, which results from focal vascular leakage from microaneurysms in the

macular capillaries, as well as diffuse vascular leakage. With time, areas of leakage progress to macular thickening associated with hard exudates or cystoid changes.

What are the different types of clinical presentation?

Patients may present with no visual symptoms, paracentral scotomata or various degrees of central visual loss. Consequently, the diagnosis and management of macular oedema depend crucially on the determination of macular thickening by fundus examination. Ophthalmoscopy detects intraretinal haemorrhages and hard exudates but does not detect substantial retinal thickening. A critical evaluation of retinal thickening requires stereoscopic examination of the retina by slit-lamp biomicroscopy with lens for retinal visualization or stereoscopic fundus photography.

SALIENT FEATURES

Patient 3 has preproliferative retinopathy which is uncommon and is caused by retinal hypoxia.

• Cottonwool spots.
• Venous dilatation, beading, looping or sausage-like segmentation.
• Arteriolar narrowing.
• Haemorrhages – large dark blots.
• Intraretinal microvascular abnormalities.

QUESTIONS

What symptoms may this patient have?

The patient is asymptomatic if the macula is spared.

How would you manage this patient?

Semiurgent referral to the ophthalmologist for close follow-up to enable early detection and treatment of proliferative retinopathy.

SALIENT FEATURES

Patient 4 has proliferative retinopathy caused by retinal hypoxia, usually seen in insulin-dependent diabetic retinopathy (Figs 75 and 76).

• Neovascularization around the disc (NVD) or away from the disc – in early stages the vessels are bare and flat and easily missed. In later stages they are elevated and may be associated with a white fibrous component.
• Presence of laser burns (in treated cases).

QUESTIONS

What symptoms may this patient have?

The patient is asymptomatic in the absence of complications.

How would you manage this patient?

Urgent referral to an ophthalmologist for laser treatment.

What are the complications of proliferative retinopathy?

• Vitreous haemorrhage.

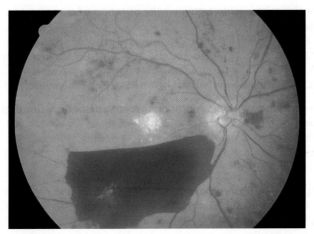

Fig. 75

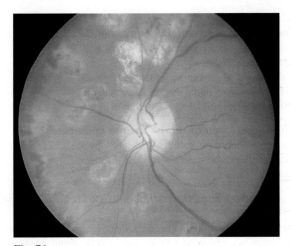

Fig. 76

- Traction retinal detachment.
- Rubeosis irides.
- Rubeotic glaucoma – some of these patients can experience partial restoration of vision by microsurgery called pars plana vitrectomy.

ADVANCED-LEVEL QUESTIONS

What is the prevalence of retinopathy in diabetes?
The overall prevalence is about 25%. It is 40% in insulin-dependent diabetes mellitus (IDDM) and 20% in non-insulin-dependent diabetes mellitus (NIDDM).

What is the relationship between the duration of diabetes and retinopathy?

There is a close relationship: in patients diagnosed as having diabetes before the age of 30 years, the incidence of retinopathy is about 50% after 10 years and 90% after 30 years. It is unusual for retinopathy to develop within 5 years of onset of diabetes; however, 5% of patients with NIDDM have background retinopathy at presentation.

What associated systemic conditions worsen diabetic retinopathy?
- Pregnancy.
- Hypertension.
- Anaemia.
- Renal failure.

What is the relationship between diabetic control and retinopathy?

The Diabetes Control and Complications Trial compared intensive treatment for blood glucose control with conventional treatment in patients with and without retinopathy at baseline who were followed for a mean of 6.5 years. Intensive treatment has profound benefits in both subgroups and was associated with a reduction in the incidence of both the development of new retinopathy and the risk of progression of existing retinopathy.

How often would you screen diabetic patients for retinopathy?
- Non-insulin-dependent diabetics: annually.
- Insulin-dependent diabetics:
  - Newly diagnosed: no screening for the first 5 years.
  - Five to ten years from initial diagnosis: annually.
  - Over 10 years after initial diagnosis: every 6 months.

What is the earliest sign of retinal change in diabetes?

An increase in capillary permeability, evidenced by the leakage of dye into the vitreous humour after fluorescein injection, is the earliest sign of retinal change in diabetes mellitus.

What do you know about the pathogenesis of retinal new vessel formation?

It is not completely understood and current theories emphasize the production of angiogenic factors by areas of ischaemic and hypoxic retina. More recently, vascular endothelial growth factor (VEGF) has been isolated from ocular fluid and is an endothelial cell-specific angiogenic factor whose production is increased by hypoxia; it has been implicated in the neovascularization seen in diabetic retinopathy and retinal vein occlusion.

What do you know about photocoagulation?

Photocoagulation is a technique whereby several thousand lesions are produced over a 2-week therapy period with lasers. Panretinal photocoagulation reduces the risk of severe visual loss. The laser is used to ablate a portion of the retina and does not directly cauterize the neovascularization. It is believed that the regression of neovascularization due to laser is a result of the destruction of ischaemic and hypoxic retina with reduction in angiogenic factors. Photocoagulation decreases the incidence of haemorrhage or scarring in proliferative retinopathy.

Photocoagulation is also useful in the treatment of microaneurysms, haemorrhages and oedema. Some loss of peripheral vision may be inevitable with this technique.

What surgical technique may be used for a non-resolving vitreous haemorrhage and retinal detachment?

Pars plana vitrectomy may be used but is often complicated by retinal tears, retinal detachment, glaucoma, infection, cataracts and loss of the eye.

Case 201

HYPERTENSIVE RETINOPATHY

INSTRUCTION

Examine this patient's eyes.
Examine this patient's fundus.

SALIENT FEATURES

History

- Usually no ocular symptoms.
- History of hypertension.

Examination (Fig. 77)

- Arteriovenous nipping.
- Arteriolar narrowing.

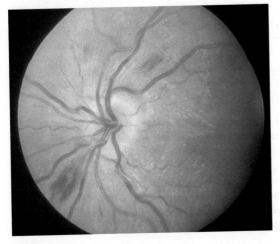

Fig. 77

- Macular star.
- Flame-shaped and blot haemorrhages.
- Cottonwool exudates.
- Papilloedema may or may not be present.

Proceed as follows:
Tell the examiner that you would like to:

- Check the blood pressure.
- Examine the urine for proteinuria.
- Examine the heart for left ventricular hypertrophy.

DIAGNOSIS

This patient has flame-shaped haemorrhages with a macular star (lesions) due to hypertension (aetiology).

ADVANCED-LEVEL QUESTIONS

How would you grade hypertensive retinopathy?
Keith–Wagner–Barker classification (*Am J Med Sci* 1939; **197**: 332–43):

- Stage I – arteriolar narrowing.
- Stage II – irregular calibre of arterioles.
- Stage III – cottonwool exudates; flame and blot haemorrhages, retinal oedema.
- Stage IV – papilloedema.

Note. Subsequent studies have shown that the clinical features and prognosis of patients with stage III and stage IV disease were similar whether or not papilloedema was present; consequently the terms 'malignant' and 'accelerated' can be used interchangeably (*BMJ* 1986; **292**: 235–7; *Q J Med* 1993; **86**: 485–93). Instead, 'hypertensive crisis' is used to refer to the syndrome of raised blood pressure complicated by end-organ damage (e.g. stroke, renal failure, myocardial ischaemia or infarction, stage III or IV hypertensive retinopathy).

Mention some causes of cottonwool spots (Lancet *1965; i: 303*).

- HIV infection *per se*.
- Anaemias.
- Infective endocarditis.
- Leukaemias.
- Diabetic retinopathy (see pp 518–23).

Mention a few causes of hypertension.

- In 90% of cases it is essential hypertension with no underlying cause, and this may represent the 'normal' spread.
- In 10% of cases there is an underlying cause:
  - Renal causes: renal artery stenosis, polycystic kidneys, chronic glomerulonephritis, polyarteritis nodosa, chronic pyelonephritis.
  - Endocrine causes: Cushing's syndrome, Conn's syndrome, phaeochromocytoma, acromegaly, diabetes mellitus.

– Eclampsia and pre-eclamptic toxaemia of pregnancy.
– Coarctation of the aorta.

How would you investigate a patient with hypertension?
• Urine for protein, glucose, casts.
• Mid-stream urine for microscopy and culture.
• Urea and electrolytes, fasting lipids.
• CXR.
• ECG.
• Urine catecholamines.
• Intravenous pyelography.
• Renal artery digital subtraction angiography (DSA).

How would you treat hypertension?
• Salt restriction.
• Drug therapy.
• First line (*BMJ* 1990; **301:** 1172):
  – In women and smokers – bendroflumethiazide (bendrofluazide).
  – In non-smoking men – beta-blockers.
• Advise the patient to stop smoking.

Sir C.T. Dollery, was Dean of the Royal Postgraduate Medical School, Hammersmith Hospital, London; his interests include clinical pharmacology, hypertension and medical education.

John Swales, contemporary Professor of Medicine, Leicester; his chief interest is hypertension.

James C. Petrie, Professor and Head of Medicine and Therapeutics, Aberdeen; his interests included hypertension and cardiovascular prevention. He was also the President of the Royal College of Physicians of Edinburgh.

Case 202

PAPILLOEDEMA

INSTRUCTION

Examine this patient's fundus.

SALIENT FEATURES

History
• Headache.
• Transient visual disturbances.
• Diplopia (due to associated sixth cranial nerve palsy).
• History of hypertension, brain tumour.
• History of ingestion of steroids, hypervitaminosis A (causes of benign intracranial hypertension).

Examination

- There is swelling of the optic disc (look for haemorrhages and soft exudates; Fig. 78).

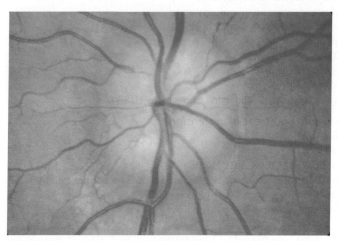

Fig. 78

Note. Remember that the common causes are:

- Intracranial space-occupying lesion.
- Hypertensive retinopathy.
- Benign intracranial hypertension.

DIAGNOSIS

This patient has bilateral papilloedema (lesion) and I would like to investigate for an intracranial space-occupying lesion (aetiology).

QUESTIONS

What do you understand by the term 'papilloedema'?

Papilloedema is the swelling of the nerve head as seen on ophthalmoscopy. The colour of the disc becomes redder, approximating to that of the rest of the retina; its contour becomes blurred and the cup and cribrosa are filled in.

What is the first manifestation of papilloedema?

The earliest manifestation of papilloedema is the engorgement of the veins.

What is the nature of the field defect in papilloedema?

Papilloedema is always associated with enlargement of the blind spot, with a consequent diminution of visual fields and gradual loss of visual acuity, but a fair degree of acuity may remain until papilloedema is marked.

ADVANCED-LEVEL QUESTIONS

Mention a few causes of papilloedema.

- Raised intracranial pressure resulting from one of the following conditions:
  - Impaired circulation of the CSF due to aqueduct stenosis.
  - Meningitis.
  - Subarachnoid haemorrhage.
- Cerebral oedema:
  - Following head injury.
  - Following cerebral anoxia.
- Metabolic causes:
  - Carbon dioxide retention.
  - Steroid withdrawal.
  - Thyroid eye disease.
  - Vitamin A intoxication.
  - Lead poisoning.
- Increased protein in the CSF due to one of the following:
  - Guillain–Barré syndrome.
  - Spinal cord tumours.
  - Any spinal block.
- Haematological and circulatory disorders:
  - Central retinal vein thrombosis.
  - Superior vena caval obstruction.
  - Polycythaemia vera.
  - Multiple myeloma.
  - Macroglobulinaemia.

Mention a few conditions simulating papilloedema.

- Deep optic cup:
  - Nasal edge appears heaped up.
  - Vessels plunge into the optic cup.
  - Temporal edge is quite normal.
- Medullated nerve fibres, seen on the disc or even on the retina. The appearance is typically flared and on focusing will reveal fibres traversing the area. Field defects are due to the retinal vessels being obscured. Since these are present from birth, the patient is unaware of the defect.
- Bergmeister's papilla, in which there is a whitish elevation of the centre of the disc with venous and arterial sheathing. It is common and seen at all ages. There is an equal sex and racial incidence.
- Pseudopapilloedema, i.e. congenitally elevated discs secondary to hyaloid tissue (drüsen) or hyperopia.

Note. Elevation or swelling of the optic disc occurs in the following conditions:

- Papilloedema.
- Papillitis.
- Drüsen.
- Infiltration of the nerve head by malignant cells.

What do you know about Foster Kennedy syndrome?

Unilateral papilloedema, with or without 'secondary' optic atrophy on the other side, suggests a tumour of the opposite side on the olfactory lobe or orbital surface of the frontal lobe or of the pituitary body.

What do you understand by the term 'papillitis'?

- Demyelination of the optic nerve (multiple sclerosis).
- Inflammation.
- Degeneration (Leber's optic atrophy).
- Vascular disorders of the nerve head.
- Malignant infiltration.

How do you differentiate papillitis from papilloedema?

Papillitis	Papilloedema
Usually unilateral	Usually bilateral
Visual acuity is considerably reduced in relation to the degree of swelling of the disc	Visual acuity only slightly reduced until late stages
Visual field defect is usually central, particularly for red and green	Peripheral constriction or enlargement of the blind spot
Marcus Gunn pupil may be present	Marcus Gunn pupil is absent
Eye movements may be painful	Eye movements are never painful

Note. A Marcus Gunn pupil is one that shows better constriction to an indirect response than to direct light.

What are the stages of papilloedema?

- Stage I – increase in venous calibre and tortuosity.
- Stage II – optic cup becomes pinker and less distinct, the vessels seeming to disappear suddenly on the surface of the disc.
- Stage III – blurring of the discs on the nasal side. (**Note.** In many normal discs the nasal edge is less distinct and one of the most frequent false-positive signs is questionable blurring of the nasal disc margins.)
- Stage IV – the whole disc becomes suffused and slightly elevated. The margins may disappear and the vessels seem to emerge from a mushy swelling. The optic cup is filled and there are haemorrhages around the disc.

What are the features of benign intracranial hypertension?

Dandy's diagnostic criteria (*Brain* 1991; **114:** 155–80):

- Patient is alert.
- Clinical features of increased intracranial pressure.
- No localizing neurological signs (except sixth cranial nerve palsy).
- Opening pressure of cerebrospinal fluid (CSF) during lumbar puncture is >20 cmH$_2$O and CSF is of normal composition.
- Normal ventricles and normal study on CT or MRI.

What treatment options are available for pseudotumor cerebri?

- Discontinuation of steroids, weight loss.
- Drugs: carbonic anhydrase inhibitors, diuretics.

- Serial lumbar punctures, lumboperitoneal shunt.
- Optic nerve fenestration, subtemporal decompression.

> Foster Kennedy (1884–1952) was born in Belfast. He was Professor of Neurology at Cornell University. He described his syndrome in 1923.

Case 203

OPTIC ATROPHY

INSTRUCTION

Examine this patient's eyes.
Examine this patient's fundus.

SALIENT FEATURES

History

- Visual loss – onset of symptoms depends on underlying aetiology.
- History of multiple sclerosis.
- History of glaucoma.
- Optic nerve tumour.
- Vitamin B_{12} deficiency.
- Paget's disease.
- Exposure to toxins: lead, methanol, arsenic.

Examination

- Pale disc with sharp margins (Fig. 79).

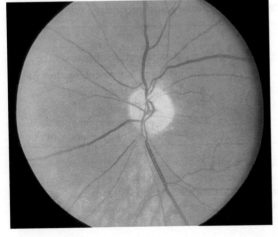

Fig. 79

- Intact consensual light reflex but impaired direct light reflex – Marcus Gunn pupillary response (seen in asymmetrical involvement of the two eyes).
- Central scotoma on testing of visual fields.

Proceed as follows:
Tell the examiner that you would like to look for cerebellar signs (remember that multiple sclerosis is the commonest cause of optic atrophy).

DIAGNOSIS

This patient has primary optic atrophy (lesion) due to multiple sclerosis (aetiology). I would like to check the visual fields for central scotoma (functional status).

QUESTIONS

What is your diagnosis?
The differential diagnosis is as follows:

- Demyelinating disorders (multiple sclerosis).
- Optic nerve compression by tumour or aneurysm.
- Glaucoma.
- Toxins: methanol, tobacco, lead, arsenical poisoning.
- Ischaemia, including central retinal artery occlusion due to thromboembolism, temporal arteritis, idiopathic acute ischaemic optic neuropathy, syphilis.
- Hereditary disorders: Friedreich's ataxia, Leber's optic atrophy (sex linked, seen in young males).
- Paget's disease.
- Vitamin B_{12} deficiency.
- Secondary to retinitis pigmentosa.

ADVANCED-LEVEL QUESTIONS

What is the difference between primary and secondary optic atrophy?

Primary	Secondary
White and flat with clear-cut edges	Greyish-white, edges indistinct
Visible lamina cribrosa	Cup filled and lamina cribrosa not visible
Arteries and veins normal	Arteries thinner than normal Veins may be dilated
Capillaries decreased in number	Capillaries decreased in number (fewer than seven) – Kestenbaum's sign

What is consecutive optic atrophy?
Consecutive optic atrophy is a controversial term and is best avoided. Some use it as an equivalent or alternative for what has been described above as secondary optic atrophy, but others use the term to indicate an atrophy complicating retinitis or, rarely, Tay–Sachs disease or retinitis pigmentosa.

What is glaucomatous optic atrophy?

Glaucomatous optic atrophy denotes loss of disc substance, referred to as increased cupping.

How would you investigate a patient with optic neuropathy?

- FBC, ESR.
- Blood glucose.
- Serology for syphilis.
- Vitamin B_{12} and B_1 levels.
- Radiography of pituitary fossa, optic foramina and sinuses, or CT scan of the brain and orbit.
- ECG.
- Pattern-stimulated visual evoked responses.
- Electroretinography.

R. Marcus Gunn (1850–1909), a Scottish ophthalmologist who worked at Moorfields Eye Hospital, London.

T. von Leber (1840–1917), Professor of Ophthalmology at the University of Heidelberg, Germany.

W. Tay (1843–1927), a British ophthalmologist, Moorfields Eye Hospital, London.

B.P. Sachs (1858–1944), a German neuropsychiatrist who worked in New York. He described this condition independent of Tay.

Case 204

RETINAL VEIN THROMBOSIS

INSTRUCTION

Examine this patient's eyes.
Examine this patient's fundus.

SALIENT FEATURES

History

- Branched retinal vein occlusion: decreased vision, floaters suggest vitreal haemorrhage.
- Central retinal vein occlusion: loss of or decreased vision, headache (associated increase in intraocular pressure), floaters.
- History of hypertension, diabetes, glaucoma, multiple myeloma or macro-globulinaemia.

Examination

Patient 1 has central retinal vein occlusion (Fig. 80), i.e. occlusion is behind the cribriform plate:

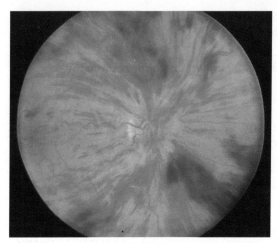

Fig. 80

- Multiple retinal and preretinal haemorrhages surround the optic nerve head. There is marked dilatation and tortuosity of the veins, hyperaemia or oedema of the nerve head and soft exudates – 'blood and thunder' appearance.
- Visual acuity is only slightly reduced.

Patient 2 has branch vein occlusion (Fig. 81); the occlusion is in front of the cribriform plate:

- Occlusion occurs just distal to the arteriovenous crossing. The superior temporal vein is most commonly involved. Haemorrhages are seen surrounding the occluded vein.
- May cause a quadrantic field defect.
- Visual prognosis is good if the haemorrhages do not extend to the macula with accompanying macular oedema.

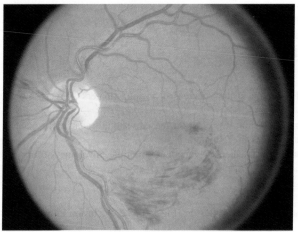

Fig. 81

Proceed as follows:
Tell the examiner that you would like to check for the following conditions:

- Diabetes (urine sugar).
- Hypertension.
- Chronic simple glaucoma.
- Hyperviscosity syndromes (Waldenström's macroglobulinaemia, multiple myeloma).

DIAGNOSIS

This patient has multiple retinal haemorrhages (lesions) due to central retinal vein occlusion with underlying diabetes mellitus (aetiology).

ADVANCED-LEVEL QUESTIONS

What are the usual sites of occlusion in branch retinal vein occlusion?

- At arteriovenous crossings, causing classical quadrantic or small macular occlusions.
- Along the main veins, as in diabetes mellitus.
- At the edges of the optic disc, resulting in occlusion of the hemisphere.
- Peripherally, as in sickle cell disease.

What are the vascular responses to retinal vein occlusion?

These include dilatation of retinal capillaries, abnormal vascular permeability and retinal capillary closure.

What is the prognosis in branch retinal vein occlusion?

It varies from complete resolution with no residual visual deficits to a progressive deterioration resulting in permanent loss of vision.

What is the clinical course in central retinal vein occlusion?

- In mild cases, there is minimal dilatation of veins and haemorrhages with little or no oedema of the macula and no visual deficit.
- In severe instances, the vision may deteriorate to hand motions, with extensive deep and superficial haemorrhages with stagnation of blood in the markedly dilated veins and several cottonwool spots.

What are the complications of central retinal vein occlusion?

These include neovascularization of the retina, rubeosis iridis (usually visible by 1 month) and rubeotic glaucoma (usually by 3 months).

How would you manage such eyes?

- Treat the underlying condition.
- Fluorescein angiography to determine areas of retinal ischaemia.
- Regular follow-up by the ophthalmologist as secondary neovascularization is a common sequela and may need laser therapy. Panretinal photocoagulation prevents the dreaded complication of neovascular glaucoma.

J.G. Waldenström (b. 1906), Professor of Medicine, Uppsala University, Sweden.

Case 205

SUBHYALOID HAEMORRHAGE

INSTRUCTION

Examine this patient's fundus.

SALIENT FEATURES

History

- Sudden, painless loss of vision.
- Sudden appearance of floaters and black spots with or without flashing lights.
- History of stroke (subarachnoid haemorrhage).
- History of diabetes, retinal tears, vitreous detachment, retinal vein occlusion.
- History of trauma.

Examination

- A large, solitary subhyaloid haemorrhage (there may be no fluid level if the patient is lying flat).
- There may be associated retinal haemorrhage.
- Twenty per cent have mild papilloedema.

Proceed as follows:
- Comment on any obvious hemiplegia.

Note. When the subhyaloid (preretinal) haemorrhage extends into the vitreous humour it is called Terson's syndrome.

DIAGNOSIS

This hemiplegic patient has a subhyaloid haemorrhage (lesion) due to subarachnoid haemorrhage (aetiology).

ADVANCED-LEVEL QUESTIONS

What is the commonest cause of subhyaloid haemorrhage?
Subarachnoid haemorrhage (*BMJ* 1990; **301:** 190).

What are the other causes of haemorrhage into the vitreous?
- Local injury.
- Blood diseases.
- Hypertension.
- Diabetes.
- Idiopathic.

Mention some causes of neck stiffness.
- Subarachnoid haemorrhage.

- Meningitis.
- Posterior fossa tumours.
- Local neck pathology such as cervical spondylosis.

What are causes of deterioration in a patient with subarachnoid haemorrhage?
- Rebleeds.
- Cerebral infarction due to reflex vasospasm of cerebral vessels (hence the rationale to use nimodipine).
- Secondary hydrocephalus.

How would you investigate such a patient?
CT head scan, and if this rules out intracranial hypertension, then a lumbar puncture to diagnose minor leaks.

Case 206

RETINITIS PIGMENTOSA

INSTRUCTION

Examine this patient's fundus.
Examine this patient's eyes.

SALIENT FEATURES

History

- Family history of blindness (can be autosomal recessive, which is more severe, or autosomal dominant, which is more benign).
- Decreased nocturnal vision.
- Altered colour vision.
- Loss of peripheral vision.
- Blurry vision.

Examination

- Peripheral retina shows perivascular 'bone spicule pigmentation' and arteriolar narrowing (Fig. 82). The retinal veins (never the arteries) often have a sheath of pigmentation for part of their course. The pigment spots that lie near the retinal veins are seen to be anterior to them, so that they hide the course of the vessel. (In this respect they differ from the pigment around the spots of choroidal atrophy in which the retinal vessels can be traced over the spots.)

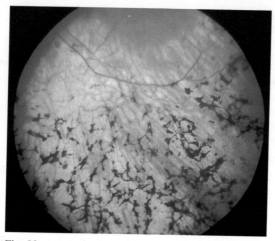

Fig. 82

- Optic disc is pale.
- Maculopathy, which is atrophic or cystoid.

Proceed as follows:
- Look for polydactyly in the hands and feet (Laurence–Moon–Biedl syndrome).
- Comment on the white walking aid (if any) used by the registered blind.
- Tell the examiner that you would like to check visual fields.

DIAGNOSIS

This patient is obese, has polydactyly and retinitis pigmentosa (lesion) due to Laurence–Moon–Biedl syndrome (aetiology) and is registered blind (functional status).

QUESTIONS

What is the prognosis in retinitis pigmentosa?
Most patients are registered blind by the age of 40 years, with central field less than 20° in diameter. Almost all patients lose central vision by the seventh decade.

What do you know about retinitis pigmentosa?
Retinitis pigmentosa is a slow degenerative disease of the retina. It occurs in both eyes, begins in early childhood, and often results in the loss of sight by middle or advanced age. The degeneration primarily affects the rods and cones, in particular the rods (*N Engl J Med* 1990; **323:** 1502).

How may it present?
It may present with defective vision at dusk (night blindness), which may occur several years before the pigment is visible in the retina.

ADVANCED-LEVEL QUESTIONS

Mention a few systemic disorders associated with retinitis pigmentosa.

- Laurence–Moon–Biedl–Bardet syndrome, which is a recessively inherited disorder characterized by mental disability, polydactyly, syndactyly, hypogonadism and obesity.
- Bassen–Kornzweig syndrome (abetalipoproteinaemia), characterized by fat malabsorption, abetalipoproteinaemia, acanthocytosis and spinocerebellar ataxia (*Ophthalmology* 1984; **91**: 991).
- Refsum's disease (phytanic acid storage disease), an autosomal recessive disorder characterized by hypertrophic peripheral neuropathy, deafness, ichthyosis, cerebellar ataxia, raised CSF protein levels in the absence of pleocytosis.
- Kearns–Sayre syndrome, a triad of retinitis pigmentosa, progressive external ophthalmoplegia and heart block (*Br J Ophthalmol* 1985; **69**: 63).
- Usher's disease, a recessively inherited disorder characterized by congenital, non-progressive, sensorineural deafness (*Arch Ophthalmol* 1983; **101**: 1367).
- Friedreich's ataxia (see pp 191–3).

Which ocular conditions are associated with retinitis pigmentosa?

- Open-angle glaucoma.
- Posterior subcapsular cataracts.
- Myopia.
- Keratoconus.

What is secondary retinitis pigmentosa?

Secondary retinitis pigmentosa is a sequela to inflammatory retinitis. It is often ophthalmoscopically indistinguishable from the primary condition; the electro-retinographic and electro-oculographic responses are slightly subnormal unless the condition is far advanced. (In the primary type the response is markedly subnormal to the electroretinogram and electro-oculogram).

What is retinitis pigmentosa sine pigmento?

A variety of retinitis pigmentosa without visible pigmentation of the retina.

What is inverse retinitis pigmentosa?

Bone corpuscles are visible in the perifoveal area, whereas the retinal periphery is normal.

How would you manage this patient?

- Refer for genetic counselling.
- Impaired vision training and aids for daily living.
- Refer for job training.
- Regular ophthalmology follow-up including visual fields, electroretinogram.

J.Z. Laurence (1830–1874), an English ophthalmologist.

R.C. Moon (1844–1914), a US ophthalmologist.

A. Biedl (1869–1933), a Czech physician.

G. Bardet (b. 1885), a French physician.

F.A. Bassen (b. 1903), physician, and A.L. Kornzweig (b. 1900), ophthalmologist, Mount Sinai Hospital, New York.

S. Refsum, a Norwegian physician.

Case 207

OLD CHOROIDITIS

INSTRUCTION

Examine this patient's fundus.

SALIENT FEATURES

History

- Decreased vision, floaters, red eye.
- History of HIV, sarcoidosis, TB.

Examination

- Old or inactive retinochoroiditis appears as white, well-defined areas of chorio-retinal atrophy with pigmented edges (due to proliferation of retinal pigment epithelium).
- The retinal blood vessels pass over the lesions undisturbed.

DIAGNOSIS

This patient has areas of retinal atrophy with pigmented edges (lesion) due to old choroiditis complicating cytomegalovirus infection (aetiology).

QUESTIONS

What may be the aetiology?

- Reactivation of congenital toxoplasmosis.
- Cytomegalovirus infection.
- AIDS.
- Sarcoidosis.
- TB.
- Syphilis.
- Behçet's disease.

What is the prognosis?

Prognosis varies according to the underlying aetiology. It is poor if the fovea is involved.

What does the presence of pigment on fundoscopy indicate?

A chronic lesion of the retina or choroid.

In which other conditions is the retinal pigment seen?

- Normally – racial (tigroid fundus).
- Retinitis pigmentosa.
- Malignant melanoma.

H. Behçet (1889–1940), Professor of Dermatology in Turkey, described this syndrome in 1937, based on three patients he observed between 1924 and 1936.

Case 208

CHOLESTEROL EMBOLUS IN THE FUNDUS

INSTRUCTION

Examine this patient's fundus.

SALIENT FEATURES

History

- Severe, acute and painless diminution or loss of vision.
- History of atherosclerosis.
- Risk factors of atherosclerosis: family history, diabetes, hypertension, ischaemic heart disease, peripheral vascular disease, cerebrovascular disease.

Examination

Presence of a cholesterol embolus (Hollenhorst plaque; Fig. 83) in one of the branches of the retinal artery.

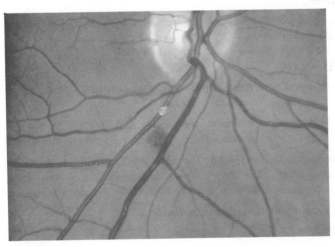

Fig. 83

Proceed as follows:

- Look for a cherry-red spot at the fovea (the ischaemic retina at the posterior pole becomes milky white and swollen, and the choroid is seen through the fovea as a cherry-red spot).
- Tell the examiner that you would like to check for visual field defects.

Remember that retinal artery occlusion results in infarction of the inner two thirds of the retina, reflex vasoconstriction of the retinal arterial tree and stasis in the retinal capillaries.

DIAGNOSIS

This patient has a cholesterol embolus in one of the branches of the retinal artery (lesion) due to underlying atherosclerotic disease (aetiology).
  Read classic review on this subject: *N Engl J Med* 1993; **329:** 427.

QUESTIONS

What are the complications of such an embolus?
Retinal artery occlusion causing field defects or loss of vision.

Where is the likely origin of this embolus?
The most likely origin is an atherosclerotic plaque in the carotid circulation.

What are the causes of retinal arterial occlusion?
The commonest cause is emboli arising from the major arteries supplying the head or from the left side of the heart. Embolic particles consist of platelet clumps, cholesterol crystals or Hollenhorst plaques and others (mixed thrombus, calcific or septic material from cardiac valves, fat, myxoma, talc in intravenous drug abusers or silicone in those who receive injections for cosmetic purposes).
  Other causes include:

* Temporal arteritis.
* Collagen vascular diseases.
* Increased orbital pressure, e.g. retrobulbar haemorrhage, Graves' exophthalmos.
* Sickle cell disease.
* Acute arteriolar spasm due to intranasal cocaine.
* Syphilis.

What do you understand by the term 'amaurosis'?
Amaurosis means blindness from any cause.

What do you understand by the term 'amblyopia'?
Amblyopia means that impaired vision is not due to refractive error or ocular disease.

What do you understand by the term 'amaurosis fugax'?
Amaurosis fugax is a retinal artery transient ischaemic attack (TIA) which manifests with a painless, unilateral loss of vision that usually lasts a few minutes.

How would you manage this patient?
* Aspirin.
* Ophthalmology opinion.
* Ultrasonography of the carotid arteries.
* Advise the patient to stop smoking.
* Control of hypertension.
* Carotid angiography with a view to performing carotid endarterectomy.

What is the effect of cholesterol crystals?
Cholesterol crystals rarely cause significant obstruction to the retinal arterioles.

What manoeuvre would you use to make the cholesterol crystals more apparent?

Mild lateral pressure on the globe may make the presence of unobtrusive crystals clearly visible when the retinal arteries pulsate.

How would you manage an acute occlusion of the retinal artery?

- Lie the patient in a supine position to ensure adequate circulation.
- Apply intermittent ocular massage for 15 minutes to dislodge the emboli, lower intraocular pressure and improve circulation.
- Intravenous acetazolamide to lower intraocular pressure.
- Inhalation of a mixture of 5% carbon dioxide and 95% oxygen.
- Anterior chamber paracentesis.

If the investigation of a patient with amaurosis fugax provides no evidence of carotid artery disease, embolism or other recognized causes of the disorder, then the diagnosis by exclusion should be vasospasm. In such cases a calcium channel blocker should be tried.

What do you know about the 'purple toe syndrome'?

This was first described with warfarin therapy by Feder and Auerbach in 1961 and was shown to be caused by showers of atheroemboli (*Ann Intern Med* 1961: **55:** 911–17). Now, with the increasing use of coronary angioplasty and thrombolytic therapy in the elderly, cholesterol emboli are increasingly reported. They result in 'purple toes' (Fig. 84), amaurosis fugax, and atheroembolic disease of kidneys, skin and gastrointestinal tract.

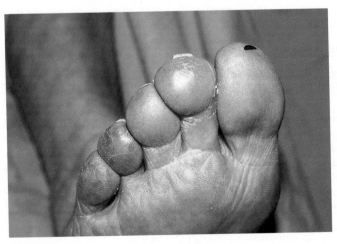

Fig. 84

Case 209

VITREOUS OPACITIES

INSTRUCTION

Examine this patient's fundus.

SALIENT FEATURES

History

- History of diplopia (monocular diplopia).
- Floaters.
- History of diabetes, hypertension.

Examination

- Small white opacities which are present in front of the retinal vessels.
- The patient may complain of diplopia (monocular diplopia).

Proceed as follows:
Tell the examiner that you would like to:

- Test for monocular diplopia.
- Check urine for sugar.
- Check the blood pressure.

DIAGNOSIS

This patient has vitreous opacities (lesions) with monocular diplopia (functional status), and has underlying diabetes mellitus (aetiology).

QUESTIONS

What are the causes of vitreous opacities?

- Blood: diabetes, retinal vein occlusion, trauma, subarachnoid haemorrhage, sickle cell retinopathy.
- Cholesterolosis bulbi, where free-floating, highly refractile crystals are seen in liquified vitreous and in patients with severe intraocular disease.
- Asteroid hyalitis (Benson's disease), where whitish yellow solid bodies, containing calcium palmitate and stearate, are suspended in normal vitreous. Prognosis for vision is good.
- Synchysis scintillans: gold or yellowish-white particles made up of cholesterol are located in the vitreous; they settle to the bottom of the eye due to gravity. Associated with previous trauma or surgery to the eye.
- Other, e.g. retinoblastoma, primary amyloidosis.

What are the other causes of monocular diplopia?

- Opacities in the lens.
- Corneal opacities.
- Retinal detachment.

Case 210

MYELINATED NERVE FIBRES

INSTRUCTION

Examine this patient's fundus.

SALIENT FEATURES

History

Asymptomatic.

Examination

White, streaky patches which extend from the disc and terminate peripherally in a feather-like pattern. It may cover the retinal vessels (Fig. 85).

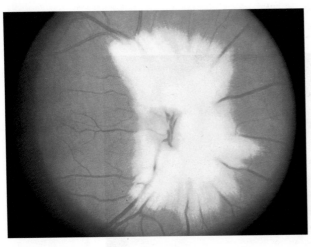

Fig. 85

DIAGNOSIS

This patient has white streaky patches in a feather-like pattern (lesion); these are medullated nerve fibres (aetiology) and are benign (functional status).

QUESTIONS

What is the pathology?

Occasionally, the myelination of the optic nerve does not stop at the lamina cribrosa but extends on to nerve fibres surrounding the optic disc. This condition is a benign congenital abnormality known as medullated or myelinated nerve fibres. It terminates peripherally in a feather-like margin with fine striations from the course of the nerve fibre layer.

Case 211

RETINAL CHANGES IN AIDS

INSTRUCTION

At a distance from the patient, the examiner will say that this patient has HIV, examine his fundus.

SALIENT FEATURES

History
- Floaters.
- Red eye.
- Impaired vision.

Examination
Patient 1: Cottonwool spots
Cottonwool spots (Fig. 86).

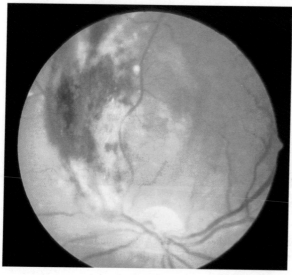

Fig. 86

Proceed as follows:
Tell the examiner that you would like to exclude diabetes and retinal vascular disease.

Patient 2: Cytomegalovirus (CMV) retinitis.
- An area of retinitis with nerve fibre layer infarcts, haemorrhages, retinal opacification and perivascular sheathing – 'pizza-pie fundus'.
- Tell the examiner that you would like to do a CD4 count (<50 in acute infection).

QUESTIONS

How would you treat cottonwool spots?
In a patient with known HIV infection, such infarcts require no specific therapy.

ADVANCED-LEVEL QUESTIONS

How would you treat the lesions of CMV retinitis?
- Therapy with intravenous ganciclovir or foscarnet is given lifelong to protect unaffected areas but does not restore functional areas already affected. The optimal treatment for patients with AIDS, normal renal function and CMV retinitis is foscarnet plus an antiretroviral nucleoside such as zidovudine. For similar patients with impaired renal function, ganciclovir would be the drug of choice, perhaps with an antiretroviral agent such as didanosine that has few overlapping side-effects. Late retinal detachment occurs despite therapy in one fifth of these patients.
- Sustained release ganciclovir implant in the pars plana of the eye. Oral ganciclovir in conjunction with an implant reduces the incidence of new cytomegalovirus disease and delays the progression of retinitis (*N Engl J Med* 1999; **340:** 1063–70).
- Intravitreal injections of ganciclovir or foscarnet.

What do you know about ganciclovir?
It is a derivative of aciclovir. It can cause bone marrow depression and hence should not be administered simultaneously with zidovudine.

What do you know about foscarnet?
It is an organic analogue of inorganic pyrophosphate. Its side-effects include renal impairment, electrolyte imbalance and seizures. It can be safely administered with zidovudine.

What are the other retinal manifestations in patients with AIDS?
- Toxoplasmosis retinochoroiditis – usually nasal to the disc, characterized by extensive whitish infarction and inflammation, with minimal associated intra-retinal haemorrhage (outer retinal involvement may show 'brush-fire' advancement of infection).
- *Pneumocystis carinii* choroiditis – characterized by scattered nodular yellowish-orange lesions deep in the retina, usually throughout the posterior pole.
- Acute retinal necrosis syndrome – with severe peripheral retinal infarction and retinal vasculitis. Atrophic retinal holes appear later in these areas.
- Progressive outer retinal necrosis syndrome – characterized by diffuse whitish opacification of the retina beneath the retinal vessels and a cherry-red spot in the fovea. It is associated with herpes zoster and the prognosis for visual acuity is dismal.
- Ocular presentations of syphilis include anterior and posterior uveitis, retinitis, retinal vasculitis and papillitis.
- Acute syphilitic posterior placoid chorioretinitis – large placoid yellowish lesions at the level of the retinal pigment epithelium in the posterior retina with inflammation of the vitreous and loss of vision.

What diagnostic tests would you perform to detect retinal manifestations of AIDS?
- Careful clinical observations.
- Serology: CD4 count (usually <50 in untreated cases of CMV retinitis).
- Culture.
- Retinal biopsy by pars plana vitrectomy.
- Fluorescein angiography: helpful in differentiating retinal lesions.
- Sequential fundus photographs: for diagnosis and monitoring of lesions.
- Testing of ocular fluid by polymerase chain reaction.

Mention some ocular non-retinal manifestations of AIDS.
- Optic neuropathy.
- Kaposi's sarcoma of the conjunctiva.
- Orbital lymphoma.
- Cranial nerve palsies.
- Nystagmus.

Case 212

RETINAL DETACHMENT

INSTRUCTION

Examine this patient's eye.

SALIENT FEATURES

History

- Patient complains of a dark curtain progressing across the visual field.
- Floaters, flashes.
- History of diabetes, hypertension.
- History of kidney disease (diabetic renal–retinal syndrome).

Examination

- The retina has lost its pink colour and appears grey and opaque.
- When the collection of subretinal fluid is large, the retina shows ballooning detachment with numerous folds (Figs 87 and 88).
- Examine visual acuity and visual fields.

Proceed as follows:
Tell the examiner that you would like to:

- Check urine for sugar.
- Check the blood pressure.
- Comment on any walking aid for the registered blind.

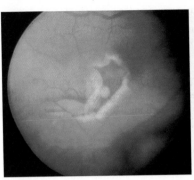

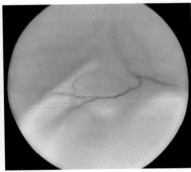

Fig. 87   Fig. 88

DIAGNOSIS

This patient has neovascularization and retinal detachment (lesion) due to under-lying diabetes mellitus (aetiology). She has a walking aid for the registered blind (functional status).

ADVANCED-LEVEL QUESTIONS

What is the pathology of retinal detachment?

It is a separation within the retina between the photoreceptors and the retinal pig-ment epithelium, characterized by collection of fluid or blood in this potential space.

What are the types of retinal detachment?

Rhegmatogenous retinal detachment

This is defined as the presence of a hole or break in the retina that allows fluid from the vitreous capacity to enter the subretinal space. It usually occurs spontaneously in those who have a predisposition to it following trauma to the eye or after intra-ocular surgery. Most of these patients develop symptoms. A break in the peripheral retina is associated with a sudden burst of flashing lights or sparks that may be followed by small floaters or spots in the field of vision. When the retina detaches, the patient perceives a dark curtain progressing across the visual field, and when the fovea detaches central vision is abruptly diminished.

It is treated surgically with a scleral buckling procedure (where all retinal breaks are localized and adhesions between the choroid and retina are performed around the break with diathermy or a cryoprobe). After draining the subretinal fluid, the detached portion of the retina is indented towards the vitreous cavity by a scleral implant or explant. This results in pushing of the retina towards the vitreous, causing closure of the retinal break (by the buckled sclera and choroid) and release of traction of vitreous.

Traction retinal detachment

The intact retina is forcibly elevated by contracting membranes on the surface of the retina or by vitreous traction on areas of retinal neovascularization. Causes include diabetes, intraocular foreign body, perforating eye injuries and loss of vitreous following cataract surgery. These retinal detachments are difficult to treat; pars plana vitrectomy is the only way to treat these lesions.

Secondary retinal detachments

These occur secondary to systemic disorders including hypertension, toxaemia of pregnancy, chronic glomerulonephritis, retinal venous occlusive disease and retinal vasculitis. Treatment is directed towards the underlying cause as these detachments are not amenable to scleral buckling surgery.

Case 213

AGE-RELATED MACULAR DEGENERATION (SENILE MACULAR DEGENERATION)

INSTRUCTION

Look at this patient's fundus.

SALIENT FEATURES

History

- Visual loss is often detected when one eye is covered for testing visual acuity.
- Loss of ability to read, recognize faces or drive a car; however, patients have enough peripheral vision to walk unaided.
- Decrease in visual acuity (severe loss suggests choroidal neovascularization).
- Metamorphosia (distortion of the shape of objects in view).
- Paracentral scotoma.
- Variable visual loss due to atrophy of a large area of retinal pigment epithelium involving the fovea.
- Family history.
- History of smoking.
- High blood pressure (increases risk of choroidal neovascularization).

Examination

- Drüsen.
- Disruption of pigment of the retinal pigment epithelium into small areas of hypopigmentation and hyperpigmentation (Fig. 89).
- Choroidal neovascularization.

Proceed as follows:

- Comment on the white walking aid by the bedside, which indicates the patient is registered blind.

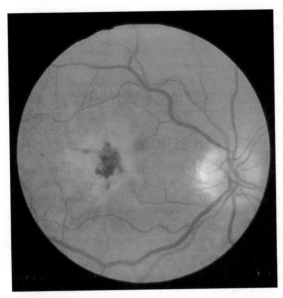

Fig. 89

- Check visual acuity and visual field (in most patients there is loss of central vision and maintenance of peripheral vision). Patients with only drüsen typically require additional magnification of text and more intense light to read small print text.

Remember that age-related macular degeneration is now the commonest cause of registrable blindness in the United Kingdom.

DIAGNOSIS

This patient has senile macular degeneration (aetiology) and is registered blind, as evidenced by the white walking aid (functional status).

QUESTIONS

What are drüsen?

Drüsen are pale yellow spots that occur individually or in clusters throughout the macula. Nearly all individuals over the age of 50 years of age have at least one small drüsen (≤ 63 μm) in one or both eyes (*Ophthalmology* 1992; **14**: 130–42). They consist of amorphous material accumulated between Bruch's membrane and the pigment epithelium. Although the exact origin is not known, it is believed that drüsen occur due to the accumulation of lipofuscin and other cellular debris derived from cells of the retinal pigment epithelium that are compromised by age and other factors. Only eyes with large drüsen (>63 μm) are at increased risk for senile macular degeneration (*Ophthalmology* 1997; **104**: 7–21).

What are the types of senile macular degeneration?

There are two types:

1. Atrophic or 'dry' type: involving the choriocapillaries, retinal pigment epithelium and the rods and cones. There is no leakage of blood or serum.
2. Neovascular exudative or 'wet' type: there is haemorrhagic or serous detachment of the retinal pigment epithelium and choroidal neovascularization resulting in leakage and fibrovascular scarring.

ADVANCED-LEVEL QUESTIONS

What do you know about neovascularization in these patients?

Substantial visual loss occurs as a result of neovascularization. Choroidal vessels proliferate across Bruch's membrane under the retinal pigment epithelium and, in certain cases, continue their extension into the subretinal space. Substantial leakage from these neovascular membranes can result in retinal detachment. The most devastating consequence is haemorrhage, which resolves forming a disciform scar.

What are the risk factors for choroidal neovascularization in the other eye of a patient with disorder in one eye?

Large drüsen (>63 μm), more than 5 drüsen, focal hyperpigmentation of the retinal pigment epithelium.

What investigations are performed to detect choroidal neovascularization?

- Rapid-sequence fluorescein angiography.
- Retinal angiography using indocyanine green and infrared photography.

How is the neovascularization treated?

- Laser photocoagulation of regions outside the foveal avascular zone.
- Subfoveal neovascularization: when photocoagulated is associated with a treatment-induced visual loss immediately but in the long term is found to be beneficial. Treatment may have to be deferred in those with good initial visual acuity because a large scotoma occurs as a result of treatment.
- Photodynamic therapy with photosensitizers such as verteporfin is currently being evaluated.
- Interferon-α is currently being evaluated.
- Submacular surgery: surgical removal of subfoveal choroidal neovascularization has been reported to be useful but the results are not as good as laser photocoagulation.
- Zinc: the use of zinc as a therapeutic agent for macular degeneration has not been evaluated in a rigorous trial.
- External beam radiation therapy.
- Thalidomide.
- Others: indocyanine green-guided laser treatment, retinal transplantation and transplantation of retinal pigment epithelium, retinal translocation, retinal prosthesis, gene therapy.

What is the difference between krypton and argon laser photocoagulation?

The krypton red photocoagulator is useful in treatment when the neovascularization is closer than 200 μm but not under the fovea, because of its ability to spare the inner retina by its virtual lack of absorption by haemoglobin (unlike the argon laser). The conventional argon laser has blue and green wavelengths. The green wavelength is absorbed by haemoglobin and thus may damage the retina, whilst the blue wavelength is absorbed by the macular xanthophyll and results in foveal damage.

Mention some drugs that can cause maculopathy.

Chloroquine, thioridazine, chlorpromazine.

EXAMINATION OF THE FOOT

INSPECTION

- Comment on deformity: hallux valgus, pes cavus.
- Skin: comment on the colour, ulcers and gangrene, hair loss (remember that hair loss is not a reliable sign of ischaemia).
- Joint: comment on the swelling, e.g. ankle joint, first metatarsophalangeal joint in gout.

PALPATION

- Ask the patient whether the foot is sore.
- Feel for temperature difference between the two feet.
- Pulses: dorsalis pedis and posterior tibials (compare with the other side).
- Sensation: check light touch, pain and joint sensation.
- Check the plantar response and the ankle jerk.

Case 214

DIABETIC FOOT

INSTRUCTION

Examine this patient's legs.
Examine this patient's feet.

SALIENT FEATURES

Neuropathic foot

History

- Whether there is pain (usually painless neuropathy, but may be painful).
- Whether there is blistering (usually due to an ill-fitting shoe).
- About a previous history of foot ulcers,
- History of diabetes.

Examination

- Dry, warm and pink with palpable pulses.
- Impaired deep tendon reflexes.
- Reduced pinprick, light touch and vibration sensation.
- Ulcers usually painless and plantar.

Ischaemic foot

History

- Ask whether there is pain (usually painful).
- Ask about rest pain and claudication.
- History of diabetes.

Examination

- Skin is shiny and atrophic with sparse hair.
- The foot is cold to touch.
- Peripheral pulses are absent (calcified arteries may make pulse examination less reliable).
- Ulcers usually painful and present on the heels and toes.
- Check all peripheral pulses.

Neuropathic and ischaemic foot present together

- Ulcer on the foot with callosities at pressure points.
- Loss of the arch of the foot.
- Stocking distribution of sensory loss of all modalities.
- Loss of dorsalis pedis and/or posterior tibial pulsations.

Proceed as follows:

Tell the examiner that you would like to check the urine for sugar.

Note. When asked to examine the feet, remember that the common conditions affecting the feet are diabetes and atherosclerosis. Pay particular attention to the pulses and the skin.

DIAGNOSIS

This patient has features of both an ischaemic and neuropathic foot (lesion) which is due to diabetes mellitus (aetiology); walking is limited by the plantar ulcer (functional status).

Read reference: *BMJ* 1991; **303:** 1053.

QUESTIONS

What are the types of diabetic foot?
- Neuropathic foot.
- Ischaemic foot.

Note. Features of both types often occur together.

ADVANCED-LEVEL QUESTIONS

What is the pathophysiology of the ischaemic foot?
Occlusive vascular disease involving both microangiopathy and atherosclerosis of large and medium-sized arteries.

Mention a few conditions in which neuropathic ulcers are seen.
- Progressive sensory neuropathy.
- Tabes dorsalis.
- Leprosy.
- Amyloidosis.
- Porphyria.

How would you manage this patient?
- Patient education: avoid cigarette smoking, inspect the feet daily for blisters, no walking barefoot, avoid tight shoes and cutting toenails straight across.
- Radiograph of the foot.
- Antibiotics.
- Removal of necrotic tissue.
- Removal of weight-bearing and friction from ulcerated areas – appropriate footwear such as moulded insoles or plaster cast, or crutches to avoid weight-bearing.
- Control hyperglycaemia.
- Chiropody.
- Surgical opinion and arteriography if reconstructive vascular surgery or angioplasty is considered. When irreversible arterial insufficiency occurs, it is often quicker and more humane for the patient to undergo early major amputation rather than be subjected to a series of debilitating conservative procedures.

How would you monitor a diabetic at annual review?
- Eyes: visual acuity, fundoscopy.
- Sensory system: touch, pinprick and vibration sense.
- Deep tendon reflexes.
- Cardiovascular system: blood pressure, peripheral pulses.
- Biochemistry: urine and blood sugar, albumin, glycosylated haemoglobin, creatinine.

What do you know about measurement of cutaneous pressure perception?

This is done with the use of Semmes–Weinstein monofilaments to assess neuropathic foot. Individuals with normal foot sensation can usually feel the 4.17 monofilament (~1 g of linear pressure). Patients who cannot feel the 5.07 monofilament (~10 g of linear pressure) before it buckles are considered to have lost protective sensation. A seven-fold increase in the risk of ulceration has been reported in patients insensitive to the 5.07 monofilament. However, up to 10% of persons who feel the mono-filament before it buckles may still have cutaneous breakdown.

Case 215

SWOLLEN LEG I: DEEP VEIN THROMBOSIS

INSTRUCTION

Look at this patient's leg.

SALIENT FEATURES

History

- Recent history of immobilization including surgery, cerebrovascular accident, myocardial infarction.
- Whether onset was acute or chronic.
- Pain.
- Past and family history of thromboses including deep venous thrombosis, pulmonary embolism.
- Drug history: oral contraceptives.
- Air travel – the evidence is circumstantial (*BMJ* 2001; **322:** 188).

Examination

- Painful calf.
- Redness.
- Engorged superficial veins.
- Unilateral swollen leg with pitting oedema.
- Pain in the calf on dorsiflexion of the foot – Homans' sign (not a diagnostic sign).

Proceed as follows:

- Check for pitting oedema on both sides (look at the patient's eyes while eliciting this sign, to ensure that you are not hurting the patient).
- Compare the temperature of both the legs (use the dorsum of your fingers to elicit this sign).
- Check the arterial pulses in the leg.
- Comment on the heparin pump by the bedside.

Remember to collect your thoughts when asked to examine the legs – do not rush in to grab the patient's legs.

DIAGNOSIS

This patient has a swollen leg resulting from deep vein thrombosis (lesion) which may be due to the oral contraceptives she is taking (aetiology); the leg is oedematous and the patient is at risk of pulmonary embolism (functional status).

Read recent reviews: *Lancet* 1999; **353:** 479–85; *BMJ* 2000; **320:** 1453–6.

QUESTIONS

What are the complications of deep vein thrombosis (DVT)?
- Pulmonary embolism.
- Venous gangrene.
- Pain, particularly in iliofemoral thrombosis.

What are the predisposing factors for venous thrombosis?
- Surgery (particularly of leg or pelvis, or after prostatectomy).
- Following cerebrovascular accident (about half of the patients develop DVT).
- Following myocardial infarction (one third of patients have DVT).
- Obesity.
- Malignancy (*Lancet* 1998; **351:** 1077–80).
- Varicose veins.
- Oral contraceptives.
- Older age (exponential increase above the age of 50 years).
- Immobilization (paralysed limbs in stroke, paraplegia).
- Previous DVT (risk increases two- to three-fold).
- Pregnancy (risk increased in postpartum period).
- Hypercoagulable states (antithrombin III deficiency, protein C deficiency, protein S deficiency, antiphospholipid syndrome, excessive plasminogen activator inhibitor, polycythaemia vera, erythrocytosis).
- Tissue trauma.

How would you investigate a patient with suspected deep vein thrombosis?
As clinical diagnosis is unreliable it is essential to perform the following investigations to assess the extent of thrombosis:

- Duplex ultrasonography scanning and colour Doppler studies.
- D-dimer.
- Venography – by injecting contrast into one of the leg veins.

What is the risk of pulmonary embolism in patients with below-knee thrombi?
The risk in such cases is low and many physicians refrain from anticoagulating these patients.

How would you treat these patients?
- Pain relief.

- Control of oedema:
  - Intermittent elevation of foot, and elevation of foot during the night above the level of the heart.
  - Avoid long periods of standing.
  - Elastic support stockings from the mid-foot to just below the knee, worn during the day.
- The main aim is to prevent pulmonary emboli and restore venous patency and valvular function in order to prevent postphlebitic syndrome.
  1. Aspirin 160 mg every day reduces the risk of pulmonary embolism and deep-vein thrombosis by at least a third particularly after hip surgery (*Lancet* 2000; **355**: 1295–302).
  2. All patients with thrombi above the knee must be anticoagulated:
     - Unfractionated heparin: initial therapy with heparin with the aim of maintaining activated partial thromboplastin time (APTT) 1.5–2.5 times the normal value within the first 24 hours. Failure to achieve this target APTT *within 24 hours* increases the risk of recurrent venous thromboembolism 15-fold. Heparin therapy is continued for about 5–10 days.
     - Low molecular weight heparin (instead of unfractionated heparin): requires subcutaneous injection but does not require bolus or laboratory monitoring. Examples include dalteparin, nadroparin and tinzaparin. Reviparin has recently been shown to be more effective than unfractionated heparin in reducing size of thrombus and prevention of recurrence (*N Engl J Med* 2001; **344**: 626–31).
     - Recent data suggest that synthetic pentasaccharide with antithrombotic effects may be superior to low molecular weight heparins in prevention of thromboembolism (*N Engl J Med* 2001; **344**: 619–25).
     - This is followed by warfarin therapy with the aim of maintaining the international normalized ratio (INR) at 2.0–3.0, recommended for the treatment of venous thromboembolic disease, but substantially less intensive anticoagulation may be effective. Remember that anticoagulants do not affect thrombus that is already present.
     - There is no consensus on duration of therapy but the following are broad guidelines: (a) a duration of 3–6 months with first episode, (b) about 6 weeks to 3 months in postoperative cases without any other risk factor, (c) 6–12 months in patients with persistent risk factors and recurrent venous thromboembolic events, and (d) lifelong only rarely.
- When anticoagulation is contraindicated, inferior vena caval filters may be required when there is a high risk of pulmonary embolism.

How would you prevent deep venous thrombosis?

- Subcutaneous low-dose heparin should be given to patients:
  - who are undergoing surgery to the leg, pelvis or prostatectomy
  - with myocardial infarction
  - with cardiac failure.
- Early ambulation within 72 hours after surgery.
- Encourage leg exercise following surgery.
- Elastic supports to patients with a history of thrombosis or obesity.

ADVANCED-LEVEL QUESTIONS

What are causes of recurrent venous thrombosis?

- Pregnancy, surgery, trauma, oral contraceptives.
- Abnormalities in antithrombin III, protein C, protein S, fibrinogen or factor V.
- Acquired conditions such as antiphospholipid antibody syndrome, occult cancer, myeloproliferative disorders, some vasculitides.
- Potential abnormalities include thrombomodulin, tissue factor pathway inhibitor, vitronectin associated with heparin and antithrombin III and fibrinolytic receptors.

What do you know of the antiphospholipid antibody syndrome?

The diagnosis of this syndrome requires that a patient have recurrent clinical events (such as thromboses or fetal loss) and an antiphospholipid antibody (such as anti-cardiolipin antibody or lupus anticoagulant). The 'primary' syndrome has no accompanying autoimmune disease, whereas it is 'secondary' if the patient also has systemic lupus erythematosus or lupus-like disease. Many patients with this syndrome have livedo reticularis, thrombocytopenia and neurological symptoms (*Lancet* 1999; **353:** 1348–53).

(**Note.** The antiphospholipid antibody can occur in certain drug reactions and infectious diseases, but only those that occur in patients with autoimmune disease are associated with the clinical syndrome.) The clinical course of the secondary syndrome is independent of the activity and severity of the lupus, but the presence of antiphospholipid antibody worsens the prognosis of the lupus. Warfarin therapy with an international normalized ratio of 3 or more offers the best protection against recurrent thrombosis for patients who have a confirmed major thrombosis.

J. Homans (1877–1954) was an American surgeon who worked at Johns Hopkins Hospital with Cushing, initially on experimental hypophysectomy and later on vascular disease. He first reported venous thrombosis related to air travel in a 54-year old physician who developed DVT after a 14-hour flight (*N Engl J Med* 1954; **250:** 148–9).

G.R.V. Hughes, contemporary London physician, Raynes Institute, St Thomas' Hospital, first described the antiphospholipid antibody syndrome (*N Engl J Med* 1995; **332:** 993–7).

Case 216

SWOLLEN LEG II: CELLULITIS

INSTRUCTION

Look at this patient's leg.

SALIENT FEATURES

History

- History of fever.
- Diabetes.

Examination

- Red, inflamed leg with a definite demarcation of erythematous area.
- Oedema.
- Increased temperature.

Proceed as follows:

- Examine the peripheral pulses.
- Varicose veins (varicose eczema should be considered in the differential diagnosis of cellulites of the leg, *BMJ* 1999; **318:** 1672–3).
- Look for superficial ulcers.

DIAGNOSIS

This patient has cellulitis of the leg (lesion) which is due to pyogenic bacterial infection (aetiology) and the leg is acutely swollen and painful (functional status).

QUESTIONS

How would you manage such a patient?

- Blood cultures.
- Intravenous antibiotics.
- Pain relief and pyretics.
- Surgical referral.
- Experimental: granulocyte-colony stimulating factor (G-CSF), particularly in diabetics.

What are the causes of bilateral swollen legs?

- Cardiac failure.
- Renal failure.
- Hypoproteinaemia (due to cirrhosis or nephrotic syndrome).

What are the causes of an acutely swollen leg?

- Deep vein thrombosis.
- Cellulitis.
- Arterial occlusion.
- Trauma.
- Arthritis.

What are the causes of a chronically swollen leg?

- Venous causes: varicose veins, postphlebitic limb.
- Lymphoedema: Milroy's disease, filariasis (in the tropics).
- Congenital.

W.F. Milroy (1855–1942) described familial lymphoedema of the legs in 1892.

Case 217

CLUBBING

INSTRUCTION

Examine this patient's hands.

SALIENT FEATURES

History

- Lung conditions (bronchogenic carcinoma; fibrosing alveolitis; mesothelioma; suppurative lung disease such as bronchiectasis, lung abscess and empyema).
- Cardiac conditions (infective endocarditis, cyanotic heart disease).
- Gastrointestinal tract conditions (cirrhosis, ulcerative colitis, Crohn's disease).
- Thyroid disease (thyroid acropachy).
- Family history (hereditary clubbing).

Examination

- Increased curvature of the nails, obliteration of the angle of the nail. When in doubt, approximate the dorsal aspects of terminal phalanges of the fingers of both hands which are flexed at the interphalangeal joints. Normally, the angle between the nails does not extend more than halfway up the nail bed. In clubbing there is a wide and deep angle – this is known as Schamroth's sign (*S Afr Med J* 1976; **50:** 297).
- The nails may have a drumstick appearance.

Proceed as follows:
- Look for the following signs:
  - Fluctuation at the nail bed.
  - Palpate the wrist joints for tenderness seen in hypertrophic pulmonary osteo-arthropathy (HPOA). Rapid painful clubbing is nearly always due to bronchogenic carcinoma.
  - Nicotine (tar) staining of fingers.
  - Central cyanosis.
  - Clubbing of the toes.
- Tell the examiner that you would like to examine the following systems:
  - Chest (bronchogenic carcinoma; fibrosing alveolitis; mesothelioma; suppurative lung disease such as bronchiectasis, lung abscess and empyema).
  - Heart (infective endocarditis, cyanotic heart disease). In infective endocarditis the fingers may be pale and their tips flushed ('pale hands, pink tipped').
  - Gastrointestinal tract (cirrhosis, ulcerative colitis, Crohn's disease).
  - Thyroid (thyroid acropachy).

DIAGNOSIS

This patient has marked clubbing of the fingernails (lesion) and tar staining, indicating that the condition may be due to an underlying bronchial neoplasm (aetiology).

QUESTIONS

How is clubbing graded?

There are four grades:

- Grade I: increased glossiness and cyanosis of the skin at the root of the nail associated with increased fluctuation at the base of the nail bed.
- Grade II: the normal angle between the base of the nail and the skin is obliterated (Lovibond's sign) and may even be reversed.
- Grade III: hypertrophy of the soft tissue of the nail pulp and the nail curves excessively longitudinally to give a 'drum-stick' or 'parrot-beak' appearance ('doigts Hippocratique').
- Grade IV: bony changes involving the wrists and ankles, and sometimes the elbows and knees (HPOA).

What do you know about pachydermoperiostitis?

This is an unusual variety of idiopathic familial HPOA, in which postpubertal clubbing and bone changes are accompanied by increased sweating of the palms and soles and marked thickening of the skin of the face, forehead and scalp.

ADVANCED-LEVEL QUESTIONS

What are the mechanisms for clubbing (Eur J Clin Invest 1993; 23: 330–8)?

- Increased blood flow in clubbed fingers due to vasodilatation rather than hyperplasia of vessels in the nail bed. The nature of the vasodilator is unclear and many contenders, such as ferritin, bradykinin, prostaglandin and 5-hydroxytryptamine (5-HT), have been implicated. The vasodilator is probably inactivated in the lung in normal persons but when this inactivation is defective, or there is a right-to-left shunt, clubbing occurs.
- Increased growth hormone in disease states causes excessive cellular tissue in the nail bed.
- Clubbing occurs whenever organs supplied by the vagus are affected. It has been shown that, in bronchogenic carcinoma, vagotomy causes reversal of clubbing.
- Tumour necrosis factor has been implicated.
- Megakaryocytes and clumps of platelets may preferentially stream into blood vessels of the digits and release platelet-derived growth factor. The resulting increased capillary permeability, fibroblastic activity and arterial smooth muscle hyperplasia could cause clubbing.

Digital clubbing was first described approximately 2400 years ago by Hippocrates (Adams F 1849 *Hippocrates. The Book of Prognostics. The Genuine Works of Hippocrates*, Vol. 1. London: Sydenham Society).

N Engl J Med 1993; **329**: 1862. Classical pictures of these conditions.

Case 218

DUPUYTREN'S CONTRACTURE

INSTRUCTION

Look at this patient's hands.

SALIENT FEATURES

History

- Family history (as there is a genetic predisposition).
- Cigarette smoking (*J Bone Joint Surg Br* 1997; **79-B:** 206–10).
- Alcohol intake (*Arch Intern Med* 1977; **129:** 561–6).
- Chronic antiepileptic medications.
- Systemic conditions: cirrhosis, diabetes, TB, epilepsy.

Examination

- Thickening of the palmar fascia, particularly along the medial aspect (Fig. 90). (Feel for thickening before you comment on it.)
- In almost all cases, the fourth finger is affected with associated involvement of fifth, third and second fingers in decreasing order of frequency.

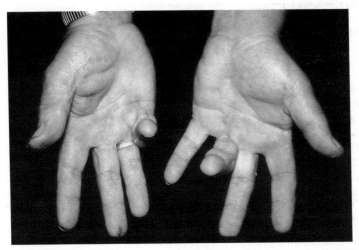

Fig. 90

Proceed as follows:
Tell the examiner that you would like to:

- Check the feet for contracture of the plantar fascia.
- Look for signs of alcoholism and cirrhosis.

DIAGNOSIS

This patient has Dupuytren's contracture (lesion) associated with chronic alcoholic liver disease (aetiology) and has developed disabling contractures (functional status).

ADVANCED-LEVEL QUESTIONS

What do you know about Dupuytren's contracture?

It is caused by the thickening and shortening of palmar fascia; the plantar fascia may also be affected. Fibrous nodules are often the earliest abnormality, resulting from a contracture of the proliferating fibroblasts in the superficial compartment of the palm. The nodules consist of mature-appearing fibroblasts surrounded by dense collagen. Ultrastructurally, many of these cells are myofibroblasts and thus may be contractile.

What other structures are involved?

There does not appear to be any direct involvement of the muscles, joints, tendons (and their sheaths), and nervous or vascular tissue. However, the dermis is frequently invaded by fibroblastic cells, resulting in fixation to deeper structures.

What is the natural history of this condition?

It is unpredictable, with little change or disability over a period of many years in some individuals. In others, the contraction of the fascia occurs rapidly, resulting in severe deformity and loss of hand function.

What do you know about the epidemiology of Dupuytren's contracture?

There may be a hereditary predisposition (usually autosomal dominant) and the disorder is about five times more frequent in men, more common in whites and in Europe. There is a gradual increase in the incidence with age.

With which other conditions is Dupuytren's contracture associated?

- Alcoholism.
- Chronic antiepileptic therapy.
- Systemic conditions such as cirrhosis, diabetes, epilepsy, tuberculosis.
- Thickening of the corpora cavernosa of the penis (Peyronie's disease).
- Garrod's knuckle pads.
- Retroperitoneal fibrosis.

Why is the deformity caused by this condition usually well tolerated?

Because it exaggerates the normal position of function of the hand.

How would you manage such patients?

Treatment depends on the severity of findings and includes:

- Periodic examination of patients in the early stages. If the palmar thickening is growing rapidly, local injections of triamcinolone into the growing nodule may be of benefit.
- Surgery is indicated when there are disabling flexion contractures, although recurrences are common (*Lancet* 1997; **350:** 1568).

Baron Guillaume Dupuytren (1777–1835), Surgeon-in-Chief, Hôtel-Dieu, Paris, is reported to have been the first to achieve successful removal of the lower jaw.

Sir A.E. Garrod (1857–1936), physician at St Bartholomew's Hospital, London, succeeded Osler as Regius Professor at Oxford.

F. de la Peyronie (1678–1747), a French surgeon who influenced Louis XVI in his decision to issue an ordinance banning barbers from practising surgery.

Case 219

CATARACTS

INSTRUCTION

Examine this patient's eyes.

SALIENT FEATURES

History

- Drug history (steroids, chloroquine, phenothiazines, chlorambucil, busulfan).
- History of gradual deterioration of vision.
- History of diabetes.
- Enquire about smoking (*JAMA* 1992; **268:** 989–94) and alcohol consumption (*Arch Ophthalmol* 1993; **111:** 1130) – both cigarette smoking and heavy alcohol consumption increase the risk of cataract formation.
- Family history: this is important even in age-related nuclear cataract as it explains about 50% variation in the severity of disease (*N Engl J Med* 2000; **342:** 1786–90).

Examination

Bilateral cataracts (shine light obliquely across the lens).

Proceed as follows:
Tell the examiner that you would like to check the urine for sugar.

DIAGNOSIS

This patient has premature bilateral cataracts (lesion) due to diabetes mellitus (aetiology) and has had a gradual deterioration of vision (functional status).

QUESTIONS

Mention a few causes of cataracts.

Common causes
- Old age (look for arcus senilis). The Framingham study reported that 13% of people aged 65–74 years and about 40% of those over the age of 75 years had cataracts.

- Diabetes mellitus (non-enzymatic glycosylation of lens protein is twice as high in diabetics as in age-matched controls and may contribute to the premature occurrence of cataracts).

Uncommon causes
- Trauma.
- Metabolic: Cushing's syndrome, Wilson's disease (stellate cataracts), galactosaemia.
- Chromosomal disorders: dystrophia myotonica, Turner's syndrome.
- Congenital infections (rubella or cytomegalovirus).
- Drugs (see above).
- Dermatological disorders: atopic dermatitis, ichthyosis.
- Radiation: infrared (glass-blower's cataract), X-ray radiation, microwave radiation.

ADVANCED-LEVEL QUESTIONS

How are cataracts treated?

Cataract extraction is performed by removing the lens nucleus and cortex from within the lens capsule. In most adults, a plastic lens is implanted within the capsule. Multifocal intraocular lens implants in some instances have reduced the need for both reading and distance spectacles. Lens extraction improves vision in 95% of instances. In the remaining cases, prior retinal disease or postoperative complications such as haemorrhage, glaucoma, infection or retinal detachment may be the cause. Recent data suggest that there is substantial benefit from bilateral cataract eye surgery in that it improves stereoacuity (*Lancet* 1998; **352**: 925–9).

How is early cataract detected using direct ophthalmoscopy?

Examination of the red reflex with +4 dioptres at approximately 20 cm from the patient will reveal a black opacity in the lens against the reddish hue of the reflex. If this opacity appears to move down on upward gaze, it is located in the posterior half of the lens, but if it appears to move up then it is located in the anterior half of the lens.

Is the use of inhaled steroids associated with cataracts?

The use of inhaled steroids is associated with nuclear and posterior subcapsular cataracts (*N Engl J Med* 1997; **337**: 8–14).

Jacques Divel of Bernay, a small town in Brittany, in 1748 devised extracapsular extraction of cataracts.

Harold Ridley, who worked at St. Thomas's and Moorfields's Eye Hospital in London, UK, was the first to champion the insertion of artificial lens after removal of a cataract over 50 years ago (*Lancet* 1999; **354**: 1912).

Case 220

ANAEMIA

PATIENT 1

Instruction

Would you like to ask this anaemic patient a few questions?

Salient features

Proceed as follows:
Ask about the following:

- Blood loss such as bleeding per rectum, melaena, haematemesis.
- Menstrual blood loss (duration of periods, the occurrence of clots, and the number of sanitary towels or tampons used).
- Drug history – NSAIDs, phenytoin, chloramphenicol.
- Associated symptoms such as weight loss, shortness of breath, chronic diarrhoea.
- Diet – in vegans, alcoholics, elderly patients.
- Past history of gastrectomy.

Diagnosis

This patient's anaemia is caused by severe melaena which indicates bleeding in the upper gastrointestinal tract and is probably due to peptic ulcer or bleeding varices (aetiology). The patient is currently receiving a blood transfusion, indicating that the anaemia was severe (functional status).

PATIENT 2

Instruction

Would you like to examine this anaemic patient?

Salient features

Proceed as follows:
- Examine the following:
  - Nails for koilonychia or iron deficiency anaemia, and (rarely) for clubbing of infective endocarditis.
  - Comment on the pallor of the face and conjunctiva, looking for the lemon-yellow hue of pernicious anaemia.
  - Tongue for glossitis of vitamin B_{12} deficiency.
  - Mouth for angular stomatitis of severe malnutrition, and ulcers of neutropenia.
  - Lymph nodes in the neck, axillae and groin (secondaries, lymphoproliferative disorders).
  - Skin for bruising associated with bone marrow depression seen in leukaemia and aplastic anaemia.
  - Abdomen for hepatomegaly, splenomegaly and other masses.
  - Legs for ulcers seen in haemoglobinopathies.

- Comment on the ethnic origin (thalassaemia).
- Tell the examiner that you would like to:
  - Perform a rectal examination and inspect the stool for occult blood.
  - Obtain a FBC including a peripheral smear and ESR.

Diagnosis

This patient has koilonychia and anaemia indicating an iron deficiency anaemia. I would like to exclude a gastrointestinal cause for the blood loss (aetiology).

QUESTIONS

Mention a few causes of anaemia.

With a low mean corpuscular volume (MCV)
- Iron deficiency anaemia.
- Thalassaemia.
- Sideroblastic anaemia.

With a high MCV
- Vitamin B_{12} deficiency (pernicious anaemia, vegans, alcoholics, coeliac disease).
- Folate deficiency (pregnancy, phenytoin, sprue, coeliac disease, malignancy, haemolysis).
- Other: myxoedema, liver disease, alcoholics.

With a normal MCV
- Uraemia.
- Malignancy.
- Rheumatoid arthritis.
- Aplastic anaemia (myelofibrosis, chloramphenicol, phenylbutazone, gold, anti-cancer drugs).

What do you know about the Paterson–Kelly syndrome?

It comprises iron deficiency anaemia and dysphagia due to oesophageal webs in middle-aged women. The clinical significance of this syndrome is uncertain. It is also known as Plummer–Vinson syndrome.

What are the common causes of iron deficiency anaemia?

Occult gastrointestinal bleeding from the following:

- Peptic ulcer.
- Carcinoma located anywhere in the gastrointestinal tract.
- Excessive anticoagulation.
- Hereditary haemorrhagic telangiectasia.
- Angiodysplasia of the colon.

How would you investigate microcytic anaemia?

- FBC.
- Serum ferritin.
- Faecal occult blood.
- Upper gastrointestinal endoscopy.
- Barium enema, colonoscopy.

- International normalized ratio (INR), prothrombin time and platelet count.
- Haemoglobin electrophoresis in susceptible ethnic groups (Asians, Afro-Caribbeans).

How would you investigate macrocytic anaemia?
- Peripheral smear.
- Vitamin B_{12} and red cell folate and serum folate concentrations.
- Serum ferritin, plasma iron and total iron-binding capacity (for associated iron deficiency).
- Schilling test.
- Gastric parietal cell and intrinsic factor antibodies.
- Upper gastrointestinal endoscopy.
- Reticulocyte count (a high MCV could be present when the reticulocyte count is over 50%).
- Bone marrow examination.

R.F. Schilling (b. 1919), Chairman of the Department of Medicine and haematologist at the University of Wisconsin.

Case 221

LYMPHADENOPATHY

INSTRUCTION

Perform a general examination.
Examine this patient's neck.

SALIENT FEATURES

History and Examination

Use the mnemonic **ALL AGES** to approach a patient with lymphadenopathy:

– **A**ge at presentation (e.g. infectious mononucleosis is commoner in younger age groups, Hodgkin's disease has a bimodal peak).
– **L**ocation(s) of lymph nodes (lymph nodes present outside the inguinal regions, for longer than one month and measuring 1 cm × 1 cm or larger without an obvious diagnosis should be considered for biopsy; *Semin Oncol* 1993; **20**: 570–82).
– **L**ength of time the lymph nodes are present.
– **A**ssociated symptoms and signs including fever ('B' symptoms: temp >38°C, drenching night sweats, unexplained weight loss >10% body weight).
– **G**eneralized lymph node enlargement.
– **E**xtranodal organ involvement.
– **S**plenomegaly (rare in metastatic cancer; consider infectious mononucleosis, lymphoma, chronic lymphocytic leukaemia, and acute leukaemia; *Cancer* 1987; **60**: 100–2).

As soon as you feel a group of lymph nodes, examine drainage areas for obvious pathology. For example:

- Inguinal lymph nodes: examine the lower limbs and external genitalia.
- Axillary lymph nodes: examine the chest, breast and upper limbs.
- Upper cervical lymph nodes: examine the chest, breast and upper limbs. Also, perform an ear, nose and throat (ENT) examination for nasopharyngeal carcinoma.
- Lower cervical and supraclavicular lymph nodes: examine the thyroid, chest, abdomen for gastric carcinoma (Virchow's nodes) and testis.
- Examine other lymph node areas in a systemic manner: submental, submandibular, deep cervical (upper and lower), occipital, posterior triangle, supraclavicular, axillary, epitrochlear and inguinal.
- Examine the mouth for the following signs:
  - Tonsillar lymph nodes.
  - Palatal petechiae and pharyngitis (glandular fever).
  - Neoplastic tumours or ulcers.
- Examine the abdomen for liver and spleen.
- Examine the chest and do a CXR (for bronchogenic carcinoma, TB).

DIAGNOSIS

This patient has generalized lymphadenopathy, probably a lymphoma – either Hodgkin's or non-Hodgkin's (aetiology) – and has severe disease as evidenced by alopecia, presumably due to chemotherapy (functional status). I would like to discuss other causes of generalized lymphadenopathy.

QUESTIONS

What are the causes of regional lymphadenopathy?

- Cervical lymphadenopathy: Causes include infections and malignancies. Infectious causes include bacterial pharyngitis, dental abscess, otitis media, infectious mononucleosis, cytomegalovirus, gonococcal pharyngitis, toxoplasmosis, hepatitis and adenovirus. Malignancies include non-Hodgkin's disease, Hodgkin's disease, and squamous cell carcinoma of head and neck.
- Virchow's node (anterior left supraclavicular lymph node). Also known as Troiser's ganglion. Suggests the presence of a thoracic or abdominal neoplasm (*Am J Surg* 1979; **138**: 703). Common causes include carcinoma of breast, bronchus, lymphomas and gastrointestinal neoplasms.
- Delphian node (a midline prelaryngeal lymph node): heralds thyroid disease, laryngeal malignancy or lymphoma.
- Axillary lymphadenopathy: Causes include infections and malignancies. Infectious causes include staphylococcal, streptococcal infections of the arm, cat-scratch fever, tularaemia and sporotrichosis. Malignant causes include Hodgkin's disease, non-Hodgkin's lymphoma, carcinoma of breast and melanoma.
- Epitrochlear lymphadenopathy: The most common causes are lymphoma/CLL and infectious mononucleosis. Other diagnoses include HIV, sarcoidosis, and connective tissue disorders. In developing countries secondary syphilis, lepromatous leprosy, leishmaniasis and rubella are important causes.

- Inguinal lymphadenopathy: In adults some degree of lymph node enlargement is not uncommon. In those who walk outdoors without footwear, benign reactive lymphadenopathy is common. Malignant causes include lymphoma, malignant melanoma, carcinoma of external genitalia. Benign causes include cellulitis, syphilis, chancroid, genital herpes, and lymphogranuloma venereum.
- Node of Cloquet (also known as Rosenmüller node): A deep inguinal lymph node located near the femoral canal. When palpable it may be mistaken for an inguinal hernia.

What are the causes of generalized lymphadenopathy?
- Lymphomas, chronic lymphatic leukaemia, acute lymphoblastic leukaemia.
- Glandular fever, cytomegalovirus.
- AIDS, toxoplasmosis.
- SLE, rheumatoid arthritis, sarcoid.
- Chronic infections such as TB, secondary syphilis, brucellosis.
- Drugs – phenytoin.

Use the mnemonic **CHICAGO**: **C**ancers, **H**ypersensitivity, **I**nfections, **C**onnective tissue disorders, **A**typical lymphoproliferative disorders, **G**ranulomatous disorders, **O**ther unusual causes.

What do you understand by the term 'Hodgkin's disease'?
Hodgkin's disease is a group of neoplasms characterized by Reed–Sternberg cells in an appropriate reactive cellular background. It is divided into several subtypes histologically: lymphocyte predominance, nodular sclerosis, mixed cellularity and lymphocyte depletion. The Reed–Sternberg cell is a giant cell with two or more nuclear lobes and huge eosinophilic inclusion-like nucleoli. The classic Reed–Sternberg cell has a symmetrical, mirror image nucleus that creates an 'owl-eye' appearance.

ADVANCED-LEVEL QUESTIONS

What is the cause of egg-shaped calcification in hilar lymph nodes?
Silicosis.

What do you know of Sister Joseph's nodule?
It is a classic sign of gastric adenocarcinoma in the umbilical area which may represent a metastatic deposit or an enlarged anterior abdominal wall lymph node.

What is the mode of presentation of Hodgkin's disease?
- Usually as a painless lymphadenopathy.
- Other presenting symptoms include systemic symptoms such as fever, weight loss, drenching night sweats, generalized pruritus or pain in the affected lymph node following the ingestion of alcohol.

How is Hodgkin's disease staged?
- Stage I: one lymph node region involved.
- Stage II: more than two lymph node regions involved on one side of the diaphragm.
- Stage III: lymph nodes involved on both sides of the diaphragm.
- Stage IV: disseminated disease with bone marrow or liver involvement.

In addition, it is designated as Stage A when systemic symptoms are absent or as Stage B when there is significant weight loss, fever or night sweats.

How is a patient with Hodgkin's disease treated?

- Localized disease (i.e. Stages IA, IIA) is treated with radiotherapy. Five-year cure rates are in excess of 80% and relapses are treated with chemotherapy.
- Disseminated disease (Stages IIIB, IV) is treated with combination chemotherapy with an ABVD (adriamycin, bleomycin, vincristine, dacarbazine) regimen alternating with a MOPP regimen (mechlorethamine (chlormethine), oncovin, procarbazine and prednisolone). Five-year survival rates are about 50%. Patients who relapse after initial chemotherapy may be cured with autologous bone marrow transplantation.
- In Stages IIB and IIIA, optimal management is controversial but current evidence suggests an advantage to combination chemotherapy (*N Engl J Med* 1993; **328:** 560).

What do you understand by the term 'non-Hodgkin's lymphomas'?

These are a heterogeneous group of cancers of lymphocytes. They are variable in their presentation and natural history, varying from a slow indolent course to a rapidly progressive illness (*N Engl J Med* 1993; **328:** 1023).

How are non-Hodgkin's lymphomas classified?

A working classification is as follows:

- Low-grade or favourable: slow, indolent course with good response to minimal therapy and long survival. These include small lymphocytic, plasmacytoid, follicular small cleaved cell and follicular mixed cell. Patients are usually treated with alkylating agents such as chlorambucil or a CVP regimen (cyclophosphamide, vincristine and prednisolone).
- High-grade or unfavourable: include immunoblastic, small non-cleaved (Burkitt's and non-Burkitt's), lymphoblastic and true histiocytic. The mainstay of therapy is combination chemotherapy; traditionally the CHOP regimen (cyclophosphamide, doxorubicin, vincristine and prednisolone) is used. In highly aggressive lymphomas autologous bone marrow transplantation may increase the chances of cure.
- Intermediate grade: follicular large cell, diffuse small cleaved cell, diffuse mixed cell, diffuse large cell.
- Other: cutaneous T-cell (mycosis fungoides, adult T-cell leukaemia/lymphoma).

What is Kimura's disease?

Kimura's disease is a chronic inflammatory condition of unknown aetiology, endemic in the Far East, and occurs predominantly in young and middle-aged adults (mean age of onset 27–40 years). Males are three times more commonly affected than females. The onset is insidious and includes adenopathy or tumour-like skin nodules. Kimura's disease usually results in generalized lymphadenopathy and major salivary glands, and chronic inflammation of the subcutaneous tissues in the head and neck. Other sites, such as mouth, axilla, groin, limbs and trunk may also be involved. There is no systemic or visceral involvement. It is commonly associated with raised serum IgE and eosinophilia. The disease has a self-limiting course and no treatment is necessary, although other causes of adenopathy must be excluded. The typical pathological features include florid germinal centres, vascularization of germinal centres, increased postcapillary venules in the paracortex, prominent eosinophilic infiltration, and sclerosis. Immunoperoxidase studies show IgE reticular networks in the germinal centres. The clinical course and pathological findings support the proposal that Kimura's disease represents an aberrant immune reaction to an unknown stimulus (*Lancet* 1998; **351:** 1098).

R.L.K. Virchow (1821–1902), successively Professor of Pathology at Würzberg and Berlin. He also described the Virchow cell (lepra cell), Virchow space (perivascular space of Virchow–Robin) and Virchow triad of the pathogenesis of thrombosis.

Thomas Hodgkin (1798–1866), an English physician at St Thomas's Hospital, London. He was the Curator of the Pathology Museum at Guy's Hospital before this.

Dorothy Reed (1874–1964) graduated from Johns Hopkins Hospital, Baltimore, and worked successively in New York and Wisconsin.

K. Sternberg (1872–1935), an Austrian pathologist who described the cells in 1898.

Burkitt's lymphoma was described by Dennis Burkitt in children in West Africa who presented with a lesion in the jaw, extranodal abdominal involvement and ovarian tumours. Most patients have Epstein–Barr antibodies in the serum.

The entity now called Kimura's disease was first described in China in 1937 by Kim and Szeto but became more widely known as Kimura's disease after a description in 1948 by Kimura and co-workers.

Case 222

CHRONIC LYMPHOCYTIC LEUKAEMIA

INSTRUCTION

Perform a general examination of this patient.

SALIENT FEATURES

History

- Asymptomatic in 70% of patients.
- Palpable lymph nodes or left upper quadrant abdominal discomfort in a fifth of patients.
- Bleeding or bruising is rare.
- Symptoms of anaemia are uncommon.
- Weight loss, fever and night sweats are unusual.

Examination

- Usually men over the age of 40 years (male:female ratio is 2:1).
- Symmetrical, painless, rubbery lymph nodes.
- Liver or spleen may be palpable.

Proceed as follows:
- Tell the examiner that you would like to do a full blood count and examine the peripheral smear (lymphocytosis >15 000/μl, with mature appearance of small lymphocytes).

- Remember that chronic lymphocytic leukaemia (CLL) manifests clinically with organ infiltration with lymphocytes, immunosuppression (hypogamma-globulinaemia) and bone marrow failure.

DIAGNOSIS

This elderly male patient with painless enlargement of lymph nodes probably has chronic lymphocytic leukaemia (lesion). He has severe pallor, indicating that he is in Binet Stage C (functional status).

QUESTIONS

What are the causes of anaemia in CLL?
Bone marrow infiltration, autoimmune (Coombs' positive) haemolysis.

How may this patient present?
About 25% of patients are asymptomatic. Some complain of general malaise, weight loss and loss of appetite, and others complain of bleeding.

ADVANCED-LEVEL QUESTIONS

What is the prognosis in chronic lymphocytic leukaemia?
Approximately one third of the patients will not require treatment and die from unrelated causes, in another third the disease is initially indolent followed by rapid progression, and in the remaining third the disease is very aggressive from the out-set and needs immediate treatment.

How is chronic lymphocytic leukaemia staged?
Binet staging (evaluates the enlargement of spleen, liver and lymph nodes in the head and neck, axillae and groin):

- Stage A – no anaemia or thrombocytopenia and less than three areas of lymphoid enlargement.
- Stage B – no anaemia or thrombocytopenia, with three or more involved areas.
- Stage C – anaemia and/or thrombocytopenia, regardless of the number of areas of lymphoid enlargement.

Rai staging:

- Stage 0 – lymphocytosis only (in blood and bone marrow).
- Stage I – lymphocytosis plus lymphadenopathy.
- Stage II – lymphocytosis with hepatic and/or splenic enlargement.
- Stage III – lymphocytosis with anaemia.
- Stage IV – lymphocytosis with thrombocytopenia.

Note. Although clinical staging is useful for prognosis, it does not provide information on the likelihood of progression in a given patient. A recent multivariate analysis reported that the presence or absence of 17p deletion, the presence or absence of an 11q deletion, Binet stage, serum lactate dehydrogenase, white cell count and age give significant prognostic information (*N Engl J Med* 2000; **343**: 1910–16).

How are patients with CLL treated?

- Specific treatment may not be indicated until Stage B or C. Patients with Stage A disease should be reassured that, despite the frightening diagnosis of leukaemia, they will be able to live a normal life for many years with a median survival of 8 years (*N Engl J Med* 1998; **338:** 1506–14).
- Patients with Stage B and C will require specific and supportive therapy, i.e. correction of anaemia and folic acid deficiency, and correction of bone marrow infiltration, initially with prednisolone and oxymetholone and subsequently with chemotherapeutic agents such as chlorambucil. Fludarabine yields higher response rates and longer duration of remission and progression-free survival than chlorambucil; overall survival is not enhanced (*N Engl J Med* 2000; **343:** 1750–7). Other purine analogues such as 2-chlorodeoxyadenosine and pentostatin are currently being investigated. Combination chemotherapy (CHOP regimen) and radiotherapy have also been used. Intravenous immunoglobulin reduces the incidence of infection.

What is Richter's syndrome?

In Richter's syndrome an isolated lymph node in CLL is transformed into an aggressive large cell lymphoma. There is a median survival of less than 1 year after its appearance.

Which lymphomas can convert to leukaemias?

- Small cell lymphoma (chronic lymphocytic leukaemia).
- Burkitt's lymphoma (B-cell acute lymphoblastic leukaemia).
- Lymphoblastic lymphoma (T-cell acute lymphoblastic leukaemia).

Case 223

CROHN'S DISEASE

INSTRUCTION

These patients have chronic diarrhoea.
Examine this patient's face (*Patient 3*).
Examine this patient's abdomen (*Patients 1 and 2*).
Comment on this patient's perianal area (*Patient 4*).

SALIENT FEATURES

History

- Loose stools or diarrhoea which is not usually bloody.
- Abdominal discomfort or pain.
- Anorexia, malaise and weight loss.
- Perianal inflammation and pain.
- Joint pains, eye complaints, skin changes.

Examination

- Mass in the right iliac fossa (*Patient 1*).
- Multiple fistulous openings in the right iliac fossa (*Patient 2*).
- Swollen lips (*Patient 3*).
- Multiple perianal fistulous tracts (*Patient 4*).

Proceed as follows:
In all four patients, examine for the following:

- The mouth for aphthous ulcers.
- Uveitis.
- Anaemia.
- Arthropathy.
- Skin lesions (erythema nodosum, pyoderma gangrenosum).
- Liver disease.

Remember that Crohn's disease may affect any part of the gastrointestinal tract from the mouth to the anus, but has a tendency to involve the terminal ileum. The inflammation is transmural (extending through all layers of bowel) with relatively normal bowel in between (skip lesions).

DIAGNOSIS

Patient 4 has multiple anal fistulas (lesions) due to Crohn's disease (aetiology), indicating that the disease is active (functional status).

QUESTIONS

What investigations would you perform?

- Sigmoidoscopy and biopsy.
- Small bowel study.
- Barium enema.
- Colonoscopy.

Mention some complications.

- Iritis.
- Arthritis.
- Erythema nodosum.
- Pyoderma gangrenosum.

Mention some associated diseases.

- Ankylosing spondylitis (HLA-B27 positive).
- Sacroiliitis.
- Cholangitis, hepatitis, cirrhosis.

ADVANCED-LEVEL QUESTIONS

Mention some ocular features of Crohn's disease.

Eye lesions are seen in about 5% of cases.

- Common: conjunctivitis, anterior uveitis.
- Rare: scleritis, keratitis, keratoconjunctivitis sicca, choroiditis, retinal vasculitis, optic neuritis and orbital pseudotumour.

How would you treat Crohn's disease?

- Sulfasalazine or rectal steroids for colonic disease.
- Oral steroids for small bowel disease.
- Metronidazole for perianal disease and fistulas.
- 6-Mercaptopurine may be useful in severe cases.
- Surgery is reserved for intestinal fistulas and intestinal obstruction that does not respond to medical management. Proctocolectomy and ileostomy is the standard operation. (**Note.** Ileorectal anastomosis or ileoanal anastomosis should be avoided in Crohn's disease.)

Burrill Bernard Crohn (b. 1884) was a physician in Mount Sinai Hospital, New York; he described the condition in 1932 and pointed out the non-tuberculous aetiology (Crohn BB, Ginzburg L, Oppenheimer GD 1932 Regional ileitis: a pathologic and clinical entity. *JAMA* **99**: 1323–9).

Anne Ferguson, contemporary Professor of Gastroenterology at the Western General Hospital in Edinburgh, whose chief interest is inflammatory bowel disease.

Case 224

DYSPHAGIA

INSTRUCTION

This patient has difficulty in swallowing; would you like to ask him a few questions and examine him?

SALIENT FEATURES

History

Ask about the following:

- The duration of symptoms: progressive dysphagia over months or weeks suggests the presence of organic narrowing (carcinoma of oesophagus, stricture from ongoing reflux oesophagitis).
- Whether the difficulty is in swallowing liquids or solids, or both.
- Nasal regurgitation.
- Whether or not the patient coughs on swallowing.
- The level at which the food sticks (suprasternal notch or mid-sternal).
- Associated heart burn.
- Weight loss.

Examination

- Examine:
  - Mouth for ulcers, thrush and pallor; check the gag reflex.
  - Neck for lymph glands and goitres.
  - For scleroderma.

- Look for an underlying neurological deficit (evidence of stroke, motor neuron disease, myasthenia gravis).

DIAGNOSIS

This patient with dysphagia is recovering from a stroke (aetiology) and his functional status is best determined by videofluoroscopy and assessment by a speech therapist.

QUESTIONS

Mention a few causes of dysphagia.
- Benign oesophageal stricture.
- Carcinoma of the oesophagus.
- Peptic ulcer of the oesophagus.
- Achalasia of the cardia.
- Pharyngeal pouch.
- Retrosternal goitre, bulbar palsy, myasthenia gravis, Plummer–Vinson syndrome (Paterson–Kelly syndrome).

Remember that oesophageal dysphagia is due either to mechanical narrowing or to a motor disorder affecting normal peristalsis.

How would you investigate such a patient?
- FBC, ESR.
- Barium swallow.
- Gastroscopy.

What do you understand by the term 'presbyoesophagus'?
It is a condition that occurs in the elderly and is characterized by impaired motor function of the oesophagus.

H.S. Plummer and P.P. Vinson, both physicians at the Mayo Clinic, Rochester, Minnesota.
D.R. Paterson and A. Brown Kelly, both British ENT surgeons.

Case 225

DIARRHOEA

PATIENT 1

Instruction

The patient has diarrhoea; would you like to ask him a few questions?

Salient features

Proceed as follows:
Ask about the following:

- Onset.
- Duration of diarrhoea.
- Frequency.
- Whether or not it is nocturnal.
- Blood (seen in ulcerative colitis, shigellosis, diverticulitis, carcinoma of the colon) and mucus in the stools; blood on the toilet paper.
- Nature of the stools (pale and bulky and difficult to flush away in steatorrhoea).
- Associated pain in the abdomen.
- Appetite (increased in thyrotoxicosis).
- Weight loss (marked in chronic diarrhoea).
- Associated nausea and vomiting.
- Drug ingestion (including antibiotics and laxatives).
- Foreign travel.

PATIENT 2

Instruction

The patient has diarrhoea, would you like to examine her?

Salient features

Proceed as follows:
- Look for the following signs:
  - Anaemia.
  - Clubbing.
  - Aphthous ulcers.
  - Abdominal tenderness, abdominal masses.
- Tell the examiner that you would like to do a rectal examination and check for faecal occult blood.

Diagnosis

This patient has chronic diarrhoea with aphthous ulcers and abdominal tenderness indicating that she has inflammatory bowel disease (aetiology).

QUESTIONS

What do you understand by the term 'diarrhoea'?
It implies passing of increased amounts of loose stool (more than 300 g per day).

How would you investigate a patient with diarrhoea?
- FBC, ESR.
- Serum albumin.
- Sigmoidoscopy.
- Stool chart, stool cultures, faecal cultures.
- Barium enema, small bowel barium studies.

ADVANCED-LEVEL QUESTIONS

What are the mechanisms of diarrhoea?

- Osmotic diarrhoea: the mucosa of the gut acts as a semipermeable membrane; the diarrhoea stops when the patient fasts, e.g. diarrhoea due to magnesium sulphate, lactulose, malabsorptive states.
- Secretory diarrhoea: there is active secretion of intestinal fluid, e.g. *Escherichia coli* diarrhoea.
- Inflammatory diarrhoea: there is mucosal damage, e.g. shigellosis, ulcerative colitis.
- Increased gut motility, e.g. irritable bowel syndrome.

What are the poor prognostic factors in ulcerative colitis?

Anaemia (Hb <10 g/dl), raised ESR (30 mm in the first hour), fever (37.5°C), increased frequency of stools (more than six per day), tachycardia (>90 beats/min) and hypoalbuminaemia (<30 g/l).

Case 226

MARFAN'S SYNDROME

INSTRUCTION

Look at this patient.
Examine this patient's heart.

SALIENT FEATURES

History

Family history.

Examination

Disproportionately long limbs compared with the trunk – the arm span will exceed the height.

Proceed as follows:

Examine the following:

- *Hands*, for hypermobile joints and spidery fingers or arachnodactyly. Confirm by:
  (1) *thumb sign* – asking the patient to clench his thumb in his fist; the thumb should not exceed the ulnar side of the hand in normal subjects but because of hypermobility and laxity of the joint in Marfan's disease it protrudes beyond his clenched fingers; and (2) *wrist sign* – put the patient's fingers around his other wrist: normal subjects cannot overlap the thumb and little finger around the wrist but in Marfan's syndrome the little finger will overlap by at least 1 cm in 80% of patients; *Arch Intern Med* 1970; **126:** 276.

- *Eyes*, for iridodonesis or ectopia lentis (subluxation upwards) – the patient may be wearing thick spectacles; blue sclera.
- *Head*, for long-headedness (dolichocephalic with bossing of frontal eminences and prominent supraorbital ridges).
- *Palate*, for high-arched palate.
- *Skin*, for small papules in the neck (Miescher's elastoma).
- *Chest,* for pectus excavatum, cystic lung disease (*Thorax* 1984; **39:** 780–4).
- *Heart*, for mitral valve prolapse, aortic aneurysm and aortic regurgitation.
- *Spine*, for scoliosis and kyphosis.

Remember that each patient should be referred for ophthalmic examination, annual echocardiography and genetic counselling to maximize the preventive potential in this disease.

DIAGNOSIS

This patient has Marfan's syndrome and aortic regurgitation (lesion) and is limited by cardiac failure (functional status).

QUESTIONS

What are the criteria for Marfan's syndrome?
- People with no family history require, apart from skeletal features (including pectus carinatum or excavatum, reduced upper–lower segment ratio, arm-span-to-height ratio >1.05, scoliosis and reduced elbow extension), involvement of at least two other systems and one of the major criteria (these include ectopia lentis, dilatation of the aortic root or aortic dissection and lumbosacral dural ectasia by CT or MRI).
- Patients with a family history need features in at least two systems.

What is your differential diagnosis?
Homocystinuria (recessively inherited inborn error of amino acid metabolism due to a deficiency of cystathionine β-synthetase) in which the skeletal features are similar.

How would you differentiate the two?
In homocystinuria the lens is dislocated downwards and there is homocystine in the urine.

ADVANCED-LEVEL QUESTIONS

Why do these patients need annual echocardiography?
To monitor aortic diameter and mitral valve function. Prophylactic replacement of the aortic root with a composite graft when the diameter reaches 50–55 mm (normal <40 mm) prolongs life. Untreated patients commonly die in the fourth or fifth decade from dissection of the aorta or from cardiac failure due to aortic regurgitation. Chronic beta-blockade to produce a negative inotropic effect retards the rate of aortic dilatation (*N Engl J Med* 1994; **330:** 1335–41). Also, patients should be advised regarding infective endocarditis prophylaxis.

What is the common cause of mortality in Marfan's syndrome?
Cardiovascular complications cause 95% of deaths in such patients and reduce mean life expectancy by 40%.

What are the ocular features of Marfan's syndrome?
- Subluxation of lens.
- Small and spherical lens.
- Glaucoma.
- Hypoplasia of dilator pupillae, making pupillary dilatation difficult.
- Flat cornea.
- Myopia.
- Retinal detachment.

What are the complications of pregnancy in women with Marfan's syndrome?
- Early premature abortion.
- Risk of maternal death from aortic dissection. Pregnancy is not dangerous when the aortic diameter is less than 40 mm.

Is there a gene implicated in Marfan's syndrome?
Marfan's syndrome appears to be caused by mutations in a single fibrillin gene (*FBN1*) on chromosome 15 (*Genomics* 1993; **17**: 468–75; *N Engl J Med* 1992; **326**: 905). Fibrillin is a glycoprotein produced by fibroblasts; it aggregates in conjunction with other proteins or alone in the extracellular matrix. The microfibrillary fibres form the framework on which elastin is deposited. These microfibrillary fibres are particularly abundant in the ciliary zonules that support the lens, in ligaments and in the aorta. Dilatation of the aorta occurs due to cystic medionecrosis.

B-J. Antoine Marfan (1858–1942), a French paediatrician, wrote his paper in 1896. He was appointed Foundation Professor of Hygiene at the Clinic of Infantile Diseases in Paris in 1914.

Victor McKusick, contemporary Professor of Medicine at Johns Hopkins Hospital, Baltimore, whose chief interest is genetics.

American President Abraham Lincoln is suspected to have had Marfan's syndrome.

Case 227

NEPHROTIC SYNDROME

INSTRUCTION

Look at this patient.

SALIENT FEATURES

History

- History of diabetes (*N Engl J Med* 1998; **338:** 1202–11).
- Hypertension.
- History of acute glomerulonephritis, streptococcal sore throat.
- Medications (NSAIDs, captopril, street heroin, gold, penicillamine, lithium, chlorpropamide, rifampicin, tolbutamide).
- History of SLE, vasculitides, amyloidosis.
- Neoplasms (Hodgkin's and other lymphomas, solid tumours).
- Familial history (sickle cell disease, partial lipodystrophy – p. 433, Alport's syndrome).
- Parasites (malaria, toxoplasmosis, schistosomiasis).

Examination

- Generalized oedema – puffiness of face, pitting oedema of legs and hands.
- Look at the nails for ridges of hypoproteinaemia.
- Comment on the pallor.

Proceed as follows:
Tell the examiner that you would like to examine:

- The abdomen for ascites.
- The urine for protein and sugar. (Urine microscopy may show oval fat bodies which consist of degenerating tubular epithelial cells having cholesteryl esters. These appear as 'grape clusters' with light microscopy and have a 'Maltese-cross' appearance under polarized light.)

DIAGNOSIS

This patient has nephrotic syndrome (lesion) due to diabetes mellitus (aetiology), and has developed gross anasarca indicating hypoalbuminaemia and marked urinary protein loss (functional status).

QUESTIONS

What do you understand by the term 'nephrotic syndrome'?

It consists of albuminuria (more than 3.5 g/day) and hypoalbuminaemia accompanied by generalized oedema, hyperlipidaemia (due to increased hepatic production) and lipiduria.

What causes this syndrome?

- Glomerular disease: minimal change glomerulonephritis, membranous glomerulonephritis, proliferative glomerulonephritis.
- Systemic disease: diabetes mellitus, SLE, amyloidosis, drugs (captopril, gold, penicillamine, street heroin), Hodgkin's disease, syphilis, malaria, HIV, cancer, hepatitis B, multiple myeloma, renal primary (AL) amyloidosis.

How would you investigate these patients?

- 24-hour urinary protein, creatinine clearance, urine electrophoresis.
- FBC, ESR.
- Urea and electrolytes, serum creatinine, albumin.
- Serum cholesterol (dyslipidaemia is due to both overproduction and impaired catabolism of apolipoprotein B-containing lipoproteins).
- DNA antibody, antinuclear factor, complement levels.
- Renal biopsy.

What complications may such a patient suffer?

- Thromboembolic events, including renal vein thrombosis and deep vein thrombosis (due to loss of antithrombin III and other proteins involved in the coagulation and fibrinolytic cascade).
- Protein malnutrition.
- Acclerated atherosclerosis.
- Infection.

ADVANCED-LEVEL QUESTIONS

What is orthostatic proteinuria?

It is usually seen in adolescents, occurs when standing and resolves on lying down. The long-term prognosis is good.

What do you know about Tamm–Horsfall protein in the urine?

Normal individuals excrete less than 150 mg protein per day. Of this, about 5–15 mg is albumin and the remainder consists of different plasma proteins and glycoproteins derived from renal cells. Tamm–Horsfall mucoprotein is the most abundant protein that is not derived from plasma but from the cells of the ascending limb of the loop of Henle, and is excreted at the rate of 50–75 mg per day. Pathological proteinuria occurs when daily excretion exceeds 150 mg protein.

What is the treatment of patients with nephrotic syndrome?

- Diuresis: furosemide (frusemide; acts in the ascending thick loop of Henle) with thiazides (reduce sodium absorption in the distal nephron) and potassium-sparing diuretics.
- Prevention of thromboemboli: heparin, anticoagulants and support stockings when patients have nephrotic proteinuria, an albumin level below 20 g/l, or both.
- Infusion of hyperoncotic albumin should only be tried if symptomatic hypovolaemia is present.
- Plasma ultrafiltration in severe cases.
- Renal ablation by bilateral nephrectomy or embolization of the renal artery may be indicated to avoid serious risks of severe hypoproteinaemia and hypovolaemia.
- Pneumococcal vaccine.

- ACE inhibitors are indicated even in normotensive patients.
- Colchicine in familial Mediterranean fever, interferon-α in hepatitis B associated nephrotic syndrome, hepatitis C associated membranoproliferative glomerulo-nephritis and cryoglobulinaemia, 8-week course of prednisone in minimal change nephropathy.

I. Tamm, scientist, Rockefeller University, New York.

F.L. Horsfall, Professor of Microbiology, Sloan Kettering Institute and Cornell University, New York.

Nephrotic syndrome was clearly described by R. Bright (1789–1858), an English physician in the 19th century. He qualified from Edinburgh and worked at Guy's Hospital, London. Chronic nephritis is known as Bright's disease. Three of his renal specimens are still preserved at Guy's Hospital.

Case 228

URAEMIA

INSTRUCTION

Would you like to ask this uraemic patient some questions and perform a relevant examination?

SALIENT FEATURES

History

- Loss of appetite, anorexia, nausea, vomiting and hiccups.
- Fatigue, malaise, loss of energy.
- Polyuria, nocturia, dysuria, haematuria, difficulty in passing urine.
- Swelling of the face and feet.
- Shortness of breath (due to secondary left ventricular failure).
- Itching.
- Restless legs (overwhelming need to alter position of legs frequently).
- Paraesthesia due to either hypocalcaemia (associated tetany) or peripheral neuropathy.
- Bone pain (due to metabolic bone disease).
- Drug history, in particular NSAIDs, tetracycline.
- History of diabetes, hypertension, recurrent urinary tract infections.
- Family history of renal disease, in particular polycystic kidneys.
- Tell the examiner that you would like to take a history for impotence in men and amenorrhoea in women.

Examination

- Pallor (due to anaemia).
- Comment on short stature (indicates uraemia from childhood).

- Examine the nails (for Lindsay's 'half-and-half' nails where the proximal portion is whitish while the distal portion is brownish red; the lunula is usually obscured).
- Comment on the lemon tinge of the skin, the pallor and scratch marks. Rarely, there may be 'uraemic frost'. Increased photosensitive skin pigmentation.
- Examine the arms for asterixis (flapping tremor), haemodialysis fistula.
- Comment on the vascular shunts, if any.
- Comment on hyperventilation of Kussmaul's respiration secondary to metabolic acidosis.
- Examine the abdomen for palpable kidneys (hydronephrosis, polycystic kidneys) and palpable bladder.
- Check for pitting leg oedema.

Proceed as follows:
Tell the examiner that you would like to:

- Check the blood pressure (hypertension, hypotension).
- Look for pericardial friction rub.
- Look for evidence of peripheral neuropathy (glove and stocking sensory loss).
- Do a rectal and vaginal examination if urinary obstruction is suspected.
- Examine the urine for sugar, albumin, specific gravity, microscopy.
- Examine the retina in diabetics.

DIAGNOSIS

This patient has chronic renal failure (aetiology) due to diabetes mellitus (aetiology), and is currently requiring dialysis as evidenced by the arteriovenous fistula in the arm (functional status).

QUESTIONS

How would you investigate a patient with renal failure?

- Urine: glucose, microscopy, specific gravity, creatinine clearance, 24-hour urinary protein, urine electrophoresis.
- Blood: FBC, ESR.
- Serum: urea, electrolytes, creatinine, protein, calcium phosphate, uric acid.
- Ultrasonography of the abdomen for kidneys, bladder.
- Special investigations: pyelography, protein electrophoresis, complement components, autoantibody screening, serum cryoglobulins, kidney biopsy.

What do you understand by the term 'azotaemia'?

Azotaemia indicates a raised level of urea and creatinine without symptoms (glomerular filtration rate (GFR) about 20–35% of normal).

What do you understand by the term 'uraemia'?

Uraemia implies a deterioration of renal function associated with symptoms (GFR below 20% of normal).

Note. Chronic renal insufficiency is defined by a serum creatinine concentration of 1.5–3.0 mg/dl (133–265 μmol/l) and chronic renal failure is serum creatinine concentration >3.0 mg/dl.

What are the common causes of chronic renal failure?
- Glomerulonephritis.
- Diabetes mellitus.
- Hypertensive nephropathy.
- Pyelonephritis.
- Polycystic kidney disease.
- Analgesic nephropathy.

ADVANCED-LEVEL QUESTIONS

Mention a few drugs that you would avoid in renal failure.
Aminoglycosides, furosemide (frusemide) with cephalosporins, potassium salts, tetracycline.

What are the consequences of renal failure?
- Metabolic: sodium imbalance, hyperkalaemia, metabolic acidosis, hyperuricaemia, hypocalcaemia, hypermagnesaemia, hyperphosphataemia.
- Cardiovascular: cardiac failure, hypertension, accelerated atherosclerosis, pericarditis. (Pericarditis is either uraemic pericarditis or dialysis pericarditis.)
- Haematological: anaemia, clotting disorders, leukocyte abnormalities.
- Skin: itching, hyperpigmentation, bruising.
- Nervous system: encephalopathy, peripheral neuropathy, autonomic neuropathy.
- Gastrointestinal: anorexia, nausea, vomiting, peptic ulcer, diarrhoea. Constipation, particularly in patients on continuous ambulatory peritoneal dialysis (CAPD).
- Endocrine: vitamin D disorders, secondary hyperparathyroidism, impotence, amenorrhoea, glucose intolerance.

When would you consider dialysis?
- Hyperkalaemia (potassium concentration >7 mmol/l).
- Bicarbonate concentration less than 12 mmol/l.
- Urea level greater than 20 mmol/l.
- Creatinine concentration greater than 500 μmol/l.
- Patients must be referred for dialysis before the above features are present because those managed close to or at end-stage renal failure have a much poorer prognosis than those managed for at least 3 months before needing dialysis or transplantation (*Am J Kidney Dis* 1995; **25:** 276–80; *Nephrol Dial Transplant* 1998; **13:** 246–50).

What are the bone changes in chronic renal failure?
- Osteomalacia (renal rickets).
- Osteitis fibrosa cystica (secondary hyperparathyroidism): subperiosteal erosions, especially of the skull (pepperpot skull), phalanges, long bones and distal end of clavicles.
- Osteosclerosis, where there is enhanced density of the bone in the upper and lower margins of vertebrae (rugger-jersey spine).

Is there any benefit in restricting dietary protein in chronic renal disease?
A large randomized controlled trial suggests no benefit from protein restriction.

What are the beneficial effects of ACE inhibitors in renal disease due to?

They are probably due to the combination of the antihypertensive and anti-proteinuric effects of these drugs (*Ann Intern Med* 1997; **127**: 337). A randomized multicentre trial demonstrated that ACE inhibitors lead to less renal failure than other antihypertensives in renal disease (*N Engl J Med* 1996; **334**: 939–45).

What is Bricker's trade-off hypothesis?

Early in the course of renal failure, the kidney fails to excrete phosphorus, causing a rise in the level of phosphorus in the body. To normalize this rise in serum levels of phosphorus and calcium, the serum parathyroid hormone level rises, but the 'trade-off' is bone disease (osteitis fibrosa cystica). This is the basis for secondary hyperparathyroidism in renal failure.

What is the intact nephron hypothesis?

There is increased solute excretion per nephron, particularly when there is depletion of extracellular fluid resulting in impaired ability of the kidney to concentrate urine. In addition, the ability of the nephrons to adjust to low and high intake of sodium, water, potassium and other dietary solutes is impaired because the nephrons are functioning at maximum capacity even during normal intake of solutes. For example, when the maximum concentrating ability is 300 mOsm and daily urine solute excretion is 600 mOsm/kg, about 2 litres of urine is required to allow this excretion whereas in a normal individual only 500 ml of urine is required to concentrate the urine to 1200 mOsm/kg.

P.G. Lindsay, an American physician.

Neil S. Bricker, a US nephrologist.

N.P. Mallick, contemporary Professor of Renal Medicine at the Manchester Royal Infirmary.

Case 229

PAGET'S DISEASE

INSTRUCTION

Examine this patient's face.
Examine this patient's legs.

SALIENT FEATURES

History

- Ask the patient whether there is an increase in hat size.
- Bone pain.
- Joint pain (due to osteoarthritis secondary to bone disease).
- Painless bowing of the bone can be the first symptom.
- Hearing loss.

- Fractures with minimal trauma.
- Nerve entrapment syndromes, including paraparesis and radiculopathy when the spine is affected.

Examination

Face
- Comment on the hearing aid, if any. Test hearing and determine whether the deafness is a conduction defect (due to involvement of the ossicle) or neural (due to compression of the eighth nerve).
- Typical appearance of the skull and increased skull diameter (more than 55 cm is abnormal).

Proceed as follows:
Tell the examiner that you would like to examine the fundus for optic atrophy or angioid streaks.

Neck
- Look for platybasia.
- Raised JVP (cardiac failure in Paget's disease is due to hyperdynamic circulation).

Spine
Deformity of the spine – kyphosis; auscultate over the vertebral bodies for bruits. In up to one third of patients the third and fourth lumbar vertebrae are involved, and in 20% the lower thoracic vertebrae are involved.

Legs
- Comment on the anterior bowing of the tibia and the lateral bowing of the femur.
- Feel the bone for warmth.
- Tell the examiner that you would like to examine the joints for osteoarthritis (limitation of hip movement, in particular abduction, and fixed flexion deformity of the knees).
- Tell the examiner that you would like to:
  - Do a urine analysis (high incidence of renal stones).
  - Measure the patient's height (for serial follow-up).
  - Compare the patient's appearance with a previous photograph.
  - Ask the patient whether there is an increase in hat size.

Remember that Paget's disease is a remodelling disease of isolated areas of the skeleton.

DIAGNOSIS

This patient has Paget's disease (lesion) with hyperdynamic cardiac failure and sensorineural deafness (functional status).

QUESTIONS

What are the complications of Paget's disease?
- Diminished mobility.
- Fractures.

- Cord compression due to basilar invagination.
- Root lesions due to vertebral damage.
- Hypercalcaemia.
- High-output cardiac failure.
- Sarcomatous changes, seen in less than 2% of patients.

ADVANCED-LEVEL QUESTIONS

Mention the neurological complications of Paget's disease.
- Headache.
- Fits.
- Platybasia.
- Hydrocephalus.
- Cerebellar signs.
- Cranial nerve palsies.
- Cord compression.

What are the mechanisms of hearing loss in such patients?
- It is usually due to the disease process involving the ossicles.
- Less commonly it is caused by the progressive closure of the skull foramina compressing the eighth cranial nerve.

What is the basic defect in bone metabolism?
Increased osteoclastic activity resulting in bone resorption and increased osteoblastic activity.

What are the radiological manifestations of this disease?
- Skull: 'honeycomb' appearance with underlying osteoporosis circumscripta, 'cottonwool' appearance.
- Pelvis: thickening of the iliopectineal line 'brim sign', enlargement of ischial and pubic bones.
- Long bones: increased trabeculation and localized bone enlargement.
- Vertebrae: sclerotic margins giving a 'picture frame' appearance.
- Remember that a bone scan is more sensitive than radiography in determining the extent of disease.

What is the prevalence of Paget's disease?
The exact prevalence is not known but several reports indicate a 3% prevalence in patients over the age of 40 years, increasing with age to reach a maximum of 10% by the ninth decade. Males predominate by a ratio of about 2:1.

What factors have been implicated in the aetiology of Paget's disease?
- Slow viral infection – measles syncytial virus, paramyxovirus (canine distemper).
- Genetic factors have been described in Italy.

What are the biochemical features of this disease?
- Serum calcium concentration is normal (except in prolonged immobilization or malignancy).
- Increased bone serum alkaline phosphatase level (indicates increased osteoblastic activity).

- Increased urinary hydroxyproline secretion (indicates increased bone resorption).

Which drugs are commonly used in the treatment of this disease?

- Diphosphonates (they inhibit osteoclast-mediated bone resorption).
- Calcitonins (act by reducing osteoclastic activity).
- Plicamycin (previously known as mithramycin; *N Engl J Med* 1997; **336(8):** 558).
- Gallium nitrate (inhibits ATP-dependent proton pump in osteoclasts).

To which patients would you offer therapy?

Treatment is offered to patients with any of the following symptoms:

- Agonizing bone pain.
- Severe deformity.
- Hypercalcaemia.
- Cardiac failure.

Sir James Paget (1814–1899), surgeon, St Bartholomew's Hospital, London. He also described Paget's disease of the nipple (carcinoma involving the areola and the nipple), Paget's disease of the skin (skin cancer involving the apocrine glands) and Paget–Schroetter syndrome (venous thrombosis of the axillary veins, of unknown cause). (Paget J 1877 On a form of chronic inflammation of bones (osteitis deformans). *Med Chir Trans* **60:** 37.)

Case 230

PAROTID ENLARGEMENT

INSTRUCTION

Look at this patient's face.

SALIENT FEATURES

History

- Ask the patient whether the parotids are painful and the mouth dry.
- Ask the patient about dry eyes or use of artificial tears.
- History of sarcoidosis.
- History of lymphoma, leukaemia.

Examination

Bilateral parotid enlargement.

Proceed as follows:

- Look for the following conditions:
  - Dry mouth.
  - Lupus pernio.
  - Rheumatoid arthritis.

- Tell the examiner that you would like to know whether the patient has gritty eyes or dry mouth.

Remember that unilateral parotid enlargement with associated facial nerve palsy is more likely to be malignant tumour of the parotids; it is very rare for facial weakness to occur with benign tumours.

DIAGNOSIS

This patient has parotid enlargement, which is painless, and has a dry mouth (lesion) probably due to Sjögren's syndrome (aetiology). The dry mouth is making swallowing difficult (functional status).

QUESTIONS

What are the causes of painless bilateral parotid enlargement?
- Sarcoidosis.
- Sjögren's syndrome or keratoconjunctivitis sicca.
- Lymphoma and leukaemia.

How would you test objectively for dry eyes?
Schirmer's test: filter paper is hooked over the lower eyelid; in normal people at least 15 mm is wet in 5 minutes whereas a value of less than 5 mm is seen in sicca syndrome.

What do you know about keratoconjunctivitis sicca?
It is a condition characterized by decreased production of tears by lacrimal glands.

ADVANCED-LEVEL QUESTIONS

Mention a few causes of keratoconjunctivitis sicca.
- Primary keratoconjunctivitis sicca is common and characterized by involvement of the lacrimal gland alone.
- Primary Sjögren's syndrome is an autoimmune disorder which is usually positive for rheumatoid factor, antinuclear antibodies and hypergammaglobulinaemia. Less frequently, autoantibodies to DNA, salivary gland, smooth muscle and gastric parietal cells are present. There may be associated dry mouth and bronchial epithelium, and the vagina may also be affected. Histopathogically, the glands show intralobar ductal epithelial hyperplasia and lymphocytic infiltration of the gland.
- Secondary Sjögren's syndrome is the presence of keratoconjunctivitis sicca in association with a systemic disorder such as the following:
  - Rheumatoid arthritis.
  - Psoriatic arthritis.
  - Connective tissue disorder.
  - Sarcoidosis.
  - Crohn's disease.

How would you manage such patients?
- Artificial tears (e.g. hypromellose) are instilled frequently for dry eyes.
- Artificial saliva for dry mouth.

Which are the other salivary glands?
These include submandibular, sublingual and minor salivary glands in the oral cavity, pharynx and larynx.

What do you know about the superficial anatomy of the salivary gland?
The gland lies on the lateral surface of the ramus of the mandible and folds itself along the posterior mandibular border. It is usually not palpable as a discrete structure. Clenching the teeth tenses the masseter and makes the anterior border of the gland more prominent (as the gland lies just behind the masseter muscle).

How are parotid secretions carried into the oral cavity?
By Stensen's duct, which opens just opposite the upper second molar tooth.

What is Mikulicz's disease?
It is the enlargement of salivary and lacrimal glands (due to sarcoidosis, lymphoma or tuberculosis) associated with dry mouth and dry eyes but not arthritis.

Which neoplasm may be associated with Sjögren's syndrome?
Usually B-cell-derived non-Hodgkin's lymphoma.

O.W.A. Schirmer (1864–1917) a German ophthalmologist.

J. von Mikulicz-Radecki (1850–1905) was successively Professor of Surgery at Könisberg and Breslau.

H.S.C. Sjögren (b. 1899), Swedish Professor of Ophthalmology in Gothenburg.

N. Stensen (1638–1686), Danish anatomist and Professor of Anatomy at Copenhagen. He was then appointed the Catholic Bishop of Titiopolis in 1677 and was an international authority on geology. He described the tetralogy of Fallot before Fallot, in 1672.

Case 231

SUPERIOR VENA CAVAL OBSTRUCTION

INSTRUCTION

Look at this patient.

SALIENT FEATURES

History

- Headache.
- Dysphagia.
- Dyspnoea.
- Wheezes.
- Blackouts.
- Oedema of the face.

Examination

- Tortuous, visible and dilated veins on the chest wall and neck.
- The neck veins are non-pulsatile.
- The face may be plethoric and suffused. The patient may be short of breath.
- Look for signs of Horner's syndrome and for radiation marks.
- Tell the examiner that you would like to examine for signs of bronchogenic carcinoma, i.e. clubbing, tar staining, lymph nodes and chest signs.

DIAGNOSIS

This patient has superior vena caval obstruction (lesion) which is usually due to bronchogenic carcinoma (aetiology), and is tachypnoeic at rest (functional status).

QUESTIONS

What are the causes of superior vena caval obstruction?
- Bronchogenic carcinoma is the commonest cause (70% of cases).
- Lymphoma – in young adults.
- Other causes:
  - Aortic aneurysm.
  - Mediastinal goitre.
  - Mediastinal fibrosis (due to methysergide, histoplasmosis or TB).
  - Constrictive pericarditis.

How would you manage this patient?
This condition is a medical emergency and an urgent CT scan of the chest should be requested (*Chest* 1993; **103** (suppl 4): 394S). Emergency treatment consists of the following:

- Intravenous furosemide (frusemide) to relieve the oedematous component of vena caval compression.
- Intravenous anticancer chemotherapy, e.g. cyclophosphamide.
- Mediastinal irradiation within 24 hours.
- More recently, expandable metal stents have been used to relieve the obstruction.
- Mechanical thrombectomy with an Amplatz thrombectomy device (*BMJ* 1994; **308**: 1697–9).

Obstruction of the superior vena cava was first described in 1757 by William Hunter in the case of syphilitic aortic aneurysm.

N Engl J Med 1993; **329**: 1007 (classical picture of this condition).

Case 232

GLASS EYE

INSTRUCTION

Look at this patient's fundus.
Examine this patient's eyes.
Check this patient's vision or visual fields.

SALIENT FEATURES

History

History of trauma.

Examination

- Glass eye, which is obvious.
- The patient is blind on the affected side.
- The light reflex is absent.

Note. Suspect malignant melanoma if you are asked to examine the abdomen and the liver is palpable (due to metastases).

DIAGNOSIS

This patient has a glass eye (lesion) which is secondary to trauma in childhood (aetiology).

ADVANCED-LEVEL QUESTIONS

What is sympathetic ophthalmitis?

It is inflammation that attacks the sound eye after injury (usually a perforating wound) of the other. It is almost always a plastic iridocyclitis; rarely it manifests as neuroretinitis or choroiditis. It never occurs after excision of an injured eye unless it has already commenced at the time of operation. Steroids improve the prognosis if such treatment is commenced early.

Mention any fungus that can invade the globe.

Rhizopus mucormycosis, originating in the paranasal sinuses and nose, occurs predominantly in patients with poorly controlled diabetes mellitus, malignancy, organ transplantation and those who are receiving long-term desferrioxamine therapy. This fungus can invade the globe or ophthalmic artery to cause blindness.

From which tissues do ocular melanomas arise?

They arise from a variety of ocular tissues including the conjunctiva, uveal tract (iris, ciliary body and choroid), eyelid, orbit and nasolacrimal ducts. Iris melanomas rarely metastasize, whereas ciliary body and choroidal melanomas readily disseminate.

What is the histology of ocular melanomas?

Unlike cutaneous melanomas, the ocular type consists of two distinct cell types – spindle and epithelioid. Lesions composed completely or predominantly of spindle cells have low aggressiveness, do not tend to metastasize and are associated with a 75% survival rate at 15 years, thus ophthalmologists tend to avoid enucleation. The epithelioid type is associated with only a 35% survival rate despite enucleation, because of late metastases.

Case 233

TURNER'S SYNDROME

INSTRUCTION

Look at this patient.

SALIENT FEATURES

- Webbing of the neck in a female patient.
- Abnormal angulation of both elbows – increased carrying angle (cubitus valgus).
- Dwarfism.
- Receding chin.
- Low-set ears.
- Epicanthal folds, double eyelashes.
- Low hairline over the back of the neck.
- Shield-shaped chest – nipples are widely separated with microthelia.
- Multiple pigmented naevi.
- Short fourth metacarpal.
- Lymphoedema of the hands and feet.
- Check for radiofemoral delay (coarctation of the aorta) and aortic stenosis.

Proceed as follows:
Tell the examiner that you would like to:

- Examine the genitalia for infantilism.
- Measure serum FSH and LH levels (these will be high, confirming primary hypogonadism).

DIAGNOSIS

This patient has Turner's syndrome (lesion) which is due to the absence of one of the X chromosomes (aetiology). She has amenorrhoea and skeletal abnormalities (functional status).

QUESTIONS

What constitutes a web?

Either a fan-like fold of skin extending from the shoulder to the neck, or an abnormal splaying out of the trapezius.

ADVANCED-LEVEL QUESTIONS

Which other cardiovascular lesions are associated with webbing of the neck?

Noonan's syndrome or Ullrich's syndrome with pulmonary stenosis.

What is the chromosomal defect in Turner's syndrome?

The syndrome results from absence of one of the X chromosomes (blood karyotype showing 46,XO). Other variants of the syndrome include 46,X (with abnormal X), 45,XO/46,XX mosaics and 45,XO/46,XY mosaics. Although this is the single most common chromosomal disorder more than 95% of the fetuses are aborted, resulting in an incidence of approximately 1 in 4000 newborns.

What are the facial features of Turner's syndrome?

Ptosis, micrognathia, low-set ears, epicanthal folds.

What are the renal abnormalities associated with Turner's syndrome?

Horseshoe kidney, hydronephrosis.

Is pregnancy possible in these patients?

Only in mosaic individuals with a normal 46,XX cell line. Sufficient follicles may persist postnatally to initiate pubertal changes and therefore cause ovulation and consequently pregnancy.

How would you manage such patients?

The treatment is supportive and includes replacement hormone therapy on attaining puberty, primarily to prevent osteoporosis and induce sexual maturation and menses.

What do you know about Lyon's hypothesis?

In 1961, the geneticist Mary Lyon postulated that only one of the X chromosomes is genetically active, whereas the other is inactive. The inactivation of either the maternal or paternal X chromosome occurs at random among all the cells of the blastocyst around the 16th day of embryonic life, and inactivation of the same X chromosome persists in all cells derived from each precursor cell.

More recent studies, however, have shown that many genes escape X chromosome inactivation and that both X chromosomes are important for normal growth, as evidenced by severe abnormalities in Turner's syndrome in which there is monosomy of the X chromosome. It is now believed that a gene which maps Xq13 serves as a master switch that is critical for 'switching off' most of the genes on the active chromosome 13. This gene is known as X-inactive-specific transcript gene (XIST).

Henry H. Turner (b. 1892), an American endocrinologist, described this condition in 1938.

Mary Lyon (b. 1925), contemporary geneticist working for the Medical Research Council in Oxford.

Case 234

YELLOW NAIL SYNDROME

INSTRUCTION

Look at this patient's hands.

SALIENT FEATURES

History

- Ask about past history of sinusitis.
- History of bronchiectasis, pleural effusion.
- History of lymphoedema.

Ask about associated disorders:

- Malignancy (melanoma, carcinoma of larynx, lung and breast, Hodgkin's disease).
- Thyroid disease (Hashimoto's thyroiditis, hypothyroidism, thyrotoxicosis).
- Hypogammaglobulinaemia.
- Rheumatoid arthritis.

Examination

Yellow discoloration of all the nails. The nails are often smooth, thickened and over-curved. There is no involvement of the skin.

Proceed as follows:
Tell the examiner that you would like to:

- Examine the chest (for pleural effusion, bronchiectasis).
- Examine the legs for lymphoedema.

DIAGNOSIS

This patient has yellow nail syndrome (lesion) complicated by severe bronchiectasis (functional status).

ADVANCED-LEVEL QUESTION

What is the pathogenesis?

The pathogenic mechanism underlying the yellow nail syndrome has not been defined. Abnormality of lymphatic vessels was suggested as the cause by Samman and White in their original description of the syndrome (*Br J Dermatol* 1964; **76:** 153–7). This theory is supported by lymphangiographic findings which in most patients showed few, hypoplastic or dilated, deficient lymphatics. Electron micro-scopy in two cases noted dilated but otherwise normal lymphatics (*J Am Acad Dermatol* 1983; **10:** 187–92).

This syndrome was first described in 1964 by P.D. Samman and W.F. White.

Case 235

OSTEOGENESIS IMPERFECTA

INSTRUCTION

Look at this patient's eyes.

SALIENT FEATURES

History

- Ask about previous fractures.
- Whether or not the condition runs in the family.

Examination

Blue sclera.

Proceed as follows:
Look for the following signs:

- Hearing loss due to otosclerosis.
- Signs of old fractures.
- Defective dentine formation in the teeth.
- Kyphosis and scoliosis.
- Joint hypermobility.
- Hernias.
- Aortic regurgitation.

DIAGNOSIS

This patient has blue sclera with abnormalities of skeleton and teeth (lesion) due to osteogenesis imperfecta tarda (aetiology), and is disabled by the condition (functional status).

QUESTIONS

Why is the sclera blue?
Because the choroid pigment is visible.

Mention other conditions in which the sclera is blue.
- Marfan's syndrome.
- Ehlers–Danlos syndrome.

ADVANCED-LEVEL QUESTIONS

What is the inheritance?
Usually autosomal dominant, although some cases may be autosomal recessive. The gene defects are in the two genes that encode the procollagen chains of type I collagen.

What is the characteristic pathology?

The most characteristic pathology is a primary reduction in bone matrix with secondary mineralization.

What are the clinical types?

– Type I: Nearly normal stature, imperfect dentition, blue sclera, fractures of variable number and minimal deformity.
– Type II: Usually fetuses die in utero or shortly after birth; multiple fractures of ribs and long bones with little mineralization of calvarium and pulmonary hypertension.
– Type III or osteogenesis imperfecta congenita (fetal type): Stature markedly diminished due to multiple fractures and deformity of long bones in utero; blue sclera, imperfect dentition and hearing loss.
– Type IV or osteogenesis imperfecta tarda: Stature usually reduced, bone deformity and fractures common, sclera bluish to normal, imperfect dentition; loss of hearing may or may not be present.

How would you manage this patient?

• Genetic counselling.
• Bisphosphonates may improve bone density and growth in children (*N Engl J Med* 1998; **339:** 947).
• Bone marrow transplantation to correct mesenchymal defect in children (*Nat Med* 1999; **5:** 309–13.

Case 236

DOWN'S SYNDROME

INSTRUCTION

Look at this patient.

SALIENT FEATURES

History

Ask the mother at what age she delivered the child (Down's syndrome occurs in 1 in 1550 live births in women under the age of 20 years, in contrast to 1 in 25 live births for mothers over the age of 45 years).

Examination

• Collapse of the bridge of the nose.
• Low-set ears.
• Epicanthic folds.
• Look at the iris for Brushfield's spots, i.e. yellow speckles seen in young children.

- Tell the examiner that you would like to:
  – Examine the hands for simian palmar crease (Fig. 91).

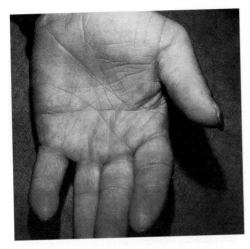

Fig. 91

  – Examine for short, inward-curving little finger (Siegert's sign).
  – Examine the heart for murmur of mitral regurgitation (endocardial cushion defects), and atrial septal defect (ASD; ostium primum type).
  – Check mental status quotient (MSQ) and perform formal IQ testing (80% have an IQ between 25 and 50).
- Tell the examiner that you would like to check for hypothyroidism and thyroid antibodies.

DIAGNOSIS

This patient has features of Down's syndrome (lesion) which is usually due to trisomy 21 (aetiology) and is associated with a reduced life expectancy (functional status).

QUESTIONS

What complications can be seen in such patients?
- Increased incidence of acute leukaemia.
- Presenile dementia of Alzheimer type (occurs in the fourth and fifth decades and reduces life expectancy).
- Atlantoaxial subluxation.
- Duodenal atresia in children.

ADVANCED-LEVEL QUESTIONS

Mention two chromosomal abnormalities seen in this condition.
- Trisomy 21 (*N Engl J Med* 1991; **324**: 872).
- Mosaicism (46,XY/47,XY, +21). Approximately 1% are mosaics due to mitotic non-dysjunction.

What are the underlying genetic mechanisms?

- Non-dysjunction (occurs during meiosis, particularly in the ovum, and correlates with maternal age).
- *De novo* translocation.
- Familial translocation, usually robertsonian translocation of the long arm of chromosome 21 to another acrocentric chromosome, e.g. 22 or 14.

Which maternal serum markers are used for prenatal screening of Down's syndrome?

Serum α-fetoprotein, chorionic gonadotrophin and oestriol.

J. Langdon Down (1828–1896) wrote an article in *Clinical Lectures and Reports of the London Infirmary* (now the Royal London Hospital) in 1866 entitled 'The ethnic classification of idiots'. The extra chromosome was discovered by Lejeune in 1959.

T. Brushfield (1858–1937), a British physician.

Ferdinand Siegert (1865–1946), a German paediatrician.

Hyman Isaac Goldstein (1887–1954), an American physician, described Goldstein's sign, which is a wide space between the great toe and the adjoining toe seen in Down's syndrome.

Mitchell in 1876 observed the increased incidence with maternal age and Penrose in 1933 confirmed it statistically.

Case 237

LATE CONGENITAL SYPHILIS

INSTRUCTION

Look at this patient.

SALIENT FEATURES

History

- Hearing loss.
- Arthritis due to Clutton's joints.
- Eye pain (due to interstitial keratitis).

Examination

- Collapsed bridge of the nose (saddle nose or Zaufal's sign).
- Corneal opacity (interstitial keratitis).
- Rhagades (linear scars at the angles of the mouth).
- Peg-shaped incisors (Hutchinson's teeth): the central incisors are widely spaced, have a central notch and are tapered like a peg.
- Perforation of the palate.
- Frontal bossing.

Proceed as follows:
- Check for deafness (nerve deafness).
- Look at the shins for sabre tibia.
- Look for Clutton's joints (bilateral knee effusions).
- Look at the fundus for optic atrophy.

Remember. (a) Cardiovascular manifestations have not been observed in this condition; (b) late congenital syphilis is defined as congenital syphilis of more than two years' duration.

DIAGNOSIS

This patient has a saddle nose and peg-shaped incisors (lesions) due to congenital syphilis caused by maternal *Treponema pallidum* infection (aetiology).

ADVANCED-LEVEL QUESTIONS

What is Hutchinson's triad?
- Interstitial keratitis.
- Deafness.
- Typical dental change, i.e. peg-shaped incisors (Hutchinson's teeth).

What are the ocular features of congenital syphilis?
- Interstitial keratitis.
- Retinopathy – fine pigmentation, 'salt and pepper fundus'.

Sir Johnathan Hutchinson (1828–1913) was simultaneously a surgeon at The London Hospital (now the Royal London Hospital), an ophthalmologist at Moorfields Hospital and a dermatologist at Blackfriars Hospital (now closed).

H. Clutton (1850–1901), an English surgeon who worked at St Thomas's Hospital, London.

Emanuel Zaufal (1833–1910), a Czechoslovakian rhinologist.

Case 238

ARTERIOVENOUS FISTULA

INSTRUCTION

Look at this patient's arms.

SALIENT FEATURES

History
- History of trauma to the limb.
- History of haemodialysis and artificial arteriovenous fistula.

Examination

- Hypertrophy of the affected arm.
- Prominent, dilated, tortuous veins.
- Continuous thrill over the fistula; listen for continuous bruit.
- Collapsing pulse; increased pulse pressure indicating hyperdynamic circulation.

Proceed as follows:

- Look for signs of cardiac failure.
- Elicit Branham's sign, i.e. slowing of the pulse on occluding the feeding vessel of the fistula.
- If the fistula is in the upper limb, perform Allen's test: the radial and ulnar arteries are occluded at the wrist and the hand is exercised; the arteries are then released one at a time to establish which is the dominant feeding vessel.
- Look for signs of chronic renal failure.

DIAGNOSIS

This patient has an arteriovenous fistula (lesion) which has been surgically created (aetiology) for haemodialysis and is functioning well.

Read the classical review: *BMJ* 1991; **303**: 1191–4.

ADVANCED-LEVEL QUESTIONS

How are arteriovenous malformations classified?

Angiographically, as follows:

- Group 1 – predominantly arterial or arteriovenous lesions: present with pain, hypertrophy of the digit or limb, deformity, distal ischaemia, venous hypertension; large lesions can cause symptoms and signs of cardiac failure.
- Group 2 – lesions affecting tiny vessels including capillaries: for example, port-wine stain, epistaxis in hereditary haemorrhagic telangiectasia, gastrointestinal haemorrhage with colonic dysplasia.
- Group 3 – predominantly venous lesions: local oedema, pain and venous ulceration; there may be a history of trauma.

How would you manage a patient with an arteriovenous malformation?

- Referral to a vascular surgeon.
- Doppler ultrasonography.
- Angiography.

When and how is an arteriovenous malformation treated?

Arteriovenous malformations are treated when they cause discomfort, disfigurement and danger to the patient. The patient should be jointly assessed by a vascular surgeon and an interventional radiologist for embolization. The temptation to ligate the feeder vessel should be resisted as subsequent embolization may be difficult. Complete excision of the fistula is accepted treatment in resistant cases.

What are the alternatives when a fistula cannot be formed in a patient requiring long-term haemodialysis?

Placement of synthetic grafts subcutaneously or of a long central line into a great vein.

Case 239

CAROTID ARTERY ANEURYSM

INSTRUCTION

Examine this patient's neck.

SALIENT FEATURES

History

- History of hypertension.
- History of diabetes.
- History of smoking.

Examination

Pulsatile swelling along the course of the carotids, usually unilateral (the swelling may be firm) and at the base of the neck.

Proceed as follows:
- Auscultate over the mass for a bruit.
- Look for Horner's syndrome.
- Tell the examiner that you would like to proceed as follows:
  - Examine all peripheral pulses.
  - Examine the heart and blood pressure.

DIAGNOSIS

This patient has a carotid artery aneurysm (lesion) due to atherosclerosis (aetiology), and may require surgery before the lesion ruptures (functional status).

ADVANCED-LEVEL QUESTIONS

How would you manage this patient?

- All patients must be referred to a vascular surgeon.
- Check urine for sugar.
- Serum lipids.
- Intravenous carotid digital subtraction angiography.

Case 240

RETRO-ORBITAL TUMOUR

INSTRUCTION

Examine this patient's eyes.

SALIENT FEATURES

History

- History of atherosclerosis.
- History of hypertension.
- History of diabetes.
- History of trauma to the eye or head.

Examination

- Unilateral exophthalmos.
- Impaired extraocular movement (due to either muscle or nerve involvement).
- Chemosis, conjunctival oedema.
- Radiation marks may be present.

Proceed as follows:
- Examine the visual acuity and visual fields.
- Look for pulsations over the globe.
- Palpate the orbital margin for erosion of the underlying bone.
- Auscultate over the globe for bruit.

DIAGNOSIS

This patient has a retro-orbital tumour with a bruit over the globe (lesion) indicating a pulsatile structure such as an arteriovenous fistula in the orbit (aetiology). The tumour is causing considerable distress to the patient (functional status).

ADVANCED-LEVEL QUESTIONS

What is your differential diagnosis?

- The commonest cause of unilateral exophthalmos is Graves' disease.
- Other causes are as follows:
  - Retro-orbital tumour (primary or metastatic).
  - Arteriovenous fistula (carotico-cavernous fistula).
  - Cavernous sinus thrombosis.
  - Orbital cellulitis.

What investigations would you do?

- T_4, TSH, free T_3.
- Orbital ultrasonography.
- Cranial CT, in particular the orbits.

How would you manage such a patient?
- Ophthalmology opinion.
- Therapy – radiation to the orbit and steroids; surgical decompression, depending on the underlying aetiology.

What are the causes of a unilateral pulsating proptosis?
- Arteriovenous fistula between the carotid artery and cavernous sinus – stops with pressure on the artery in the neck.
- Aneurysm of the ophthalmic artery.
- Cirsoid aneurysm of the orbit.
- Vascular neoplasms in the orbit growing rapidly.

Case 241

ACHONDROPLASIA

INSTRUCTION

Look at this patient.

SALIENT FEATURES

History
- Family history (autosomal dominant inheritance; however, 80% are new mutations).
- Paternal age (increases in frequency with increasing paternal age).

Examination
- Dwarfism.
- Bulging forehead.
- Depression of the root of the nose.
- Midface hypoplasia.
- Shortened proximal extremities; hands have a 'trident' shape.
- Trunk of normal size.
- Exaggerated lumbar lordosis.

DIAGNOSIS

This patient with short stature and normal trunk size has achondroplasia (lesion), which is due to mutation of the fibroblast growth factor receptor gene (aetiology).

QUESTIONS

Is the lifespan reduced in these subjects?
No, they have a normal lifespan. More recently this has been disputed in the literature (*Lancet* 1998; **352:** 1950).

How is the IQ affected in these patients?

The IQ in these patients is normal.

Is the reproductive status affected?

No, people with achondroplasia have normal reproductive status.

What are the complications of this condition?

Hydrocephalus or compression of brainstem, spinal cord or nerve roots. Impingement by an osteophyte or disk on the small spinal canal can cause neurological disturbance.

ADVANCED-LEVEL QUESTIONS

What do you know about the genetics of achondroplasia?

It is inherited as an autosomal dominant trait with complete penetrance. Mutations of the fibroblast growth factor receptor 3 (FGFR-3) gene on human chromosome 4 with the transition from guanine to adenine or a guanine to cytosine transversion at nucleotide 1138 is the defect in these patients (*Cell* 1994; **78:** 335–42; *Nature* 1994; **371:** 252).

What do you know about Crouzon syndrome?

Crouzon syndrome is an autosomal dominant condition characterized by premature fusion of the cranial sutures (craniosynostosis). It has been shown to map to chromosome 10 and is associated with mutations of the fibroblast growth factor receptor 2 gene (FGFR-2).

This syndrome has been depicted by artists in several paintings including the painter Velasquez in his portrait of Don Sebastian de Morra, a courtier of the Spanish King Phillip V.

Case 242

BREAST LUMP

INSTRUCTION

Examine this patient's breasts.

SALIENT FEATURES

History

- History of weight loss.
- History of a palpable mass in breast and/or axilla.
- Breast pain (present in 10% of breast cancer patients) unrelated to menstrual cycle.
- Nipple discharge, erosion, enlargement or itching of the nipple.
- Back or bone pain, jaundice or weight loss (indicate systemic metastases).

- Family history (20% of breast cancer patients have family history).
- Some forms of mammary dysplasia.
- History of cancer in the other breast.
- History of endometrial cancer.
- Nulliparous or late first pregnancy.

Examination

Breast lump which is non-tender and has poorly delineated margins. Asymmetry of the breasts and retraction or dimpling of the skin can often be accentuated by having the patient raise her arms overhead or press her hands on her hips to contract the pectoralis muscle.

Proceed as follows:
- Examine axillary and supraclavicular lymph nodes.
- Look for oedema of the ipsilateral arm (due to metastatic infiltration of regional lymphatics).
- Examine the chest (metastases, lymphangitis carcinomatosa).
- Examine for hepatomegaly (metastases).

DIAGNOSIS

This patient has a breast lump which is infiltrating the skin and axillary lymph nodes (lesion) indicating malignant breast carcinoma (aetiology).

QUESTIONS

How would you investigate such a patient?
- FBC and ESR (ESR is consistently raised).
- Urea and electrolytes, liver function tests (hypercalcaemia, raised alkaline phosphatase level indicates bone or liver metastases).
- Biopsy: large needle core biopsy, fine-needle aspiration or open biopsy under local anaesthesia.
- Carcinoembryonic antigen (CEA) could be a marker for recurrence.
- Imaging for metastases:
  - Chest radiograph for lung secondaries.
  - CT scan of liver or brain when metastasis is suspected in these areas.
  - Bone scanning (if patient has bone pain or raised alkaline phosphatase level).

ADVANCED-LEVEL QUESTIONS

How would you investigate a patient with a suspicious mammogram but no clinical evidence of mass?
Although a mass cannot be palpated, the patient should undergo a mammographic localization biopsy.

What are the histological types of breast cancer?
They are of two main types, which may be invasive or *in situ*:

- Ductal: arising from the epithelial lining of large or intermediate-sized ducts. Most arise from intermediate ducts and are invasive (e.g. invasive ductal, infiltrating ductal). When ductal carcinoma has not invaded extraductal tissue, it is intra-ductal or *in situ* ductal.

- Lobular: arising from the epithelium of the terminal ducts of the lobules.

How are patients with breast cancer managed?

Surgery

- *Breast-conserving surgery* (lumpectomy, axillary dissection and radiation therapy) is usually offered to patients with single tumours less than 4 cm in diameter, because the cosmetic outcome of excising larger tumours is poor. However, in 80% of patients with large tumours and in 25% of those with locally advanced breast cancers, breast conservation is possible if the size of the tumour is reduced by a course of primary systemic treatment (such as combination chemotherapy and hormonal therapy).
- *Modified radical mastectomy* (total mastectomy, removal of the overlying skin and nipple as well as the underlying pectoralis fascia with axillary lymph node dissection). The major advantage is that radiation is not necessary, but many patients suffer from the psychological trauma of breast loss.

Adjuvant therapy

- CMF regimen: cyclophosphamide, methotrexate and fluorouracil.
- MMM regimen: mitoxantrone (mitozantrone), methotrexate and mitomycin C.
- Doxorubicin and cyclophosphamide.
- Tamoxifen.

Palliative therapy

Radiotherapy (may be complicated by brachial plexus neuropathy), hormonal treatment (tamoxifen, diethylstilboestrol, megestrol acetate, aminoglutethimide), chemotherapy (doxorubicin, paclitaxel, docetaxel or trastuzumab).

Which breast cancers are suitable for treatment by conservative breast surgery?

- Single clinical and mammographic lesion.
- Tumours less than 4 cm in diameter (or those greater than 4 cm in a large breast).
- No sign of local advancement.

Which patients are best treated by mastectomy?

- Those who prefer mastectomy.
- Those in whom breast conservation would produce an unacceptable cosmetic result.
- Those with either clinical or mammographic evidence of more than one focus of cancer in the breast.

What factors are associated with increased rates of local recurrence after mastectomy?

Axillary lymph node involvement, lymphatic or vascular invasion by cancer, grade III carcinoma or tumours greater than 4 cm in diameter.

What are the prognostic factors in 'node-negative' breast cancer?

Tumour size, oestrogen and progesterone receptor status, histologic grade, percentage of cells in S phase (i.e. synthesizing DNA) and the *HER-2/neu* (c-erb-B2) oncogene. The *HER-2/neu* (c-erb-B2) oncogene is expressed by 25% of breast cancers and is associated with a poorer prognosis but a better response to doxorubicin and trastuzumab therapy.

Which patients are more likely to respond to hormone therapy?

Women with high levels of oestrogen receptors in the tumour, those in whom there is a long interval from initial surgery to time of relapse, and those with metastatic disease in bone and soft tissue (unlike those with liver metastases or lymphangitis carcinomatosa).

Are women with fibroadenomas at increased long-term risk of breast cancer?

Not all patients with fibroadenomas are at increased risk, but those with a family history of breast cancer, complex fibroadenomas or proliferative disease have an increased long-term risk of breast cancer.

What is the role of implants for breast augmentation?

In breast cancer, silicone gel implants were used for augmentation, but doctors have stopped using these implants as there is new evidence that they may cause auto-immune reactions or connective tissue disorders. Saline implants do not work well for reconstruction after surgery for breast cancer or for very thin women. If silicone gel implants are removed from the market, these patients will have no alternative.

Which genes have been implicated in familial breast cancer?

There may be more than five genes causing familial breast cancer; the most important of these is *BRCA1* located on the long arm of chromosome 17. The gene *p53* on the short arm of chromosome 17 has been implicated in the rare breast cancer family syndrome (Li–Fraumeni syndrome, in which breast cancer occurs at a younger age associated with soft tissue sarcoma, osteosarcoma, adrenal tumours, gliomas and other childhood tumours).

What are the factors associated with increased rates of local recurrence after mastectomy?

Axillary lymph node involvement, lymphatic or vascular invasion by cancer, grade III carcinoma, tumour >4 cm in diameter.

In 1894, William Halsted published his seminal report on radical mastectomy for the cure of cancer of the breast.

In 1896, George Beaston published his seminal report that bilateral oophorectomy resulted in the remission of breast cancer in premenopausal women (Beaston GT. On the treatment of inoperable cases of carcinoma of the mamma: suggestions for a new method of treatment, with illustrative cases. *Lancet* 1896; **2**: 104–7).

Marc Lippman, Professor and Chair of Medicine, University of Michigan, successively worked at NIH and Georgetown University Medical Center. He has made a major contribution to the cell biology of breast cancer. His laboratory was one of the first to characterize the effect of tamoxifen on cultured breast cancer cell lines.

RAGE (Radiotherapy Action Group Exposure) is a pressure group formed by patients who suffered the side-effects of radiotherapy, including brachial plexus neuropathy, often resulting in severe pain and the loss of use of the arm.

Case 243

GINGIVAL HYPERTROPHY

INSTRUCTION

Look at this patient's mouth.

SALIENT FEATURES

History

- Drugs (phenytoin, ciclosporin, nifedipine).
- Leukaemia (myelomonocytic leukaemia).

Examination

Hypertrophy of the gums.

Proceed as follows:
Look for other features of chronic phenytoin therapy (coarsening of facial features, hypertrichosis, hirsutism, generalized lymphadenopathy, rash, cerebellar syndrome, peripheral lymphadenopathy).

DIAGNOSIS

This patient has poor oral hygiene and gingival hypertrophy (lesion) due to chronic ingestion of phenytoin (aetiology).

QUESTIONS

What are the other long-term side-effects of phenytoin?
Coarsening of facial features, rashes, systemic lupus erythematosus, blood dyscrasias, generalized lymphadenopathy, induction of hepatic microsomal enzymes, folic acid deficiency, peripheral neuropathy, cerebellar syndrome (ataxia, nystagmus and dysarthria), hypertrichosis, osteomalacia and encephalopathy. When taken during pregnancy, phenytoin may result in cleft lip and palate in the child.

For which types of seizure is phenytoin generally used?
Generalized clonic–tonic seizures.

A classical picture of gingival hypertrophy: *N Engl J Med* 1994; **330**: 826.

Case 244

HAEMOPHILIA A

INSTRUCTION

Examine this patient's knee (or elbow) joint; he has a bleeding disorder.

SALIENT FEATURES

History

- Family history of bleeding (X-linked recessive disorder): draw the family tree.
- Recurrent bleeding into the joints.
- Intramuscular haematomas (after trauma, such as injections).
- Retroperitoneal bleeds.
- Bleeding from mucous membranes.
- Haematuria, haemospermia.
- Intracranial bleeds (second most common cause of death in haemophiliacs after HIV).

Examination

- Male patient.
- Fixed deformity of the joint (haemarthrosis causes bone and joint destruction).

DIAGNOSIS

This patient has a fixed deformity of the elbow (lesion) due to bleeding into the joint as a complication of haemophilia A (aetiology). The joint is now undergoing osteo-arthritic changes (functional status).

QUESTIONS

What is the inheritance of haemophilia?

One third of cases are sporadic and the rest are X-linked (defects include deletions, point mutations and insertions on the X chromosome).

What is deficient in haemophilia?

Factor VIII:C – the clinical manifestations depend on its level. Levels lower than 1% are associated with spontaneous bleeding, whereas patients with levels lower than 5% have severe bleeding after trauma and occasionally spontaneous bleeding. When levels are above 5%, bleeding occurs after trauma.

ADVANCED-LEVEL QUESTIONS

How are bleeding episodes treated?

- Factor VIII concentrates: for minor bleeding, factor VIII concentrates should be raised to 20–30% of normal, and for severe bleeding to at least 50%. For major surgery, levels should be raised to 100% and maintained at over 50% until healing has occurred. Patients can stock factor VIII in domestic refrigerators for self-administration to start treatment immediately on bleeding. It is given twice daily and intravenously.

- DDAVP, administered intravenously, can increase factor VIII levels, depending on the initial level.

What is the commonest cause of mortality?

Currently, it is HIV infection, transmitted by contaminated factor VIII concentrate administered in the past. HIV-associated immune thrombocytopenia may worsen the bleeding tendency.

Queen Victoria's descendants are said to have suffered from haemophilia (*BMJ* 1995; **311**: 1106–7).

In 1803, John Conrad Otto emphasized its inheritance as an X-linked disorder in his description of a New Hampshire family.

In 1964, Pool and co-workers discovered that factor VIII is concentrated in cryoprecipitate.

In 1984, the factor VIII gene was cloned and expressed in tissue culture.

Robert Gwyn Macfarlane, Professor at Oxford, did pioneering work on the care of haemophiliacs and was the first to propose the cascade hypothesis of blood coagulation.

Case 245

KLINEFELTER'S SYNDROME

INSTRUCTION

Examine this patient and give us your diagnosis.

SALIENT FEATURES

History

- Infertility (commonest cause of male infertility).
- Mentally subnormal.
- Ask about sensation of smell (to exclude Kallman's syndrome).

Examination

- Male patient with eunuchoid body habitus with abnormally long legs.
- Elongated body with an increase in length between the soles and pubic bone.
- Lack of a beard, and the voice is not masculine.

Proceed as follows:

Tell the examiner that you would like to:

- Examine the external genitalia (small atrophic testes, lack of male distribution of pubic hair).

- Test the IQ (usually lower than normal, although mental disability is uncommon).
- Check for hypo-osmia (Kallman's syndrome).

DIAGNOSIS

This patient has Klinefelter's syndrome (lesion) due to an excess of X and Y chromosomes (aetiology), and has infertility (functional status).

QUESTIONS

How would you investigate such a patient?

- Plasma gonadotrophins (FSH levels are consistently raised).
- Plasma testosterone concentration (variably reduced).
- Plasma oestradiol level (raised).
- Chromosomal analysis (two or more X chromosomes and one or more Y chromosomes).

What is the commonest karyotype?

Eighty-two per cent of patients have 47,XXY, which results from non-dysjunction during meiosis in one of the parents.

Are the patients fertile?

No; however, some men having chromosomal mosaicism (46,XY/47,XXY) are fertile. A recent report suggested that births after intracytoplasmic injection of sperm may be possible in non-mosaic Klinefelter's syndrome (*N Engl J Med* 1998; **338:** 588).

ADVANCED-LEVEL QUESTIONS

What is Kallman's syndrome?

It is idiopathic hypogonadotrophic hypogonadism with involvement of the hypothalamus. Patients have hypo-osmia and other defects of the rhinencephalon (cleft lip/palate, congenital deafness and blindness). Replacement therapy with both gonadotrophins and gonadotrophin-releasing hormone (GnRH) ensures fertility in many of the affected individuals.

Harry F. Klinefelter (1912–1990), an American physician who worked at Johns Hopkins Hospital in Baltimore. He described this syndrome with Fuller Albright (1900–1969) and Edward Reifenstein while he was a visiting fellow at Massachusetts General Hospital and Harvard Medical School (Klinefelter HF Jr, Reifenstein EC Jr, Albright F 1942 Syndrome characterized by gynecomastia, aspermatogenesis with a Leydigism and increased excretion of follicle stimulating hormone, *J Clin Endocrinol* **2:** 615–27). Fifteen years after their description, A. Jacobs and J.A. Strong confirmed the association between the extra X chromosome and Klinefelter's syndrome (*Nature* 1959; **183:** 302–3; *Lancet* 2000; **356:** 333–5).

Albright described Albright's syndrome; he was stricken with Parkinson's disease at the age of 36 years, and was rendered invalid in 1953 following surgical attempts to improve his Parkinson's disease.

Case 246

MACROGLOSSIA

INSTRUCTION

Examine this patient's mouth.

SALIENT FEATURES

History

• Ask whether there is any difficulty in breathing or swallowing.
• Look for an underlying cause such as hypothyroidism or acromegaly.

Examination

Protrusion of the resting tongue beyond the teeth or alveolar ridge. The impressions of the teeth may be obvious along the edges of the tongue on either side.

DIAGNOSIS

This patient has macroglossia (lesion) of which the cause is not obvious by clinical examination (aetiology), and which is complicated by heavy breathing (functional status).

Read: *BMJ* 1994; **309:** 1386.

QUESTIONS

What do you understand by the term 'macroglossia'?

It is a resting tongue that protrudes beyond the teeth or alveolar ridge. It is usually used to indicate long-term painless enlargement rather than the rapid growth of acute parenchymatous glossitis.

What are the types of macroglossia?

• True macroglossia – definitive histopathological findings:
  Primary – characterized by hypertrophy or hyperplasia of tongue muscles.
  Secondary – the result of infiltration of normal tissue with anomalous elements.
• Pseudomacroglossia – relative enlargement secondary to a small mandible with no histological abnormalities.

ADVANCED-LEVEL QUESTIONS

What are the causes of true macroglossia?

~~~ dren
  thyroidism.
  hangioma.
  angioma.

- Idiopathic hyperplasia.
- Metabolic disorders.
- Beckwith–Wiedemann syndrome.

Secondary macroglossia
- Amyloidosis.
- Acromegaly.
- Angio-oedema.
- Lymphoma.
- Chronic infections: TB, syphilis.
- Space-occupying lesions: cystic hygroma, cysts in lingual thyroglossal ducts, rhabdomyosarcoma.

What are the causes of pseudomacroglossia?
Down's syndrome, Pierre Robin syndrome, cerebral palsy.

What are the complications of macroglossia?
- Prolonged exposure can cause ulceration and necrosis of the mouth and tip of the tongue.
- Noisy breathing, drooling and unsightly appearance, particularly in children.
- Maxillofacial defects such as anterior open bite, prognathism.
- Difficulty in swallowing and, as a consequence, poor weight gain.
- Difficulty in the articulation of consonants requiring the tip of the tongue to be in contact with the alveolar ridge or roof of the mouth.
- Airway obstruction, which can be life threatening.

How would you manage macroglossia?

Medical
- Treatment of the underlying systemic cause, e.g. thyroxine in hypothyroidism, bromocriptine in acromegaly.
- Steroids – in life-threatening airway obstruction or postoperative oedema.

Surgical
- Reduction glossectomy for symptomatic macroglossia.
- Excision for neoplastic lesions.

Rehabilitation of physical and psychological problems
- Secondary orthodontic care and speech therapy.
- Psychological and psychiatric support.

Case 247

OSTEOPOROSIS OF THE SPINE (DOWAGER'S HUMP)

INSTRUCTION

Examine this patient's spine.

SALIENT FEATURES

History

- History of back pain (usually the onset is sudden with severe pain in the dorsal spine).
- Spontaneous fractures and loss of height.
- Long-term corticosteroid or heparin therapy.
- Postmenopausal or has had an oophorectomy.
- Does the patient smoke and consume alcohol.
- Is there a family history.
- Associated conditions: rheumatoid arthritis, uncontrolled diabetes mellitus, multiple myeloma, Cushing's syndrome, thyrotoxicosis, oestrogen deficiency in women and androgen deficiency in men, Marfan's syndrome, Ehlers–Danlos syndrome, homocystinuria.

Examination

- Elderly patient (usually a woman).
- Marked kyphosis.
- Loss of height.
- Protuberant abdomen.

Proceed as follows:
Look for spinal tenderness, demonstrate straight-leg rising sign.

DIAGNOSIS

This elderly patient with marked kyphosis (lesion) has postmenopausal osteoporosis (aetiology) complicated by frequent fractures and loss of height (functional status).

QUESTIONS

What do you understand by the term 'osteoporosis'?
It is 'a systemic skeletal disorder characterised by low bone mass and micro-architectural deterioration of bone tissue, with a consequent increase in bone fragility and susceptibility to fracture' (*Am J Med* 1993; **94:** 646–50).

ADVANCED-LEVEL QUESTIONS

What are the types of osteoporosis?
- Type I: results from accelerated bone loss, particularly trabecular bone, and is probably due to oestrogen deficiency. It typically results in fractures of vertebral bodies and the distal forearm in women in their 60s and 70s.

- Type II: results from age-related bone loss and is much slower. It occurs in both sexes and typically results in fracture of the proximal femur in the elderly.
- Secondary osteoporosis: accounts for about 20% of cases in women and 40% of cases in men.

What are the typical sites of fracture in osteoporosis?
Vertebrae, neck of femur, distal radius (Colles' fracture).

What are the clinical consequences of osteoporosis?
Increased mortality rate (increases by 20% in the first year after hip fracture), pain, deformities (kyphosis, loss of height and abdominal protrusion) and loss of independence.

What are the risk factors for osteoporosis?
Smoking, high alcohol consumption, thin body type in women, heredity, premature menopause, prolonged secondary amenorrhoea, primary hypogonadism, corticosteroid therapy, anorexia nervosa, malabsorption, primary hyperparathyroidism, organ transplantation, chronic renal failure, hyperthyroidism, prolonged immobilization.

How would you investigate such a patient?
- Radiography and bone scans to look for fractures and to exclude metastases.
- Serum calcium and phosphates, alkaline phosphatase and creatinine (remember, osteoporosis is not a disorder of calcium metabolism).
- 24-hour urinary calcium and creatinine excretion.
- Urinary Bence-Jones protein concentration and serum protein electrophoresis.
- Thyroid-stimulating hormone concentrations.
- Serum testosterone level in men.
- Dual-energy X-ray absorptiometry (DEXA) scanning, which determines bone density.

What are the recommendations to measure bone mineral density?
Bone mineral density measurements are recommended for the following indications where assessment would influence management:

- Radiographic evidence of osteopenia and/or vertebral deformity.
- Loss of height, thoracic kyphosis (after radiographic confirmation of vertebral deformity).
- Previous fragility fracture.
- Prolonged corticosteroid therapy (prednisolone >7.5 mg daily for 6 months or more).
- Premature menopause (age <45 years).
- Prolonged secondary amenorrhoea (>1 year).
- Primary hypogonadism.
- Chronic disorders associated with osteoporosis.
- Maternal history of hip fracture.
- Low body mass index (<19 kg/m^2).

Is general population screening recommended?
Screening for osteoporosis is not recommended until issues about long-term treatment have been resolved (*BMJ* 1999; **319**: 1148–9).

How would you prevent osteoporosis?

- The goal of therapy is to halve the risk of fracture.
- Lifestyle advice: exercise, stop smoking and reduce alcohol consumption.
- Replacement oestrogen therapy in postmenopausal women should be administered for at least five years.
- Raloxifene (a selective oestrogen receptor modulator) can be used in postmenopausal women.
- Dietary calcium intake increased to 1.5 g per day and vitamin D.
- Alendronate is a new bisphosphonate. It is 1000 times more potent than etidronate in inhibiting bone resorption and hence is able to provide effective inhibition at a dosage that does not affect bisphosphonates. Residronate significantly reduces the risk of hip fracture among elderly women with confirmed osteoporososis but not prophylactically (*N Engl J Med* 2001; **344:** 333–40). Another new bisphosphonate currently being evaluated is tiludronate.
- Calcitonin nasal spray results in decreased bone resorption.
- Sodium fluoride.
- Future treatments: parathyroid hormone, vitamin D analogues, strontium salts, ipriflavone.

What is the pathology of osteoporosis?

It is characterized by a decrease in the amount of bone present, so that the structural integrity of the skeleton is compromised. The rate of bone formation is normal but the rate of bone resorption is increased. This results in greater loss of trabecular bone than compact bone, accounting for the clinical features of the disease.

> A. Colles (1773–1843), Professor of Anatomy and Surgery at the College of Surgeons (Ireland).

Case 248

PRESSURE SORES (BEDSORES)

INSTRUCTION

Look at this leg.

SALIENT FEATURES

History

- Prolonged bed rest.
- Diabetes mellitus.
- Anaemia.
- Malnutrition.
- General debility.

Examination

Pressure sore over the sacrum.

Proceed as follows:

- Look for pressure sores elsewhere, particularly the skin overlying the occiput, ears, elbows, hips and ankles.
- Comment on any obvious paralysis or incontinence (the latter contributes to ulcers in the sacral areas).
- Comment on skin traction or any orthopaedic splints (as 70% are orthopaedic patients).
- Tell the examiner that you would like to culture and biopsy the ulcer if it has not been healing properly or looks suspicious.

DIAGNOSIS

This patient has a large non-healing ulcer (lesion) over the sacral region due to pressure (aetiology) requiring special nursing care to allow the pressure sore to heal (functional status).

QUESTIONS

What are the causes of pressure sores?

- Loss of sensation, and when circulation or nutrition to the skin and underlying tissue are compromised: diabetes mellitus, malnutrition, peripheral vascular disease, oedema, arthritis, anaemia, general debility.
- Others: urinary or faecal incontinence, sedation and anaesthesia.

How are pressure sores best prevented?

- Good nursing care, nutrition and maintenance of skin hygiene.
- Moribund, paralysed patients should be turned frequently (at least every hour) and pressure points should be inspected for areas of redness and tenderness.
- Water beds, alternating pressure mattresses and sheepskins are useful.

ADVANCED-LEVEL QUESTIONS

How are pressure sores graded?

- Grade I: erythema, skin intact.
- Grade II: skin loss, epidermis or dermis (abrasion, blister, shallow crater).
- Grade III: full thickness loss and damage to subcutaneous tissues.
- Grade IV: extensive destruction, tissue necrosis or damage to the underlying muscle or bone.

Case 249

SICKLE CELL DISEASE

INSTRUCTION

Examine the hands of this patient who has recurrent episodes of abdominal pain, precipitated by infection.

SALIENT FEATURES

History

Ask about:

- Bone pain.
- Past history of strokes, fits.
- Priapism.
- Family history of similar problem.
- Precipitating factors (infection, dehydration, cold, acidosis or hypoxia).
- Recurrent painful episodes.

Examination

- Afro-Caribbean patient.
- Anaemia.
- Digits of varying lengths (may be painful).
- Tell the examiner that you would like to examine the:
  - Urine for haematuria (renal papillary necrosis).
  - Leg for arterial ulcers.
  - Abdomen for hepatomegaly.
  - Heart for cardiomegaly and hyperdynamic circulation.
  - Retina (for neovascularization which may cause blindness).

DIAGNOSIS

This African black patient has evidence of old dactylitis (lesions) due to sickle cell anaemia (aetiology) which has caused severe deformity of the hand. She has difficulty buttoning her clothes (functional status).

QUESTIONS

What is the abnormality in this patient?

This patient has a structural abnormality of the haemoglobin chain in which there is a single base mutation from adenine to thymine which produces a substitution of valine for glutamine at the sixth codon of the β-globin chain. This results in the characteristic sickle appearance of haemoglobin. Sickling can produce shortened red cell survival and impaired passage of cells through the microcirculation, leading to obstruction of small vessels and tissue infarction.

What do you know about the genetics of this syndrome?

In the homozygous state, i.e. sickle cell anaemia, both genes are abnormal (Hb SS), whereas in the heterozygous state, i.e. sickle cell trait, only one chromosome carries the gene (Hb AS). The disease does not manifest until the Hb F decreases to adult levels at about 6 months of age.

Does the haemoglobin level fall during a sickle cell crisis?

The patient has 'steady state' anaemia and the haemoglobin level does not fall unless there is parvovirus-induced bone marrow aplasia, drug-induced haemolysis or sequestration of sickle cells in the liver and spleen.

Is the spleen enlarged in these patients?

The spleen may be enlarged in childhood, due to haemolysis, but in adult life patients often undergo autosplenectomy (due to infarcts) which increases their susceptibility to infection by *Streptococcus pneumoniae* (pneumonia, meningitis) and salmonella osteomyelitis.

What are the other complications of this disease?

Chronic leg ulcers (due to ischaemia), pigmentary gallstones (due to persistent haemolysis), aseptic necrosis of femoral heads and chronic renal disease.

How would you investigate these patients?

- FBC: haemoglobin 6–8 g/dl, with raised reticulocyte count.
- Blood smear shows signs of hyposplenism (Howell–Jolly bodies, target cells).
- Sickling of red cells can be induced by sodium metabisulphite.
- Haemoglobin electrophoresis: there is no haemoglobin A, 80–95% Hb SS, and 2–20% Hb F. High Hb F levels are associated with a more benign progress. The parents of the patient will show features of sickle cell trait (remember that sickle cell trait protects against *Plasmodium falciparum* malaria).

How would you manage an acute sickle cell crisis?

Supportive therapy with intravenous fluids, oxygen, antibiotics and analgesia. Folic acid is given to those with severe haemolysis.

Is there any long-term treatment?

- Hydroxyurea and erythropoietin are given to increase synthesis of Hb F.
- Allogeneic bone marrow transplantation is being investigated as a possible 'cure' in severely affected individuals.
- Experimental therapy: induction of haemoglobin F by short-chain fatty acids, membrane-active drugs and other experimental treatments.

What is the role of blood transfusion in these patients?

Steady-state anaemia requires no treatment, and regular blood transfusions are given only when the anaemia is severe or if the patient has frequent episodes of crisis, particularly during pregnancy (to suppress endogenous production of Hb S). Exchange transfusion for intractable pain crises, priapism and stroke.

What is the prognosis of this condition?

It is variable: some have a normal lifespan while others succumb in the first few years of life to infection or episodes of sequestration. Median age of death is 42 years for homozygotes. The acute chest syndrome is the leading cause of death and its cause is unknown. The syndrome is precipitated by fat embolism and infection, particularly community-acquired pneumonia (*N Engl J Med* 2000; **342:** 1855–65).

> W.H. Howell (1860–1945), Professor of Physiology at Johns Hopkins Hospital, Baltimore, who also discovered and isolated heparin.
>
> J.M.J. Jolly (1870–1953), French Professor of Histology.

Case 250

THRUSH

INSTRUCTION

Look at this patient's tongue.

SALIENT FEATURES

History

- Ask the patient about dysphagia (oesophagitis).
- Diabetes mellitus.
- Leukaemia, anticancer therapy or immunosuppressive drugs (cause neutropenia).
- Drugs (steroids, broad-spectrum antibiotics and oral contraceptives).
- HIV infection.

Examination

Superficial white patches or large fluggy membranes that are easily detachable, e.g. by a tongue depressor, leaving underlying erythema.

Proceed as follows:

- Look for other sites of candidal infection (eczematoid lesions in moist areas of the skin, such as inframammary folds, inguinal creases, between the fingers and toes).
- Look for id reactions (hypersensitivity cutaneous reactions remote from the site of infection).
- Ask the patient about dysphagia (oesophagitis).
- Tell the examiner that you would like to investigate for underlying:
  - Diabetes mellitus.
  - Neutropenia (secondary to chronic granulomatous disease, leukaemia, anticancer therapy or immunosuppressive drugs).
  - Drugs (steroids, broad-spectrum antibiotics and oral contraceptives).
  - HIV infection.
  - Polyendocrine deficiencies (including hypoparathyroidism, hypoadrenalism and hypothyroidism).

DIAGNOSIS

This patient has oral thrush or candidal infection (lesion), which is a complication of the use of the broad-spectrum antibiotic tetracycline (aetiology), and has dysphagia (functional status).

QUESTIONS

What is the most common species that causes human infection?
Candida albicans.

How would you confirm your diagnosis?
- Wet preparation of a smear with potassium hydroxide will confirm spores and may show non-septate mycelia.
- Biopsy will show intraepithelial pseudomycelia.

With which type of antibiotics is candidal infection common?
Broad-spectrum antibiotics, e.g. tetracycline, chloramphenicol.

Which candidal species usually colonizes skin?
C. parapsilosis.

How would you treat candidal infection?
Effective antifungal therapy may be achieved with fluconazole, ketoconazole, clotrimazole or nystatin.

What are the features of disseminated candidiasis?
Disseminated candidiasis manifests with systemic features including fever, toxicity, pulmonary involvement, endocarditis and retinal abscesses. Very rarely, it may cause focal manifestations including pustular skin abscesses, osteomyelitis, myositis, brain abscess or meningitis. It often causes sepsis associated with intravenous catheterization. Patients whose blood cultures demonstrate *Candida* should receive intravenous amphotericin B.

INDEX